Recent volumes in PROGRESS IN BRAIN RESEARCH

PROGRESS IN BRAIN RESEARCH

VOLUME 90

# GABA IN THE RETINA AND CENTRAL VISUAL SYSTEM

EDITED BY

R.R. MIZE

*Department of Anatomy and The Neuroscience Center, Louisiana State University Medical Center,
1901 Perdido Street, New Orleans, LA 70112, USA*


R.E. MARC

*Sensory Science Center, University of Texas, 6420 Lamar Fleming Avenue, Houston, TX 77030, USA*


A.M. SILLITO

*Department of Visual Science, Institute of Ophthalmology, University of London, Judd Street,
London WC1H 9QS, England, UK*

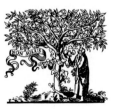

ELSEVIER
AMSTERDAM · LONDON · NEW YORK · TOKYO
1992

MF

ISBN 0-444-81446-9 (volume)
ISBN 0-444-80104-9 (series)

Published by
Elsevier Science Publishers BV
P.O. Box 211
1000 AE Amsterdam
The Netherlands

Library of Congress Cataloging in Publication Data

GABA in the retina and central visual system / edited by R.R. Mize,
  R.E. Marc, A.M. Sillito.
      p.   cm. -- (Progress in brain research ; v. 90)
   Includes bibliographical references and index.
   ISBN 0-444-81446-9 (alk. paper)
   1. GABA--Physiological effect. 2. Visual pathways. 3. Visual
cortex. 4. Retina. 5. GABA receptors.   I. Mize, R. Ranney.
II. Marc, R.E. III. Sillito, A.M. IV. Series.
   [DNLM: 1. GABA--physiology. 2. Receptors, GABA-Benzodiazepine-
-physiology. 3. Retina--growth & development. 4. Visual Cortex-
-growth & development. 5. Visual Pathways--growth & development.
W1 PR667J y. 90 / WW 270 G1115]
QP376.P7 vol. 90
[QP563.G32]
612.8'2 s--dc20
[612.8'4]
DNLM / DLC
for Library of Congress                                                91-46934
                                                                          CIP

Printed in The Netherlands on acid-free paper

2-11-93

# List of Contributors

Y. Arimatsu, Laboratory of Neuromorphology, Mitsubishi Kasei Institute of Life Sciences, II Minamiooya, Machida-shi, Tokyo, Japan

R. Baker, Department of Physiology and Biophysics, NYU Medical Center, 550 First Avenue, New York, NY 10016, USA

C.J. Barnstable, Department of Ophthalmology and Visual Science, Yale University School of Medicine, P.O. Box 3333, New Haven, CT 06510, USA

N.J. Berman, MRC Anatomical Neuropharmacology Unit, Mansfield Road, Oxford OX1 3TM, England, UK

N.C. Brecha, University of California, Los Angeles, Wadworth VA Center, Bldg. 115, Room 217, Los Angeles, CA 90073, USA

R.K. Carder, Department of Anatomy and Neurobiology, University of California, Irvine, CA 92717, USA

B.W. Connors, Section of Neurobiology, Division of Biology and Medicine, Brown University School of Medicine, Providence, RI 02912, USA

V. Crunelli, Department of Physiology, University of Wales, College of Cardiff, Museum Avenue, Cardiff CF1 1SS, Wales, UK

J.B. Cucchiaro, Department of Neurobiology and Behavior, SUNY, Grad Biology Building, Stony Brook, NY 11794, USA

P. Dean, Department of Psychology, University of Sheffield, Sheffield S102 TN, England, UK

R.J. Douglas, MRC Anatomical Neuropharmacology Unit, Mansfield Road, Oxford OX1 3TM, England, UK

U.T. Eysel, Department of Neurophysiology, Ruhr Universitat Bochum, Universitätsstrasse 150, D-4630 Bochum 1, FRG

D. Ferster, Department of Neurobiology and Physiology, Northwestern University, 2153 Sheridan Road, Evanston, IL 60201, USA

M.A. Freed, Laboratory of Neurophysiology, National Institute of Neurological Diseases and Stroke, NIH, Building 36, Room 2C02, Bethesda, MD 20892, USA

D.W. Godwin, Department of Physiological Optics, University of Alabama, School of Optometry, Birmingham, AL 35294, USA

S. Hendry, Department of Anatomy and Neurobiology, University of California, Irvine, CA 92717, USA

A.T. Ishida, Department of Animal Physiology, University of California, Davis, CA 95616, USA

Z.F. Kisvárday, Department of Neurophysiology, Ruhr Universitat Bochum, Universitätsstrasse 150, D-4630 Bochum, FRG

T. Kosaka, Department of Anatomy, Faculty of Medicine, Kyushu University, Higashiku, Fukuoka 812, Japan

R.E. Marc, Sensory Science Center, University of Texas, 6420 Lamar Fleming Avenue, Houston, TX 77030, USA

K.A.C. Martin, MRC Anatomical Neuropharmacology Unit, Mansfield Road, Oxford OX1 3TM, England, UK

R.R. Mize, Department of Anatomy, Louisiana State University Medical Center, 1901 Perdido Street, New Orleans, LA 70112, USA

J.R. Naegele, Department of Ophthalmology, Yale University School of Medicine, 330 Cedar Street, New Haven, CT 06510, USA

T.T. Norton, Department of Physiological Optics, University of Alabama, School of Optometry, Birmingham, AL 35294, USA

J.J. Nunes Cardozo, Department of Morphology, Netherlands Ophthalmic Research Institute, P.O. Box 12141, 1100 AC Amsterdam, The Netherlands

Y. Okada, Department of Physiology, Kobe University School of Medicine, Kusunoki-cho 7-5-1, Chuo-Ku, Kobe 650, Japan

Z.-H. Pan, Departments of Biophysical Sciences and Ophthalmology, SUNY School of Medicine, 118 Cary Hall, Buffalo, NY 14214, USA

J.G. Parnavelas, Department of Anatomy and Embryology, University College London, Gower Street, London WC1E 6BT, England, UK

D.A. Redburn, Department of Neurobiology and Anatomy, University of Texas Medical School, P.O. Box 20708, Houston, TX 77225, USA

P. Redgrave, Department of Psychology, University of Sheffield, Sheffield S102 TN, England, UK

A.M. Sillito, Department of Visual Science, Institute of Ophthalmology, University of London, Judd Street, London, WC1H 9QS, England, UK

M.M. Slaughter, Departments of Biophysical Sciences and Ophthalmology, SUNY School of Medicine, 118 Cary Hall, Buffalo, NY 14214, USA

I. Soltesz, Department of Visual Science, Institute of Ophthalmology, University of London, Judd Street, London, WC1H 9QS, England, UK

R.F. Spencer, Department of Anatomy, Medical College of Virginia, P.O. Box 906, Richmond, VA 23298, USA

C. van der Togt, Department of Morphology, Netherlands Ophthalmic Research Institute, P.O. Box 12141, 1100 AC, Amsterdam, The Netherlands

D.J. Uhlrich, Department of Anatomy, University of Wisconsin, 1300 University Avenue, Madison, WI 53706, USA

S.-F. Wang, Department of Anatomy, Medical College of Virginia, P.O. Box 906, Richmond, VA 23298, USA

J.J.L. van der Want, Department of Morphology, Netherlands Ophthalmic Research Institute, P.O. Box 12141, 1100 AC, Amsterdam, The Netherlands

S.M. Wu, Baylor College of Medicine, Cullen Eye Institute, Houston, TX 77030, USA

# Introduction

Gamma-aminobutyric acid (GABA) is the most prevalent inhibitory neurotransmitter in the visual system. It plays an essential role in gating signal transmission, either spatially or temporally, in retina and each of the major central projection sites of the visual system. Although the inhibitory role of GABA in the visual system has been recognized for some time, important new insights into the function of GABA have been made in the last few years. We now have accurate morphological descriptions of the various types of GABA neuron that are present in the visual system. Considerable information about the synaptic organization of these cells is also available. The role that GABA plays in the construction of receptive fields and other physiological properties remains controversial, but considerable headway is being made in elucidating these mechanisms. Much progress also has been made in defining GABA receptor subtypes and describing how ion channels operate in GABA transmission in the retina, lateral geniculate nucleus and visual cortex. Finally, there is important new information about the development of GABA in the neonatal visual system, the role that GABA plays in plasticity, and the effects on GABA of sensory deprivation and activity-dependent modifications of the environment.

Much of the recent progress in our understanding of GABA comes from technical advances in the field of neurotransmission. Thus, the development of specific antibody probes to GABA and its metabolic enzymes has made it possible to study the morphology and synaptic organization of identifiable GABA neurons. Computer morphometry techniques have allowed us to reconstruct more easily GABAergic networks in three dimensions and to measure the distributions and morphologies of GABA neurons and receptors quite precisely. The availability of more specific ligands and antibodies to GABA receptor subtypes have greatly advanced our understanding both of the selective distribution of receptor subtypes and their roles in gating the actions of GABA in various pathways. The use of these ligands in iontophoresis experiments is yielding new insights into the physiological action of GABA on receptive field structure. Finally the recent advent of patch clamp techniques in cell culture has made it possible to study the channel properties of GABA cells and to assist in modeling the biophysical properties of GABA interneurons. Each of these techniques has advanced our knowledge of how GABA cells are organized within the visual system and how GABA functions in signal transmission.

This book attempts to bring together into one volume a summary of our current understanding of the organization and function of GABA in the visual system. We have organized the book into separate sections on *Retina, Subcortical Visual Structures* and *Visual Cortex*. Each section includes, where possible, chapters on: (**1**) the distributions and functional characteristics of GABA receptor subtypes; (**2**) the contribution of GABA mediated processes to receptive field and other properties of visual cells; (**3**) the basic morphological organization and synaptic circuitry of GABAergic neurons; and (**4**) the development of GABA in the visual system and its role in plasticity.

The division of the book into three morphological components follows a long-established tradition. This organization has the advantage of combining into one section sequential chapters on the morphology, synaptic organization, physiology, pharmacological actions, receptor and channel mechanisms, and development of GABA in a single brain region. However, the book also reveals inhibitory mechanisms which are common among all of these visual structures which we believe deserves as much emphasis as descriptions of each structure's unique properties. In the final analysis, we chose to subdivide the book by structure because so many vision scientists think of them separately. At the least, the book provides a comprehensive overview of GABA function for the entire visual system and illustrates the similarities and differences in GABA organization in different regions of the visual brain.

It is our hope that the foundations for understanding GABA organization and function in the visual system are laid out in these chapters and that they provide a comprehensive analysis of this complex field. Another decade from now we expect to possess a complete set of GABAergic circuit maps, a further molecular description of GABA receptors, a complete analysis of biophysical transfer functions for GABA activated channels, and a detailed understanding of the role of GABA in establishing neural circuits in the developing retina and visual brain. It is both our current progress and this future promise which leads us to continue study of GABA in the visual system.

**Retina**

GABA has been recognized as an important inhibitory neurotransmitter in the retina for many years. However, the detailed synaptic circuitry and receptor mechanisms of GABA in the retina are just beginning to be understood. GABAergic neurons account for well over half the inhibitory neurons and over three-quarters of the inhibitory synapses in the retina of most vertebrates. GABA plays a fundamental role in feature extraction in the retina, largely mediated by lateral inhibitory elements (horizontal and amacrine cells) which modulate the vertical flow of information from photoreceptor to retinal ganglion cell. GABAergic neurons mediate a range of spectral, spatial and temporal processes and are essential elements in networks that isolate 'trigger features' in visual space.

Although the basic features of GABA circuits in the retina are fairly well understood, recent studies have shown that the GABA cell types and networks are much more elaborate than presumed by traditional models of lateral inhibition. The molecular machinery of GABAergic transmission also is sophisticated and includes a heterogeneous assembly of receptors, ion channels and other regulatory elements. The mechanism of GABA receptors in retina is reviewed by Nicholas Brecha who discusses the basic biochemical and pharmacological properties of GABA receptors. He also reports on the distribution and molecular biology of GABA receptors in the retina of a variety of vertebrates. The distribution and biophysics of $GABA_A$ receptors in retina is discussed by Andrew Ishida who has established the existence of $GABA_A$ type conductances upon isolated retinal ganglion cells and at the synaptic terminals of cone photoreceptors and bipolar cells. The biophysics and pharmacology of the $GABA_B$ receptor, a receptor with distinct pharmacological, ionic and kinetic properties, is described by Malcolm Slaughter and Zhuo-Hua Pan.

The distribution of glutamic acid decarboxylase, GABA and GABA symporters is reviewed by Robert Marc, with a summary of the degree of correspondence among these markers. He also reviews some features of vesicular and non-vesicular release.

Sam Wu then describes the physiology of horizontal cell feedback to cone photoreceptors in his chapter on ectotherm retinal circuitry. These authors also review the evidence that some retinal cells can release GABA either by $Ca^{2+}$-dependent or -independent processes. Michael Freed describes the physiology and structure of GABA circuitry in mammals. Finally, Dianna Redburn summarizes the development of GABAergic retinal neurons and explores how these neurons may interact with other cells in determining the final structure of the retinal mosaic.

## Subcortical visual pathways

Our understanding of GABA in the central visual pathways has advanced substantially in recent years. The morphology and function of GABA interneurons in the lateral geniculate nucleus (LGN) and superior colliculus (SC) are understood in some detail. The channel properties of GABA interneurons in the LGN are also under intensive study. Ivan Soltesz and Vincenzo Crunelli summarize experiments on the $Cl^-$- and $K^+$-dependent inhibitory potentials that are evoked by GABAergic interneurons in the LGN and show in vitro that GABA released from slices can generate both $GABA_A$ and $GABA_B$ receptor-mediated IPSPs in LGN relay cells. Dan Uhlrich and Josephine Cucchiaro describe the synaptic circuitry which underlies the inhibitory neural elements involved in feed-forward and feed-backward inhibition and how this circuitry might operate physiologically. They also present evidence for a number of GABAergic extrinsic pathways to the LGN. Thomas Norton and Dwayne Godwin report on how GABA alters synaptic transmission within the LGN. This review of the effects of GABA on receptive field properties suggests that GABA inhibition serves to attenuate the visual signal in the pathway from retina to visual cortex by reducing the transfer ratio from retinal to LGN cells.

GABA is also an important neurotransmitter in the oculomotor system. The basic types and synaptic organization of GABA interneurons and receptors within the mammalian superior colliculus are reviewed by Ranney Mize, who also shows that some GABA cells co-localize other neuroactive substances. Unlike visual cortex, however, GABA and calbindin, a calcium binding protein, are not affected by prolonged monocular deprivation. A chapter by Yasuhiro Okada describes the biochemical distribution of GABA in the superior colliculus and reports the effects that GABA has on the response properties of tectal cells. He also discusses the role of GABA in long-term potentiation and seizures within the colliculus. Paul Dean and Peter Redgrave describe the effects of GABA on visuomotor behavior studied by manipulating GABA neurotransmission in the midbrain. J.J.L. van der Want, J.J. Nunes Cardozo and C. van der Togt report on the synaptic organization of GABA neurons in the pretectum and accessory optic system, regions important in generating the pupillary light reflex and other visual reflexes. Finally, Robert Spencer, Shwu-Fen Wang and Robert Baker describe the basic organization of GABA pathways within the oculomotor system and then show how these GABA systems may be involved in the control of eye movements.

## Visual cortex

The visual cortex contains GABAergic neurons with remarkably heterogeneous properties and these cell types participate in a variety of inhibitory functions. The physiology of two types of inhibitory postsynaptic potential and the effects mediated by $GABA_A$ and $GABA_B$ receptors in the visual cortex are discussed by Barry Connors. The physiological effects of GABA in both the lateral geniculate nucleus and visual cortex are addressed by Adam Sillito, who discusses evidence linking GABAergic mechanisms to particular aspects of receptive field organization. He also elucidates the role of the corticogeniculate pathway in modulating LGN activity. The detailed structure and synaptic organization of GABAergic basket neurons in visual cortex are described by Zoltán Kisvárday.

Ulf Eysel introduces data showing that blocking cortical sites which are lateral to recorded cells in areas 17 and 18 reveals inhibitory influences on direction and orientation sensitivity which are mediated by horizontally distributed circuits. David Ferster, on the other hand, discusses the observation that intracellular recordings do not pick up inhibitory postsynaptic potentials driven by the types of visual stimuli that other studies of GABA processes predict.

Neil Berman, Rodney Douglas and Kevan Martin describe a theoretical canonical microcircuit that is the minimum set of connections which would be required to explain some GABA-mediated phenomena in visual cortex. The detailed morphology of GABA neurons is described by Stewart Hendry and Renee Carder who have found that morphological subtypes can be distinguished by the calcium binding proteins which they co-localize. They also show that both GABA and the calcium binding proteins can be regulated by visually driven activity in adult animals. Colin Barnstable, Toshio Kosaka, Janice Naegele and Yasuyoshi Arimatsu provide evidence that subtypes of GABA cell can be distinguished by antibodies or lectins that recognize specific membrane proteins or sugar moieties unique to these cells. The possible relation of these membrane components to cell function is also discussed in this chapter as are alterations that occur in these components during development or visual deprivation. Finally, John Parnavelas describes the ontogenesis of GABA neurons in visual cortex and the role of GABA in establishing a template for cortical organization in the prenatal brain.

# Contents

## Section III. Visual cortex

# SECTION I

# Retina

R.R. Mize, R.E. Marc and A.M. Sillito (Eds.)
Progress in Brain Research, Vol. 90

3

CHAPTER 1

# Expression of GABA$_A$ receptors in the vertebrate retina

Nicholas C. Brecha

*Department of Medicine, Department of Anatomy and Cell Biology, CURE, Brain Research Institute and Jules Stein Eye Institute, UCLA School of Medicine, UCLA, Los Angeles, CA 90024 and Veterans Administration Medical Center — West Los Angeles, Los Angeles, CA 90073, USA*

## Introduction

γ-Aminobutyric acid (GABA), which mediates neuronal inhibition at GABA receptors, is one of several neurotransmitters that have been localized in the vertebrate retina (see Brecha, 1983; Massey and Redburn, 1987; Yazulla, 1986; Ehinger and Dowling, 1987, for reviews). In the retina, as in other regions of the nervous system, GABA acts at two different and distinct membrane sites, which have been classified as GABA$_A$ and GABA$_B$ receptors on the basis of pharmacological, physiological and structural criteria (Hill and Bowery, 1981; Bowery et al., 1984; Bormann, 1988). GABA$_A$ receptors are characterized by their bicuculline sensitivity and are modulated by a wide variety of drugs including benzodiazepines, barbiturates, picrotoxin and picrotoxin-related convulsants (Bowery et al., 1984; see Olsen, 1981; Olsen and Venter, 1986; Stephenson, 1988, for reviews). Several compounds have proved to be particularly useful for investigating GABA$_A$ receptors. These include muscimol and benzodiazepines, which bind at different recognition sites on the GABA$_A$ receptor (Olsen and Venter, 1986; Stephenson, 1988; Olsen and Tobin, 1990; Möhler et al., 1990). Less is known about GABA$_B$ receptors, which are bicuculline insensitive and are characterized by specific, high affinity baclofen binding and by a lack of sensitivity to benzodiazepines and barbiturates (Hill and Bowery, 1981; Bowery et al., 1984; Bormann, 1988).

Molecular cloning studies have demonstrated that the GABA$_A$ receptor is a member of the ligand-gated ion channel superfamily of receptors (Schofield et al., 1987). This receptor is composed of a complex of several structurally distinct membrane polypeptides that form a ligand-gated Cl$^-$ channel (see Möhler et al., 1990 and Olsen and Tobin, 1990, for reviews). The exact relationship and number of polypeptides making up a GABA$_A$ receptor in vivo are unknown, and currently this receptor is believed to be composed of four or five polypeptide subunits (Mamalaki et al., 1987; Schofield et al., 1987; Olsen and Tobin, 1990).

There are several lines of evidence indicating the existence of multiple GABA$_A$ receptors. To date, twelve cDNAs related to the GABA$_A$ receptor complex have been identified and in situ hybridization studies have demonstrated marked regional variations in the distribution of their mRNAs in the nervous system (Levitan et al., 1988a; Séquier et al., 1988; Wisden et al., 1988; Shivers et al., 1989; Ymer et al., 1989a; see Möhler et al., 1990 and Olsen and Tobin, 1990, for reviews). Furthermore, immunohistochemical findings based on the use of GABA$_A$ polypeptide-specific antibodies (Richards et al., 1987; de Blas et al., 1988) together with in vitro receptor autoradiography data obtained with different

4

GABA$_A$ receptor ligands (Unnerstall et al., 1981; Young et al., 1981; Olsen et al., 1990), photoaffinity labeling of the GABA$_A$ receptor complex with muscimol or flunitrazepam (Möhler et al., 1980; Fuchs et al., 1988; Fuchs and Sieghart, 1989; Bureau and Olsen, 1990) and electrophysiological studies (Yasui et al., 1985; Akaike et al., 1986) are all suggestive of multiple GABA$_A$ receptors, each having specific pharmacological properties and distinct distributions in the nervous system.

In the retina, GABA has a major role in the processing of visual information, and the major site of action of GABA is at GABA$_A$ receptors (see Yazulla, 1986 and various Chapters in this volume for reviews). Initial investigations using in vitro receptor autoradiography indicated that specific, high affinity GABA$_A$ binding sites are abundant in the inner plexiform layer (IPL) (Brecha, 1983; Zarbin et al., 1986). More recently, in situ hybridization and immunohistochemical approaches have demonstrated that different GABA$_A$ mRNAs or polypeptides are expressed by a variety of cell populations in the retina (Mariani et al., 1987; Richards et al., 1987; Hughes et al., 1989; Yazulla et al., 1989; Brecha et al., 1990, 1991; Brecha and Weigmann, 1991). These observations, together with molecular cloning, RNA hybridization, biochemical and pharmacological findings that indicate GABA$_A$ receptor heterogeneity in the nervous system (Levitan et al., 1988a; see Stephenson, 1988; Möhler et al., 1990; Olsen and Tobin, 1990, for reviews), are consistent with the presence of multiple GABA$_A$ receptors in the retina. The aim of this chapter is to review evidence of the distribution and localization of GABA$_A$ receptors in the vertebrate retina.

**GABAergic microcircuitry in the vertebrate retina**

Comprehensive descriptions and reviews of the distribution of GABAergic cell populations, which are based on high affinity uptake of GABA and GABA-related compounds, and on the distribution of GABA and its biosynthetic enzyme, L-glutamate decarboxylase (GAD; EC 4.1.1.15) have been presented (Brandon, 1985; Yazulla, 1986; Mosinger et al., 1986; Massey and Redburn, 1987; Ehinger and Dowling, 1987; see various Chapters in this volume). The following summary is intended to acquaint the reader with some details of the localization patterns of GABA and GAD immunoreactivity and other evidence of GABA's action in those species for which most data concerning the localization of GABA$_A$ receptors are available.

*Teleost retina*

Several experimental approaches have convincingly demonstrated that H1 cone horizontal cells of the teleost retina are GABAergic (Lam et al., 1978, 1979; Marc et al., 1978; Brandon, 1985; Mosinger et al., 1986). This horizontal cell type is characterized by (1) ascending dendrites that form contacts with cone photoreceptors and (2) an axonal process that forms both gap junctions with other horizontal cells and conventional synaptic contacts with bipolar and interplexiform cell processes (Stell et al., 1975; Marc and Liu, 1984; Marshak and Dowling, 1987). Horizontal cells have an inhibitory feedback onto cone photoreceptors (Baylor et al., 1971; Burkhardt, 1977), which is likely to be mediated by GABA at GABA$_A$ receptors in several species (Murakami et al., 1982a,b; Tachibana and Kaneko, 1984; Kaneko and Tachibana, 1986; see Wu, Chapter 4). Specifically, in carp, catfish and goldfish retina, electrophysiological and pharmacological investigations provide good evidence that GABA hyperpolarizes, whereas the GABA antagonists, picrotoxin and bicuculline, depolarize cone photoreceptors (Wu and Dowling, 1980; Murakami et al., 1982a,b; Lasater and Lam, 1984a). Other studies have shown that GABA is released by horizontal cells under appropriate physiological conditions (Ayoub and Lam, 1984, 1985; Yazulla, 1985; Schwartz, 1987). All of these findings provide strong evidence that GABA is an H1 horizontal cell transmitter and that cone feedback inhibition is likely to be mediated at GABA$_A$ receptors.

Goldfish retina is characterized by multiple GABAergic amacrine cell populations (Marc et al., 1978; Yazulla and Brecha, 1980; Yazulla et al., 1986, 1987; Brandon, 1985; Mosinger et al., 1986). GABAergic processes have a laminar distribution in the IPL (Brandon, 1985; Mosinger et al., 1986; Yazulla et al., 1986; Muller and Marc, 1990). Ultrastructural studies have shown that one group of amacrine cells (Ab pyriform amacrine cells) forms prominent synaptic contacts with the axonal terminals of mixed rod-cone bipolar cells (Marc et al., 1978; Yazulla et al., 1987; Studholme and Yazulla, 1988). GABAergic amacrine cell processes also form presynaptic contacts with bipolar cell terminals, amacrine cell processes, and ganglion cell dendrites and somata (Zucker et al., 1984; Yazulla et al., 1987; Studholme and Yazulla, 1988; Muller and Marc, 1990). These morphological observations are consistent with electrophysiological findings reporting the presence of $GABA_A$ receptors on bipolar cells (Kondo and Toyoda, 1983; Tachibana and Kaneko, 1988; see Wu, Chapter 4). GABA and muscimol are equally effective in hyperpolarizing isolated rod ON-type bipolar cells and small axonal terminal-type bipolar cells (Kaneko and Tachibana, 1987; Tachibana and Kaneko, 1987, 1988). Interestingly, the highest sensitivity to GABA is at their axonal terminals, and there is little sensitivity to GABA at their somata or dendrites. Furthermore, this GABA-evoked response is antagonized by bicuculline and picrotoxin, and potentiated by diazepam (Tachibana and Kaneko, 1988) providing some pharmacological evidence for $GABA_A$ receptors.

The identification of GABAergic amacrine cell contacts onto ganglion cells also is consistent with electrophysiological evidence that (1) $GABA_A$ receptors are located on isolated goldfish ganglion cell bodies (Ishida and Cohen, 1988; see Ishida, Chapter 2) and (2) GABA influences cyprinid ganglion cell activity (Glickman et al., 1982; Lasater and Lam, 1984b). Finally, a GABAergic influence has been reported on dopamine-containing interplexiform cells (Negishi et al., 1983;

O'Connor et al., 1987). Together, all of these studies indicate GABAergic amacrine cell participation in multiple IPL pathways.

*Bird retina*

There are few studies of the GABAergic system in bird retina. Chick horizontal cells accumulate GABA or GABA-related compounds, and contain GAD and GABA immunoreactivity (Yazulla and Brecha, 1980; Brandon, 1985; Yazulla, 1986; Mosinger et al., 1986). Immunoreactive processes form distinct bands along the inner and outer margins of the outer plexiform layer (OPL), and GABA immunoreactive horizontal cell processes invaginate photoreceptor terminals (Mosinger et al., 1986). GABAergic processes have a laminar distribution in the IPL (Yazulla and Brecha, 1980; Brandon, 1985; Mosinger et al., 1986). In addition, numerous GABAergic amacrine, and perhaps ganglion cells are present in the avian retina (Yazulla and Brecha, 1980, 1981; Mosinger et al., 1986).

*Rat, rabbit and primate retina*

Rat, rabbit and primate horizontal cells do not accumulate GABA or GABA-related compounds (Yazulla, 1986), and most, but not all studies agree that they are not stained with GAD antibodies (Brandon et al., 1979; Vaughn et al., 1981; Brandon, 1985; Hendrickson et al., 1985; Mosinger and Yazulla, 1985, 1987; Nishimura et al., 1985; Mariani and Caserta, 1986; Agardh et al., 1987; Hughes et al., 1989). Recently, several investigations have reported that GABA antibodies label some bipolar and horizontal cells in these retinas (Nishimura et al., 1985; Mosinger et al., 1986; Osborne et al., 1986; Agardh et al., 1987; Mosinger and Yazulla, 1987; Grünert and Wässle, 1990; Koontz and Hendrickson, 1990). In addition, in these species GAD and GABA immunoreactive interplexiform cells have been described (Brandon, 1985; Mosinger et al., 1986; Mosinger and Yazulla, 1987; Ryan and Hendrickson, 1987). These morphological observations are suggestive of an action of GABA in the OPL.

In rat, rabbit and primate retina, there are several distinct GABAergic amacrine cell populations (Osborne and Beaton, 1986; Brecha et al., 1988; Kosaka et al., 1988; Wässle and Chun, 1988; Vaney, 1989). In these species, GAD and GABA immunoreactive processes display a laminar distribution in the IPL (Brandon et al., 1979; Vaughn et al., 1981; Hendrickson et al., 1985; Mosinger and Yazulla, 1985, 1987; Mosinger et al., 1986; Mariani and Caserta, 1986; Grünert and Wässle, 1990; Koontz and Hendrickson, 1990). The ultrastructural features of the GAD immunoreactive patterns in these retinas are comparable. GAD immunoreactivity is localized to amacrine cells and their processes, which form the majority of their synaptic contacts with bipolar cell terminals and with other amacrine cell processes. In rat and rabbit retina, but not in monkey retina, some GAD immunoreactive presynaptic contacts also are located on ganglion cell bodies and dendrites (Brandon et al., 1980; Vaughn et al., 1981; Mosinger and Yazulla, 1985; Mariani and Caserta, 1986). Recent investigations employing GABA antibodies in the macaque monkey retina have confirmed these general observations (Grünert and Wässle, 1990; Koontz and Hendrickson, 1990). These studies also show significant GABA immunoreactive amacrine cell presynaptic contacts onto ganglion cell dendrites and some contacts onto amacrine and ganglion cell bodies (Grünert and Wässle, 1990; Koontz and Hendrickson, 1990).

GABA hyperpolarizes isolated bipolar cells of the rodent retina. This response is antagonized by bicuculline and picrotoxin (Karschin and Wässle, 1990; Suzuki et al., 1990; Yeh et al., 1990) and potentiated by pentobarbitone (Suzuki et al., 1990), providing both electrophysiological and pharmacological evidence for $GABA_A$ receptors. The highest sensitivity to GABA is found at bipolar cell axonal terminals (Karschin and Wässle, 1990; Suzuki et al., 1990; but see Yeh et al., 1990), similar to observations of goldfish bipolar cells (Tachibana and Kaneko, 1988). Isolated juvenile rat ganglion cells also are hyperpolarized

by GABA, and this response is antagonized by bicuculline and picrotoxin (Tauck et al., 1988). Electrophysiological recordings of the intact mammalian retina further illustrate a critical role for GABA in the formation of many ganglion cell receptive field properties (Caldwell and Daw, 1978; Caldwell et al., 1978; Ariel and Daw, 1982; Bolz et al., 1985). For instance, in vivo application of picrotoxin to the rabbit ocular vascular system abolishes complex receptive field properties of ganglion cells, including directional sensitivity and size specificity of ON- and ON-OFF-directional-sensitive ganglion cells, and orientation specificity of orientation-sensitive ganglion cells (Caldwell and Daw, 1978; Caldwell et al., 1978; Ariel and Daw, 1982).

Other experimental approaches also have provided evidence for GABAergic modulation of retinal neurons (see Massey and Redburn, 1987, for review). For instance, in the rat retina, GABA, GABA agonists and antagonists, and benzodiazepines have complex modulatory influences on dopaminergic cell function (Morgan and Kamp, 1980; Kamp and Morgan, 1981, 1982; Marshburn and Iuvone, 1981). In rabbit retina, GABA and muscimol inhibit, and bicuculline and picrotoxin potentiate, the light-evoked release of acetylcholine from amacrine cells (Massey and Neal, 1979; Massey and Redburn, 1982). These findings, along with anatomical studies, are consistent with the action of GABA at $GABA_A$ receptors associated with different IPL pathways.

## $GABA_A$ binding sites in the retina

### Homogenate binding

Specific, sodium-independent, low and high affinity GABA binding sites were initially detected in membrane preparations of rat, cow, pig and sheep retina, and in synaptosomal fractions prepared from cow retina (Enna and Snyder, 1976; Redburn et al., 1979, 1980; Redburn and Mitchell, 1980, 1981; Guarneri et al., 1981). Furthermore, GABA binding sites in the retina and in other regions of the mammalian central nervous system have a similar order of potency for displacement by GABA agonists and antagonists including muscimol, bicuculline and picrotoxin (Enna and Snyder, 1976; Redburn et al., 1979, 1980; Redburn and Mitchell, 1980). These investigations have firmly established the presence of GABA binding sites in the retina and have shown that their binding characteristics and pharmacological properties are comparable to GABA binding sites in the central nervous system (Enna and Snyder, 1976, 1977; Olsen et al., 1981).

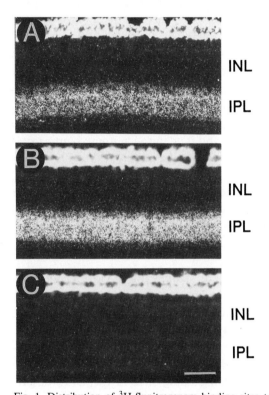

Fig. 1. Distribution of $^3$H-flunitrazepam binding sites to the inner plexiform layer (IPL) of the pigeon retina. A. Retinal section incubated with $3.3 \times 10^{-9}$ M $^3$H-flunitrazepam. B. Adjacent section incubated with $3.3 \times 10^{-9}$ M $^3$H-flunitrazepam with 100 $\mu$M muscimol, illustrating an enhancement of benzodiazepine binding in the presence of muscimol. C. Adjacent control section incubated with $3.3 \times 10^{-9}$ M $^3$H-flunitrazepam and $1 \times 10^{-6}$ M clonazepam demonstrating the inhibition of specific flunitrazepam binding sites. These sections were processed simultaneously using in vitro receptor autoradiographic techniques. Darkfield photomicrographs. Adapted from Fig. 11 of Brecha (1983). INL, inner nuclear layer. Scale bar = 100 $\mu$m.

Homogenate binding studies using muscimol and flunitrazepam have provided strong evidence for the existence of specific, high affinity GABA$_A$ binding sites in a wide variety of vertebrate retinas (Howells et al., 1979; Borbe et al., 1980; Howells and Simon, 1980; Osborne, 1980a,b; Paul et al., 1980; Redburn and Mitchell, 1980; Regan et al., 1980; Schaeffer, 1980, 1982; Skolnick et al., 1980; Yazulla and Brecha, 1980; Altstein et al., 1981; Sieghart et al., 1982). Muscimol and flunitrazepam binding affinities and the order of potency for displacement of flunitrazepam by unlabeled benzodiazepines in the retina and brain are comparable (Möhler and Okada, 1977; Williams and Risley, 1978; Howells et al., 1979; Borbe et al., 1980; Redburn and Mitchell, 1980; Schaeffer, 1980; Altstein et al., 1981; Sieghart et al., 1982). In addition, both muscimol and GABA increase benzodiazepine binding affinity, but not the number of binding sites in retinal homogenates (Howells and Simon, 1980; Paul et al., 1980; Regan et al., 1980; Altstein et al., 1981; Sieghart et al., 1982; but see Osborne, 1980b) as also observed in other regions of the central nervous system (Tallman et al., 1978; Karobath and Sperk, 1979; Unnerstall et al., 1981). An enhancement of specific flunitrazepam binding by GABA and muscimol has been demonstrated in the IPL of goldfish, pigeon (Fig. 1) and human retinas using in vitro receptor autoradiographic approaches (Brecha, 1983; Zarbin et al., 1986; Lin et al., 1991).

Changes in GABA and benzodiazepine binding properties associated with light and dark conditions have been reported. In rat, binding affinities, but not the number of GABA, diazepam and flunitrazepam binding sites are higher in dark-adapted as compared to light-adapted retinas (Biggio et al., 1981; Rothe et al., 1985). The basis for these changes is unknown.

*In vitro receptor autoradiography*

Light and electron microscopic studies using in vitro receptor autoradiography have provided direct evidence for GABA$_A$ binding sites in the OPL and IPL (Young and Kuhar, 1979; Yazulla, 1981; Yazulla and Brecha, 1981; Altstein et al., 1981; Brecha, 1983; Zarbin et al., 1986; Lin et al., 1991).

### Goldfish retina

In goldfish retina, GABA and muscimol binding sites are present in the OPL, and GABA, muscimol and flunitrazepam binding sites are distributed in a homogeneous band across the IPL (Yazulla, 1981; Lin et al., 1991). Muscimol binding sites are mainly associated with amacrine-amacrine synaptic specializations distributed to distal and mid regions of the IPL, while amacrine-bipolar synaptic specializations located in the proximal IPL (Yazulla, 1981).

### Bird retina

In chicken retina, GABA and muscimol binding sites are distributed to the OPL and to the IPL in a broad, homogeneous band (Fig. 2) (Yazulla and Brecha, 1981). In the OPL, muscimol

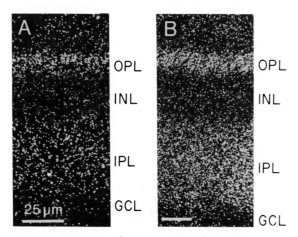

Fig. 2. Distribution of $^3$H-muscimol and $^3$H-GABA binding sites to the outer plexiform layer (OPL) and IPL of the chicken retina. Retinal section incubated with $0.29 \times 10^{-6}$ M $^3$H-muscimol (A) or with $0.8 \times 10^{-6}$ M $^3$H-GABA (B). These sections were processed by in vitro receptor autoradiographic techniques. Darkfield photomicrographs. From Brecha (1983) and originally adapted from Yazulla and Brecha (1981). GCL, ganglion cell layer. Scale bar = 25 $\mu$m.

binding is associated with (1) membranes located at horizontal cell processes and cone photoreceptor terminals and (2) specialized junctions located proximal to photoreceptor terminals (Yazulla and Brecha, 1981). In the IPL, muscimol binding is primarily associated with amacrine-amacrine and amacrine-bipolar synaptic specializations that are preferentially distributed to laminae 2 and 4 of the IPL (Yazulla and Brecha, 1981). In contrast, flunitrazepam binding sites only appear to be associated with the IPL, where they form a continuous band across this layer in the chicken and pigeon retina (Fig. 1) (Altstein et al., 1981; Brecha, 1983).

### Rat and primate retina

In rat and human retina, a low density of muscimol and flunitrazepam binding sites is observed in the OPL (Young and Kuhar, 1979; Zarbin et al., 1986). In rat, monkey (*Macaca fascicularis*) and human retina, these binding sites are distributed in a band across the IPL. A very low density of binding sites also is associated with cells located in the proximal inner nuclear layer (INL) and with scattered cells in the ganglion cell layer (GCL) (Zarbin et al., 1986).

### Summary

Homogenate binding and in vitro receptor autoradiography have been critical for establishing the presence of GABA$_A$ binding sites in the vertebrate retina. In the goldfish and bird OPL, the presence of muscimol binding sites is indicative of GABA$_A$ receptors. Reasons for the lack of flunitrazepam binding sites in the OPL, despite the presence of GABA and muscimol binding sites, and of GAD, GABA and GABA$_A$ receptor immunoreactivities, are unknown (Altstein et al., 1981; Yazulla and Brecha, 1981; Brecha, 1983; Brandon, 1985; Mosinger et al., 1986; Yazulla et al., 1989; Lin et al., 1991). The failure to detect benzodiazepine binding sites in the OPL may be due to (1) a very low density of benzodiazepine binding sites, (2) low affinity benzodiazepine binding sites or (3) the presence of GABA$_A$ receptors that lack a benzodiazepine binding site. This latter possibility also has been suggested from other in vitro receptor autoradiographic studies (Unnerstall et al., 1981; Olsen et al., 1990).

The low density of muscimol and flunitrazepam binding sites in the rat and human OPL, and the presence of GAD and GABA immunoreactivities in the rat and macaque monkey OPL (Brandon, 1985; Mosinger et al., 1986; Zarbin et al., 1986; Ryan and Hendrickson, 1987; Grünert and Wässle, 1990) are congruent with an action of GABA in this region. However, as discussed in detail below, in the primate OPL there are species differences in the distribution of these ligands, and GABA$_A$ receptor, GABA and GAD immunoreactivities (Zarbin et al., 1986; Mariani et al., 1987; Richards et al., 1987; Ryan and Hendrickson, 1987; Hughes et al., 1989; Grünert and Wässle, 1990). There are multiple possibilities for these differences. Furthermore, some of these discrepancies could be due to our limited understanding of GABA$_A$ receptor composition and number, and with the limited repertoire of reagents that are now available for studying this receptor.

In the IPL of all species investigated to date, the localization of muscimol and benzodiazepine binding sites, and of GABA and GAD immunoreactivities, is indicative of an action of GABA in this layer. These observations together with electrophysiological (Tachibana and Kaneko, 1988; Ishida and Cohen, 1988; Tauck et al., 1988; Karschin and Wässle, 1990; Suzuki et al., 1990; Yeh et al., 1990) and ultrastructural (Brandon et al., 1980; Vaughn et al., 1981; Mariani and Caserta, 1986; Yazulla et al., 1987; Grünert and Wässle, 1990; Koontz and Hendrickson, 1990; Muller and Marc, 1990) investigations clearly suggest that GABA$_A$ receptors are located at amacrine-amacrine, amacrine-bipolar and amacrine-ganglion synaptic specializations.

However, in vitro receptor autoradiographic investigations do not provide exact information as to the cellular localization or possible synaptic relationships of GABA$_A$ receptors in the retina.

Ligand binding techniques are limited due to such factors as ligand specificities and affinities, and the low anatomical resolution of the radioactive signal. Experimental approaches using in situ hybridization and immunohistochemistry are now being employed in an attempt to overcome some of these limitations and to provide a better understanding of the cellular localization of GABA$_A$ receptors. These studies are beginning to provide more detailed information regarding the distribution of GABA$_A$ receptors and additional clues regarding GABA$_A$ receptor heterogeneity in the retina.

## Expression of GABA$_A$ receptor subunits in the retina

### Background information

GABA$_A$ receptors are composed of several related polypeptides, and to date six alpha ($\alpha$), three beta ($\beta$) and two gamma ($\gamma$) cDNAs and a single delta ($\delta$) cDNA related to this receptor have been cloned and sequenced (Schofield et al., 1987; Levitan et al., 1988a; Ymer et al., 1989a,b; Shivers et al., 1989; Pritchett et al., 1989b; Khrestchatisky et al., 1989, 1991; Lüddens et al., 1990; Malherbe et al., 1990a,b; Pritchett and Seeburg, 1990; Möhler et al., 1990). Different combinations of these polypeptides are thought to form functionally distinct GABA$_A$ receptor subtypes and are theoretically associated with different GABA$_A$ sites as suggested by receptor binding and pharmacological studies (Unnerstall et al., 1981; Young et al., 1981; Olsen et al., 1990; see Olsen and Tobin, 1990 and Möhler et al., 1990, for reviews). Several investigations have examined the properties of these receptor polypeptides, whether expressed alone or in combination with other receptor polypeptides in heterologous cells. For instance, receptors expressed from bovine or human $\alpha$ and $\beta$ mRNAs have many of the electrophysiological characteristics of native GABA$_A$ receptors, although other features such as benzodiazepine sensitivity and GABA cooperativity are weak or absent (Schofield et al., 1987; Levitan et al., 1988a,b; Pritchett et al., 1988). Recently, electrophysiological and pharmacological studies have reported that the co-expression of $\alpha$, beta$_1$ ($\beta_1$) and gamma$_2$ polypeptides is required for obtaining recombinant receptors that have most of the properties of the native GABA$_A$ receptor, including benzodiazepine responses and binding (Pritchett et al., 1989a,b; Sigel et al., 1990; Verdoon et al., 1990). Interestingly, differences in benzodiazepine pharmacology may be directly related to the heterogeneity of the $\alpha$ polypeptides (Pritchett et al., 1989a; Pritchett and Seeburg, 1990; Sigel et al., 1990).

GABA$_A$ alpha$_1$ ($\alpha_1$) mRNA is the most abundant $\alpha$ variant reported to date with a widespread distribution along the neuraxis (Levitan et al., 1988a; Séquier et al., 1988; Wisden et al., 1988, 1989a; Khrestchatisky et al., 1989, 1991; Ymer et al., 1989b; MacLennan et al., 1991). GABA$_A$ alpha$_2$ ($\alpha_2$) mRNA is less abundant compared to GABA$_A$ $\alpha_1$ mRNA as determined by both Northern blot and in situ hybridization histochemical analyses (Levitan et al., 1988a; Wisden et al., 1988, 1989a; MacLennan et al., 1991). GABA$_A$ $\alpha$ variants have distinct distributions within the nervous system (Wisden et al., 1988, 1989a; MacLennan et al., 1991), consistent with the suggestion that they are associated with different GABA$_A$ receptor subtypes.

GABA$_A$ $\beta$ mRNAs also have a widespread and differential distribution in the rat central nervous system (Schofield et al., 1987; Lolait et al., 1989; Ymer et al., 1989a; Zhang et al., 1991). Beta$_2$ ($\beta_2$) and beta$_3$ ($\beta_3$) mRNAs are more abundant than the $\beta_1$ mRNA as revealed by Northern blot analysis (Schofield et al., 1987; Ymer et al., 1989a). In situ hybridization histochemical studies show an extensive distribution of these $\beta$ subunits along the neuraxis with individual differences in their location and level of expression (Zhang et al., 1991). The $\beta$ and $\alpha$ mRNAs have a partial overlap in their distribution (Séquier et al., 1988; Wisden et al., 1988,

1989a; MacLennan et al., 1991; Zhang et al., 1991).

GABA$_A$ receptors are likely to be comprised of at least one $\alpha$ and one $\beta$ polypeptide (Möhler et al., 1980; Häring et al., 1985; Schoch et al., 1985; Mamalaki et al., 1987; Schofield et al., 1987; Fuchs and Sieghart, 1989; Olsen and Tobin, 1990; Möhler et al., 1990). Therefore, it should be possible to provide a reasonably accurate description of the distribution and localization patterns of GABA$_A$ receptors using in situ hybridization histochemistry and immunohistochemistry with probes to the $\alpha$ and $\beta$ subunits. The following sections review recent investigations of the distribution of GABA$_A$ receptors based on the localization of GABA$_A$ $\alpha_1$ and $\alpha_2$ mRNAs, and GABA$_A$ $\alpha_1$, $\beta_2$ and $\beta_3$ polypeptides in the retina.

*Distribution of GABA$_A$ receptor mRNAs*

To date, information about the tissue distribution and cellular localization of GABA$_A$ receptor mRNAs is limited to some of the $\alpha$ variants in the bovine and rat retina (Wisden et al., 1989b; Brecha et al., 1990, 1991). GABA$_A$ $\alpha_1$, $\alpha_2$ and $\alpha_3$ mRNAs are present in bovine retinal extracts, with GABA$_A$ $\alpha_1$ mRNA being the most abundant (Wisden et al., 1989b).

As for the cellular localization of GABA$_A$ $\alpha$ mRNAs in the retina, the only information available so far concerns GABA$_A$ $\alpha_1$ and $\alpha_2$ mRNAs, which we have demonstrated in the rat retina using in situ hybridization histochemistry with $^{35}$S-labeled rat GABA$_A$ $\alpha_1$ and $\alpha_2$ RNA probes (Brecha et al., 1990, 1991). In all retinal regions, GABA$_A$ $\alpha_1$ and $\alpha_2$ mRNAs are expressed in neurons located in the INL and GCL. Labeling is not observed in the outer nuclear layer (ONL). GABA$_A$ $\alpha_1$ mRNA-containing cells are distributed across the entire INL, and some discretely labeled cells are present in the GCL (Fig. 3). In contrast, GABA$_A$ $\alpha_2$ mRNA has a more limited distribution, and labeled cells are confined to the proximal INL and to the GCL (Fig. 4).

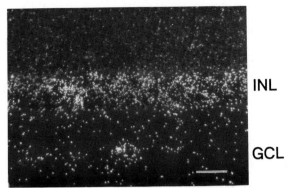

Fig. 3. Distribution of GABA$_A$ $\alpha_1$ mRNA in a transverse section of the rat retina. Cells expressing GABA$_A$ $\alpha_1$ mRNA are distributed across the INL and occasionally are observed in the GCL. On the basis of their distribution, it is likely that labeled cells in the INL are bipolar and amacrine cells, and that labeled cells in the GCL are ganglion and displaced amacrine cells. Section was incubated with a $^{35}$S-labeled GABA$_A$ $\alpha_1$ antisense RNA probe. Darkfield photomicrograph. Adapted from Fig. 3 of Brecha et al. (1991). Scale bar = 25 $\mu$m.

The position and distribution of GABA$_A$ $\alpha_1$ mRNA-containing cells in the INL and GCL suggest they are bipolar and amacrine cells, and displaced amacrine and ganglion cells, respectively (Brecha et al., 1990, 1991). Similarly, the

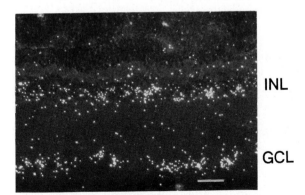

Fig. 4. Distribution of GABA$_A$ $\alpha_2$ mRNA in a transverse section of the rat retina. Cells expressing GABA$_A$ $\alpha_2$ mRNA are located in the proximal INL and in the GCL. Labeling pattern suggests that amacrine, displaced amacrine and ganglion cells express this mRNA. Section was incubated with a $^{35}$S-labeled GABA$_A$ $\alpha_2$ antisense RNA probe. Darkfield photomicrograph. Scale bar = 25 $\mu$m.

position and distribution of GABA$_A$ $\alpha_2$ mRNA-containing cells in the proximal INL and GCL suggest they are amacrine, displaced amacrine and ganglion cells. The localization of GABA$_A$ $\alpha_1$ mRNA to bipolar cells is consistent with electrophysiological evidence of GABA$_A$ receptor expression by bipolar cells (Karschin and Wässle, 1990; Suzuki et al., 1990; Yeh et al., 1990). The expression of GABA$_A$ $\alpha_1$ and $\alpha_2$ mRNAs by amacrine cells is congruent with the presence of high affinity muscimol and flunitrazepam binding sites in the IPL (Zarbin et al., 1986) and the localization of GABA$_A$ $\beta_2$ and $\beta_3$ polypeptide immunoreactivity to amacrine cells in the rat retina (Richards et al., 1978). Autoradiographic techniques using $^{35}$S-labeled probes lack high anatomical resolution, and therefore it is not possible from these experiments to determine if ganglion, interplexiform or horizontal cells also express GABA$_A$ $\alpha_1$ or $\alpha_2$ mRNAs.

The cellular labeling pattern of GABA$_A$ $\alpha_1$ or $\alpha_2$ mRNA in the GCL provides little information as to the identity of the cells expressing GABA$_A$ $\alpha$ polypeptides. There is some evidence for ganglion cells having GABA$_A$ receptors from electrophysiological evidence for the presence of GABA$_A$ receptors on all isolated, juvenile rodent ganglion cell bodies (Tauck et al., 1988). On the other hand, because of the large number of displaced amacrine cells in the GCL of the rat retina (Perry, 1981), the possibility that GABA$_A$ $\alpha$ polypeptides also are expressed by displaced amacrine cells cannot be ruled out.

*Summary*

The majority of GABA$_A$ $\alpha_1$ mRNA-containing neurons are likely to be amacrine and bipolar cells on the basis of their somal locations. Similarly, the distribution of GABA$_A$ $\alpha_2$ mRNA-containing cells is consistent with their identification as amacrine, displaced amacrine or ganglion cells. These observations extend in vitro receptor autoradiographic studies of the rat retina (Zarbin et al., 1986) and are in agreement with electrophysiological investigations (Karschin and Wässle, 1990; Suzuki et al., 1990; Yeh et al., 1990). Finally, these different GABA$_A$ $\alpha$ mRNA labeling patterns are consistent with GABA$_A$ receptor heterogenity in the retina.

*Localization of GABA$_A$ receptor polypeptide immunoreactivity*

Three monoclonal antibodies directed to either GABA$_A$ $\alpha_1$ or to GABA$_A$ $\beta_2$ and $\beta_3$ polypep-

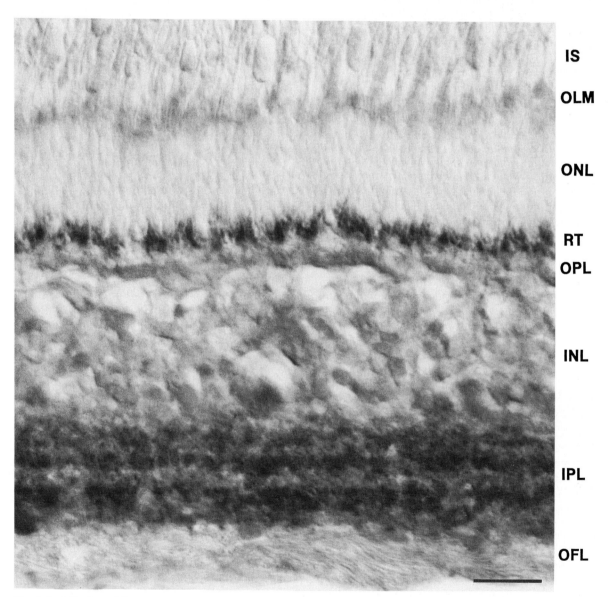

Fig. 5. Localization of GABA$_A$ $\beta_2$ and $\beta_3$ polypeptide immunoreactivity in the goldfish retina as visualized by monoclonal antibody 62-3G1. Immunoreactivity is mainly localized to photoreceptor terminals (RT), amacrine cell bodies and processes distributed to the IPL. Immunostaining is absent in the outer nuclear layer (ONL). Bright field photomicrograph. IS, inner segments; OFL, optic fiber layer; OLM, outer limiting membrane. Relabeled from Fig. 1 of Yazulla et al., (1989). Scale bar = 25 $\mu$m.

tides are presently available (Häring et al., 1985; Schoch et al., 1985; Möhler et al., 1990; Vitorica et al., 1988). Mouse monoclonal antibody bd-24 is directed to GABA$_A$ $\alpha_1$ and recognizes this $\alpha$ polypeptide in several species, except the rat (Schoch et al., 1985; Richards et al., 1987; Möhler et al., 1990). The other two monoclonal antibodies (bd-17 and 62-3G1) cross react with the GABA$_A$ $\beta_2$ and $\beta_3$ polypeptides in several species (Möhler et al., 1990; A.L. de Blas, personal communication).

*Goldfish retina*

In goldfish retina, GABA$_A$ $\beta_2$ and $\beta_3$ polypeptide immunoreactivity visualized by antibody 62-3G1 is mainly localized to photoreceptor terminals, amacrine cell bodies and processes distributed across the IPL (Fig. 5) (Yazulla et al., 1989). In the IPL, three bands contain a high density of immunoreactive processes, and they correspond best with the pattern of high affinity uptake of muscimol and of GAD immunoreactivity, rather than with the high affinity uptake of GABA or with GABA immunoreactivity (Brandon, 1985; Mosinger et al., 1986; Yazulla et al., 1986, 1989; Muller and Marc, 1990; see Marc, Chapter 5). In addition, some lightly immunolabeled amacrine cell bodies, horizontal cell bodies and their axons, and ganglion cell bodies are observed.

Cone photoreceptors have light GABA$_A$ $\beta_2$ and $\beta_3$ polypeptide immunoreactive staining around their nuclei and heavy staining of their terminals. Cone terminals are characterized by immunolabeling of (1) intracellular structures and (2) the cytoplasmic side of the plasma membrane, most prominently in regions located away from the synaptic ribbons and horizontal cell dendrites (Fig. 6). The association of GABA$_A$ receptor immunoreactivity with intracellular structures also has been described in other regions of the nervous system (Somogyi et al., 1989; Soltesz et al., 1990). The localization of GABA$_A$ $\beta_2$ and $\beta_3$ polypeptide immunoreactivity to cone photoreceptor terminals is in agreement with a large

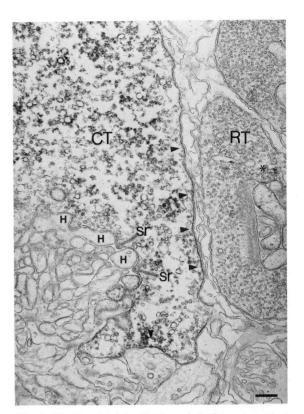

Fig. 6. Ultrastructural localization of GABA$_A$ $\beta_2$ and $\beta_3$ polypeptide immunoreactivity in the goldfish OPL. The cone photoreceptor terminal (CT) is characterized by immunostaining of intracellular structures and the plasma membrane. The heaviest plasma membrane staining (arrowheads) is located away from horizontal cell dendrites (H) and synaptic ribbons (sr). Note some light intracellular staining (*) in the rod terminal (RT). Electron micrograph. Relabeled from Fig. 2 of Yazulla et al., (1989). Scale bar = 1 $\mu$m.

body of evidence showing a GABAergic input to cone photoreceptors originating from H1 horizontal cells (see Yazulla, 1986, for review) and with the recent description of muscimol binding sites in the OPL (Lin et al., 1991). The location of prominent GABA$_A$ $\beta_2$ and $\beta_3$ polypeptide immunoreactivity on the plasma membrane at a distance from synaptic ribbons and horizontal cell dendrites suggests that the site of action of GABA on photoreceptor terminals is more laterally placed than previously thought (Stell et al., 1975; Yazulla et al., 1989). Some rod terminals are characterized by light immunolabeling of intracellular structures, but their plasma membranes are unstained (Fig. 6). Finally, although horizontal cells are lightly stained at the light microscopic level, immunoreactivity is not detected in horizontal cell dendrites at the ultrastructural level (Yazulla et al., 1989).

Interestingly, ultrastructural studies have only identified a few bipolar cell axonal terminals that are GABA$_A$ $\beta_2$ and $\beta_3$ polypeptide immunoreactive (Yazulla et al., 1989). Reasons for the apparently very modest number of immunolabeled bipolar cell terminals are unknown despite (1) ultrastructural evidence that bipolar cells including their axonal terminals are a major recipient of

GABAergic input (Marc et al., 1978; Yazulla et al., 1987; Studholme and Yazulla, 1988; Muller and Marc, 1990), (2) the association of bipolar cell synaptic specializations with muscimol binding sites (Yazulla, 1981), and (3) electrophysiological and pharmacological evidence for the presence of GABA$_A$ receptors on bipolar cell axonal terminals (Kondo and Toyoda, 1983; Tachibana and Kaneko, 1988). Perhaps, in view of the strong evidence for GABA$_A$ receptor heterogeneity, most goldfish bipolar cells express GABA$_A$ receptor types that do not contain GABA$_A$ $\beta_2$ and $\beta_3$ polypeptides.

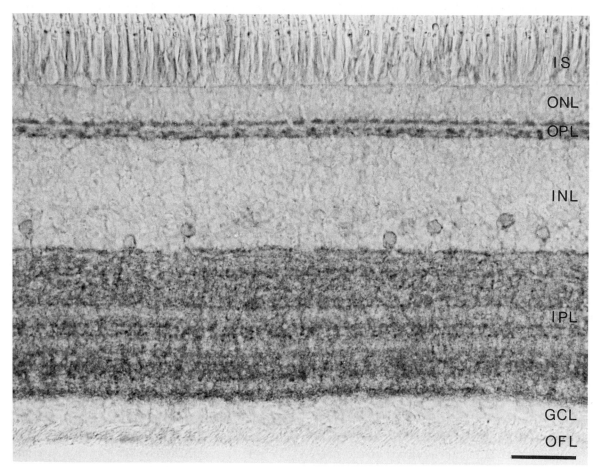

Fig. 7. GABA$_A$ $\beta_2$ and $\beta_3$ polypeptide immunoreactivity in the chicken retina as revealed by monoclonal antibody 62-3G1. Immunoreactivity is mainly localized to the OPL, amacrine cell bodies and processes distributed to the IPL. The labeling pattern in the OPL suggests that photoreceptor terminals express GABA$_A$ receptors. The prominent immunolabeling of amacrine cell bodies and processes in the IPL also indicate that many amacrine cells express GABA$_A$ receptors. Bright field photomicrograph. Relabeled from Fig. 5 of Yazulla et al., (1989). Scale bar = 50 $\mu$m.

Amacrine cell processes also display prominent immunolabeling of (1) amorphous intracellular structures and (2) the region of the plasma membrane which is located postsynaptic to either amacrine cell processes or very rarely to bipolar cell terminals (Yazulla et al., 1989). The localization of GABA$_A$ $\beta_2$ and $\beta_3$ polypeptide immunoreactivity to the IPL is consistent with the presence of muscimol and flunitrazepam binding sites in the IPL (Yazulla, 1981; Lin et al., 1991).

Finally, it is worth pointing out that a few ganglion cells are lightly positive for GABA$_A$ $\beta_2$ and $\beta_3$ polypeptide immunoreactivity (Yazulla et al., 1989), whereas nearly all isolated ganglion cell bodies have GABA$_A$ receptors on the basis of electrophysiological evidence (Ishida and Cohen, 1988). Furthermore, GABAergic amacrine cell processes are presynaptic to ganglion cell dendrites located in all regions of the IPL (Muller and Marc, 1990). Together, these findings argue that most and perhaps all ganglion cells possess GABA$_A$ receptors, which leads to the suggestion that most ganglion cells, like bipolar cells, express GABA$_A$ receptor types that do not contain GABA$_A$ $\beta_2$ and $\beta_3$ polypeptides.

*Chicken retina*

The GABA$_A$ $\beta_2$ and $\beta_3$ polypeptide immunoreactive patterns are similar in chicken and goldfish retinas, with immunolabeling of the OPL, some amacrine cells and a dense plexus of processes distributed across the IPL (Fig. 7) (Yazulla et al., 1989). The immunolabeling pattern in the OPL is suggestive of labeled photoreceptor terminals, but not bipolar or horizontal cell dendrites. GABA$_A$ receptor immunoreactivity in the IPL has a complex laminar distribution with the highest density of immunoreactive processes found in multiple bands located in all regions of the IPL. Overall, the distribution of GABA$_A$ $\beta_2$ and $\beta_3$ polypeptide immunoreactivity has little correspondence with high affinity GABA and muscimol uptake, or GABA and GAD immunoreactive patterns except for the labeling of a narrow band in the IPL adjacent to the GCL (Yazulla and

Brecha, 1980; Brandon, 1985; Mosinger et al., 1986; Yazulla et al., 1989). Immunolabeled cells are not observed in the middle and distal INL or in the GCL.

The presence of GABA$_A$ $\beta_2$ and $\beta_3$ polypeptide immunoreactivity in the OPL and IPL is generally consistent with the localization of muscimol and flunitrazepam binding sites to these layers (Altstein et al, 1981; Yazulla and Brecha, 1981; Brecha, 1983). As mentioned above, the lack of flunitrazepam binding sites in the OPL could be due to the presence of a GABA$_A$ receptor type that lacks a benzodiazepine recognition site in this layer. Together, these investigations provide good evidence for GABA$_A$ receptor localization to the OPL and IPL, consistent with the presumed GABA influence upon photoreceptor, amacrine and bipolar cells from GABAergic horizontal and amacrine cells (Yazulla and Brecha, 1980; Brandon, 1985; Mosinger et al., 1986).

*Rat retina*

In rat retina, GABA$_A$ $\beta_2$ and $\beta_3$ polypeptide immunoreactivity detected by antibody bd-17 is localized to a few amacrine cell bodies and to processes distributed in a relatively dense, homogeneous manner across the IPL (Richards et al., 1987). An increased density of GABA$_A$ $\beta_2$ and $\beta_3$ polypeptide immunoreactive processes is found in three bands, corresponding best to laminae 2, 3 and 5 of the IPL (Richards et al., 1987). Some immunoreactive cell bodies also are reported in the GCL, although from published descriptions it is not possible to determine if these cells are of the size of displaced amacrine cells or ganglion cells. In addition, immunolabeled cells are not observed in the ONL or the middle and distal INL.

GABA$_A$ $\beta_2$ and $\beta_3$ polypeptide immunoreactivity does not appear to be localized to bipolar cells. However, GABA$_A$ receptors are likely to be expressed by these cells based on both in situ hybridization (Brecha et al., 1990) and electrophysiological (Karschin and Wässle, 1990; Suzuki et al., 1990; Yeh et al., 1990) findings. A possible explanation for these observations is the presence of GABA$_A$ receptors on bipolar cells that lack GABA$_A$ $\beta_2$ and $\beta_3$ polypeptides.

GABA, GAD and GABA$_A$ $\beta_2$ and $\beta_3$ polypeptide immunoreactive processes, and muscimol and flunitrazepam binding sites are localized to the IPL with some differences in their laminar distribution (Vaughn et al., 1981; Brandon, 1985; Mosinger et al., 1986; Zarbin et al., 1986; Richards et al., 1987). A comprehensive comparison of the laminar distribution of these immunoreactive processes in the IPL has not been conducted, although some correspondence between the GABA$_A$ $\beta_2$ and $\beta_3$ polypeptide and the GAD immunoreactive patterns has been noted (Richards et al., 1987). GABA$_A$ receptors are likely to be present at amacrine-ama-

crine synaptic specializations since (1) GABA$_A$ $\alpha$ mRNAs are localized to amacrine cell bodies (Brecha et al., 1990) and (2) GAD immunoreactive amacrine processes are presynaptic to other amacrine cell processes (Vaughn et al., 1981).

Since the combinations and relationships of $\alpha$ and $\beta$ variants that form native GABA$_A$ receptors are poorly understood (see Olsen and Tobin, 1990 and Möhler et al., 1990 for reviews), it is not possible to speculate if the retinal cells expressing GABA$_A$ $\alpha$ mRNAs or GABA$_A$ $\beta_2$ and $\beta_3$ polypeptide immunoreactivity are the same or are different amacrine cell populations. A double-label study using in situ hybridization and immunohistochemistry could address this issue.

There is inconclusive immunohistochemical (Richards et al., 1987) and in situ hybridization histochemical evidence (Brecha et al., 1990) for

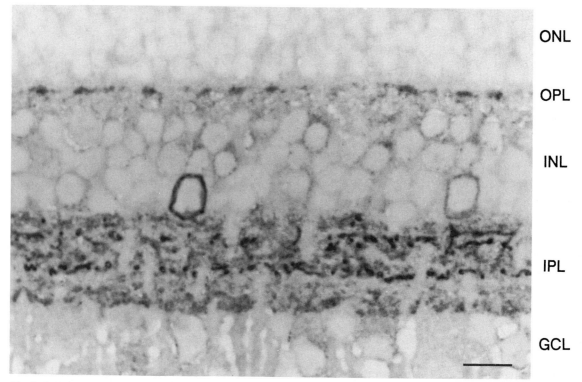

**ONL**

**OPL**

**INL**

**IPL**

**GCL**

Fig. 8. GABA$_A$ $\alpha_1$ polypeptide immunoreactivity in the rabbit retina as visualized by monoclonal antibody bd-24. Immunoreactivity is localized to bipolar cell dendrites in the OPL, bipolar cell bodies, amacrine cells and processes in the IPL. Lightly labeled bipolar cells are seen in the distal INL and prominent labeled amacrine cells are seen in the proximal INL. Bright field photomicrograph of a 1 $\mu$m section. Scale bar = 10 $\mu$m.

the expression of GABA$_A$ receptors by ganglion cells in the rat retina. However, there is electrophysiological evidence for the presence of these receptors on isolated juvenile ganglion cell bodies (Tauck et al., 1988). It is possible that the failure to convincingly demonstrate GABA$_A$ receptors by immunohistochemical approaches is due to the presence of receptors that lack GABA$_A$ $\beta_2$ and $\beta_3$ polypeptides. Some support for this speculation is derived from in situ hybridization histochemical observations showing GABA$_A$ $\alpha$ mRNA-containing cells in the GCL (Brecha et al., 1990).

*Rabbit retina*

In the rabbit retina, all three monoclonal antibodies have been used to determine the distribution of GABA$_A$ receptor immunoreactivity (Brecha and Weigmann, 1990). Monoclonal antibody (bd-24) directed to the GABA$_A$ $\alpha_1$ polypeptide labels bipolar cell bodies and dendrites, amacrine cell bodies, and processes distributed in the IPL (Figs. 8 and 9). Most immunolabeled amacrine cells are characterized by a prominently labeled plasma membrane (Figs. 9 and 10). A few lightly stained amacrine cells also are visualized with this antibody. Immunolabeled bipolar cell bodies are numerous and are characterized by an absence of cytoplasmic staining and light immunolabeling of the somatic plasma membrane (Figs. 8 and 11).

Monoclonal antibody bd-17 directed to the GABA$_A$ $\beta_2$ and $\beta_3$ polypeptides also labels bipolar cells (Fig. 12). Similar to observations using antibody bd-24, bipolar cell dendrites are well stained and bipolar cell bodies are more lightly stained. Monoclonal antibody 61–3G1, which also cross reacts with GABA$_A$ $\beta_2$ and $\beta_3$ polypeptides, faintly labels processes in the OPL (Fig. 13) and a few cell bodies in the distal INL, which may be bipolar cell bodies. Both of these monoclonal antibodies label amacrine cells and processes distributed to the IPL (Figs. 12, 13 and 14). The immunostaining of bipolar and amacrine cells and their processes was consistently stronger with

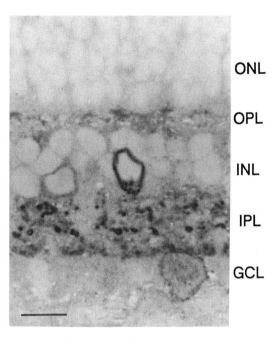

Fig. 9. Localization of GABA$_A$ $\alpha_1$ polypeptide immunoreactivity in the rabbit retina. In addition to the distribution of immunoreactivity described in Fig. 8, an immunolabeled cell in the GCL is illustrated. Bright field photomicrograph of a 1 $\mu$m section. Scale bar = 10 $\mu$m.

antibody bd-17. Reasons for these variations in staining are unknown, but they may be due to some differences in the immunological characteristics of these monoclonal antibodies.

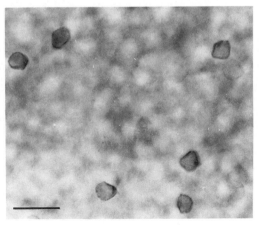

Fig. 10. GABA$_A$ $\alpha_1$ polypeptide immunoreactive amacrine cells in a whole mount preparation of the rabbit retina. Brightfield photomicrograph. Scale bar = 20 $\mu$m.

18

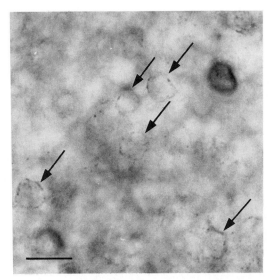

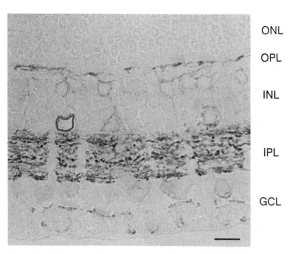

Fig. 11. Lightly labeled GABA$_A$ $\alpha_1$ polypeptide immunoreactive bipolar cells (arrows) in a whole mount preparation of the rabbit retina. Note that the immunostaining is primarily associated with the plasma membrane. The out-of-focus cell in this figure is a heavily labeled amacrine cell. Brightfield photomicrograph. Scale bar = 10 $\mu$m.

Fig. 12. GABA$_A$ $\beta_2$ and $\beta_3$ polypeptide immunoreactivity in the rabbit retina detected by monoclonal antibody bd-17. Immunoreactivity is localized to bipolar cell dendrites in the OPL, bipolar cell bodies, amacrine cell bodies, processes in the IPL and cells in the GCL. Brightfield photomicrograph of a 1 $\mu$m section. Scale bar = 10 $\mu$m.

Finally, all three monoclonal antibodies immunolabel some medium to large cells located in the GCL, which are likely to be ganglion cells (Figs. 9, 12 and 13). These cells have a granular cytoplasmic staining and a light staining plasma membrane.

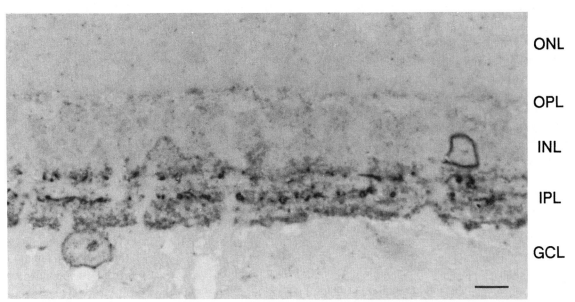

Fig. 13. GABA$_A$ $\beta_2$ and $\beta_3$ polypeptide immunoreactivity in the rabbit retina detected by monoclonal antibody 62-3G1. Immunoreactivity is localized to amacrine cell bodies, processes distributed to the IPL and to a cell in the GCL. Brightfield photomicrograph of a 1 $\mu$m section. Scale bar = 10 $\mu$m.

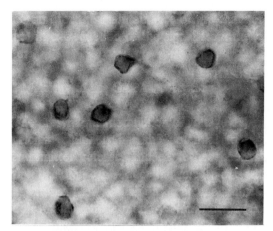

Fig. 14. GABA$_A$ $\beta_2$ and $\beta_3$ immunoreactive amacrine cells in a whole mount preparation of the rabbit retina as visualized by monoclonal antibody 62-3G1. Brightfield photomicrograph. Scale bar = 20 $\mu$m.

GABA immunoreactive interplexiform cell processes are present in the OPL and there is some evidence for GABA and GAD immunoreactive horizontal cells (Mosinger et al., 1986; Mosinger and Yazulla, 1987). These observations, with the presence of GABA$_A$ $\alpha_1$, and $\beta_2$ and $\beta_3$ polypeptide immunoreactivity in the OPL, suggest an action of GABA at GABA$_A$ receptors in this layer. However, ultrastructural studies are needed to better define the processes expressing GABA$_A$ polypeptides, since presently it has not been conclusively established if this immunoreactive staining is only associated with bipolar cell dendrites, or if it is also associated with interplexiform cell processes and photoreceptor terminals, as reported for the goldfish and chicken retina (Yazulla et al., 1989).

Numerous bipolar cell bodies express GABA$_A$ $\alpha_1$, and $\beta_2$ and $\beta_3$ polypeptides. At this time it is unknown how many or which type of bipolar cells express these GABA$_A$ polypeptides.

Similar to observations in other vertebrate retinas, the GABA$_A$ polypeptide immunoreactive pattern in the rabbit IPL has partial overlap with the GAD and GABA immunolabeling patterns (Brandon, et al., 1979, 1980; Brandon, 1985; Mosinger and Yazulla, 1985, 1987; Mosinger et al., 1986; Brecha and Weigmann, 1991). The strongly immunolabeled amacrine cells identified by these GABA$_A$ antibodies have moderate densities across the retina. To date, double label studies have not been conducted and therefore it is unknown if any of the several histochemically identified amacrine cell populations described in the rabbit retina (Vaney, 1990) express these GABA$_A$ subunits. In addition, because of the dense plexus of processes in the IPL, it is not possible to determine the laminar distribution of individual cell processes. In the GCL, immunolabeled cells identified as ganglion cells on the basis of their size are observed. These light microscopic observations together with ultrastructural studies (Brandon et al., 1980; Mosinger and Yazulla, 1985) are indicative of GABA$_A$ receptors at amacrine-bipolar, amacrine-amacrine and amacrine-ganglion cell synaptic specializations. Finally, the differential staining observed with these antibodies further supports the argument for multiple GABA$_A$ receptors in the retina.

*Primate retina*

In the retina of *Saimiri sciureus*, a New World monkey, GABA$_A$ $\beta_2$ and $\beta_3$ polypeptide immunoreactivity, as visualized by antibody 61–3G1, is localized to some sparsely occurring and nonoverlapping processes distributed to the vitreal margin of the OPL, perhaps originating from interplexiform or flat bipolar cells (Hughes et al., 1989). Immunoreactivity also is localized to some amacrine and ganglion cell bodies, and to processes distributed across the IPL with an increased density of processes in laminae 2 and 4 of the IPL (Fig. 15). The presence of GABA$_A$ $\beta_2$ and $\beta_3$ polypeptide immunoreactive ganglion cells was directly demonstrated by experimental approaches using retrograde labeling techniques (Hughes et al., 1989). In contrast, an earlier study of the Old World monkey *Macaca mulatta* (Mariani et al., 1987) employing monoclonal antibodies bd-17 and bd-24 and immunofluorescence techniques did not reveal GABA$_A$ receptor immunoreactivity in the OPL, but did describe immunolabeling of some small cells in the proximal INL and in the GCL, and of processes distributed to the IPL. These cells are likely to be amacrine and displaced amacrine cells (Mariani et al., 1987).

Overall, there are numerous discrepancies in the presence or absence of muscimol and fluni-trazepam binding sites, and $GABA_A$ $\beta_2$ and $\beta_3$ polypeptide, GAD and GABA immunoreactivities in the primate OPL (Zarbin et al., 1986; Mariani et al., 1987; Ryan and Hendrickson, 1987; Hughes et al., 1989; Grünert and Wässle, 1990). For instance, in the macaque retina there is an absence of muscimol and flunitrazepam binding sites and $GABA_A$ $\beta_2$ and $\beta_3$ polypeptide immunoreactivity, but there are GABA immunoreactive interplexiform and horizontal cell processes in this layer. There are many possible explanations for the discrepancies reported in the

primate OPL, including (1) species differences in $GABA_A$ receptor expression, (2) a low density of muscimol and benzodiazepine binding sites, (3) low affinity muscimol and benzodiazepine binding sites, (4) the presence of $GABA_A$ receptors that lack $GABA_A$ $\alpha_1$, $\beta_2$ and $\beta_3$ polypeptides, (5) a density of $GABA_A$ receptors below the level of detectability of immunofluorescence techniques, (6) the presence of $GABA_B$ receptors, rather than $GABA_A$ receptors, (7) transmitter-transmitter receptor mismatch (see Herkenham, 1987, for review).

In the IPL of *Saimiri sciureus* or *Macaca mulatta* direct comparisons of the distribution of GAD and $GABA_A$ polypeptide immunolabeling patterns showed little correspondence (Mariani et al., 1987; Hughes et al., 1989). Similar to observations in other species, a limited number of amacrine cells express this receptor in the pri-

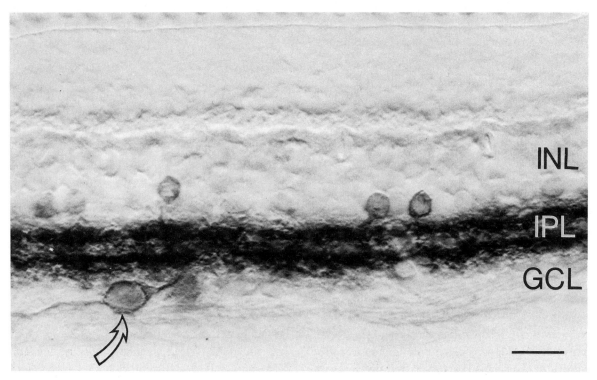

Fig. 15. Localization of $GABA_A$ $\beta_2$ and $\beta_3$ polypeptide immunoreactivity in the *Saimiri sciureus* retina using monoclonal antibody 62-3G1. Immunoreactivity is mainly localized to amacrine and ganglion cell bodies and processes distributed to the IPL. Labeled fibers are also seen in the optic fiber layer. Peripheral retina. Brightfield photomicrograph. From Fig. 1 of Hughes et al., (1989). Scale bar = 50 µm.

mate retina. Furthermore, in primate retina there is little evidence for GABA$_A$ receptor expression by bipolar cells. Finally, in *Saimiri sciureus* retina, GABA$_A$ $\beta_2$ and $\beta_3$ polypeptide immunoreactivity is present in a limited number of ganglion cells that are likely to ramify in laminae 2 and 4 of the IPL (Hughes et al., 1989). These cells have a well stained axon that could be traced to the optic nerve head.

*Summary*

Investigations using GABA$_A$ receptor subunit specific antibodies provide strong evidence for the presence of GABA$_A$ receptors in both the OPL and IPL. In the goldfish and chicken OPL, GABA$_A$ receptors are associated with photoreceptor terminals. In goldfish retina, there is good evidence that this receptor participates in a feedback circuit from horizontal cells to cone photoreceptor terminals (Wu and Dowling, 1980; Murakami et al., 1982a,b; Lasater and Lam, 1984a).

In rat and primate OPL, the presence of sparsely occurring GAD and GABA immunoreactive fibers (Vaughn et al., 1981; Brandon, 1985; Mosinger et al., 1986; Grünert and Wässle, 1990; Koontz and Hendrickson, 1990) and a low density of muscimol and flunitrazepam binding sites (Zarbin et al., 1986) are indicative of GABA$_A$ receptors in this layer. However, GABA$_A$ $\beta_2$ and $\beta_3$ polypeptide immunoreactivity is absent in the rat and primate OPL (except for the few fibers reported in the *Saimiri sciureus* retina) (Mariani et al., 1987; Richards et al., 1987; Hughes et al., 1989). Therefore, it is not possible to speculate as to the cellular localization of these presumed GABA$_A$ receptors. As mentioned above, there are many possibilities for these discrepant observations, and some of these differences can be explained by the presence of a GABA$_A$ receptor type in this layer that lacks $\beta_2$ and $\beta_3$ polypeptides in these species. In contrast, in rabbit retina GABA$_A$ $\alpha_1$, and $\beta_2$ and $\beta_3$ polypeptides are associated with bipolar cell dendrites (Brecha and Weigmann, 1991), although the possibility that

interplexiform and perhaps photoreceptor terminals also express these polypeptides has not been completely ruled out.

At the present time there is limited morphological evidence, in contrast to electrophysiological evidence (Tachibana and Kaneko, 1988; Karschin and Wässle, 1990; Suzuki et al., 1990; Yeh et al., 1990), for GABA$_A$ receptor localization to bipolar cells. In situ hybridization histochemical findings indicate GABA$_A$ $\alpha_1$ mRNA expression by rat bipolar cells (Brecha et al., 1990) and immunohistochemical observations demonstrate GABA$_A$ $\alpha_1$, and $\beta_2$ and $\beta_3$ polypeptide immunoreactivity in rabbit bipolar cells (Brecha and Weigmann, 1991). The expression of GABA$_A$ polypeptide immunoreactivity by rabbit bipolar cells is consistent with ultrastructural studies showing that GABAergic amacrine cell processes are presynaptic to bipolar cell axonal terminals (Brandon et al., 1980; Mosinger and Yazulla, 1985).

In all species studied to date, GABA$_A$ receptor immunoreactivity is prominently expressed by some amacrine cells. These findings are in agreement with in situ hybridization studies of the rat retina (Brecha et al., 1990) and earlier studies reporting both muscimol and flunitrazepam binding sites in the IPL (Yazulla, 1981; Yazulla and Brecha, 1981; Altstein et al., 1981; Brecha, 1983; Zarbin et al., 1986; Lin et al., 1991). These observations also are consistent with ultrastructural evidence showing some GABAergic presynaptic input to amacrine cell processes (Brandon et al., 1980; Vaughn et al., 1981; Mariani and Caserta, 1986; Yazulla et al., 1987; Grünert and Wässle, 1990; Koontz and Hendrickson, 1990; Muller and Marc, 1990).

Finally, GABA$_A$ receptor immunoreactive ganglion cells in the *Saimiri sciureus* retina and likely in the goldfish and rabbit retina have been reported (Hughes et al., 1989; Yazulla et al., 1989; Brecha and Weigmann, 1991). The presence of immunolabeled ganglion cells in these retinas is consistent with ultrastructural evidence showing that GABAergic amacrine cell processes are presynaptic to ganglion cell dendrites and somata (Brandon et al., 1980; Grünert and Wässle, 1990; Koontz and Hendrickson, 1990; Muller and Marc, 1990). In addition, these observations are in agreement with electrophysiological studies describing GABA$_A$ receptors on isolated ganglion cells (Ishida and Cohen, 1988; Tauck et al., 1988).

**Conclusions**

In vitro receptor autoradiographic, in situ hybridization histochemical and immunohistochemical studies provide strong evidence that GABA$_A$ receptors have an extensive distribution in the retina. Initial studies showed the localization of high affinity muscimol and benzodiazepine binding sites indicative of these receptors in both the OPL and IPL in most species. Subsequent investigations have shown that GABA$_A$ receptors are expressed by numerous retinal cell types. Furthermore, these recent studies provide evidence for multiple GABA$_A$ receptors in the retina.

GABA$_A$ receptors are expressed by goldfish and likely by chicken photoreceptors (Yazulla et al., 1989). This observation in goldfish retina is in agreement with several electrophysiological investigations that indicate the presence of GABA$_A$ receptors on fish cone photoreceptor terminals (Wu and Dowling, 1980; Murakami et al., 1982a,b; Lasater and Lam, 1984a; see Wu, Chapter 4). In mammals, to date there is no evidence for the localization of GABA$_A$ receptors at photoreceptor terminals.

Electrophysiological studies have provided strong evidence that isolated goldfish and rodent bipolar cells express GABA$_A$ receptors and furthermore, they suggest that these receptors are concentrated to the axonal terminal (Tachibana and Kaneko, 1988; Karschin and Wässle, 1990; Suzuki et al., 1990; but see Yeh et al., 1990; see Wu, Chapter 4). These electrophysiological observations, along with the expression of (1) GABA$_A$ $\alpha_1$ mRNA by rat bipolar cells and (2) GABA$_A$ $\alpha_1$, and $\beta_2$ and $\beta_3$ polypeptide im-

munoreactivity by rabbit bipolar cells, suggest that many and perhaps all bipolar cells express GABA$_A$ receptors. However, quite clearly, additional studies using other GABA$_A$ receptor probes are required for a better understanding of bipolar cell expression of this receptor in other vertebrate retinas. Overall, these investigations with ultrastructural studies (Brandon et al., 1980; Vaughn et al., 1981; Mariani and Caserta, 1986; Yazulla et al., 1987; Grünert and Wässle, 1990; Koontz and Hendrickson, 1990; Muller and Marc, 1990; see Marc, Chapter 5 and Freed, Chapter 6) indicate that GABA$_A$ receptors are localized to amacrine-bipolar synaptic specializations.

There also is strong morphological evidence that GABA$_A$ receptors are expressed by some amacrine cells. The expression of GABA$_A$ receptor immunoreactivity by amacrine cells (Mariani et al., 1987; Richards et al., 1987; Hughes et al., 1989; Yazulla et al., 1989; Brecha and Weigmann, 1991) is in agreement with in situ hybridization studies of the rat retina (Brecha et al., 1990). Furthermore, these observations are consistent with the localization of GABA$_A$ binding sites to the IPL (Altstein et al., 1981; Yazulla, 1981; Yazulla and Brecha, 1981; Brecha, 1983; Zarbin et al., 1986). All of these studies, together with ultrastructural observations (Brandon et al., 1980; Vaughn et al., 1981; Mariani and Caserta, 1986; Yazulla et al., 1987; Grünert and Wässle, 1990; Koontz and Hendrickson, 1990; Muller and Marc, 1990), are consistent with the presence of GABA$_A$ receptors at amacrine-amacrine synaptic specializations.

Different experimental approaches indicate that GABA$_A$ receptors are likely to be expressed by ganglion cells (Ishida and Cohen, 1988; Tauck et al., 1988; Hughes et al., 1989; Yazulla et al., 1989; Brecha and Weigmann, 1991). Electrophysiological investigations report the presence of GABA$_A$ receptors on isolated ganglion cells (Ishida and Cohen, 1988; Tauck et al., 1988), and an action of GABA on ganglion cells has been suggested in studies of the intact retina (see Yazulla, 1986, for review). These observations with the demonstration of GABAergic amacrine cell contacts on ganglion cell dendrites and somata (Brandon et al., 1980; Grünert and Wässle, 1990; Koontz and Hendrickson, 1990; Muller and Marc, 1990) provide evidence that GABA inhibits ganglion cell responses, in part by a direct action through GABA$_A$ receptors on these cells.

In situ hybridization and immunohistochemical investigations using GABA$_A$ receptor probes indicate a heterogeneity of GABA$_A$ receptor expression in the retina. GABA$_A$ receptors are localized to a variety of retinal cell populations and the differential expression patterns of the GABA$_A$ $\alpha$ and $\beta$ variants illustrate the likely existence of multiple GABA$_A$ receptors. At this time, it is unknown if only one GABA$_A$ receptor subtype is associated with a particular cell population or if multiple GABA$_A$ receptor subtypes are localized to the same cell population. Both alternatives are possible. The presence of multiple GABA$_A$ receptors in the retina, together with investigations that indicate that GABA$_A$ receptor subtypes are likely to have distinct electrophysiological and pharmacological properties, illustrate the complexity of GABA's action in the retina. Clearly, the advances gained from the use of GABA$_A$ receptor subunit specific probes are beginning to clarify the site of action of GABA at GABA$_A$ receptors in the retina.

## Acknowledgements

I wish to thank K. Anderson, K. Bhakta, M. Lai and C. Weigmann for their important contributions to the present studies. I am grateful to Drs. M. Khrestchatisky, J. MacLennan, and A.J. Tobin for providing the rat GABA$_A$ cDNAs, Dr. J.G. Richards for providing monoclonal antibodies bd-17 and bd-24 and Dr. A.L. de Blas for providing monoclonal antibody 61–3G1, and Drs. T. Hughes and S. Yazulla for providing some of the figures used in this review. I also wish to thank D. Rickman and C. Weigmann, and Drs. G. Casini, T. Hughes, L. Kruger and C. Sternini for their helpful comments on the manuscript. Supported by National Institutes of Health grants EY 04067 and VA Medical Research Funds.

## References

Agardh, E., Ehinger, B. and Wu, J.-Y. (1987) GABA- and GAD-like immunoreactivity in the primate retina. *Histochemistry,* 86: 485–490.

Akaike, N., Inoue, M. and Krishtal, O.A. (1986) 'Concentration-clamp' study of $\gamma$-aminobutyric-acid-induced chloride current kinetics in frog sensory neurones. *J. Physiol. (London),* 379: 171–185.

Altstein, M., Dudai, Y. and Vogel, Z. (1981) Benzodiazepine receptors in chick retina: Development and cellular localization. *Brain Res.,* 206: 198–202.

Ames, A. and Pollen, D.A. (1969) Neurotransmission in central nervous tissue: a study of isolated rabbit retina. *J. Neurophysiol.,* 32: 424–442.

Ariel, M. and Daw, N.W. (1982) Pharmacological analysis of directionally sensitive rabbit retinal ganglion cells. *J. Physiol. (London),* 324: 161–185.

Ayoub, G.S. and Lam, D.M.K. (1984) The release of $\gamma$-aminobutyric acid from horizontal cells of the goldfish (*Carassius auratus*) retina. *J. Physiol. (London),* 355: 191–214.

Ayoub, G.S. and Lam, D.M.K. (1985) The content and release of endogenous GABA in isolated horizontal cells of the goldfish retina. *Vision Res.,* 25: 1187–1193.

Baylor, D.A., Fuortes, M.G.F. and O'Bryan, P.M. (1971) Receptive fields of cones in the retina of the turtle. *J. Physiol. (London),* 214: 265–294.

Biggio, G., Guarneri, P. and Corda, M.G. (1981) Benzodiazepine and GABA receptors in the rat retina: effect of light and dark adaptation. *Brain Res.,* 216: 210–214.

Bolz, J., Frumkes, T., Voigt, T. and Wässle, H. (1985) Action and localization of $\gamma$-aminobutyric acid in the cat retina. *J. Physiol. (London),* 362: 369–393.

Borbe, H.O., Müller, W.E. and Wollert, U. (1980) The identification of benzodiazepine receptors with brain-like specificity in bovine retina. *Brain Res.,* 182: 466–469.

Bormann, J. (1988). Electrophysiology of GABA$_A$ and GABA$_B$ receptor subtypes. *Trends Neurosci.,* 11: 112–116.

Bowery, N.G., Price, G.W., Hudson, A.L., Hill, D.R., Wilkin, G.P. and Turnbull, M.J. (1984) GABA receptor multiplicity. Visualization of different receptor types in the mammalian CNS. *Neuropharmacol.,* 23: 219–231.

Brandon, C. (1985) Retinal GABA neurons: Localization in vertebrate species using an antiserum to rabbit brain glutamate decarboxylase. *Brain Res.,* 344: 286–295.

Brandon, C., Lam, D.M.K. and Wu, J.-Y. (1979) The $\gamma$-aminobutyric acid system in rabbit retina: Localization by immunocytochemistry and autoradiography. *Proc. Natl. Acad. Sci. USA,* 76: 3557–3561.

Brandon, C., Lam, D.M.K., Su, Y.Y.T. and Wu, J.-Y. (1980) Immunocytochemical localization of GABA neurons in the rabbit and frog retina. *Brain Res. Bull.,* 5: 21–29.

Brecha, N. (1983) Retinal neurotransmitters: Histochemical and biochemical studies. In: P.C. Emson (Ed.), *Chemical Neuroanatomy*, Raven Press, New York, pp. 85–129.

Brecha, N. and Weigmann, C. (1990) GABA$_A$ $\alpha$ and $\beta$ subunit immunoreactivities in the rabbit retina. *Soc. Neurosci. Abstr.*, 16: 1075.

Brecha, N. and Weigmann, C. (1991) GABA$_A$ receptor subunit immunoreactivities in the rabbit retina. *Invest. Ophthal. Vis. Sci. Suppl.*, 32: 1189.

Brecha, N., Johnson, D., Peichl, L. and Wässle, H. (1988) Cholinergic amacrine cells of the rabbit retina contain glutamate decarboxylase and $\gamma$-aminobutyrate immunoreactivity. *Proc. Natl. Acad. Sci. USA*, 85: 6187–6191.

Brecha, N., Lai, M. and Sternini, C. (1990) Differential expression of GABA$_A$ $\alpha_1$ and $\alpha_2$ receptor mRNAs in the rat retina. *Invest. Ophthal. Vis. Sci. Suppl.*, 31: 330.

Brecha, N., Sternini, C. and Humphrey, M.F. (1991) Cellular distribution of GAD and GABA$_A$ receptor mRNAs in the retina. *Cell. Mol. Neurobiol.*, 11: 497–509.

Bureau, M. and Olsen, R.W. (1990) Multiple distinct subunits of the $\gamma$-aminobutyric acid-A receptor protein show different ligand-binding affinities. *Mol. Pharmacol.*, 37: 497–502.

Burkhardt, D.A. (1977) Responses and receptive-field organization of cones in perch retinas. *J. Neurophysiol.*, 40: 53–62.

Caldwell, J.H. and Daw, N.W. (1978) Effects of picrotoxin and strychnine on rabbit retinal ganglion cells: changes in centre surround receptive fields. *J. Physiol. (London)*, 276: 299–310.

Caldwell, J.H., Daw, N.W. and Wyatt, H.J. (1978) Effects of picrotoxin and strychnine on rabbit retinal ganglion cells: lateral interactions for cells with more complex receptive fields. *J. Physiol. (London)*, 276: 277–298.

de Blas, A.L., Vitorica, J. and Friedrich, P. (1988) Localization of the GABA$_A$ receptor in the rat brain with a monoclonal antibody to the 57,000 $M_r$ peptide of the GABA$_A$ receptor/benzodiazepine receptor/Cl$^-$ channel complex. *J. Neurosci.*, 8: 602–614.

Ehinger, B. and Dowling, J.E. (1987) Retinal neurocircuitry and transmission. In: A. Bjorklund, T. Hökfelt and L.W. Swanson (Eds.), *Handbook of Chemical Neuroanatomy, Vol 5: Integrated Systems of the CNS, Part 1*, Elsevier Science Publishers, Amsterdam, New York, pp. 389–446.

Enna, S.J. and Snyder, S.H. (1976) Gamma-aminobutyric acid (GABA) receptor binding in mammalian retina. *Brain Res.*, 115: 174–179.

Enna, S.J. and Snyder, S.H. (1977) Influences of ions, enzymes, and detergents on $\gamma$-aminobutyric acid receptor binding in synaptic membranes of rat brain. *Mol. Pharm.*, 13: 442–453.

Fuchs, K. and Sieghart, W. (1989) Evidence for the existence of several different $\alpha$- and $\beta$-subunits of the GABA/benzodiazepine receptor complex from rat brain. *Neurosci. Lett.*, 97: 329–333.

Fuchs, K., Möhler, H. and Sieghart, W. (1988) Various proteins from rat brain, specifically and irreversibly labeled by [$^3$H]flunitrazepam, are distinct $\alpha$-subunits of the GABA-benzodiazepine receptor complex. *Neurosci. Lett.*, 90: 314–319.

Glickman, R.D., Adolph, A.R. and Dowling, J.E. (1982) Inner plexiform circuits in the carp retina: effects of cholinergic agonists, GABA, and substance P on the ganglion cells. *Brain Res.*, 234: 81–99.

Grünert, U., and Wässle, H. (1990) GABA-like immunoreactivity in the macaque monkey retina: A light and electron microscopic study. *J. Comp. Neurol.*, 297: 509–524.

Guarneri, P. Corda, M.G., Concas, A. and Biggio, G. (1981) Kainic acid-induced lesion of rat retina: Differential effect on cyclic GMP and benzodiazepine and GABA receptors. *Brain Res.*, 209: 216–220.

Häring, P., Stähli, P., Schoch P., Takács, B., Staehelin, T. and Möhler, H. (1985) Monoclonal antibodies reveal structural homogeneity of $\gamma$-aminobutyric acid/benzodiazepine receptors in different brain areas. *Proc. Natl. Acad. Sci. USA*, 82: 4837–4841.

Hendrickson, A., Ryan, M., Noble, B. and Wu, J.-Y. (1985) Colocalization of [$^3$H]muscimol and antisera to GABA and glutamic acid decarboxylase within the same neurons in monkey retina. *Brain Res.*, 348: 391–396.

Herkenham, M. (1987) Mismatches between neurotransmitter and receptor localizations in brain: Observations and implications. *Neuroscience*, 23: 1–38.

Hill, D.R. and Bowery, N.G. (1981) $^3$H-baclofen and $^3$H-GABA bind to bicuculline-insensitive GABA$_B$ sites in rat brain. *Nature (London)*, 290: 149–152.

Howells, R.D., Hiller, J.M. and Simon, E.J. (1979) Benzodiazepine binding sites are present in retina. *Life Sci.*, 25: 2131–2136.

Howells, R.D. and Simon, E.J. (1980) Benzodiazepine binding in chicken retina and its interaction with $\gamma$-aminobutyric acid. *Europ. J. Pharmacol.*, 67: 133–137.

Hughes, T.E., Carey, R.G., Vitorica, J., de Blas, A.L. and Karten, H.J. (1989) Immunohistochemical localization of GABA$_A$ receptors in the retina of the new world primate *Saimiri sciureus*. *Vis. Neurosci.*, 2: 565–581.

Ishida, A.T. and Cohen, B.N. (1988) GABA-activated whole-cell currents in isoated retinal ganglion cells. *J. Neurophysiol.*, 60: 381–396.

Kamp, C.W. and Morgan, W.W. (1981) GABA antagonists enhance dopamine turnover in the rat retina in vivo. *Eur. J. Pharmacol.*, 69: 273–279.

Kamp, C.W. and Morgan, W.W. (1982) Benzodiazepines suppress the light response of retinal dopaminergic neurons in vivo. *Eur. J. Pharmacol.*, 77: 343–346.

Kaneko, A. and Tachibana, M. (1986) Effects of $\gamma$-aminobutyric acid on isolated cone photoreceptors of the turtle retina. *J. Physiol. (London)*, 373: 443–461.

Kaneko, A. and Tachibana, M. (1987) GABA mediates the negative feedback from amacrine to bipolar cells. *Neurosci. Res. Suppl.*, 6: S239-S252.

Karobath, M. and Sperk, G. (1979) Stimulation of benzodiazepine receptor binding by $\gamma$-aminobutyric acid. *Proc. Natl. Acad. Sci. USA*, 76: 1004–1006.

Karschin, A. and Wässle, H. (1990) Voltage- and transmitter-gated currents in isolated rod bipolar cells of rat retina. *J. Neurophysiol.*, 63: 860–876.

Khrestchatisky, M., MacLennan, A.J., Chiang, M.-Y., Xu, W., Jackson, M.B., Brecha, N., Sternini, C., Olsen, R.W. and

Tobin, A.J. (1989) A novel α subunit in rat brain GABA_A receptors. *Neuron,* 3: 745–753.

Khrestchatisky, M., MacLennan, A.J., Tillakaratne, N.J.K., Chiang, M.-Y. and Tobin, A.J. (1991) Sequence and regional distribution of the mRNA encoding the alpha 2 polypeptide of rat GABA_A receptors. *J. Neurochem.,* 56: 1717–1722.

Kondo, H. and Toyoda, J.-I. (1983) GABA and glycine effects on the bipolar cells of the carp retina. *Vision Res.,* 23: 1259–1264.

Koontz, M.A. and Hendrickson, A.E. (1990) Distribution of GABA-immunoreactive amacrine cell synapses in the inner plexiform layer of macaque monkey retina. *Vis. Neurosci.,* 5: 17–28.

Kosaka, T., Tauchi, M. and Dahl, J.L. (1988) Cholinergic neurons containing GABA-like and/or glutamic acid decarboxylase-like immunoreactivities in various brain regions of the rat. *Exp. Brain Res.,* 70: 605–617.

Lam, D.M., Lasater, E.M. and Naka, K.-I. (1978) γ-Aminobutyric acid: A neurotransmitter candidate for cone horizontal cells of the catfish retina. *Proc. Natl. Acad. Sci. USA,* 75: 6310–6313.

Lam, D.M.K., Su, Y.Y.T., Swain, L., Marc, R.E., Brandon, C. and Wu, J.-Y. (1979) Immunocytochemical localisation of L-glutamic acid decarboxylase in the goldfish retina. *Nature (London),* 278: 565–567.

Lasater, E.M. and Lam, D.M.K. (1984a) The identification and some functions of GABAergic neurons in the distal catfish retina. *Vision Res.,* 24: 497–506.

Lasater, E.M. and Lam, D.M.K. (1984b) The identification and some functions of GABAergic neurons in the proximal retina of the catfish. *Vision Res.,* 24: 875–881.

Levitan, E.S., Schofield, P.R., Burt, D.R., Rhee, L.M., Wisden, W., Köhler, M., Fujita, N., Rodriguez, H.F., Stephenson, A., Darlison, M.G., Barnard, E.A. and Seeburg, P.H. (1988a) Structural and functional basis for GABA_A receptor heterogenity. *Nature (London),* 335: 76–79.

Levitan, E.S., Blair, L.A.C., Dionne, V.E. and Barnard, E.A. (1988b) Biophysical and pharmacological properties of cloned GABA_A receptor subunits expressed in xenopus oocytes. *Neuron,* 1: 773–781.

Lin, Z., Studholme, K. and Yazulla, S. (1991) Evidence for subtypes of GABA_A receptors in goldfish retina. *Invest. Ophthal. Vis. Sci. Suppl.,* 32: 1262.

Lolait, S.J., O'Carroll, A.-M., Kusano, K. and Mahan, L.C. (1989) Pharmacological characterization and region-specific expression in brain of the β_2- and β_3-subunits of the rat GABA_A receptor. *FEBS Lett.,* 258: 17–21.

Lüddens, H., Pritchett, D.B., Köhler, M., Killisch, I., Kainänen, K., Monyer, H., Sprengel, R. and Seeburg, P.H. (1990) Cerebellar GABA_A receptor selective for a behavioural alcohol antagonist. *Nature (London),* 346: 648–651.

MacLennan, A.J., Brecha, N., Khrestchatisky, M., Sternini, C., Tillakaratne, N.J.K., Chiang, M.-Y., Anderson, K., Bhakta, K., Lai, M. and Tobin, A.J. (1991) Independent cellular and ontogenetic expression of mRNAs encoding three a polypeptides of the rat GABA_A receptor. *Neuroscience,* 43: 369–380.

Malherbe, P., Sigel, E., Baur, R., Persohn, E., Richards, J.G. and Möhler, H. (1990a) Functional expression and sites of gene transcription of a novel α subunit of the GABA_A receptor in rat brain. *FEBS Lett.,* 260: 261–265.

Malherbe, P., Sigel, E., Baur, R., Persohn, E., Richards, J.G. and Möhler, H. (1990b) Functional characteristics and sites of gene expression of the α_1, β_1, γ_2-isoform of the rat GABA_A receptor. *J. Neurosci.,* 10: 2330–2337.

Mamalaki, C., Stephenson, F.A. and Barnard, E.A. (1987) The GABA_A/benzodiazepine receptor is a heterotetramer of homologous α and β subunits. *EMBO J.,* 6: 561–565.

Marc, R.E., Stell, W.K., Bok, D. and Lam, D.M.K. (1978) GABA-ergic pathways in the goldfish retina. *J. Comp. Neur.,* 182: 221–243.

Marc, R.E. and Liu, W.-L.S. (1984) Horizontal cell synapses onto glycine-accumulating interplexiform cells. *Nature (London),* 312: 266–269.

Mariani, A.P. and Caserta, M.T. (1986) Electron microscopy of glutamate decarboxylase (GAD) immunoreactivity in the inner plexiform layer of the rhesus monkey retina. *J. Neurocytol.,* 15: 645–655.

Mariani, A.P., Cosenza-Murphy, D. and Barker, J.L. (1987) GABAergic synapses and benzodiazepine receptors are not identically distributed in the primate retina. *Brain Res.,* 415: 153–157.

Marshak, D.W. and Dowling, J.E. (1987) Synapses of cone horizontal cell axons in goldfish retina. *J. Comp. Neur.,* 256: 430–443.

Marshburn, P.B. and Iuvone, P.M. (1981) The role of GABA in the regulation of the dopamine/tyrosine hydroxylase-containing neurons of the rat retina. *Brain Res.,* 214: 335–347.

Massey, S.C. and Neal, M.J. (1979) The light evoked release of acetylcholine from rabbit retina in vivo and its inhibition by γ-aminobutyric acid. *J. Neurochem.,* 32: 1327–1329.

Massey, S.C. and Redburn, D.A. (1982) A tonic γ-aminobutyric acid-mediated inhibition of cholinergic amacrine cells in rabbit retina. *J. Neurosci.,* 2: 1633–1643.

Massey, S.C. and Redburn, D.A. (1987) Transmitter circuits in the vertebrate retina. *Progr. Neurobiol.,* 28: 55–96.

Möhler, H. and Okada, T. (1977) Benzodiazepine receptor: Demonstration in the central nervous system. *Science,* 198: 849–851.

Möhler, H., Battersby, M.K. and Richards, J.G. (1980) Benzodiazepine receptor protein identified and visualized in brain tissue by a photoaffinity label. *Proc. Natl. Acad. Sci. USA,* 77: 1666–1670.

Möhler, H., Malherbe, P., Draguhn, A. and Richards, J.G. (1990) GABA_A-receptors: structural requirements and sites of gene expression in mammalian brain. *Neurochem. Res.,* 15: 199–207.

Morgan, W.W. and Kamp, C.W. (1980) A GABAergic influence on the light-induced increase in dopamine turnover in the dark-adapted retina in vivo. *J. Neurochem.,* 34: 1082–1086.

Mosinger, J.L. and Yazulla, S. (1985) Colocalization of GAD-like immunoreactivity and ³H-GABA uptake in amacrine cells of rabbit retina. *J. Comp. Neurol.,* 240: 396–406.

26

Mosinger, J.L., Yazulla, S. and Studholme, K. (1986) GABA-like immunoreactivity in the vertebrate retina: a species comparison. *Exp. Eye Res.,* 42: 631–644.

Mosinger, J.L. and Yazulla, S. (1987) Double-label analysis of GAD- and GABA-like immunoreactivity in the rabbit retina. *Vision Res.,* 27: 23–30.

Muller, J.F. and Marc, R.E. (1990) GABA-ergic and glycinergic pathways in the inner plexiform layer of the goldfish retina. *J. Comp. Neurol.,* 291: 281–304.

Murakami, M., Shimoda, Y., Nakatani, K., Miyachi, E. and Watanabe, S. (1982a) GABA-mediated negative feedback from horizontal cells to cones in carp retina. *Jpn. J. Physiol.,* 32: 911–926.

Murakami, M., Shimoda, Y., Nakatani, K., Miyachi, E. and Watanabe, S. (1982b) GABA-mediated negative feedback and color opponency in carp retina. *Jpn. J. Physiol.,* 32: 927–935.

Negishi, K., Teranishi, T. and Kato, S. (1983) A GABA antagonist, bicuculline, exerts its uncoupling action on external horizontal cells through dopamine cells in carp retina. *Neurosci Lett.,* 37: 261–266

Nishimura, Y., Schwartz, M.L. and Rakic, P. (1985) Localization of $\gamma$-aminobutyric acid and glutamic acid decarboxylase in rhesus monkey retina. *Brain Res.,* 359: 351–355.

O'Connor, P.M., Zucker, C.L. and Dowling, J.E. (1987) Regulation of dopamine release from interplexiform cell processes in the outer plexiform layer of the carp retina. *J. Neurochem.,* 49: 916–920.

Olsen, R.W. (1981) GABA-benzodiazepine-barbiturate receptor interactions. *J. Neurochem.,* 37: 1–13.

Olsen, R.W. and Tobin, A.J. (1990) Molecular biology of GABA$_A$ receptors. *FASEB J.,* 4: 1469–1480.

Olsen, R.W. and Venter, J.C. (Eds.) (1986) Benzodiazepine/GABA receptors and chloride channels: structural and functional properties. *Receptor Biochemistry and Methodology, Vol. 5,* A.R. Liss, New York.

Olsen, R.W., Bergman, M.O., Van Ness, P.C., Lummis, S.C., Watkins, A.E., Napias, C. and Greenlee, D.V. (1981) $\gamma$-aminobutyric acid receptor binding in mammalian brain. Heterogeneity of binding sites. *Mol. Pharmacol.,* 19: 217–227.

Olsen, R.W., McCabe, R.T. and Wamsley, J.K. (1990) GABA$_A$ receptor subtypes: autoradiographic comparison of GABA, benzodiazepine, and convulsant binding sites in the rat central nervous system. *J. Chem. Neuroanatomy,* 3: 59–76.

Osborne, N.N. (1980a) Binding of [$^3$H]-muscimol, a potent $\gamma$-aminobutyric acid receptor agonist, to membranes of the bovine retina. *Br. J. Pharmac.,* 71: 259–264.

Osborne, N.N. (1980b) Benzodiazepine binding to bovine retina. *Neurosci. Lett.,* 16: 167–170.

Osborne, N.N. and Beaton, D.W. (1986) Direct histochemical localisation of 5,7-dihydroxytryptamine and the uptake of serotonin by a subpopulation of GABA neurones in the rabbit retina. *Brain Res.,* 382: 158–162.

Osborne, N.N., Patel, S., Beaton, D.W. and Neuhoff, V. (1986) GABA neurones in retinas of different species and their postnatal development in situ and in culture in the rabbit retina. *Cell Tissue Res.,* 243: 117–123.

Paul, S.M., Zatz, M. and Skolnick, P. (1980) Demonstration of brain-specific benzodiazepine receptors in rat retina. *Brain Res.,* 187: 243–246.

Perry, V.H. (1981) Evidence for an amacrine cell system in the ganglion cell layer of the rat retina. *Neuroscience,* 6: 931–944.

Pritchett, D.B. and Seeburg, P.H. (1990) $\gamma$-Aminobutyric acid$_A$ receptor $\alpha_5$-subunit creates novel type II benzodiazepine receptor pharmacology. *J. Neurochem.,* 54: 1802–1804.

Pritchett, D.B., Sontheimer, H., Gorman, C.M., Kettenmann, H., Seeburg, P.H. and Schofield, P.R. (1988) Transient expression shows ligand gating and allosteric potentiation of GABA$_A$ receptor subunits. *Science,* 242: 1306–1308.

Pritchett, D.B., Lüddens, H. and Seeburg, P.H. (1989a) Type I and type II GABA$_A$-benzodiazepine receptors produced in transfected cells. *Science,* 245: 1389–1392.

Pritchett, D.B., Sontheimer, H., Shivers, B.D., Ymer, S., Kettenmann, H., Schofield, P.R. and Seeburg, P.H. (1989b) Importance of a novel GABA$_A$ receptor subunit for benzodiazepine pharmacology. *Nature (London),* 338: 582–585.

Redburn, D.A. and Mitchell, C.K. (1980) GABA receptor binding in bovine retina. *Brain Res. Bull.,* 5: 189–193.

Redburn, D.A. and Mitchell, C.K. (1981) GABA receptor binding in bovine retina: effects of triton X-100 and perchloric acid. *Life Sci.,* 28: 541–549.

Redburn, D.A., Kyles, C.B. and Ferkany, J. (1979) Subcellular distribution of GABA receptors in bovine retina. *Exp. Eye Res.,* 28: 525–532.

Redburn, D.A., Clement-Cormier, Y. and Lam, D.M.K. (1980) GABA and dopamine receptor binding in retinal synaptosomal fractions. *Neurochem.,* 1: 167–181.

Regan, J.W., Roeske, W.R. and Yamamura, H.I. (1980) $^3$H-Flunitrazepam binding to bovine retina and the effect of GABA thereon. *Neuropharm.,* 19: 413–414.

Richards, J.G., Schoch, P., Häring, P., Takacs, B. and Möhler, H. (1987) Resolving GABA$_A$/benzodiazepine receptors: cellular and subcellular localization in the CNS with monoclonal antibodies. *J. Neurosci.,* 7: 1866–1886.

Rohte, T., Schliebs, R. and Bigl, V. (1985) Benzodiazepine receptors in the visual structures of monocularly deprived rats. Effect of light and dark adaptation. *Brain Res.,* 329: 143–150.

Ryan, M.K. and Hendrickson, A.E. (1987) Interplexiform cells in macaque monkey retina. *Exp Eye Res.,* 45: 57–66.

Schaeffer, J.M. (1980) [$^3$H] Muscimol binding in the rat retina. *Life Sci.,* 27: 1199–1204.

Schaeffer, J.M. (1982) Biochemical characterization of isolated rat retinal cells: The $\gamma$-aminobutyric system. *Exp. Eye Res.,* 34: 715–726.

Schoch, P., Richards, J.G., Häring, P., Takács, B., Stähli, C., Staehelin, T., Haefely, W. and Möhler, H. (1985) Co-localization of GABA$_A$ receptors and benzodiazepine receptors in the brain shown by monoclonal antibodies. *Nature (London),* 314: 168–171.

Schofield, P.R., Darlison, M.G., Fujita, N., Burt, D.R., Stephenson, F.A., Rodriguez, H., Rhee, L.M., Ramachandran, J., Reale, V., Glencorse, T.A., Seeburg, P.H. and

Barnard, E.A. (1987) Sequence and functional expression of the GABA$_A$ receptor shows a ligand-gated receptor super-family. *Nature (London)*, 328: 221–227.

Schwartz, E.A. (1987) Depolarization without calcium can release γ-aminobutyric acid from a retinal neuron. *Science*, 238: 350–355.

Séquier, J.M., Richards, J.G., Malherbe, P., Price, G.W., Mathews, S. and Möhler, H. (1988) Mapping of brain areas containing RNA homologous to cDNAs encoding the α and β subunits of the GABA$_A$ γ-aminobutyrate receptor. *Proc. Natl. Acad. Sci. USA*, 85: 7815–7819.

Shivers, B.D., Killisch, I., Sprengel, R., Sontheimer, H., Köhler, M., Schofield, P.R. and Seeburg, P.H. (1989) Two novel GABA$_A$ receptor subunits exist in distinct neuronal subpopulations. *Neuron*, 3: 327–337.

Sieghart, W., Drexler, G., Supavilai, P. and Karobath, M. (1982) Properties of benzodiazepine receptors in rat retina. *Exp. Eye Res.*, 34: 961–967.

Sigel, E., Baur, R., Trube, G., Möhler, H. and Malherbe, P. (1990) The effect of subunit composition of rat brain GABA$_A$ receptors on channel function. *Neuron*, 5: 703–711.

Skolnick, P., Paul, S., Zatz, M. and Eskay, R. (1980) "Brain-specific" benzodiazepine receptors are localized in the inner plexiform layer of rat retina. *Eur. J. Pharmacol.*, 66: 133–136.

Soltesz, I., Roberts, J.D.B., Takagi, H., Richards, J.G., Möhler, H. and Somogyi, P. (1991) Synaptic and nonsynaptic localization of benzodiazepine/GABA$_A$ receptor/Cl$^-$ channel complex using monoclonal antibodies in the dorsal lateral geniculate nucleus of the cat. *Eur. J. Neurosci.*, 2: 414–429.

Somogyi, P., Takagi, H., Richards, J.G. and Möhler, H. (1989) Subcellular localization of benzodiazepine/GABA$_A$ receptors in the cerebellum of rat, cat, and monkey using monoclonal antibodies. *J. Neurosci.*, 9: 2197–2209.

Stell, W.K., Lightfoot, D.O., Wheeler, T.G. and Leeper, H.F. (1975) Goldfish retina: Functional polarization of cone horizontal cell dendrites and synapses. *Science*, 190: 989–990.

Stephenson, F.A. (1988) Understanding the GABA$_A$ receptor: a chemically gated ion channel. *Biochem. J.*, 249: 21–32.

Studholme, K.M. and Yazulla, S. (1988) Localization of GABA and glycine in goldfish retina by electron microscopic postembedding immunohistochemistry: improved visualization of synaptic structures with LR White resin. *J. Neurocyt.*, 17: 859–870.

Suzuki, S., Tachibana, M. and Kaneko, A. (1990) Effects of glycine and GABA on isolated bipolar cells of the mouse retina. *J. Physiol. (London)*, 421: 645–662.

Tachibana, M. and Kaneko, A. (1984) γ-Aminobutyric acid acts at axon terminals of turtle photoreceptors: Difference in sensitivity among cell types. *Proc. Natl. Acad. Sci. USA*, 81: 7961–7964.

Tachibana, M. and Kaneko, A. (1987) γ-Aminobutyric acid exerts a local inhibitory action on the axon terminal of bipolar cells: Evidence for negative feedback from amacrine cells. *Proc. Natl. Acad. Sci. USA*, 84: 3501–3505.

Tachibana, M. and Kaneko, A. (1988) Retinal bipolar cells receive negative feedback input from GABAergic amacrine cells. *Vis. Neurosci.*, 1: 297–305.

Tallman, J.F., Thomas, J.W. and Gallager, D.W. (1978) GABAergic modulation of benzodiazepine binding site sensitivitiy. *Nature (London)*, 274: 383–385.

Tauck, D.L., Frosch, M.P. and Lipton, S.A. (1988) Characterization of GABA- and glycine-induced currents of solitary rodent retinal ganglion cells in culture. *Neuroscience*, 27: 193–203.

Unnerstall, J.R., Kuhar, M.J., Niehoff, D.L. and Palacios, J.M. (1981) Benzodiazepine receptors are coupled to a subpopulation of γ-aminobutyric acid (GABA) receptors: Evidence from a quantitative autoradiographic study. *J. Pharmacol. Exp. Ther.*, 218: 797–804.

Vaney, D.I. The mosaic of amacrine cells in the mammalian retina. (1990) In: N. Osborne and J. Chader (Eds.), *Progress in Retinal Research, Vol. 9*, Pergamon Press, Oxford, pp. 49–100.

Vaughn, J.E., Famiglietti, E.V. Jr., Barber, R.P., Saito, K., Roberts, E. and Ribak, C.E. (1981) GABAergic amacrine cells in rat retina: Immunocytochemical identification and synaptic connectivity. *J. Comp. Neurol.*, 197: 113–127.

Verdoorn, T.A., Draguhn, A., Ymer, S., Seeburg, P.H. and Sakman, B. (1990) Functional properties of recombinant rat GABA$_A$ receptors depend upon subunit composition. *Neuron*, 4: 919–928.

Vitorica, J., Park, D., Chin, G. and de Blas, A.L. (1988) Monoclonal antibodies and conventional antisera to the GABA$_A$ receptor/benzodiazepine receptor/Cl$^-$ channel complex. *J. Neurosci.*, 8: 615–622.

Wässle, H., and Chun, M.H. (1988) Dopaminergic and indoleamine-accumulating amacrine cells express GABA-like immunoreactivity in the cat retina. *J. Neurosci.*, 8: 3383–3394.

Williams, M. and Risley, E.A. (1978) Characterization of the binding of [$^3$H]muscimol, a potent γ-aminobutyric acid antagonist, to rat brain synaptosomal membranes using a filtration assey. *J. Neurochem.*, 32: 713–718.

Wisden, W., Morris, B.J., Darlison, M.G., Hunt, S.P. and Barnard, E.A. (1988) Distinct GABA$_A$ receptor a subunit mRNAs show differential patterns of expression in bovine brain. *Neuron*, 1: 937–947.

Wisden, W., Morris, B.J., Darlison, M.G., Hunt, S.P. and Barnard, E.A. (1989a) Localization of GABA$_A$ receptor α-subunit mRNAs in relation to receptor subtypes. *Mol. Brain Res.*, 5: 305–310.

Wisden, W., Morris, B.J., Darlison, M.G., Hunt, S.P. and Barnard, E.A. (1989b) Differential distribution in bovine brain of distinct γ-aminobutyric acid$_A$ receptor α-subunit mRNAs. *Biochem. Soc. Trans.*, 17: 566–567.

28

Wu, S.M. and Dowling, J.E. (1980) Effects of GABA and glycine on the distal cells of the cyprinid retina. *Brain Res.,* 199: 401–414.

Yasui, S., Ishizuka, S. and Akaike, N. (1985) GABA activates different types, of chloride-conducting receptor-ionophore complexes in a dose-dependent manner. *Brain Res.,* 344: 176–180.

Yazulla, S. (1981) GABAergic synapses in the goldfish retina: An autoradiographic study of $^3$H-muscimol and $^3$H-GABA binding. *J. Comp. Neurol.,* 200: 83–93.

Yazulla, S. (1985) Evoked efflux of [$^3$H]GABA from goldfish retina in dark. *Brain Res.,* 325: 171–180.

Yazulla, S. (1986) GABAergic mechanisms in the retina. In: N.N. Osborne and G.J. Chader (Eds.), *Progress in Retinal Research, Vol. 5,* Pergamon Press, Oxford, pp. 1–52.

Yazulla, S. and Brecha, N. (1980) Binding and uptake of the GABA analogue, $^3$H-muscimol, in the retinas of goldfish and chicken. *Invest. Ophthal. Vis. Sci.,* 19: 1415–1426.

Yazulla, S. and Brecha, N. (1981) Localized binding of [$^3$H]muscimol to synapses in chicken retina. *Proc. Natl. Acad. Sci. USA,* 78: 643–647.

Yazulla, S., Studholme, K. and Wu, J.-Y. (1986) Comparative distribution of $^3$H-GABA uptake and GAD immunoreactivity in goldfish retinal amacrine cells: A double label analysis. *J. Comp. Neurol.,* 244: 149–162.

Yazulla, S., Studholme, K. and Wu, J.-Y. (1987) GABAergic input to the synaptic terminals of mb$_1$ bipolar cells in the goldfish retina. *Brain Res.,* 411: 400–405.

Yazulla, S., Studholme, K.M., Vitorica, J. and de Blas, A.L. (1989) Immunocytochemical localization of GABA$_A$ receptors in goldfish and chicken retina. *J. Comp. Neurol.,* 280: 15–26.

Yeh, H.H., Lee, M.B. and Cheun, J.E. (1990) Properties of GABA-activated whole-cell currents in bipolar cells of the rat retina. *Vis. Neurosci.,* 4: 349–357.

Ymer, S., Schofield, P.R., Draguhn, A., Werner, P., Köhler, M. and Seeburg, P.H. (1989a) GABA$_A$ receptor $\beta$ subunit heterogeneity: functional expression of cloned cDNAs. *EMBO J.,* 8: 1665–1670.

Ymer, S., Draguhn, A., Köhler, M., Schofield, P.R. and Seeburg, P.H. (1989b) Sequence and expression of a novel GABA$_A$ receptor a subunit. *FEBS Lett.,* 258: 119–122.

Young, W.S. III and Kuhar, M.J. (1979) Autoradiographic localisation of benzodiazepine receptors in the brains of humans and animals. *Nature (London),* 280: 393–395.

Young, W.S. III, Niehoff, D., Kuhar, M.J., Beer, B. and Lippa, A.S. (1981) Multiple benzodiazepine receptor localization by light microscopic radiohistochemistry. *J. Pharm. Exp. Ther.,* 216: 425–430.

Zarbin, M.A., Wamsley, J.K., Palacios, J.M. and Kuhar, M.J. (1986) Autoradiographic localization of high affinity GABA, benzodiazepine, dopaminergic, adrenergic and muscarinic cholinergic receptors in the rat, monkey and human retina. *Brain Res.,* 374: 75–92.

Zhang, J.H., Sato, M. and Tohyama, M. (1991) Region-specific expression of the mRNAs encoding $\beta$ subunits ($\beta_1$, $\beta_2$, and $\beta_3$) of GABA$_A$ receptor in the rat brain. *J. Comp. Neurol.,* 303: 637–657.

Zucker, C., Yazulla, S. and Wu, J.-Y. (1984) Non-correspondence of [$^3$H]GABA uptake and GAD localization in goldfish amacrine cells. *Brain Res.,* 298: 154–158.

R.R. Mize, R.E. Marc and A.M. Sillito (Eds.)
Progress in Brain Research, Vol. 90
© 1992 Elsevier Science Publishers B.V. All rights reserved

CHAPTER 2

# The physiology of GABA$_A$ receptors in retinal neurons

## A.T. Ishida

*Department of Animal Physiology, University of California Davis, CA 95616, USA*

## Introduction

GABA (gamma-aminobutyric acid) is one of several neurotransmitters which exert inhibitory electrophysiological effects on many vertebrate neurons (for reviews, see Alger, 1985; Bormann, 1988). In the vertebrate retina, the identification of GABA as a neurotransmitter used by specific cell types is widely accepted (see Marc, Chapter 4), and GABA figures prominently in several proposed synaptic circuits (see Wu, Chapter 5; Freed, Chapter 6).

As is true of several neurotransmitters (recall acetylcholine, L-glutamate, dopamine, serotonin), more than one type of receptor can mediate neuronal responses to GABA. The two most well-known of these are termed "GABA$_A$" and "GABA$_B$" (see also Slaughter and Pan, Chapter 3). The former denotes receptor-ionophore complexes identified biochemically and electrophysiologically by their ability to both (1) bind several classes of ligands (especially GABA, bicuculline, benzodiazepines, and barbiturates: see Olsen, 1982), and (2) mediate changes in membrane permeability to anions (especially Cl$^-$: see Bormann et al., 1987). These complexes are sometimes referred to simply as either "GABA$_A$ receptors" or "GABA$_A$ channels", without implying that GABA or barbiturates affect only Cl$^-$ channels, that all Cl$^-$ channels are coupled to GABA binding sites, or that all GABA$_A$ receptor-channels are identical electrophysiologically or structurally. Recently, several different poly-

peptides which can either form functional GABA$_A$ receptor-channels, or which impart certain biochemical and electrophysiological properties to expressed GABA$_A$ receptor-channels, have been described (Schofield et al., 1987; Blair et al., 1988; Pritchett et al., 1988, 1989; Shivers et al., 1989; Verdoorn et al., 1990). This chapter reviews the electrophysiological effects of GABA mediated by GABA$_A$ receptor-channels in single retinal neurons. Six aspects will be addressed: their distribution, pharmacology, ion selectivity, elementary properties, modulation, and possible functions.

## Distribution

Three experimental approaches have demonstrated the presence of GABA$_A$ receptors in specific types of retinal neurons: (1) measurement of electrophysiological responses to GABA and related chemicals in situ after blockade of synaptic transmission (e.g., using cobaltous (Co$^{2+}$) ion); (2) measurement of electrophysiological responses to GABA and related chemicals in vitro in single cells physically isolated from the retina; and (3) localization of GABA$_A$ receptors in situ using immunocytochemical methods. These studies have yielded two types of information. First, cells with and without GABA-sensitivity and/or GABA receptors have been identified. Second, regions of high GABA-sensitivity have been localized within some cell types.

GABA$_A$ receptors in cone photoreceptors were first demonstrated unequivocally by the patch-clamp measurements of Tachibana and Kaneko (turtle: 1984). GABA$_A$ receptors have since been localized in cones with a monoclonal antibody (goldfish and chick: Yazulla et al., 1989; see Brecha, Chapter 2). These results corroborate those of Murakami et al. (carp: 1978) and of Wu and Dowling (carp: 1980). Whether all cone GABA receptors are type A, or for that matter, whether all cones possess GABA receptors of any sort, is not certain (mudpuppy: Miller et al., 1981; primate: Mariani et al., 1987; salamander: Eliasof and Werblin, 1989; Barnes and Hille, 1989). Rod photoreceptors show little GABA sensitivity (Tachibana and Kaneko, 1984), and no surface membrane labeling with the GABA$_A$-receptor antibody which stains cones (Yazulla et al., 1989). In concert with these results, rod horizontal cells show no GABA uptake (goldfish: Marc et al., 1978).

Horizontal cells can be depolarized by GABA in situ in the presence of Co$^{2+}$ (turtle: Laufer, 1982; Perlman and Normann, 1990; roach: Hankins and Ruddock, 1984; *Xenopus*: Witkovsky and Stone, 1987; urodeles: Stockton et al., 1988). Whether these responses are mediated by a single mechanism in all horizontal cells, or even in individual horizontal cells, is unclear. Bicuculline reduces GABA-activated whole-cell currents in isolated skate (Lasater et al., 1984) and salamander (Gilbertson et al., 1990) horizontal cells, and rabbit horizontal cells display GABA$_A$ receptor $\alpha$-subunit-like immunoreactivity (Brecha and Weigmann, 1990). However, a bicuculline-insensitive response in isolated skate horizontal cells has recently been identified as due to sodium-dependent GABA-transport (Malchow and Ripps, 1990). Some horizontal cells are reportedly GABA-insensitive (Miller et al., 1981; carp: Lasater and Dowling, 1982).

Voltage responses of bipolar cells to GABA can also be recorded in situ after block of synaptic transmission with Co$^{2+}$ (Miller et al., 1981; carp: Kondo and Toyoda, 1983). Bipolar cell GABA-sensitivity resides largely, if not entirely, in their axon terminals (Kondo and Toyoda, 1983). These responses were first analyzed under voltage clamp by Tachibana and Kaneko (carp: 1987, 1988), and similar responses have been identified in several species (goldfish: Schwartz, 1987; mouse: Suzuki et al., 1990; rat: Karschin and Wässle, 1990; Yeh et al., 1990). Although both rod and rod/cone bipolar cells clearly possess GABA$_A$ receptors (skate: Lasater et al., 1984; axolotl: Attwell et al., 1987; carp, goldfish, mouse, and rat as cited above), it is unclear whether all bipolar cells do (Miller et al., 1981; Kondo and Toyoda, 1983). Some bipolar cells possess GABA$_B$ receptors (salamander: Maguire et al., 1989), while other bipolar cells possess GABA receptors which are neither GABA$_A$ nor sensitive to typical GABA$_B$ agonists (goldfish: Heidelberger and Matthews, 1991).

Both dopaminergic and glycinergic interplexiform cells probably possess GABA receptors, given the morphological synapses from GABA-ergic horizontal cells onto these cells (see Marc, Chapter 4). Although these receptors are likely to be GABA$_A$ in dopaminergic interplexiform cells (carp: Negishi et al., 1983; O'Connor et al., 1986; turtle: Piccolino et al., 1984), it is not yet known which type(s) exist in glycinergic units.

Similar results suggest that at least some amacrine cells possess GABA receptors. It would not be surprising if all amacrine cells were GABA-sensitive, given that so many amacrine cells seem GABA-ergic (Marc, Chapter 4; Freed, Chapter 6), and given the widespread interconnections among amacrine cells in general (Dowling and Boycott, 1966; Kolb and Nelson, 1984). The immunocytochemical studies of Richards et al. (1987), Yazulla et al. (1989), Hughes et al. (1989), and of Brecha and Weigmann (1990), indicate that at least some amacrine cells possess GABA$_A$ receptors. Whether all amacrine cell GABA receptors are type A is not certain (see Slaughter and Pan, Chapter 3). The possibility that more than one type of GABA$_A$ receptor may be present in amacrine cells has been raised

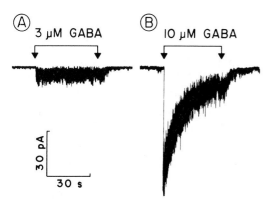

Ⓐ 3 μM GABA

Ⓑ 10 μM GABA

30 pA

30 s

Fig. 1. Current elicited in a single retinal ganglion cell by two concentrations of GABA. The response of this cell to 3 μM GABA (A) remains constant in amplitude during the entire GABA application, whereas the response to 10 μM GABA (B) fades by approximately 90% within 10–15 s after onset of the maintained GABA application. Substantial increases in clamp current noise accompany both responses to GABA. Holding potential ($E_{hold}$) = −60 mV. Here, as in Figs. 2–6, currents were measured with the tight-seal, whole-cell patch-clamp method (Hamill et al., 1981) from individual retinal ganglion cell somata dissociated from adult goldfish. Currents are plotted conventionally (left to right; downward deflections representing inward current, viz. Cl⁻ efflux). In Figs. 1–5, patch electrodes filled with (in mM; pH 7.5): 148 CsCl, 17 NaOH, 0.5 CaCl₂, 4.7 EGTA, and 10 Hepes; control bath saline contained (in mM; pH 7.5): 135 NaCl, 2.5 KCl, 1.0 CaCl₂, 10 tetraethylammonium Cl, 10 D-glucose, 21 sucrose, and 3 Hepes, plus 30 nM tetrodotoxin. Drugs applied by microperfusion (see Fenwick et al., 1982) or by bath application. (From Ishida and Cohen, 1988; methods described in detail therein.)

recently by the results of Friedman and Redburn (1990).

GABA$_A$ receptors have been found in all types of ganglion cells in several species (carp: Negishi et al., 1978; Glickman et al., 1982; goldfish: Ishida and Cohen, 1988; Cohen et al., 1989; mudpuppy: Miller et al., 1981; Belgum et al., 1984; rat and mouse: Tauck et al., 1988; rabbit: Wyatt and Daw, 1976; cat: Bolz et al., 1985; see Fig. 1). GABA$_B$ receptors have not been found in ganglion cells (Ishida and Cohen, 1988; Tauck et al., 1988; Ishida, 1989) with the possible exception of some units in mudpuppy (see Slaughter and Pan, Chapter 3). Whether all ganglion cells possess GABA$_A$ receptors in all vertebrates, or whether all ganglion cell GABA$_A$ receptors are identical in all respects, remains to be clarified (see below).

The results summarized above indicate that GABA$_A$ receptors exist in at least some members of each basic type of retinal neuron, except rod photoreceptors. These receptors have been found localized to specific regions of individual cells. In cone photoreceptors (Tachibana and Kaneko, 1984) and bipolar cells (Kondo and Toyoda, 1983; Tachibana and Kaneko, 1987; Karschin and Wässle, 1990), GABA$_A$ receptors seem to reside largely, if not only, in the axon terminals (however, see Suzuki et al., 1990; Yeh et al., 1990), while in ganglion cells GABA$_A$ receptors are found on somata (Mariani et al., 1987; Ishida and Cohen, 1988; Hughes et al., 1989) and dendrites (Lukasiewicz and Werblin, 1990). There is ample precedent for the existence of GABA$_A$ receptors in axon terminals (e.g., Dudel and Kuffler, 1961) and somata (e.g., Gray and Johnston, 1985), and GABA receptors on ganglion cell dendrites (rat: Vaughn et al., 1981; salamander: Lukasiewicz and Werblin, 1990; goldfish: Muller and Marc, 1990) could account for at least some of the dense labeling by GABA$_A$ receptor antibodies in the inner plexiform layer (Richards et al., 1987; Yazulla et al., 1989; Hughes et al., 1989; Brecha and Weigmann, 1990).

## Pharmacology

GABA$_A$ receptor-channel function can be isolated, antagonized, and modulated by a variety of pharmacological agents. Here, agents which are useful for "blocking" GABA$_A$ responses, and ionic conditions under which responses mediated by GABA$_A$ receptors can be studied with minimal interference from other membrane currents, will be described.

Bicuculline inhibits GABA-receptor binding competitively in preparations derived from retina (bovine: Enna and Snyder, 1976) as well as other tissues. It has therefore been used universally to inhibit electrophysiological responses to exogenously applied GABA (e.g., Fig. 2) as well as

32

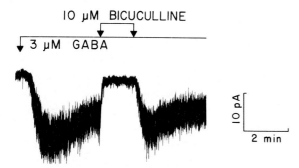

Fig. 2. Antagonism of response to 3 $\mu$M GABA by 10 $\mu$M bicuculline. Continuous bath application of GABA begins at first arrow; microperfusion of 10 $\mu$M bicuculline + 3 $\mu$M GABA (at paired arrows) produces decrease in current amplitude and noise. Note that the response to GABA here (unlike those in Figs. 1, 4, and 6) fades before the application of bicuculline. $E_{hold} = -75$ mV. (From Ishida and Cohen, 1988.)

synaptically released GABA (e.g., Belgum et al., 1984; Bolz et al., 1985). Consistent with its effect on GABA binding, bicuculline produces parallel rightward shifts of the dose-response curves for GABA-activated currents in cones and bipolar cells (Kaneko and Tachibana, 1986a; Suzuki et al., 1990). Furthermore, bicuculline can reduce GABA-activated currents in ganglion cells without drastically affecting their kinetics (Ishida and Cohen, 1988). Although bicuculline thus appears to be an appropriate antagonist, certain precautions must be exercised to achieve useful results with it. First, bicuculline hydrochloride is remarkably unstable in saline solutions at neutral pH, hydrolyzing to bicucine, particularly at elevated temperatures (Olsen et al., 1975). Methyl-halides of bicuculline are more stable, have pharmacological properties similar to those of bicuculline-HCl, and may therefore be used in place of bicuculline (Johnston et al., 1972). Elevating the dose of bicuculline, rather than preparing fresh mixtures of bicuculline or using the more expensive methyl-halides, would be ill-advised because high bicuculline concentrations block not only GABA responses, but also responses to other neurotransmitters, e.g., serotonin (Mayer and Straughan, 1981) and glycine (Biscoe et al., 1972). Cohen et al. (1989) recently showed that such nonselective effects can be avoided by using bicu-

culline at no more than 3 $\mu$M. This emphasizes the need to apply pharmacological agents at known concentrations.

A variety of other substances are known to inhibit GABA responses. Picrotoxin is perhaps the most widely used of these. Like bicuculline, picrotoxin is capable of inhibiting GABA responses while sparing glycine responses (Wyatt and Daw, 1976; Hamill et al., 1983; Belgum et al., 1984). However, the modes of action of bicuculline and picrotoxin differ, because picrotoxin does not displace GABA from GABA-binding sites (Zukin et al., 1974; Enna and Snyder, 1976). Although the mechanism underlying the effect of picrotoxin on retinal cell GABA responses is not known, studies in crayfish muscle and mammalian spinal neurons suggest interference with GABA-activated channel open (and perhaps closed) states (Takeuchi and Takeuchi, 1969; Twyman et al., 1989). Consistent with this, the inhibition of cone and bipolar cell GABA responses by picrotoxin is not competitive (Kaneko and Tachibana, 1986a; Suzuki et al., 1990). Antagonists usually associated with entirely different receptors can also block GABA responses, e.g., the cholinergic antagonist curare (Nicoll, 1975) and the opiate antagonist naloxone (Dingledine et al, 1978). This emphasizes the need to utilize more than one pharmacological agent to characterize neurotransmitter receptor-channels.

As discussed below in more detail, GABA$_A$ receptors are typically coupled to ion channels selectively permeable to anions. GABA$_A$ responses can therefore be elicited in cells whose cationic currents are suppressed, and thus studied over ranges of membrane potentials which normally activate voltage-gated cation currents. For example, GABA$_A$ responses can be elicited in isolation from sodium and potassium currents, by including tetrodotoxin, tetraethylammonium, cesium, and 4-aminopyridine in the bathing medium (Schwartz, 1987; Ishida and Cohen, 1988; Karschin and Wässle, 1990). GABA responses of retinal bipolar and ganglion cells can also be measured in the absence of extracellular and intracellular Na$^+$ and K$^+$ ions (see Fig. 6; see also Karschin and Wässle, 1990) in order to minimize extraneous cationic currents, as well as the possibility of current due to GABA transport (Malchow and Ripps, 1990). Finally, at least with retinal bipolar and ganglion cells, it is also possible to study GABA$_A$ responses after blockade of their Ca$^{2+}$ currents (Tachibana and Kaneko, 1987; Schwartz, 1987; Ishida and Cohen, 1988; Suzuki et al., 1990). In contrast, GABA$_A$ responses of isolated cones (turtle: Kaneko and Tachibana, 1986b) are blocked by certain divalent cations (Co$^{2+}$, Ni$^{2+}$, Cd$^{2+}$). This may partly explain why horizontal cell *hyperpolarizations* during GABA application to whole carp retina (Wu and Dowling, 1980), and bipolar cell responses to ionophoretic GABA applications near their dendrites in situ (Kondo and Toyoda, 1983), can be inhibited by Co$^{2+}$.

## Ion selectivity

The ion selectivity of the bicuculline-sensitive GABA-activated conductances examined so far in all retinal cell-types of all species is anionic (cones: Tachibana and Kaneko, 1984; Kaneko and Tachibana, 1986a; bipolar cells: Lasater et al., 1984; Tachibana and Kaneko, 1987; Attwell et al., 1987; Schwartz, 1987; Suzuki et al., 1990; Karschin and Wässle, 1990; Yeh et al., 1990; ganglion cells: Ishida and Cohen, 1988; Tauck et al., 1988; Cohen et al., 1989; Müller cells: Malchow et al., 1989). These results are all based on comparisons of GABA response reversal potentials with chloride ion equilibrium potentials ($E_{Cl}$; see Fig. 3) using whole-cell or cell-free patch-clamp methods (Hamill et al., 1981). In these experiments, bath and patch-electrode Cl$^-$ concentrations were altered by equimolar replacement of Cl$^-$ with large organic anions: acetate (Attwell et al., 1987), aspartate (Tauck et al., 1988; Lipton, 1989), gluconate (Karschin and Wässle, 1990; Yeh et al., 1990), glutamate (Tachibana and Kaneko, 1984), isethionate (Malchow et al., 1989; Cohen et al., 1989), and

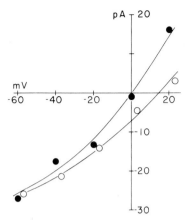

Fig. 3. Peak amplitude of the whole-cell current elicited in a single cell by 3 $\mu$M GABA, plotted against holding potential, in bath saline containing either 100% (filled circles) or 50% (open circles) of the Cl$^-$ concentration in the recording electrode (see legend to Fig. 1). Cl$^-$ concentration reduced by equimolar replacement of NaCl by NaCH$_3$SO$_3$. Holding potentials compensated for change in junction potential at ground electrode due to change in bath Cl$^-$ concentration. Curves drawn through points by eye; both curves show slight outward rectification, particularly at voltages more positive than $-20$ mV. In control bath ($E_{Cl} = 0$ mV), the GABA response reverses near zero mV; in the $\frac{1}{2}$-Cl$^-$ bath, the GABA response reverses at $+16$ mV. (From Ishida and Cohen, 1988.)

methanesulfonate (Kaneko and Tachibana, 1986a; Tachibana and Kaneko, 1987; Ishida and Cohen, 1988; Suzuki et al., 1990). None of these anions appear to permeate the GABA-activated channels of cones, bipolar and ganglion cells to any large extent, because the reversal potentials differed by no more than 5 mV from the $E_{Cl}$ values calculated from the bath and pipette Cl$^-$ concentrations used. Such findings are no mean feat given the complicated geometry of some of the cells examined, and given that substantial drifts in $E_{Cl}$ can occur with reduced intracellular Cl$^-$ concentrations (see below). In any event, these results corroborate earlier observations that responses of retinal neurons to GABA are sensitive to Cl$^-$-loading (Miller et al., 1981), and agree with the ionic selectivities of GABA$_A$ channels (see Bormann et al., 1987), as well as of most other known anion-permeable channels, in other cells. To substantiate the extent of this similarity will require measuring the relative permeabilities of smaller, inorganic anions (e.g., $F^-$, $Br^-$, $I^-$) in retinal cells. Nevertheless, although ion selectivity measurements are not yet available for horizontal, interplexiform, or amacrine cells, it would be surprising if their bicuculline-sensitive GABA-activated currents were not anionic.

## Elementary properties

The elementary properties (i.e., amplitude and kinetics) of single-channel currents activated in retinal neurons by GABA are known at a rudimentary level. The single-channel conductance of $GABA_A$ currents in retinal neurons were first estimated from whole-cell current fluctuations (see Neher and Stevens, 1977) in bipolar cells (Attwell et al., 1987) and ganglion cells (Ishida and Cohen, 1988), yielding values of 4 pS and 16 pS, respectively. Although the value obtained from bipolar cells has not yet been confirmed by direct measurement of single-channel currents (cf. Hamill et al., 1981), it should be relatively easy to do so using the large bulbous axon terminals of certain fish bipolar cells (Cajal, 1972; Ishida et al., 1980; Tachibana and Kaneko, 1987; Schwartz, 1987). On the other hand, the amplitude of single-channel currents activated in ganglion cells by GABA has recently been measured in the outside-out configuration of the patch-clamp method (cf. Hamill et al., 1981).

One study (goldfish: Cohen et al., 1989) showed that GABA activates channels whose most frequently observed conductance level is 16 pS, matching the single-channel conductance estimated in the same cells by noise analysis (Ishida and Cohen, 1988; see Fig. 4). Transitions between this main conductance level and a subconductance state of roughly 11 pS were seen in some (but not all) of these GABA-activated single channels (Cohen et al., 1989). No spontaneous openings of these channels (i.e., no openings of these channels in the absence of GABA) were described.

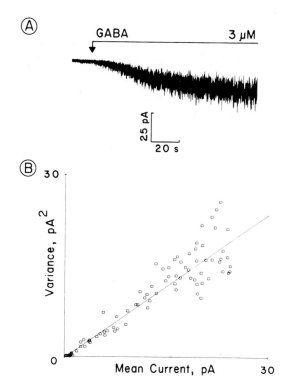

Fig. 4. Estimate of single-channel conductance from GABA-activated whole-cell current fluctuations ('noise'). A. Increase in mean current and noise during rise of the response to bath-application of GABA (starts at arrow; concentration at steady-state, 3 $\mu$M); $E_{hold} = -60$ mV. B. Increase in variance of clamp current noise during response in A plotted against mean current amplitude. Line through points is linear regression; division of its slope by response driving force (60 mV) yields single-channel conductance of 13 pS. Mean from 6 cells = $16 \pm 2$ pS. (From Ishida and Cohen, 1988.)

The only other measurements of single-channel currents activated by GABA in ganglion cells are those of Lipton (rat: 1989). This study showed currents of several different amplitudes, including transitions between the closed state and conductance levels of 10, 20, 30, and 45 pS. These were interpreted as different conductance states of single-channel currents similar to those demonstrated by Bormann et al. (1987). An alternative explanation could be that the 20- and 30-pS events consist of simultaneous occurrences (in pairs and triplets) of 10-pS events. This would imply that the unitary conductances activated by GABA in this study were 10 and 45 pS.

Although the values of GABA-activated single-channel conductance measured in rat and fish ganglion cells might appear to differ, it should be kept in mind that the latter were measured at 10–12 °C, whereas the former were measured at 33–35 °C. If the GABA-activated conductances of all retinal ganglion cells are as temperature-sensitive as that described by Mathers and Barker (1981) (viz., if their $Q_{10} = 1.3$), then at least the largest GABA-activated conductance level observed in membrane patches of fish and rodent ganglion cells should agree. Similar arguments may explain differences between the single-channel current amplitudes described in ganglion cells and those examined at room temperature in several other preparations (see discussion in Cohen et al., 1989).

However, until demonstrated otherwise, the possibility that the main state of GABA-activated channels in fish retinal ganglion cells could measure less than 20 pS under the same conditions that rodent ganglion cell GABA channels exceed 40 pS can not be excluded. Differences of such magnitude have, in fact, been known for several years from recordings in mammalian hippocampal and spinal cord cells (Bormann et al., 1983; Hamill et al., 1983; Gray and Johnston, 1985; Bormann et al., 1987). Recently, differences of similar magnitude have also been measured in GABA-activated channels expressed from different combinations of cloned subunit-specific cDNAs (Verdoorn et al., 1990). The latter results suggest that large differences in Cl$^-$ flux (seen as differences in main-state conductance levels) could result from differences in receptor-channel subunit composition. These results, together with those collected from hippocampal and spinal cord cells, also indicate that particular GABA-activated single-channel current amplitudes are not unique to a particular vertebrate class.

In any event, the GABA-activated single-channel conductances for both fish and rodent retinal ganglion cells appear to be linear at membrane potentials more negative than −20 mV (Ishida and Cohen, 1988; Cohen et al., 1989; Lipton,

1989). In fact, the GABA-activated single-channel current-voltage curves for rodent ganglion cells appear linear between −60 and +60 mV (Lipton, 1989), as in spinal cord (Bormann et al., 1987) and astrocytes (Bormann and Kettenmann, 1988). Because the GABA-activated *whole-cell* current *also* varies linearly with membrane potential in rodent ganglion cells (Tauck et al., 1988), the gating of GABA-activated channels in these cells is likely to be voltage-insensitive. It is less clear whether the gating of GABA-activated channels in fish ganglion cells is voltage-sensitive or not. At membrane potentials between −20 and −80 mV, the single-channel conductance is linear, and voltage-sensitive kinetics are not obvious (Ishida and Cohen, 1988; Cohen et al., 1989). However, the GABA-activated whole-cell current in these cells exhibits a slight outward rectification, particularly at membrane potentials more positive than −20 mV (Ishida and Cohen, 1988; Cohen et al., 1989). If the single-channel conductance remains linear over these voltages, or if it rectifies inwardly, then the gating of GABA channels in these cells is likely to be voltage-sensitive. It would therefore be of interest to measure single-channel current amplitudes and kinetics at voltages more positive than −20 mV. However, Cohen et al. (1989) have reported that GABA-activated single-channel currents fade irreversibly before records can be obtained at various membrane potentials. This is unfortunate because GABA-activated channels in fish ganglion cells otherwise seem well-suited for this sort of analysis: their conductance is large enough to provide good signal-to-noise ratios, and they show few subconductance states (if any). Two reasons why the results summarized above may be of interest are that expressed GABA receptors consisting of different subunit combinations have been found to yield whole-cell current-voltage curves rectifying to different extents (Verdoorn et al., 1990), and because some GABA-activated single-channel currents rectify even with identical Cl$^-$ concentrations in the solutions bathing the cytoplasmic and external membrane faces (hip-

36

pocampus: Gray and Johnston, 1985; adrenal chromaffin cells: Bormann and Clapham, 1985; dorsal root ganglion: Yasui et al., 1985; expressed GABA channels: Blair et al., 1988). Recently, a variety of $GABA_A$ receptor forms have been characterized in the vertebrate retina by in situ hybridization techniques (see Brecha, Chapter 1).

Although the GABA-activated whole-cell current in turtle cones (Kaneko and Tachibana, 1986a) and rat bipolar cells (Yeh et al., 1990) also display a slight outward rectification, whether or not the underlying single channel currents vary linearly with voltage is unknown.

Apart from the above considerations, the kinetics of GABA-activated currents in retinal cells have been characterized by noise analysis (Attwell et al., 1987; Ishida and Cohen, 1988; see Fig. 5). These studies showed that sums of two Lorentzian curves fit the power spectra of the

GABA-induced current noise increases in both bipolar and ganglion cells, consistent with the possibility that the underlying channels pass through more than two kinetic states (see Colquhoun and Hawkes, 1977). The time constants for the slower components were relatively long in both cell types (20 ms for bipolar cells (calculated from the data of Attwell et al., 1987), and 30 ms for ganglion cells), in agreement with the slow time constants measured by noise analysis in other preparations (spinal neurons: McBurney and Barker, 1978; cerebellar neurons: Cull-Candy and Ogden, 1981). These slow time constants probably correspond to the duration of bursts of single-channel openings (Sakmann et al. 1983; Macdonald et al., 1989). The time constants for the faster components measured roughly 1–2 ms in both bipolar and ganglion cells. Whole-cell currents passing through the expressed GABA

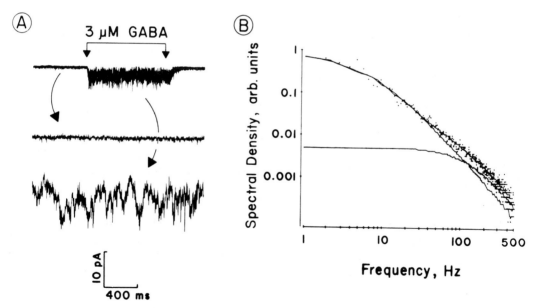

Fig. 5. Power spectrum of GABA-induced current noise. A. Upper trace shows response from which power spectrum in B was measured; recorded from same cell as in Fig. 1 ($E_{hold}$ (−60 mV), GABA dose (3 $\mu M$), and response amplitude (6 pA) identical to those in Fig. 1A). Duration of GABA application (paired arrows) is 45 s. Middle and lower traces (separated for clarity) plot control and response currents, respectively, digitized at 1 kHz from portions of upper trace (arrows). Calibration applies to digitized traces only. B. Difference of spectra calculated from several control and response current segments. Fit by eye through points in B is sum of the two single Lorentzian curves plotted underneath the data points. Time constants for these slow and fast component Lorentzians are 32 and 1.5 ms, respectively. (From Ishida and Cohen, 1988.)

channels of Verdoorn et al. (1990) exhibit both slow and fast components similar to those described here.

## Modulation

Patch-clamp studies have shown that cone, bipolar, and ganglion cell responses to GABA can undergo various types of modulation, e.g., diminution by receptor desensitization, and enhancement by benzodiazepines and barbiturates.

The GABA-activated whole-cell currents of cone, bipolar and ganglion cells all decline during the maintained application of elevated doses of GABA. At least in part, these declines seem to result from receptor desensitization (Katz and Thesleff, 1957), because background applications of low GABA doses produce decreases in response amplitude (see Kaneko and Tachibana, 1986a), and because it can be observed even in cells dialyzed against electrode salines containing elevated $Cl^-$ concentrations (see Fig. 1, and below). Desensitization appears to be dose-dependent, both in degree and rate of onset (see Fig. 1; also, compare Fig. 5A of Kaneko and Tachibana, 1986a; Fig. 3B of Ishida and Cohen 1988; and Fig. 6C of Tachibana and Kaneko, 1987). GABA-activated currents have been reported to decline exponentially, with time constants of roughly 4–6 s in ganglion cells (Tauck et al., 1988; Lipton, 1989), and 2–2.5 s in horizontal cells (Gilbertson et al., 1990). Although the rates at which both whole-cell and single-channel GABA-activated currents desensitize in ganglion cells have been reported to be voltage-insensitive (Tauck et al., 1988; Lipton, 1989), it is not clear whether this is also true in bipolar cells (see Fig. 3 of Tachibana and Kaneko, 1987; Fig. 4 of Karschin and Wässle, 1990). Additional time constants of desensitization have not yet been described (cf. Bormann and Clapham, 1985), although a slow, irreversible "run-down" has been observed in ganglion cells (Lipton, 1989; Cohen et al., 1989).

After prolonged GABA applications are terminated, GABA-activated whole-cell currents of control amplitude can be recorded in bipolar cells within 3–5 minutes (see Fig. 5A of Kaneko and Tachibana, 1986a). After washout of high doses of GABA (30 $\mu$M), Cohen et al. (1989) showed that recovery of ganglion cell GABA-sensitivity occurs within 3–5 min if ATP (complexed with $Mg^{2+}$) is included in the patch-electrode solution and/or intracellular $Ca^{2+}$ is well-buffered. The latter observations are in accord with the findings of Stelzer et al. (1988) in hippocampal neurons. Unfortunately, the presence of these substances does not ameliorate the run-down of GABA-activated single-channel currents (Cohen et al., 1989). Whether similar solutions would facilitate recovery from desensitization in cone, horizontal, or bipolar cells is not yet known.

Desensitization has several consequences. For example, because intense desensitization is provoked by GABA concentrations less than one log unit above the minimum dose which elicits reliably measurable responses (Ishida and Cohen, 1988; Suzuki et al., 1990; see Fig. 1), desensitization almost certainly depresses both the slope and maxima of dose-response curves. Although the extent of this distortion has not been fully assessed in retinal cells, Gilbertson et al. (1990) have recently reported that Hill coefficients may be significantly underestimated as a result of desensitization. Similar effects have been seen in responses of other cells to GABA (Feltz, 1971; Akaike et al., 1987). These results emphasize the need to consider amplitudes of GABA-activated currents in terms of channels entering and leaving their open states via closed as well as desensitized states, before using these currents to estimate ligand-receptor stoichiometry and receptor-channel density.

Whether rates and extents of desensitization differ significantly with cell type (e.g., cone vs. bipolar cell) or GABA dose (cf. Akaike et al., 1987; Verdoorn et al., 1990) remains to be examined in detail in retinal neurons. These characterizations are likely to be tedious, because the extent to which currents activated by single doses of GABA decline varies from cell to cell even within single cell types (compare Figs. 3 and 5 of Ishida and Cohen, 1988; Fig. 6 of Cohen et al., 1989), as has also been observed in mouse spinal cord neurons (Mathers, 1987) and transiently expressed $GABA_A$ receptor-channels of different subunit compositions (Verdoorn et al., 1990). The results obtained so far from retinal neurons are of interest for two reasons. First, variations in levels of desensitization are consistent with the possibility of $GABA_A$-receptor structural heterogeneities (cf. Verdoorn et al., 1990). Secondly, a complete collapse of currents during maintained applications of elevated GABA doses has not been seen in isolated retinal neurons (Kaneko and Tachibana, 1986a; Ishida and Cohen, 1988; Cohen et al., 1989; Suzuki et al., 1990). Unless the residual current seen under these conditions corresponds to electrogenic GABA transport (Malchow and Ripps, 1990), the inhibitory effect of GABA on retinal neurons in situ should persist even if GABA reaches high concentrations, or is released tonically, at synaptic clefts.

In homogeneous populations of receptor-channels, receptor desensitization has been found to alter gating kinetics (Sakmann et al., 1980) and not channel ionic selectivity (Katz and Miledi, 1977). Thus, response reversal potentials would not be expected to change as a result of receptor desensitization. However, responses can fade (i.e., appear to desensitize) for reasons other than receptor desensitization. For example, GABA-activated whole-cell $Cl^-$ fluxes can be so large that intracellular $Cl^-$ concentrations change (Takeuchi and Takeuchi, 1967). The result of these $Cl^-$ fluxes is that $E_{Cl}$ will shift in the direction which reduces the difference between $E_{Cl}$ and cell membrane potential, i.e., $Cl^-$ will exit cells whose membrane potential is negative with respect to $E_{Cl}$, and enter cells whose membrane potential is positive with respect to $E_{Cl}$. This will undermine the driving force sustaining GABA responses at a given membrane potential, causing the response to fade (e.g., Adams and

Brown, 1975). Although such problems can be minimized by internally dialyzing cells with salines containing elevated $Cl^-$ concentrations, $E_{Cl}$ can shift by 10–15 mV if internal $Cl^-$ levels are low and $Cl^-$ fluxes are high (Huguenard and Alger, 1986; Akaike et al., 1987).

$GABA_A$ receptor-channel function can also be modulated by various ligands which bind to sites other than those which primarily bind GABA and bicuculline. As alluded to above, a picrotoxin-binding site may reside within the channel itself, or close to it (see Olsen, 1987). Patch-clamp studies have recently shown that picrotoxin reduces the mean channel open time, number of openings per burst, and probability of opening, of GABA-activated channels, without altering their conductance (Twyman et al., 1989). A $Ca^{2+}$ ion-binding site appears to be accessible from the cytoplasmic side of the channel, because increases in intracellular $Ca^{2+}$ levels diminish the inhibitory effect of GABA in some cells (Inoue et al., 1986; Feltz et al., 1987) and enhance it in other cells (Llano et al., 1991). Extracellularly-applied $Zn^{2+}$, and some other divalent cations, can block $GABA_A$ channels in some preparations, consistent with a third binding site (see Draguhn et al., 1990). A fourth type of binding site are phosphorylation sites for protein kinases (e.g., Schofield et al., 1987). Activators of both protein kinase A and C reduce GABA-activated currents in certain preparations (Sigel and Baur, 1988; Porter et al., 1990). The possibility that $GABA_A$ receptor function is regulated in retinal neurons by cytoplasmic factors remains to be explored systematically.

A fifth locus binds barbituates, such as pentobarbital and phenobarbital. Because all four major types of $GABA_A$ receptor subunits described to date (alpha, beta, delta, and gamma) bind barbiturates (Blair et al., 1988; Pritchett et al., 1988; Shivers et al., 1989), it is not surprising that the $GABA_A$ response of bipolar (Suzuki et al., 1990) and ganglion (Fig. 6A,B) cells are barbiturate-sensitive. Although the mechanism underlying the effect of barbiturates on retinal neurons is

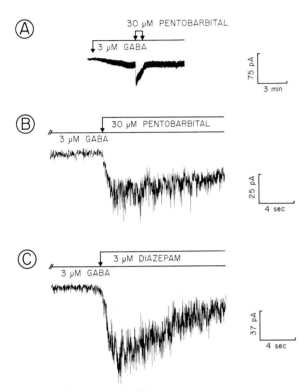

Fig. 6. Enhancement of GABA-activated whole-cell current by benzodiazepine and barbiturate. A. Pen-record of current elicited by 3 $\mu$M GABA (bath application starting at first arrow), and by subsequent addition of 30 $\mu$M pentobarbital (microperfused with 3 $\mu$M GABA, at paired arrows). Mean steady-state current prior to pentobarbital is $-18$ pA; mean current peaks at $-62$ pA after onset of pentobarbital. B. 20-s segment of A, showing current in 3 $\mu$M GABA before and just after pentobarbital application. Note change in time-scale and gain from A. C. Enhancement by 3 $\mu$M diazepam of response of a different ganglion cell to 3 $\mu$M GABA, formatted as in B. Mean steady-state current prior to diazepam is $-30$ pA; mean current peaks at $-115$ pA after onset of diazepam. In B and C, note that GABA-activated currents increase upon application of both pentobarbital and diazepam, then fade even though superfusion of latter are maintained. In A, current fluctuations increase in amplitude as GABA-activated current rises, as in Figs. 1, 2, and 4; current fluctuations also increase with drug-elicited increases in mean current. In A, this increase is not obvious due to damping by pen-recorder; in B and C, this increase is exaggerated because sampling frequency here produces larger (roughly 2-fold) decrement of current noise in GABA alone than in drug-enhanced currents. In these records, bath contains (in mM, pH 7.5): 140 $N$-methyl-D-glucamine Cl, 2.5 CaCl$_2$, 10 D-glucose; patch electrode contains (in mM, pH 7.5): 140 CsCl, 16 CsOH, 0.5 CaCl$_2$, 5 EGTA, 5 Hepes. $E_{hold} = -70$ mV.

not known, the enhancement by pentobarbital of retinal bipolar and ganglion cell GABA$_A$ responses is consistent with voltage-clamp studies of other neurons which have shown that bursts of GABA-activated channels (see above) are prolonged by pentobarbital (Study and Barker, 1981; Mathers, 1987; Twyman et al., 1989).

A sixth modulatory binding site on GABA$_A$ receptors is that for benzodiazepines (see Olsen, 1982). This site is particularly interesting because electrophysiological (see Haefely and Polc, 1986), biochemical (see Olsen, 1982), autoradiographic (e.g., Unnerstall et al., 1981), and immunocytochemical (e.g., de Blas et al., 1988) evidence indicate that not all GABA$_A$ receptor-channels possess this type of site. That this site differs from those binding GABA, bicuculline, picrotoxin, and barbiturates, is suggested by findings of benzodiazepine-insensitive, but bicuculline-, picrotoxin- and barbiturate-sensitive currents mediated by expressed GABA$_A$ receptors (see Pritchett et al., 1988; Pritchett et al., 1989; Malherbe et al., 1990). The presence of benzodiazepine binding sites in the retina has been known for several years (see Zarbin et al., 1986 and references therein). Furthermore, GABA-activated whole-cell currents in both retinal bipolar cells (Suzuki et al., 1990) and ganglion cells (Fig. 6C) can be enhanced by the widely studied benzodiazepine, diazepam. However, it would probably be premature to conclude that all GABA-sensitive retinal neurons possess benzodiazepine receptors (see Robbins and Ikeda, 1989; Friedman and Redburn, 1990). Resolution of this ambiguity with electrophysiological methods may not be simple because benzodiazepines may promote desensitization in addition to potentiating GABA-activated currents (see Bormann and Clapham, 1985; see also Fig. 6C).

## Possible functions and future steps

The results reviewed above show that at least some cells of each major class in the retina (except rods) possess GABA$_A$ receptor-channels, and that most of these receptor-channels share several features: they are selectively permeable to anions; their single-channel conductance is moderate (tens of pS); their kinetics resemble those of other neurons ($\tau_{slow}$ = tens of ms); and they are sensitive to bicuculline, benzodiazepines, and barbiturates. Activation of these receptor-channels in situ should in all cases shunt membrane resistance, and therefore be inhibitory. However, the polarity and size of the membrane potential changes elicited by GABA may vary from cell to cell, because intracellular $Cl^-$ concentrations have been found to differ with cell type (Miller and Dacheux, 1983). In any event, the distribution of these receptors should allow them to mediate inhibition both pre-synaptically (in cones and bipolar cells) and post-synaptically (in ganglion cells). The inhibition exerted on single bipolar cell axon terminals may allow bipolar input to ganglion cells to be attenuated locally, while the direct effects of GABA on ganglion cell dendrites and somata could shunt the response to bipolar and certain amacrine cell inputs more diffusely.

There are several hints of heterogeneity among $GABA_A$ receptors in the retina. First, different minimum effective doses of GABA have been found, e.g., 1–3 $\mu$M for ganglion cells (Ishida and Cohen, 1988; Tauck et al., 1988; Cohen et al., 1989), versus 0.3 $\mu$M for bipolar cells (Suzuki et al., 1990). Second, cells vary in the extent of desensitization induced by GABA (Ishida and Cohen, 1988; Cohen et al., 1989). Third, benzodiazepines do not affect GABA responses in all cells (Friedman and Redburn, 1990; see also Robbins and Ikeda, 1989). Fourth, some cells show linear current-voltage curves (Tauck et al., 1988), whereas others do not (Kaneko and Tachibana, 1986a; Ishida and Cohen, 1988; Cohen et al., 1989; Yeh et al., 1990; Karschin and Wässle, 1990). Finally, the bicuculline-sensitive GABA responses of some cells are picrotoxin-insensitive (Hankins and Ruddock, 1984; Cohen, 1985; Cohen et al, 1989), while others are picrotoxin-sensitive (Kaneko and Tachibana, 1986a; Tauck et al., 1988; Suzuki et al., 1990; Karschin

and Wässle, 1990). It is interesting that some of the combinations of electrophysiological properties seen in retinal neurons (e.g., weakly rectifying current-voltage curves in association with a Hill coefficient of 2 (Kaneko and Tachibana, 1986a) and with strong desensitization by 10 $\mu$M GABA (Ishida and Cohen, 1988)) have not yet been seen in expressed $GABA_A$ channels (see Verdoorn et al., 1990).

Results obtained recently with monoclonal antibodies directed against benzodiazepine receptors and against specific $GABA_A$ receptor subunits are also consistent with the possibility that $GABA_A$ receptors in the retina may be heterogeneous. For example, the scant staining of ganglion cell somata (Mariani et al., 1987; Richards et al., 1987; Hughes et al., 1989) contrasts with the high percentage of cells which respond electrophysiologically to GABA (Negishi et al., 1978; Miller et al., 1981; Bolz et al., 1985; Ishida and Cohen, 1988; Tauck et al., 1988; Cohen et al., 1989). That this does not reflect vagaries of immunocytochemistry is suggested by the widespread staining of cones observed by Yazulla et al. (1989). However, it would obviously be of interest to determine whether only receptor-immunoreactive somata bear receptor-immunoreactive dendrites.

The distribution of different $GABA_A$ receptors among the different cell types of the retina is not yet known in detail, and whether individual cells possess more than one subtype of $GABA_A$ receptor remains to be investigated. It would also be of interest to find both $GABA_A$ and $GABA_B$ receptors in single cells. One consequence of such a colocalization would be that neither $GABA_A$ antagonists alone, nor $GABA_B$ antagonists alone, could block all of the effects of GABA on such cells. One possible advantage of having both $GABA_A$ and $GABA_B$ receptors in single cells would be for activation of the $GABA_B$ receptor to produce a decrease in $Ca^{2+}$ permeability (see Feltz et al., 1987; Bormann, 1988), and thus minimize $Ca^{2+}$ influx into cells depolarized by $GABA_A$ receptor-mediated $Cl^-$ efflux or by other inputs. Without the GABA$_B$ receptor, a voltage-activated Ca$^{2+}$ influx could produce increases in intracellular Ca$^{2+}$ levels large enough to *reduce* the Cl$^-$ currents activated via certain GABA$_A$ receptors (Inoue et al, 1986; Feltz et al., 1987). This may not be the only advantage gained by cells bearing both GABA$_A$ and GABA$_B$ receptors, because responses mediated by some GABA$_A$ receptors are enhanced by internal Ca$^{2+}$ (see above), and not all GABA$_B$ receptors are coupled to Ca$^{2+}$ channels (Feltz et al., 1987; Bormann, 1988). How these receptors work in concert, if at all, is likely to be of broad interest because GABA$_A$ and GABA$_B$ receptors coexist in at least some single neurons in central as well as peripheral nervous system (e.g., Newberry and Nicoll, 1985; Désarmenien et al., 1984), and recently, it has been reported that single retinal bipolar cells possess some GABA receptors coupled to Cl$^-$ channels, together with other GABA receptors coupled to Ca$^{2+}$ channels (Heidelberger and Matthews, 1991).

In summary, GABA$_A$ receptors appear to be ubiquitously distributed in all vertebrate retinas, and the electrophysiological responses they mediate seem to share at least some basic properties. To clarify whether heterogeneous GABA receptors exist in all types of retinal neuron, to unveil how such receptor distributions arise developmentally, and to comprehend the functional advantages such heterogeneities confer, will no doubt require future anatomical, electrophysiological, immunocytochemical, and molecular biological studies, both in situ and in vitro.

## Note added in proof

We have found that voltage-gated calcium current in fish retinal ganglion cells can be inhibited by GABA and the GABA$_B$ receptor agonist, baclofen (Bindokas and Ishida, in press).

## Acknowledgements

Supported by National Institutes of Health grant EY 08120.

## References

Adams, P.R. and Brown, D.A. (1975) Actions of gamma-aminobutyric acid on sympathetic ganglion cells. *J. Physiol.*, 250: 85–120.

Akaike, N., Inomata, N. and Tokutomi, N. (1987) Contribution of chloride shifts to the fade of gamma-butyric acid-gated currents in frog dorsal root ganglion cells. *J. Physiol.*, 391: 219–234.

Akaike, N., Inoue, M. and Krishtal, O.A. (1986) "Concentration-clamp" study of gamma-aminobutyric-acid-induced chloride current kinetics in frog sensory neurones. *J. Physiol.*, 379: 171–185.

Alger, B.E. (1985) GABA and glycine: Postsynaptic actions. In: M.A. Rogawski and J.L. Barker (Eds.), *Neurotransmitter Actions in the Vertebrate Nervous System*, Plenum Press, New York, pp. 33–69.

Attwell, D., Mobbs, P., Tessier-Lavigne, M. and Wilson, M. (1987) Neurotransmitter-induced currents in retinal bipolar cells of the axolotl, *Ambystoma mexicanum*. *J. Physiol.*, 387: 125–161.

Barnes, S. and Hille, B. (1989) Ionic channels of the inner segment of tiger salamander cone photoreceptors. *J. Gen. Physiol.*, 94: 719–743.

Belgum, J.H., Dvorak, D.R. and McReyonolds, J.S. (1984) Strychnine blocks transient but not sustained inhibition in mudpuppy retinal ganglion cells. *J. Physiol.*, 354: 273–286.

Biscoe, T.J., Duggan, A.W. and Lodge, D. (1972) Antagonism between bicuculline, strychnine, and picrotoxin and depressant amino-acids in the rat nervous system. *Comp. Gen. Pharmacol.*, 3: 423–433.

Blair, L.A.C., Levitan, E.S., Marshall, J., Dionne, V.E. and Barnard, E.A. (1988) Single subunits of the GABA$_A$ receptor form ion channels with properties of the native receptor. *Nature*, 242: 577–579.

Bolz, J., Frumkes, T., Voigt, T. and Wässle, H. (1985) Action and localization of gamma aminobutyric acid in the cat retina. *J. Physiol.*, 362: 369–393.

Bormann, J. (1988) Electrophysiology of GABA$_A$ and GABA$_B$ receptor subtypes. *Trends Neurosci.*, 11: 112–116.

Bormann, J. and Clapham, D.E. (1985) Gamma-aminobutyric acid receptor channels in adrenal chromaffin cells: A patch-clamp study. *Proc. Natl. Acad. Sci. USA*, 82: 2168–2172.

Bormann, J., Hamill, O.P. and Sakmann, B. (1987) Mechanism of anion permeation through channels gated by glycine and gamma-aminobutyric acid in mouse cultured spinal neurones. *J. Physiol.*, 385: 243–286.

Bormann, J. and Kettenmann, H. (1988) Patch-clamp study of gamma-aminobutyric acid receptor Cl$^-$ channels in culture astrocytes. *Proc. Natl. Acad. Sci. USA*, 85: 9336–9340.

Bormann, J., Sakmann, B. and Seifert, W. (1983) Isolation of GABA-activated single-channel Cl$^-$ currents in the soma membrane of rat hippocampal neurons. *J. Physiol.*, 341: 9–10P.

Brecha, N. and Weigmann, C. (1990) GABA$_A$ $\alpha$ and $\beta$ subunit immunoreactivities in the rabbit retina. *Soc. Neurosci. Abstr.*, 16: 1075.

42

Bruun, A., Ehinger, B. and Sytsma, V.M. (1984) Neurotransmitter localization in the skate retina. *Brain Res.*, 295: 233–248.

Cajal, S.R. y (1972) *The Structure of the Retina*. Translated by S.A. Thorpe and M. Glickstein, C.C. Thomas, Springfield.

Cohen, B.N., Fain, G.L. and Fain, M.J. (1989) GABA and glycine channels in isolated ganglion cells from the goldfish retina. *J. Physiol.*, 417: 53–82.

Cohen, J.L. (1985) Effects of glycine and GABA on the ganglion cells of the retina of the skate Raja erinacea. *Brain Res.*, 332: 169–173.

Colquhoun, D. and Hawkes, A.G. (1977) Relaxation and fluctuations of membrane currents that flow through drug-operated channels. *Proc. R. Soc. London B*, 199: 231–262.

Cull-Candy, S.G. and Ogden, D.C. (1981) Ion channels activated by L-glutamate and GABA in cultured cerebellar neurons of the rat. *Proc. R. Soc. London B*, 224: 367–373.

de Blas, A.L., Vitorica, J. and Friedrich, P. (1988) Localization of the GABA$_A$ receptor in the rat brain with a monoclonal antibody to the 57000 M$_r$ peptide of the GABA$_A$ receptor/benzodiazepine/Cl$^-$ channel complex. *J. Neurosci.*, 8: 602–614.

Désarmenien, M., Feltz, P., Occhipinti, G., Santangelo, F. and Schlichter, R. (1984) Coexistence of GABA$_A$ and GABA$_B$ receptors on A$\delta$ and C primary afferents. *Brit. J. Pharmacol.*, 81: 327–333.

Dingledine, R., Iversen, L.L. and Breuker, E. (1978) Naloxone as a GABA antagonist: Evidence from iontophoretic, receptor binding and convulsant studies. *Eur. J. Pharmacol.*, 47: 19–27.

Dowling, J.E. and Boycott, B.B. (1966) Organization of the primate retina: Electron microscopy. *Proc. R. Soc. London B*, 166: 80–111.

Draguhn, A., Verdoorn, T.A., Ewert, M., Seeburg, P.H. and Sakmann, B. (1990) Functional and molecular distinction between recombinant rat GABA$_A$ receptor subtypes by Zn$^{2+}$. *Neuron*, 5: 781–788.

Dudel, J. (1975) Kinetics of postsynaptic action of glutamate pulses applied iontophoretically through high resistance micropipettes. *Pflügers Arch.*, 356: 329–346.

Dudel, J. and Kuffler, S.W. (1961) Presynaptic inhibition at the crayfish neuromuscular junction. *J. Physiol.*, 155: 543–562.

Eliasof, S. and Werblin, F.S. (1989) GABA$_A$ and GABA$_B$ mediated synaptic transmission to cones in the tiger salamder retina. *Invest. Ophthal. Vis. Sci.*, 30: 163.

Enna, S.J. and Snyder, S.H. (1976) Gamma-aminobutyric acid (GABA) receptor binding in mammalian retina. *Brain Res.*, 115: 174–179.

Feltz, A. (1971) Competitive interaction of $\beta$-guanidino propionic acid and gamma aminobutyric acid on the muscle fibre of the crayfish. *J. Physiol.*, 216: 391–401.

Feltz, A., Demeneix, B., Feltz, P., Taleb, O., Trouslard, J., Bossu, J.-L. and Dupont, J.-L. (1987) Intracellular effectors and modulators of GABA-A and GABA-B receptors: A commentary. *Biochimie*, 69: 395–406.

Fenwick, E.M., Marty, A. and Neher, E. (1982) A patch-clamp study of bovine chromaffin cells and of their sensitivity to acetylcholine. *J. Physiol.*, 331: 577–597.

Friedman, D.L. and Redburn, D.A. (1990) Evidence for functionally distinct subclasses of gamma-aminobutyric acid receptors in rabbit retina. *J. Neurochem.*, 55: 1189–1199.

Gilbertson, T.A., Borges, S. and Wilson, M. (1990) Horizontal cells contain two types of inhibitory amino acid receptors. *Soc. Neurosci. Abstr.*, 16: 465.

Glickman, R.D., Adolph, A.R. and Dowling, J.E. (1982) Inner plexiform layer circuits in the carp retina: Effects of cholinergic agonists, GABA, and substance P on the the ganglion cells. *Brain Res.*, 234: 81–99.

Gray, R. and Johnston, D. (1985) Rectification of single GABA-gated chloride channels in adult hippocampal neurons. *J. Neurophysiol.*, 54: 134–142.

Haefely, W. and Polc, P. (1986) Physiology of GABA enhancement by benzodiaxepines and barbiturates. In: R.W. Olsen and J.C. Venter (Eds.), *Benzodiazepine / GABA Receptors and Chloride Channels: Structural and Functional Properties*, A.R. Liss, New York, pp. 97–133.

Hamill, O.P., Bormann, J. and Sakmann, B. (1983) Activation of multiple-conductance state chloride channels in spinal neurones by glycine and GABA. *Nature*, 305: 805–808.

Hamill, O.P., Marty, A., Neher, E., Sakmann, B. and Sigworth, F. (1981) Improved patch clamp techniques for high resolution current recording from cells and cell-free membrane patches. *Pflügers Arch.*, 391: 85–100.

Hankins, M.W. and Ruddock, K.H. (1984) Electrophysiological effects of GABA on fish retinal horizontal cells are blocked by bicuculline but not by picrotoxin. *Neurosci. Lett.*, 44: 1–6.

Heidelberger, R. and Matthews, G. (1991) GABA reduces calcium current of retinal bipolar neurons. *Biophys. J.*, 59: 83a.

Hughes, T.E., Carey, R.G., Vitorica, J., de Blas, A.L. and Karten. H.J. (1989) Immunocytochemical localization of GABA$_A$ receptors in the retina of the new world primate Saimiri sciureus. *Visual Neurosci.*, 2: 565–581.

Huguenard, J.R. and Alger, B.E. (1986) Whole-cell voltage-clamp study of the fading of GABA-activated currents in acutely dissociated hippocampal neurons. *J. Neurophysiol.*, 56: 1–18.

Inoue, M., Oomura, Y., Yakushiji, T. and Akaike, N. (1986) Intracellular calcium ions decrease the affinity of the GABA receptor. *Nature*, 324: 156–158.

Ishida, A.T. (1989) Voltage-activated sodium and calcium currents in goldfish retinal ganglion cells. *Soc. Neurosc. Abstr.*, 15: 968.

Ishida, A.T. and Cohen, B.N. (1988) GABA-activated whole-cell currents in isolated retinal ganglion cells. *J. Neurophysiol.*, 60: 381–396.

Ishida, A.T., Stell, W.K. and Lightfoot, D.O. (1980) Rod and cone inputs to bipolar cells in goldfish retina. *J. Comp. Neurol.*, 191: 315–335.

Johnston, G.A.R., Beart, P.M., Curtis, D.R., Game, C.J.A., McCulloch, R.M. and Maclachlan, R.M. (1972) Bicuculline methochloride as a GABA antagonist. *Nature New Biol.*, 240: 219–220.

Kaneko, A. and Tachibana, M. (1986a) Effects of gamma-aminobutyric acid on isolated cone photoreceptors of the turtle retina. *J. Physiol.*, 373: 443–461.

Kaneko, A. and Tachibana, M. (1986b) Blocking effects of cobalt and related ions on the gamma-aminobutyric acid-induced current in turtle retinal cones. *J. Physiol.*, 373: 463–479.

Karschin, A. and Wässle, H. (1990) Voltage- and transmitter-gated currents in isolated rod bipolar cells of rat retina. *J. Neurophysiol.*, 63: 860–876.

Katz, B. and Miledi, R. (1977) The reversal potential at the desensitized endplate. *Proc. R. Soc. London B*, 199: 329–334.

Katz, B. and Thesleff, S. (1957) A study of the "desensitization" produced by acetylcholine at the motor end-plate. *J. Physiol.*, 138: 63–80.

Kolb, H. and Nelson, R. (1984) Neural architecture of the cat retina. *Progr. Retinal Res.*, 3: 21–60.

Kondo, H. and Toyoda, J.-I. (1983) GABA and glycine effects on the bipolar cells of the carp retina. *Vision Res.*, 23: 1259–1264.

Lasater, E.M. and Dowling, J.E. (1982) Carp horizontal cells in culture respond selectively to L-glutamate and its agonists. *Proc. Natl. Acad. Sci. USA*, 79: 936–940.

Lasater, E.M., Dowling, J.E. and Ripps, H. (1984) Pharmacological properties of isolated horizontal and bipolar cells from the skate retina. *J. Neurosci.*, 4: 1966–1975.

Laufer, M. (1982) Electrophysiological studies of drug actions on horizontal cells. In: B.D. Drujan and M. Laufer (Eds.), *The S-Potential*, A.R. Liss, New York, pp. 257–279.

Lipton, S.A. (1989) GABA-activated single channel currents in outside-out membrane patches from rat retinal ganglion cells. *Visual Neurosci.*, 3: 275–279.

Llano, I., Leresche, N. and Marty, A. (1991) Calcium entry increases the sensitivity of cerebellar Purkinje cells to applied GABA and decreases inhibitory synaptic currents. *Neuron*, 6: 565–574.

Lukasiewicz, P. and Werblin, F.S. (1990) The spatial distribution of excitatory and inhibitiory inputs to ganglion cell dendrites in the tiger salamander retina. *J. Neurosci.*, 10: 210–221.

Macdonald, R.L., Rogers, C.J. and Twyman, R.E. (1989) Kinetic properties of the GABA$_A$ receptor main conductance state of mouse spinal cord neurones in culture. *J. Physiol.*, 410: 479–499.

Maguire, G., Maple, B., Lukasiewicz, P. and Werblin, F. (1989) Gamma-aminobutyrate type B receptor modulation of L-type calcium channel current at bipolar cell terminals in the retina of the tiger salamander. *Proc. Natl. Acad. Sci. USA*, 86: 10144–10147.

Malchow, R.P., Qian, H. and Ripps, H. (1989) Gamma-aminobutyric acid (GABA)-induced currents of skate Muller (glial) cells are mediated by neuronal-like GABA$_A$ receptors. *Proc. Natl. Acad. Sci. USA*, 86: 4326–4330.

Malchow, R.P. and Ripps, H. (1990) Effects of gamma-aminobutyric acid on skate retinal horizontal cells: Evidence for an electrogenic uptake mechanism. *Proc. Natl. Acad. Sci. USA*, 87: 8945–8949.

Malherbe, P., Sigel, E., Baur, R., Persohn, E., Richards, J.G., and Möhler, H. (1990) Functional characteristics and sites of gene expression of the $\alpha_1$, $\beta_1$, gamma$_2$-isoform of the rat GABA$_A$ receptor. *J. Neurosci.*, 10: 2330–2337.

Marc, R.E., Stell, W.K., Bok, D. and Lam, D.M.K. (1978) GABA-ergic pathways in the goldfish retina. *J. Comp. Neurol.*, 182: 221–246.

Mariani, A.P., Cosenza-Murphy, D. and Barker, J.L. (1987) GABAergic synapses and benzodiazepine receptors are not identically distributed in the primate retina. *Brain Res.*, 415: 153–157.

Mathers, D.A. (1987) The GABA$_A$ receptor: New insights from single-channel recording. *Synapse*, 1: 96–101.

Mathers, D.A. and Barker, J.L. (1981) GABA- and glycine-induced Cl$^-$ channels in cultured mouse spinal neurons require the same energy to close. *Brain Res.*, 224: 441–445.

Mayer, M.L. and Straughan, D.W. (1981) Effects of 5-hydroxytryptamine on central neurones antagonized by bicuculline and picrotoxin. *Neuropharmacology*, 20: 347–350.

McBurney, R.N. and Barker, J.L. (1978) GABA-induced conductance fluctuations in cultured spinal neurones. *Nature*, 274: 596–597.

Miller, R.F. and Dacheux, R.F. (1983) Intracellular chloride in retinal neurons: Measurement and meaning. *Vision Res.*, 23: 399–411.

Miller, R.F., Frumkes, T.E., Slaughter, M.M. and Dacheux, R.F. (1981) Physiological and pharmacological basis of GABA and glycine action on neurons of mudpuppy retina. I. Receptors, horizontal cells, bipolars, and G-cells. *J. Neurophysiol.*, 45: 743–763.

Muller, J.F. and Marc, R.E. (1990) GABA-ergic and glycinergic pathways in the inner plexiform layer of the goldfish retina. *J. Comp. Neurol.*, 291: 281–304.

Murakami, M., Shimoda, Y., Nakatani, K., Miyachi, E.-I. and Watanabe, S.-I. (1982) GABA-mediated negative feedback from horizontal cells to cones in carp retina. *Jpn. J. Physiol.*, 32: 911–926.

Negishi, K., Kato, S., Teranishi, T. and Laufer, M. (1978) Dual actions of some amino acids on spike discharges in the carp retina. *Brain Res.*, 148: 67–84.

Negishi, K., Teranishi, T. and Kato, S. (1983) A GABA antagonist, bicuculline, exerts its uncoupling action of external horizontal cells through dopamine cells in carp retina. *Neurosci. Lett.*, 37: 261–266.

Neher, E. and Stevens, C.F. (1977) Conductance fluctuations and ionic pores in membranes. *Ann. Rev. Biophys. Bioeng.*, 6: 345–381.

Newberry, N.R. and Nicoll, R.A. (1985) Comparison of the action of baclofen with gamma aminobutyric acid on rat hippocampal pyramidal cells in vitro. *J. Physiol.*, 360: 161–185.

Nicoll, R.A. (1975) The action of acetylcholine antagonists on amino acid responses in the frog spinal cord in vitro. *Br. J. Pharmacol.*, 55: 449–458.

O'Connor, P., Dorison, S.J., Watling, K.J. and Dowling, J.E. (1986) Factors affecting release of [3]H-dopamine from perfused carp retina. *J. Neurosci.*, 6: 1857–1865.

Olsen, R.W. (1982) Drug interactions at the GABA receptor-ionophore complex. *Ann. Rev. Pharmacol. Toxicol.*, 22: 245–277.

Olsen, R.W. (1987) GABA-drug interactions. *Progr. Drug Res.*, 31: 223–241.

Olsen, R.W., Ban, M., Miller, T. and Johnston, G.A.R. (1975) Chemical instability of the GABA antagonist bicuculline under physiological conditions. *Brain Res.*, 98: 383–387.

Perlman, I. and Normann, R.A. (1990) The effects of GABA and related drugs on horizontal cells in the isolated turtle retina. *Visual Neurosci.*, 5: 469–477.

Piccolino, M., Neyton, J., Witkovsky, P. and Gerschenfeld, H.M. (1984) Decrease of gap junction permeability induced by dopamine and cyclic adenosine 3',5'-monophosphate in horizontal cells of the turtle retina. *J. Neurosci.*, 4: 2477–2488.

Porter, N.M., Twyman, R.E., Uhler, M.D. and Macdonald, R.L. (1990) Cyclic AMP-dependent protein kinase decreases $GABA_A$ receptor current in mouse spinal neurons. *Neuron*, 5: 789–796.

Pritchett, D.B., Sontheimer, H., Gorman, C.M., Kettenmann, H., Seeburg, P.H. and Schofield, P.R. (1988) Transient expression shows ligand gating and allosteric potentiation of $GABA_A$ receptor subunits. *Science*, 242: 1306–1308.

Pritchett, D.B., Sontheimer, H., Shivers, B.D., Ymer, S., Kettenmann, H., Schofield, P.R. and Seeburg, P.H. (1989) Importance of a novel $GABA_A$ receptor subunit for benzodiazepine pharmacology. *Nature*, 338: 582–585.

Richards, J.G., Schoch, P., Häring, P., Takacs, B. and Möhler, H. (1987) Resolving $GABA_A$/benzodiazepine receptors: Cellular and subcellular localization in the CNS with monoclonal antibodies. *J. Neurosci.*, 7: 1866–1886.

Robbins, J. and Ikeda, H. (1989) Benzodiazepines and the mammalian retina. II. Actions on retinal ganglion cells. *Brain Res.*, 479: 323–333.

Sakmann, B., Hamill, O.P. and Bormann, J. (1983) Patch-clamp measurements of elementary chloride currents activated by the putative inhibitory transmitters GABA and glycine in mammalian spinal neurons. *J. Neural Transm.*, 18: 83–95.

Sakmann, B., Patlak, J. and Neher, E. (1980) Single acetylcholine-activated channels show burst-kinetics in presence of desensitizing concentrations of agonist. *Nature*, 286: 71–73.

Schofield, P.R., Darlison, M.G., Fujita, N., Burt, D.R., Stephenson, F.A., Rodriguez, H., Rhee, L.M., Ramachandran, J., Reale, V., Glencorse, T.A., Seeburg, P.H. and Barnard, E.A. (1987) Sequence and functional expression of the $GABA_A$ receptor shows a ligand-gated receptor super-family. *Nature*, 328: 221–227.

Schwartz, E.A. (1987) Depolarization without calcium can release gamma-aminobutyric acid from a retinal neuron. *Science*, 238: 350–355.

Shivers, B.D., Killisch, I., Sprengel, R., Sontheimer, H.,

Köhler, M., Schofield, P.R. and Seeburg, P.H. (1989) Two novel $GABA_A$ receptor subunits exist in distinct neuronal subpopulations. *Neuron*, 3: 327–337.

Sigel, E. and Baur, R. (1988) Activation of protein kinase C differentially modulates neuronal $Na^+$, $Ca^{2+}$, and gamma-aminobutyrate type A channels. *Proc. Natl. Acad. Sci. USA*, 85: 6192–6196.

Stelzer, A., Kay, A.R. and Wong, R.K.S. (1988) $GABA_A$-receptor function in hippocampal cells is maintained by phosphorylation factors. *Science*, 241: 339–341.

Stockton, R.A., Bai, S.H. and Slaughter, M.M. (1988) Depolarizing actions of GABA and glycine upon retinal horizontal cells of mudpuppy and tiger salamander. *Invest. Ophthal. Vis. Sci.*, 29: 101.

Study, R.E. and Barker, J.L. (1981) Diazepam and (−) pentobarbital: fluctuation analysis reveals different mechanisms for potentiation of gamma-aminobutyric acid and responses in cultured central neurones. *Proc. Natl. Acad. Sci. USA*, 78: 7180–7184.

Suzuki, S., Tachibana, M. and Kaneko, A. (1990) Effects of glycine and GABA on isolated bipolar cells of the mouse retina. *J. Physiol.*, 421: 645–662.

Tachibana, M. and Kaneko, A. (1984) Gamma-aminobutyric acid acts at axon terminals of turtle photoreceptors: Difference in sensitivity among cell types. *Proc. Natl. Acad. Sci. USA*, 81: 7961–7964.

Tachibana, M. and Kaneko, A. (1987) Gamma-aminobutyric acid exerts a local inhibitory action on the axon terminal of bipolar cells: Evidence for negative feedback from amacrine cells. *Proc. Natl. Acad. Sci. USA*, 84: 3501–3505.

Tachibana, M. and Kaneko, A. (1988) Retinal bipolar cells receive negative feedback input from GABAergic amacrine cells. *Visual Neurosci.*, 1: 297–305.

Takeuchi, A. and Takeuchi, N. (1967) Anion permeability of the inhibitory postsynaptic membrane of the crayfish neuromuscular junction. *J. Physiol.*, 191: 575–590.

Takeuchi, A. and Takeuchi, N. (1969) A study of the action of picrotoxin on the inhibitory neuromuscular junction of the crayfish. *J. Physiol.*, 205: 377–391.

Tauck, D.L., Frosch, M.P. and Lipton, S.A. (1988) Characterization of GABA- and glycine induced currents of solitary rodent retinal ganglion cells in culture. *Neuroscience*, 27: 193–203.

Twyman, R.E., Rogers, C.J. and Macdonald, R.L. (1989) Pentobarbital and picrotoxin have reciprocal actions on single $GABA_A$ receptor channels. *Neurosci. Lett.*, 96: 89–95.

Unnerstall, J.R., Kuhar, M.J., Niehoff, D.L. and Palacios, J.M. (1981) Benzodiazepine receptors are coupled to a subpopulation of gamma-aminobutyric acid (GABA) receptors: evidence from a quantitative autoradiographic study. *J. Pharmacol. Exp. Ther.*, 218: 797–804.

Vaughn, J.E., Famiglietti, E.V. Jr., Barber, R.P., Saito, K., Roberts, E. and Ribak, C.E. (1981) GABAergic amacrine cells in rat retina: Immunocytochemical identification and synaptic connectivity. *J. Comp. Neurol.*, 197: 113–127.

Verdoorn, T.A., Draguhn, A., Ymer, S., Seeburg, P.H. and

Sakmann, B. (1990) Functional properties of recombinant rat GABA$_A$ receptors depend upon subunit composition. *Neuron*, 4: 919–928.

Witkovsky, P. and Stone, S. (1987) GABA and glycine modify the balance of rod and cone inputs to horizontal cells in the Xenopus retina. *Exp. Biol.*, 47: 13–22.

Wu, S.M. and Dowling, J.E. (1980) Effects of GABA and glycine on the distal cells of the cyprinid retina. *Brain Res.*, 199: 401–414.

Wyatt, H.J. and Daw, N.W. (1976) Specific effects of neurotransmitter antagonists on ganglion cells in rabbit retina. *Science*, 191: 204–205.

Yasui, S., Ishizuka, S. and Akaike, N. (1985) GABA activates different types of chloride conducting receptor-ionophore complexes in a dose-dependent manner. *Brain Res.*, 344: 176–180.

Yazulla, S., Studholme, K.M., Vitorica, J. and de Blas, A.L. (1989) Immunocytochemical localization of GABA$_A$ receptors in goldfish and chicken retinas. *J. Comp. Neurol.*, 280: 15–26.

Yeh, H.H., Lee, M.B. and Cheun, J.E. (1990) Properties of GABA-activated whole-cell currents in bipolar cells of the rat retina. *Visual Neurosci.*, 4: 349–357.

Zarbin, M.A., Wamsley, J.K., Palacios, J.M. and Kuhar, M.J. (1986) Autoradiographic localization of high affinity GABA, benzodiazepine, dopaminergic, adrenergic and muscarinic cholinergic receptors in the rat, monkey and human retina. *Brain Res.*, 374: 75–92.

Zukin, S.R., Young, A.B. and Snyder, S.H. (1974) Gamma-aminobutyric acid binding to receptor sites in the rat central nervous system. *Proc. Natl. Acad. Sci. USA*, 71: 4802–4807.

R.R. Mize, R.E. Marc and A.M. Sillito (Eds.)
Progress in Brain Research, Vol. 90

CHAPTER 3

# The physiology of GABA$_B$ receptors in the vertebrate retina

## Malcolm M. Slaughter and Zhuo-Hua Pan

*Departments of Biophysical Sciences and Ophthalmology, School of Medicine, State University of New York, Buffalo, NY 14214, USA*

## Introduction

The discovery of GABA$_B$ receptors in the retina offers a solution to several mysteries. For example, in the amphibian retina, many horizontal cells contain and release GABA, but classical GABA antagonists do not block a primary horizontal cell function, namely surround antagonism. What is the function of these GABAergic horizontal cells and how do they work? In the inner retina, GABA and glycine are widespread but clearly separated anatomically and have different physiological roles. Yet both of these transmitters seem to do essentially the same thing, namely open chloride channels and mediate inhibition. Why create and segregate two transmitter systems when one might be sufficient? The GABA$_B$ receptor, unsuspected until recently, plays a role in both of these functions and begins to offer an answer to these questions. It has recently become clear that GABA and glycine do more than open chloride channels. The discovery of the GABA$_B$ receptor (Bowery et al., 1980) with its unique properties, and the allosteric glycine binding site on the NMDA receptor (Johnson and Ascher, 1987) provide new avenues for inhibitory amino acid pharmacology and indicate that these two transmitters are not redundant. This chapter explores the role of the GABA$_B$ receptor in the vertebrate retina. Although the data are still preliminary, it is already

clear that GABA$_B$ receptors are important in generating center-surround antagonism in the outer retina and also control of transient and sustained signals in the inner retina.

## GABA$_B$ receptor pharmacology

The prototypical GABA$_B$ agonist is baclofen, which is a GABA analog that contains a *p*-chlorinated phenol on the beta carbon, as illustrated in Fig. 1. Baclofen activity is generally used as the

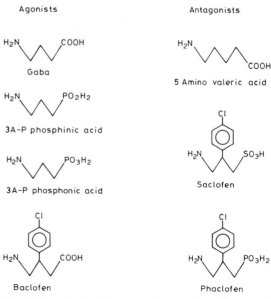

Fig. 1. The chemical structure of several GABA$_B$ receptor agonists (left) and antagonists (right); 3A-P, 3-aminopropyl.

sine qua non identifier of $GABA_B$ receptors. This analog has no activity at the $GABA_A$ receptor. The chloride atom is important for the ligand's activity, which is diminished if the chloride is located at any other position in the ring. Without the chloride, the ligand has no activity at the $GABA_B$ receptor. Phosphate analogs of GABA also act as $GABA_B$ agonists. 3-Aminopropyl phosphinic acid is the most potent analog, being about an order of magnitude more potent than baclofen itself (Hills et al., 1989; Ong et al., 1990). The equivalent phosphonic analog (3-aminopropyl phosphonic acid) is also a selective $GABA_B$ receptor agonist, although significantly less potent (Kerr et al., 1989). Although 3-aminopropyl phosphinic acid is more potent than baclofen, it does not always produce the same effect as baclofen.

Unfortunately, $GABA_B$ antagonist pharmacology has yet to develop a potent and selective antagonist. One often used antagonist is 5-aminovaleric acid, which has the unappealing property of being both a $GABA_B$ antagonist and a $GABA_A$ agonist. When used to study $GABA_B$ receptors, tissues are commonly pretreated with $GABA_A$ antagonists. 5-Aminovaleric acid is ineffective in some preparations (Bowery et al., 1983), although it has proven valuable in the retina. Phaclofen (Kerr et al., 1987) was the first selective $GABA_B$ receptor antagonist developed. It is very similar in structure to baclofen, replacing only the terminal carboxyl group with a phosphonic acid. It is a little surprising that this substitution produces an antagonist, since phosphonic acid analogs of GABA are agonists. However, the combination of the phenol group and the large, strongly acidic phosphonic group result in a ligand which apparently can bind but not activate the receptor. Kerr et al. (1988) used these properties to synthesize other $GABA_B$ antagonists, replacing the phosphonic acid with a sulphonic acid to make saclofen. Saclofen and 2-hydroxy saclofen are each more potent than phaclofen, the former being the most potent selective $GABA_B$ antagonist yet available (Kerr et al.,

1989). The sulphonic antagonists have been developed very recently and their utility has not yet been established. Phaclofen is weak, requiring millimolar concentrations for effective antagonism, and does not work at all sites where $GABA_B$ receptors are thought to be located. Dutar and Nicoll (1988b) have suggested that phaclofen is only effective at postsynaptic receptors which are linked to potassium channels. We have found that neither phaclofen nor 2-hydroxy saclofen are effective baclofen antagonists in the proximal retina.

The cumulative data on $GABA_B$ pharmacology indicates that there are two classes of $GABA_B$ receptors. The phaclofen data implies this dichotomy. Binding studies indicate that there are two $GABA_B$ sites, with affinity constants of 60 and 229 nM. The ratio of these two binding sites differs slightly between brain regions and lesioning of noradrenergic fibers in the cerebral cortex selectively decreases the low affinity sites (Karbon et al., 1983). A comparison of the effects of baclofen and 3-aminopropyl phosphinic acid also suggests that there are two receptor subtypes. In some tissues, where there exists a forskolin stimulated cAMP system, both baclofen and 3-aminopropyl phosphinate reduce the levels of cAMP. However, in other tissues where beta adrenergic drugs cause an increase in cAMP, baclofen potentiates this effect but 3-aminopropyl phosphinate acts as only a partial agonist (Pratt et al., 1989). Furthermore, 3-aminopropyl phosphonic acid inhibits the forskolin system but has no effect on the beta adrenergic system (Scherer et al., 1988). Pertussis toxin and phaclofen block the former system, but not the latter. All of this data can be interpreted to mean that there are two $GABA_B$ receptors, which cannot be distinguished by baclofen. However, the evidence in favor of two receptors is only circumstantial and other interpretations could be used to explain these differences, such as nonspecific effects or divergent second messenger system pathways.

In studies of the $GABA_B$ receptor's pharmacophore, the structure-activity relationship of

GABA$_B$ ligands revolves around substitutions for the carboxyl group. GABA is a three carbon chain with terminal carboxyl and amino groups, both of which are ionized under physiological conditions. These two charged groups apparently represent the binding sites for the receptor. Addition of a 4-chlorinated phenol to the beta carbon creates a GABA$_B$ selective ligand, whether an agonist (baclofen) or antagonist (phaclofen or saclofen). Two effects of this substitution are steric hindrance at the receptor protein and conformational restraints on the GABA backbone. A family of straight chain analogs of GABA, in which the carboxylic acid is replaced by a phosphate moiety, show selectivity for the GABA$_B$ receptor. The phosphinic substitution forms the most potent agonist (3-aminopropyl phosphinic acid), the analogous phosphonic analog is a less potent agonist and shows some antagonist activity as well, while the incremental lengthening of the carbon chain (4-aminobutyl phosphonic acid) results in formation of an antagonist (Kerr et al., 1989). The fact that the phosphate substitutions and the phenol addition each confer GABA$_B$ receptor specificity suggests that restriction in conformation, rather than steric interference at the receptor site, is the critical parameter in conferring receptor selectivity. Both of these GABA$_B$ analogs would favor the extended form of GABA. In this respect it is interesting to compare these ligands with analogs that are effective at other types of GABA receptor. Based on the activity of conformationally restricted GABA analogs such as muscimol and THIP (4,5,6,7-tetrahydroisoxazolo[5,4-C]pyridin-3-ol), GABA$_A$ receptors bind to the partially extended and planar structure of GABA (Krogsgaard-Larsen et al., 1977, 1979; Andrews and Johnston, 1979). A third receptor subtype, termed the GABA$_C$ receptor, has been proposed because some GABA binding sites are not blocked by GABA$_A$ or GABA$_B$ analogs (Johnston, 1986). Analogs that are effective at this proposed receptor are analogous to a folded conformation of GABA.

## Ionic channels linked to the GABA$_B$ receptor

The GABA$_B$ receptor mediates two different conductances, the opening of a potassium channel and the closing of a calcium channel. Both of these conductances tend to reduce synaptic transmission, the former by hyperpolarizing and inhibiting the cell, the latter by decreasing calcium influx which can mediate chemical neurotransmission. However, experimental evidence suggests that these two conductances do not work in concert on the same neuron. The closing of the calcium conductance seems to be restricted to presynaptic sites. This is reasonable since calcium's most important function is as a second messenger, not a current carrier, and therefore calcium regulation is most critical at presynaptic release sites. This mechanism of action of GABA$_B$ receptors was first described in embryonic sensory neurons (Dunlap, 1981) and has since been found in other tissues, notably dorsal root ganglion (Dolphin and Scott, 1986), hippocampus (Lanthorn and Cotman, 1981; Harrison, 1990) and the bipolar axon terminals in retina (Maguire et al., 1989). The regulation of potassium appears to be a direct effect on post-synaptic sites (Newberry and Nicoll, 1984). In some ways this is similar to the classical inhibitory action of the GABA$_A$ receptor which opens a chloride conductance. Potassium always, and chloride usually, have reversal potentials which are more negative than the resting membrane potential. Therefore, opening these channels tends to hyperpolarize the cell. However, the reversal potential for potassium is generally $-90$ to $-100$ mV, while that of chloride varies significantly from cell to cell but often is $-65$ to $-70$ mV. Therefore, if the resting membrane potential of a cell is $-60$ mV, the driving force (the difference between the membrane potential and the ion's reversal potential) for potassium is 3–6-fold greater than that for chloride. This means that a change in potassium conductance will produce a much larger voltage response compared to an equivalent chloride conductance. Conversely, a small change in potassium conductance can produce as big a voltage response as a large change in chloride conductance. In most tissues, it appears that this second scenario is the one used by neurons. This means that $GABA_A$ receptor activation involves a large change in conductance and shunting of the cell while $GABA_B$ receptor activation produces a significant hyperpolarization but comparatively little shunting. Both types of channel regulation are found in the retina.

$GABA_B$ receptors appear to regulate several types of voltage dependent calcium channels. Nowycky al. (1985) have identified three cardiac calcium channels termed the L, T, and N channels. The L-type has a comparatively large single channel conductance (25 pS) and shows little inactivation. The T-type has a small conductance (8 pS) and quickly inactivates. Therefore the L-type can generate sustained macroscopic currents while the T-type produces transient calcium currents. In addition, the T-type is activated by small depolarizations (activation at $-60$ mV, inactivation at $-40$ mV) while the L-type requires greater depolarizations ($-10$ mV). The third, N-type channel has a intermediate conductance (13 pS), a high threshold, and prominent inactivation. The L-type has proven the most tractable, it can be blocked by dihydropyridines and enhanced by BAY K 8644. The N-type is often thought to be most important for neurotransmitter release, but there is little compelling evidence to limit this function to only a single type of calcium channel.

The $GABA_B$ receptor down regulates all three types of calcium channels (Tsien et al., 1988). The $GABA_B$ receptor is not unique in this capacity: dopamine, serotonin, adenosine, muscarine, and some peptides also close calcium channels. These receptors may act convergently. For example, in chick sensory neurons, activation of $GABA_B$, serotonin, dopamine, and noradrenaline receptors all close calcium channels in the same cell and their effects are not additive. Nor is this unique to the calcium channel, a similar interaction has been reported for opioid, muscarinic, and $GABA_B$ receptor agonists regulating a

potassium conductance in rat lateral parabrachial neurons (Christie and North, 1988). Apparently they all act through guanine nucleotide binding protein intermediates.

*Second messengers*

The link between the $GABA_B$ receptor and the channel seems to involve a second messenger system. When GABA binds to the $GABA_B$ receptor, this promotes the exchange of GTP for GDP on a binding site in the G-protein. The G-protein then dissociates and the activated alpha subunit can bind and activate a channel protein. In many tissues, pertussis toxin, which ADP-ribosylates and inactivates the alpha subunit of some G-proteins, blocks the effects of baclofen or GABA on channel conductance. The presynaptic site in the hippocampus is a notable exception. Dolphin et al. (1989) found that baclofen modestly increases the levels of inositol phosphate, but this did not appear to play a role in the regulation of the calcium channel. $GABA_B$ agonists can regulate the calcium channel through modulations in both protein kinase A and C (Kamatchi and Ticku, 1990). Thus there seem to be at least three second messenger pathways controlled by $GABA_B$ receptors: a G-protein mediated receptor action that opens potassium channels and closes calcium channels and decreases the levels of cAMP; a protein kinase A system that up regulates cAMP; and an inositol phosphate system. The first two pathways may correlate with the depression of forskolin stimulated cAMP and the potentiation of transmitter stimulated production of cAMP respectively, but the relationship to the potassium and calcium channels is not well understood. The link between the actions of G-proteins and channels regulated by $GABA_B$ receptors is further clouded by the observation that GTP alters the affinity of $GABA_B$ receptors and that GTP-$\gamma$-S prevents the rundown of L-type calcium channels (Yatani et al., 1987). This means that in studies that show that GTP-$\gamma$-S potentiates baclofen regulation of calcium currents, the second messenger may be important for the maintainance of the channel, and not in transduction of the signal from the receptor.

## Physiology of the GABA$_B$ receptor

The presynaptic modulation of voltage dependent calcium channels has the potential to regulate transmitter release. Indeed it has been shown that baclofen can reduce the release of a number of transmitters, such as catecholamines, indoleamines, and excitatory amino acids (Potashner, 1978; Bowery et al., 1980). This presumably represents a mechanism in which GABAergic neurons are presynaptic to the synaptic endings of other neurons. This is an important pathway in the retina. It has also been shown that GABA$_B$ receptors can serve as autoreceptors on GABAergic neurons, providing negative feedback to limit GABA release. Neal and Shah (1989) find that this may be an important regulatory mechanism in the cortex and spinal cord, but not in the retina.

The postsynaptic activation of the GABA$_B$ receptor causes an increase in potassium conductance, which always produces a hyperpolarization. There are several examples of synapses in which GABA activates both GABA$_A$ and GABA$_B$ postsynaptic receptors. The GABA$_A$ receptor mediates a fast onset, short duration, chloride mediated hyperpolarization while the GABA$_B$ receptor induces a slow onset, long lasting, potassium mediated hyperpolarization (Soltesz et al., 1988; Connors et al., 1988; Dutar and Nicoll, 1988a). The difference in time course presumably reflects the second messenger intermediates in the GABA$_B$ system.

## Retina

Most of the types and mechanisms of action of the GABA$_B$ receptors described above can be found in the retina. This includes the opening of potassium channels and the closing of calcium channels, and mediation through second messen-

ger systems. GABA$_B$ receptors have been most extensively studied in the amphibian retina, where they modulate photoreceptor transmitter release, close calcium channels in bipolar cells, and open potassium channels in amacrine and ganglion cells.

### Outer plexiform layer

GABA is contained in horizontal cells in most, if not all, vertebrate retinas and appears to act at three distal sites: on photoreceptor terminals, on bipolar cells, and at autoreceptors on the horizontal cells (see Wu, Chapter 5; Marc, Chapter 4). The synaptic input from horizontal cells to bipolar cells was the first to be identified yet remains the most poorly documented. Initially, this was thought to be the primary output pathway for horizontal cells because (1) physiological studies showed that bipolar cells have surround responses (presumed input from horizontal cells) while photoreceptors do not and (2) anatomical evidence indicates that bipolar cells receive synaptic input from something other than photoreceptors (presumably horizontal cells). However, more recent evidence has shown that photoreceptors do receive feedback from horizontal cells and the "other input" to bipolars could also be interplexiform cell synapses. Nevertheless, this pathway remains one branch in horizontal cell synaptic circuitry. A second circuit is the autoreceptor feedback pathway to horizontal cells, described extensively by Yang and Wu (1989). Based on evidence in brain, we might expect that these autoreceptors would be the GABA$_B$ type. Experiments indicate, however, that they are GABA$_A$ receptors (Stockton and Slaughter, 1991). This makes some sense in that GABA$_B$ autoreceptors work by closing calcium channels, thereby cutting off transmitter release. Horizontal cell neurosecretion is a calcium independent process, so this mechanism would be ineffective. The third horizontal cell synaptic pathway is feedback to photoreceptors and this may be the principal pathway for surround antagonism in the outer retina. In many cases this feedback is mediated through

GABA$_A$ receptors. However, in amphibia, GABA$_A$ antagonists do not block surround responses, while a GABA$_B$ antagonist (5-amino-valerate) does (Hare and Owen, 1990). Eliasof and Werblin (1988) have reported that baclofen decreases photoreceptor transmitter release. Coupled with the observations of Hare and Owen (1990), this would suggest that GABA$_B$ receptors could mediate surround antagonism. A fly in the ointment is that baclofen does not block bipolar cell surround responses (Bai and Slaughter, 1989). An explanation may be that 5-aminovalerate acts on both GABA$_A$ and GABA$_B$ receptors. This would mean that the effectiveness of 5-amino-valerate is based on suppression of both types of GABA receptors. Possible mechanisms include: (1) surround is generated by a GABA$_B$ receptor action on photoreceptors and a GABA$_A$ receptor action on bipolar cells or (2) photoreceptors possess both GABA$_A$ and GABA$_B$ receptors and both are involved in formation of surround responses. The latter scenario is supported by evidence of a bicuculline-sensitive feedback to tiger salamander cones (see Wu, Chapter 5). In either case, when baclofen or bicuculline is used alone, only one pathway is blocked and some surround responses persist.

*Inner plexiform layer*

The action of GABA$_B$ receptors in the inner retina has been much more extensively studied. In the tiger salamander retina, the experiments of Maguire et al. (1989b) show that GABA receptors close calcium channels in a subset of bipolar cells while studies by Slaughter and Bai (1989) indicate that GABA$_B$ receptors open potassium channels on most amacrine and ganglion cells. The studies on bipolar cells utilized the retinal slice preparation and whole cell voltage clamp techniques. Two types of voltage gated calcium channels where observed in bipolar cells, similar to the L and T types described by Nowycky et al. (1985). Staining with Lucifer yellow indicated that bipolar cells which had their axon terminals trimmed off only exhibited T type responses, indi-

cating that the L type channels were restricted to the terminal regions. This in turn suggests that the L type channel is involved in neurosecretion. When baclofen was applied to an intact bipolar cell, the L type current was blocked. When GTP-$\gamma$-S was dialyzed into the cell, the baclofen effect was magnified. This indicates that a GTP binding protein is involved in baclofen's action. This conclusion is also supported by the finding that GDP-$\beta$-S blocks the baclofen effect.

Maguire et al. (1989a) pursued the ramifications of these results for third order neurons. Still using whole cell voltage clamping in the amphibian retinal slice, they now recorded from amacrine cells. They found two morphological types, one that had a narrow dendritic tree (about 150 $\mu$m) and terminated in either sublamina a or b of the inner plexiform layer (Famiglietti and Kolb, 1976), and a wide field type that had processes up to a millimeter in length. These different morphologies could be correlated with discrete physiologies and pharmacologies. The narrow field cell appears to be GABAergic and the wide field cell is glycinergic. The small field amacrine cells had comparatively sustained light responses while the wide field amacrine's responses were more transient. The authors point out that slow and fast might be better descriptors, since the responses of the narrow field cells had a slower time to peak and a longer decay time. The synaptic input to the sustained cells appears to be a simple excitatory input, probably from bipolar cells. But in the transient cells there was a fast, transient excitatory input followed by a GABAergic inhibitory input which could be blocked by GABA$_A$ antagonists. A key finding was that transient excitatory input to the wide field amacrine cells could be blocked by baclofen, leaving only the delayed inhibitory input. Responses of narrow field amacrines were not affected by baclofen. Consistent with this observation, when 5-aminovalerate was applied, the light response of the wide field amacrine cell became more prolonged. In addition, the subset of bipolar cells that were sensitive to baclofen terminated in the middle of the inner plexiform layer, coinciding with the dendritic position of the wide field amacrine cells. These results indicate that $GABA_B$ receptors function to abbreviate the EPSPs of wide field amacrine cells. There seems to be a dual and redundant GABAergic system at work, since GABA feedback to $GABA_B$ receptors on bipolar cell terminals curtails presynaptic input to the wide field amacrine, while delayed postsynaptic input onto $GABA_A$ receptors of the wide field amacrine truncates the EPSPs (Fig. 2). The authors speculate that this mechanism could be responsible for the formation of transient response properties, which first appears in the inner retina. This baclofen feedback would therefore create a cell that was responsive to change, or the derivative of the illumination. Carrying this one step further, Werblin et al. (1988) modelled these mechanisms in the formation of directional response properties in ganglion cells (Fig. 3). The key element in this model is local, transient input (generated by

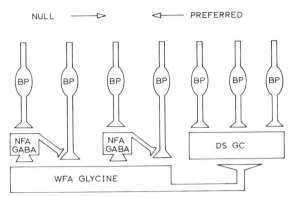

Fig. 3. The postulates of Werblin et al.'s model of directional selectivity based on the circuit elements in Fig. 2. In the preferred direction, bipolar cells (right side) excite directionally selective ganglion cells (DS GC). Inhibition from the glycinergic widefield amacrine cells (WFA) arrives too late to block this excitation. However, movement in the null direction produces an early excitation of the widefield amacrines (left side), resulting in a early inhibition of the direction selective ganglion cell. The inhibition coincides with the direct excitation from bipolar cells, cancelling the excitatory response. (Adapted from Werblin et al. (1988) *Visual Neurosci.*, 1: 317–329.)

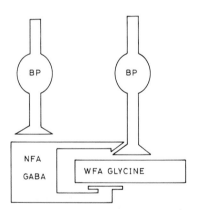

Fig. 2. The synaptic circuitry responsible for the formation of transient responses in the proximal retina, as proposed by Maguire et al. (1989). The bipolar cells (BP) generate sustained responses to light. The bipolar on the left stimulates a GABAergic narrow field amacrine (NFA) cell. This results, after a delay, in GABAergic input to some bipolar cells, turning off their synaptic calcium current. The result is transient transmitter release by the bipolar cell on the right. The difference between the two types of bipolars could account for the generation of sustained and transient inputs to the inner retina. There is also a delayed direct inhibitory input from the GABAergic narrow field amacrine cell to $GABA_A$ receptors on the wide field amacrine (WFA) cell. (Adapted from Maguire et al. (1989) *J. Neurosci.*, 9: 726–735.)

the $GABA_B$ feedback pathway) onto an asymmetric, widefield amacrine cell. The local transient synaptic potentials form a set of inputs that only respond to change, thereby maximizing their response to a moving stimulus. The widefield amacrine cell which integrates this transient input is thought to be inhibitory (glycinergic). If this amacrine cell is asymmetric, it will provide inhibition during movement in one direction, but will have little or no effect during movement in other directions. This is similar to the asymmetric inhibitory model of directionality postulated by Barlow and Levick (1965) and corresponds to observations on the role of inhibition in directional responses described by Caldwell et al. (1978) in rabbit retina. In this model, the $GABA_B$ receptors are not responsible for directionality, but form a necessary early step in this process.

It is interesting that at the same time the above experiments were performed, Pan and Slaughter (1991) took a very different path, encountered a disparate set of observations, but also arrived at the conclusion that $GABA_B$ re-

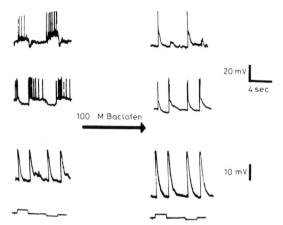

20 mV

4 sec

100 μM Baclofen

10 mV

Fig. 4. The effect of baclofen on third order neurons. The upper row shows a sustained ON cell before (left) and during (right) application of 100 μM baclofen. Baclofen produced a slight hyperpolarization and the sustained response was suppressed, leaving a large transient ON and small transient OFF EPSP. The middle row of traces shows a sustained OFF cell in which baclofen produced a hyperpolarization, eliminated the sustained spiking in the dark, and caused the cell to produce large, transient EPSPs at light onset and offset. In a transient cell (lowest row), baclofen produced a large hyperpolarization and enhanced the transient ON and OFF responses. The square pulse at the bottom indicates the timing of a diffuse light stimulus. (From Slaughter and Bai (1988) *Neurosci. Res. Suppl.*, 8: S217–S229.)

ceptors can play an important role in discerning direction of motion. Initially, Slaughter and Bai (1989) performed standard, intracellular recordings in the superfused eyecup preparation of two amphibia, the mudpuppy and the tiger salamander. They found that when baclofen was added to the retina, the cells of the distal retina (photoreceptors, bipolars, and horizontal cells) were little affected. However, the light responses of third order neurons (amacrine and ganglion cells) were dramatically altered (Fig. 4). In amacrine and ganglion cells which were normally phasic, the light responses were enhanced. In contrast, those neurons which normally responded with tonic light responses had their responses suppressed. What was particularly interesting was that in many of these sustained cells, a phasic light response appeared. This conversion from sustained to transient did not result from a temporal shortening of the tonic response, nor did it evolve de

novo. Instead, it appears that transient responses were present but hidden within the envelop of the sustained responses. When the sustained responses were suppressed, the transient response components were revealed. In many cases, a sustained ON (or OFF) neuron would show both transient ON and OFF responses after baclofen. Thus, the net effect of baclofen application is to make sustained cells more transient. Overall, the light responses in the inner retina become dominated by phasic signals.

Ikeda et al. (1990) found a similar phenomenon in cat, at least in the OFF system. When they ionotophoresed baclofen while recording sustained OFF ganglion cell spike activity, they found that the light evoked activity became more transient. When the antagonist phaclofen was applied, they found that the spike activity became more sustained. This indicates that GABA is normally acting on GABA$_B$ receptors of OFF cells to abbreviate the light response. There is also indirect evidence for an enhancement of transient responses in the rabbit retina, where Cunningham and Neal (1983) found that baclofen increased the light evoked release of acetylcholine. Since acetylcholine is released transiently at ON and OFF, this suggests that transient responses are enhanced.

Baclofen hyperpolarizes both amacrine and ganglion cells. This effect appears to be due to a direct action on third order neurons since it persists even after synaptic transmission is blocked by cobalt. The hyperpolarization is due to an opening of a potassium conductance. When the GABA$_A$ receptor is blocked by picrotoxin or bicuculline, then GABA mimics the effect of baclofen (Fig. 5). Comparing the effects of GABA on the two receptor subtypes, activation of GABA$_A$ receptors produces a large conductance increase to chloride ions, while activation of the GABA$_B$ receptor population produces only about a quarter of the conductance change. (Redburn et al., 1989 reported that about one fourth of the GABA binding sites in rabbit retina are GABA$_B$, therefore the conductance difference may reflect

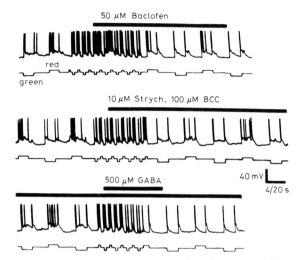

Fig. 5. GABA and baclofen have similar effects on GABA$_B$ receptors. Initially the cell responded to diffuse green or red lights with a sustained depolarization and prolonged spike activity at light ON and OFF. Baclofen made the responses, particularly the EPSPs, more transient. After recovery from baclofen, strychnine and bicuculline were applied to block both GABA$_A$ and glycine receptors. When GABA was applied in the presence of these antagonists it made the responses very transient (bottom trace). (From Bai and Slaughter (1989) *J. Neurophysiol.*, 61: 374–381.)

a population difference.) GABA$_B$ receptor activation usually produces a larger membrane hyperpolarization because of the more negative reversal potential of potassium. This difference in conductance means that when GABA$_A$ analogs are applied to the retina, third order neurons are shunted and all their light responses are suppressed. But when GABA$_B$ analogs are used, there is only a modest shunting and significant light responses can still be seen. In addition, the GABA$_B$ linked hyperpolarization means that remaining EPSPs have a larger driving force. Since the membrane properties of third order neurons are non-linear, the amplitude of the EPSP is often larger after baclofen treatment. This is one factor that accounts for the enhancement of transient responses during baclofen treatment. Another factor is a network effect. When baclofen suppresses sustained amacrine cells, tonic inhibition in the inner retina is reduced. This also contributes to the enhancement of transient signals (Bai and Slaughter, 1989). It is peculiar that an inhibitory transmitter causes the enhancement of some synaptic responses.

There is a fundamental and unresolved disparity between these results and those of Maguire et al. (1989a). Maguire et al. conclude from their experiments that GABA$_B$ receptors turn off transmitter release in some bipolar cells, resulting in the formation of a transient signal. According to this model, if GABA$_B$ receptors were constantly activated then transmitter release from these bipolars would be permanently shut off and transient responses would be eliminated. Instead, Slaughter and Bai (1989) find that transient responses are enhanced in the presence of baclofen. From our perspective, the two sets of data would be consistent if GABA$_B$ receptors turned off transmitter release from bipolars responsible for sustained (rather than transient) signals, thereby accounting for baclofen's suppression of sustained responses. But this is not consistent with Maguire et al.'s data showing that baclofen suppresses transient responses in the slice. Differences between the eyecup and the retinal slice may account for part of the discrepancy, but it is likely that properties as fundamental as phasic and tonic signalling have several layers of complexity and redundancy that have yet to be resolved.

The observation that tonically responding neurons become more phasic during baclofen treatment led Pan and Slaughter (1991) to speculate that retinal information coding might be altered by GABA$_B$ receptor activation. This was based on the difference in properties of transient and sustained signals. By their very nature, transient responses are good at signalling change but ineffective a relaying steady state conditions. Sustained signals do convey steady state information. Thus transient cells can be used to detect the onset or offset of a light stimulus, while sustained cells can be used to determine if a light stimulus is present. When baclofen enhances transient responses, it may augment the retina's ability to detect changes in illumination. Like Werblin et al. (1988), Pan and Slaughter (1991) focused on directional response properties since these are visually important and well documented responses that are dependent on change detectors. We found that baclofen "induced" directional responses in some third order neurons which did not exhibit directionality under control conditions. This effect was particularly marked when baclofen was used in conjunction with 2-amino-4-phosphonobutyrate (APB). APB is an analogue of glutamate which eliminates the light responses of ON bipolar cells and consequently eliminates ON responses throughout the retina (Slaughter and Miller, 1981).

The experiments consisted of using narrow, long bars of light that were moved in different directions across the retina. Under control conditions, some third order neurons (amacrine and ganglion cells were not distinguished) were directional, but most neurons responded about equally to all directions of movement. In about a third of these non-directional cells, application of APB and baclofen together resulted in the *appearance* of directional responses (Fig. 6). In about 20% of these neurons, baclofen alone made the cells directional. GABA$_A$ antagonists blocked directionality in only half of the cells studied, while a combination of glycine and GABA$_A$ antagonists blocked directionality in almost all cases. This differs from the findings in rabbit and turtle, where GABA$_A$ antagonists always block directionality. This implies a role for glycine in formation of directionality in at least some cells, similar to the hypothesis of Werblin et al. (1988).

The cumulative evidence seems to indicate that these directional responses are not created by baclofen treatment. Instead, like the emergence of transient responses from sustained cells, the appearance of directionality probably represents the unmasking of a small signal that normally exists in these cells. This conclusion is suggested by similarities between the characteristics of induced and normal directionality. For example, hyperpolarizing and silent inhibition are found in both cases. Picrotoxin suppresses directionality in

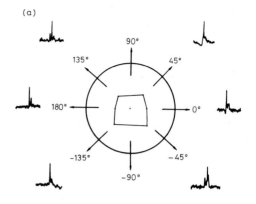

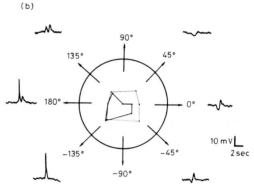

Fig. 6. The effect of baclofen and APB on direction coding in a third order neuron in the tiger salamander retina. A. The upper figure shows the responses of the cell to a narrow light slit moving in the directions indicated by the arrows. The polar plot in the center maps the peak EPSP amplitude in the various directions. There is no indication that this cell encodes directional information. B. After application of APB and baclofen, the same cell shows a directional preference, with the peak EPSP in the −135 degree direction and a small IPSP in the opposite direction. The dark polar plot represents the response amplitudes in the various directions, the dotted polar plot is the superposition of the results in control (A). (From Pan and Slaughter (1991) *J. Neurosci.*, 11: 1810–1821.)

about half the cells of each type. Baclofen enhances normal directionality as well as revealing "induced" directionality. The most parsimonious explanation of these similarities is that induced and normal directionality emerge from the same sources.

The fact that APB is required in most cases to see a baclofen induced directionality probably reflects interactions between the ON and OFF pathways. We found several indications that the

ON and the OFF pathways were not directionally aligned in the induced directional cells. For example, in some cells baclofen alone induced directionality in the OFF response but not in the ON response. In a few cells, baclofen produced almost opposite directional preferences in the ON and the OFF pathways. Thus, when viewed together, the neuron showed no directionality. This merging of signals and obscuring of directionality may be an artefact of somal recordings. At the level of individual dendrites, the two pathways may be handled discretely. The ON and OFF sublamina are anatomically distinct, so that most dendrites may receive directional information from either the ON or OFF pathway, not both. At the level of the soma these signals merge, but at the level of the individual dendrites these signals can be detected in isolation and processed separately. Our recordings from the soma may not be indicative of the neuron's full processing capability.

*GABA$_B$ receptors and selective attention*

If the retina is able to alter its response characteristics, this could be used for a number of functions. We have speculated that the GABA$_B$ system could serve as a model for selective attention. Baclofen reduces membrane noise, enhances one set of signals, and modifies another set of responses so that they also relay the selected signals. This matches the profile for a selective attention mechanism, where the response to attended signals is enhanced while the response to unattended signals is diminished. GABA has often been linked with selective attention, assuming that an action at the GABA$_A$ receptor would serve to suppress responses to unattended signals, thereby improving the signal to noise ratio of the desired signal. The GABA$_B$ system would appear to be much more powerful because it would not only act as a noise suppressor, but would also recruit cells to carry the designated responses, thereby augmenting the attended signal.

We originally offered this as a heuristic model based on the interesting properties of the GABA$_B$ receptor and thought it might have primary relevance for central brain systems. However, as pointed out to us by Dr. A.K. Ball, selective attention may also be applicable to the retina if higher brain centers can control GABA$_B$ systems. One of the exciting new trends in retinal research is the focus on efferent connections. Long known in birds, centrifugal fibers have recently been described in fish, amphibia, reptiles, and mammals. Their functions are not clear but they arise from multiple brain regions and synapse on a variety of retinal cells. In fish, Zucker and Dowling (1987) reported that efferents synapse on the dopaminergic interplexiform cell, signifying that this pathway may play a role in dark/light adaptation. In a mechanism for selective attention, we would expect that efferents would control the activation of GABA$_B$ receptors. Stell et al. (1984) and Ball et al. (1989) have shown that LHRH and FMRFamide immunoreactive efferent fibers contact GABAergic neurons in the fish inner plexiform layer. To explore this pathway, we attempted to reproduce the effects of baclofen by stimulating the optic nerve. This was ineffective, perhaps because of the poor viability of this nerve. Using another approach, we applied putative efferent fiber transmitters and compared their effects to baclofen. FMRFamide had no effect, but 1 $\mu$M LHRH mimicked the effects of baclofen in that it hyperpolarized third order neurons and made their light responses more transient. This suggests that efferent fibers may be able to regulate the responses of retinal neurons, although obviously more studies must be performed to substantiate this idea.

*Epilepsy and baclofen*

In one set of experiments, we wanted to examine the effects of baclofen on amacrine and ganglion cells after GABA$_A$ and glycine receptors had been blocked. Many times, when picrotoxin (or bicuculline) and strychnine are used for this purpose, the responses of third order neurons show spontaneous or bursting activity. When this occurs the synaptically mediated light responses disappear. If baclofen was applied under these conditions, the spontaneous activity was suppressed and synaptically driven light responses (at least transient responses) returned (Slaughter and Bai, 1988). Not only is this a rather remarkable effect, but it may be relevant to epileptiform activity. In the hippocampus $GABA_A$ or glycine antagonists are often used to generate epileptiform-like activity, which is very similar to the neuronal activity we observed in the retina. There is also some indication that baclofen may reduce epileptiform-like activity in hippocampus (Ogata et al., 1986; Swartzwelder et al., 1986), although proepileptic effects have also been reported (Mott et al., 1989). The similarities raise the possibility that the retina could be used in studies of epilepsy. The advantage, as illustrated in this case, is that relevant synaptic activity and signal processing can be evaluated. The results in the retina indicate that sustained excitatory input, in the absence of compensatory tonic inhibitory control, produces this spontaneous activity.

## Summary

Writing a chapter on retinal $GABA_B$ receptors is premature, as evidenced by the paucity of citations more than two years old. Despite that, this area of retinal pharmacology has made significant strides and, although it is a story without an ending, it has had an exciting beginning. To date, the experiments indicate that horizontal cell feedback to cones is mediated, at least in part, by the $GABA_B$ receptor system which probably regulates a potassium conductance. In the inner retina, $GABA_B$ receptors are found on bipolar cells, amacrines, and ganglion cells. Here, the actions are a subtle regulation of channel conductance, but the effects are a dramatic reorganization of a fundamental coding property of the retina, namely the distinction between tonic and phasic responses to light. In both the distal and proximal retina, the $GABA_B$ receptor does not appear to work alone, but instead works in concert with the $GABA_A$ receptor. The full significance of these interactions has yet to be determined. Although the discovery of the $GABA_B$ receptor has led to the resolution of several retinal mysteries, the case is far from closed. At this juncture, what can be said is that the $GABA_B$ receptor represents a unique and ubiquitous system that reveals the power of regulating calcium and potassium conductances, as opposed to the more familiar properties of the glutamate/acetylcholine regulated cationic conductances or the $GABA_A$/glycine controlled chloride channels.

## References

Andrews, P.R. and Johnston, G.A.R. (1979) GABA agonists and antagonists. *Biochem. Pharmacol.*, 28: 2697–2702.

Bai, S-H. and Slaughter, M.M. (1989) Effects of baclofen on transient neurons in the mudpuppy retina: Electrogenic and network actions. *J. Neurophysiol.*, 61: 382–390.

Ball, A.L., Stell, W.K., and Tutton, D.A. (1989) Efferent projections to the goldfish retina. In *Neurobiology of the Inner Retina*, Weiler, R. and Osborne, N.N., (Eds.) Springer-Verlag, Berlin, pp. 103–116.

Barlow, H.B. and Levick, W.R. (1965) The mechanism of directionally selective units in rabbit's retina. *J. Physiol. (London)*, 178: 477–504.

Bowery, N.G., Hill, D.R., and Hudson, A.L. (1983) Characteristics of $GABA_B$ receptor binding sites on rat whole brain synaptic membranes. *Br. J. Pharmacol.*, 78: 191–206.

Bowery, N.G., Hill, D.R., Hudson, A.L., Doble, A., Middlemiss, D.N., Shaw, J. and Turnbull, M.J. (1980) (-)Baclofen decreases neurotransmitter release in the mammalian CNS by an action at a novel GABA receptor. *Nature*, 283: 92–94.

Caldwell J.H., Daw, N.W., and Wyatt, H.J. (1978) Effects of picrotoxin and strychnine on rabbit retinal ganglion cells: Lateral interactions for cells with more complex receptive fields. *J. Physiol. (London)*, 276: 277–298.

Christie, M.J. and North, R.A. (1988) Agonists at mu-opioid, M2 muscarinic, and $GABA_B$-receptors increase the same potassium conductance in rat lateral parabrachial neurones. *Br. J. Pharmacol.*, 95: 896–902.

Connors, B.W., Malenka, R.C., and Silva, L.R. (1988) Two inhibitory postsynaptic potentials and $GABA_A$ and $GABA_B$ receptor-mediated responses in neocortex of rat and cat. *J. Physiol. (London)*, 406: 443–468.

Cunningham,, J.R. and Neal, M.J. (1983) Effect of $\gamma$-aminobutyric acid agonists, glycine, taurine, and neuropeptides on acetylcholine release from the rabbit retina. *J. Physiol. (London)*, 336: 563–577.

Dolphin, A.C. and Scott, R.H. (1986) Inhibition of calcium currents in cultured rat dorsal root ganglion neurones by (-)baclofen. *Br. J. Pharmacol.*, 88: 213–220.

Dunlap, K. (1981) Two types of gamma-aminobutyric acid receptor on embryonic sensory neurones. *Br. J. Pharmacol.*, 74: 579–585.

Dutar, P. and Nicoll, R.A. (1988) A physiological role for $GABA_B$ receptors in the central nervous system. *Nature*, 332: 156–158.

Dutar, P. and Nicoll, R.A. (1988) Pre- and postsynaptic $GABA_B$ receptors in the hippocampus have different pharmacological properties. *Neuron*, 1: 585–591.

Eliasof, S. and Werblin, F. (1988) $GABA_B$ modulation of synaptic release from photoreceptors in the tiger salamander. *Invest. Ophthal. Vis. Sci.*, 29(suppl.): 103.

Famiglietti, E.V., Jr. and Kolb, H. (1976) Structural basis for on- and off-center responses in retinal ganglion cells. *Science*, 194: 193–195.

Hare, W.A. and Owen, W.G. (1990) Spatial organization of the bipolar cell's receptive field in the retina of the tiger salamander. *J. Physiol. (London)*, 421: 223–245.

Harrison, N.L. (1990) On the presynaptic action of baclofen at inhibitory synapses between cultured rat hippocampal neurones. *J. Physiol. (London)*, 422: 433–446.

Hills, J.M., Dingsdale, R.A., Parsons, M.E., Dolle, R.E. and Howson, W. (1989) 3-Aminopropylphosphinic acid - a potent, selective $GABA_B$ receptor agonist in the guinea-pig ileum and rat anococcygeus muscle. *Br. J. Pharmacol.*, 97; 1292–1296.

Ikeda, H., Hankins, M.W., and Kay, C.D. (1990) Actions of baclofen and phaclofen upon ON- and OFF-ganglion cells in the cat retina. *Eur. J. Pharmacol.*, 190: 1–9.

Johnson, J.W. and Ascher, P. (1987) Glycine potentiates the NMDA response in cultured mouse brain neurons. *Nature*, 325: 529–531.

Johnston, G.A.R. (1986) Multiplicity of GABA receptors. In: *Benzodiazepine / GABA receptors and chloride channels: Structural and Functional Properties*, Olsen, R.W. and Venter, J.C. (Eds.), Alan Liss Inc., New York, pp. 57–71.

Kamatchi, G.L. and Ticku, M.K. (1990) Functional coupling of presynaptic $GABA_B$ receptors with voltage-gated $Ca^{2+}$ channel: Regulation by protein kinases A and C in cultured spinal cord neurons. *Mol. Pharmacol.*, 38: 342–347.

Kamatchi, G.L. and Ticku, M.K. (1990) $GABA_B$ receptor activation inhibits $Ca^{2+}$-activated Rb-efflux in cultured spinal cord neurons via G-protein mechanism. *Brain Res.*, 506: 181–186.

Karbon, E.W., Duman, R., Enna, S.J. (1983) Biochemical identification of multiple $GABA_B$ binding sites: Association with noradrenergic terminals in rat forebrain. *Brain Res.*, 274: 393–396.

Kerr, D.I., Ong, J., Johnston G.A.R., Abbenante, J. and Prager R.H. (1988) 2-Hydroxy-saclofen: An improved antagonist at central and peripheral $GABA_B$ receptors. *Neurosci. Lett.*, 92: 92–96.

Kerr, D.I., Ong, J., Johnston G.A.R., Abbenante, J. and Prager R.H. (1989) Antagonism at $GABA_B$ receptors by saclofen and related sulphonic analogues of baclofen and GABA. *Neurosci. Lett.*, 107: 239–244.

Kerr, D.I., Ong J., Johnston, G.A.R., Prager, R.H. (1989) $GABA_B$ receptor mediated actions of baclofen in rat isolated neocortical slice preparations: antagonism by phosphono-analogues of GABA. *Brain Res.*, 480: 312–316.

Kerr, D.I., Ong J., Prager, R.H., Gynther, B.D. and Curtis, D.R. (1987) Phaclofen: A peripheral and central baclofen antagonist. *Brain Res.*, 405: 150–154.

Krogsgaard-Larsen, P, Johnston, G.A.R., Lodge, D., Curtis, D.R. (1977) A new class of GABA agonist. *Nature*, 268: 53–55.

Krogsgaard-Larsen, P., Hjeds, H., Curtis, D.R., Lodge, D. and Johnston, G.A.R. (1979) Dihydromuscimol, thiomuscimol, and related heterocyclic compounds as GABA analogues. *J. Neurochem.*, 32: 1717–1724.

Lanthorn, T.H. and Cotman, C.W. (1981) Baclofen selectively inhibits excitatory synaptic transmission in the hippocampus. *Brain Res.*, 225: 171–178.

Maguire G., Lukasiewicz, P., and Werblin F. (1989a) Amacrine cell interactions underlying the response to change in the tiger salamander retina. *J. Neurosci.*, 9: 726–735.

Maguire, G., Maple, B., Lukasiewicz, P. and Werblin, F. (1989b) Gamma-aminobutyrate type B receptor modulation of L-type calcium channel current at bipolar cell terminals in the retina of the tiger salamander. *Proc. Natl. Acad. Sci. USA*, 86: 10144–10147.

Mott, D.D., Bragdon, A.C., Lewis, D.V., and Wilson, W.A. (1989) Baclofen has a proepileptic effect in the rat dentate gyrus. *J. Pharmacol. Exp. Ther.*, 249: 721–725.

Neal, M.J. and Shah, M.A. (1989) Baclofen and phaclofen modulate GABA release from slices of rat cerebral cortex and spinal cord but not from retina. *Br. J. Pharmacol.*, 98: 105–112.

Newberry, N.R. and Nicoll, R.A. (1984) Baclofen directly hyperpolarizes hippocampal cells. *Nature*, 308: 450–452.

Nowycky, M.C., Fox, A.P., and Tsien, R.W. (1985) Three types of calcium channel with different calcium agonist sensitivity. *Nature*, 316: 440–449.

Ogata, N., Matsuo, T., and Inoue, M. (1986) Potent depressant action of baclofen on hippocampal epileptiform activity in vitro: possible use in the treatment of epilepsy. *Brain Res.*, 377: 362–367.

Ong, J., Harrison, N.L., Hall, R.G., Barker, J.L., Johnston, G.A.R., Kerr, D.I. (1990) 3-Aminopropanephosphinic acid is a potent agonist at peripheral and central presynaptic $GABA_B$ receptors. *Brain Res.*, 526: 138–142.

Pan, Z-H. and Slaughter, M.M. (1991) Control of retinal information coding by $GABA_B$ receptors. *J. Neurosci.*, 11: 1810–1821.

Potashner, S.J. (1978) Baclofen: Effects on amino acid release. *Can. J. Physiol. Pharmacol.*, 56: 150–154.

Pratt, G.D., Knott, C., Davey, R. and Bowery, N.G. (1989) Characterization of 3-aminopropylphosphinic acid as a $GABA_B$ agonist in rat brain tissue. *Br. J. Pharmacol.*, 96: 141P.

Redburn, D.A., Friedman, D.L., and Massey, S.C. (1989) The function of multiple subclasses of GABA receptors in rabbit retina. In: *Neurobiology of the Inner Retina*. Weiler, R. and Osborne, N.N. (Eds.), Springer-Verlag, Berlin, pp 41–52.

60

Scherer, R.W., Ferkany, J.W., and Enna, S.J. (1988) Evidence for pharmacologically distinct subsets of GABA$_B$ receptors. *Brain Res. Bull.*, 21: 439–443.

Scott, R.H. and Dolphin, A.C. (1989) G-protein regulation of neuronal voltage-activated calcium currents. *Gen. Pharmacol.*, 20: 715–720.

Slaughter, M.M. and Bai, S-H. (1988) Baclofen's suppression of epileptiform-like activity: A retinal model. *Neurosci. Res. Suppl.*, 8: S217–S229.

Slaughter, M.M., Bai, S-H., and Pan, Z.H. (1989) Desegregation: Bussing of signals through the retinal network. In: *Neurobiology of the Inner Retina*, Weiler, R. and Osborne, N.N. (Eds.), Springer Verlag, Berlin. p. 335–347.

Slaughter, M.M. and Bai, S-H. (1989) Differential effects of baclofen on sustained and transient cells in the mudpuppy retina. *J. Neurophysiol.*, 61: 374–381.

Slaughter, M.M. and Miller, R.F. (1981) 2-Amino-4-phosphonobutyric acid: A new pharmacological tool for retina research. *Science*, 211: 182–185.

Soltesz, I., Haby, M., Leresche, N. and Crunelli, V.(1988) The GABA$_B$ antagonist phaclofen inhibits the late K$^+$-dependent IPSP in the cat and rat thalamic and hippocampal neurones. *Brain Res.*, 448: 351–354.

Stell W.K., Walker, S.E., Cholan, K.S. and Ball, A.K. (1984) The goldfish nervus terminalis: A luteinizing hormone-releasing hormone and molluscan cardioexcitatory peptide immunoreactive olfactoretinal pathway. *Proc. Natl. Acad. Sci. USA*, 81: 940–944.

Stockton, R.A. and Slaughter, M.M. (1991) Depolarizing actions of GABA and glycine upon amphibian retinal horizontal cells. *J. Neurophysiol.*, 65: 680–692.

Stirling, J.M., Cross, A.J., Robinson, T.N. and Green, A.R. (1989) The effects of GABA$_B$ receptor agonists and antagonists on potassium stimulated $[Ca^{2+}]_i$ in rat brain synaptosomes. *Neuropharmacology*, 28: 699–704.

Swartzwelder, H.S., Bragdon, A.C., Sutch, C.P., Ault, B. and Wilson, W.A. (1986) Baclofen suppresses hippocampal epileptiform activity at low concentrations without suppressing synaptic transmission. *J. Pharmacol. Exp. Ther.*, 237: 881–886.

Tsien, R.W., Lipscombe, D., Madison, D.V., Bley, K.R., and Fox, A.P. (1988) Multiple types of neuronal calcium channels and their selective modulation. *TINS*, 11: 431–438.

Werblin, F., Maguire, G., Lukasiewicz, P., Eliasof, S, and Wu, S.M. (1988) Neural interactions mediating the detection of motion in the retina of the tiger salamander. *Vis. Neurosci.*, 1: 317–329.

Yatani, A., Codina, J., Imoto, Y., Reeves, J.P., Birnbaumer, L. and Brown, A.M. (1987) A G-protein directly regulates mammalian cardiac channels. *Science*, 238: 1288–1292.

Yang, X-L and Wu, S.M. Effects of prolonged light exposure, GABA, and glycine on horizontal cell responses in tiger salamander retina. *J. Neurophysiol.*, 61: 1025–1035.

Zucker C.L. and Dowling, J.E. (1987) Centrifugal fibres synapse on dopaminergic interplexiform cells in the teleost retina. *Nature*, 330: 166–168.

R.R. Mize, R.E. Marc and A.M. Sillito (Eds.)
Progress in Brain Research, Vol. 90

CHAPTER 4

# Structural organization of GABAergic circuitry in ectotherm retinas

Robert E. Marc

*University of Texas Graduate School of Biomedical Sciences, Sensory Sciences Center, Houston, TX, USA*

## Introduction

Lateral inhibitory processes are the means by which signal transforming systems draw distinctions between or among parallel signal channels (Ratliff, 1971; Marmarelis and Marmarelis, 1977). The basic vertical signal channels in the retina are the photoreceptor → bipolar cell → ganglion cell chains. The ectotherm photoreceptor stage is complex. The retinas of most ectotherms have more than three cone types and their circuitries are richer than those depicted in simple models of mammalian trichromacy (e.g., Walls, 1942; Crescitelli, 1972; Scholes, 1975; Marc and Sperling, 1976a,b; Stell and Hárosi, 1976). Bipolar cells are those vertical elements that sample from this diverse sensor matrix, some types selecting rod-rich connections, others preferentially contacting one or more subsets of cone types (Ramon y Cajal, 1893; Scholes, 1975; Ishida et al., 1980; Van Haesendonck and Missotten, 1984; Kalloniatis and Marc, 1990a). Thus the output array to the ganglion cells of the retina may be comprised of ten, twenty or more varieties of bipolar cells, each with its own unique photoreceptor cohort and a distinctive arrangement of signal distribution sites manifested as telodendria and varicosities positioned in specific sublayers of the inner plexiform layer (e.g., Scholes, 1975; Kalloniatis and Marc, 1990a). The impression we have, then, is of a great many varieties of photoreceptor →

bipolar cell → ganglion cell chains. In this review, my intent is to emphasize the simplifying idea that each of these different channels is endowed with surround properties conferred predominantly through the actions and connectivities of horizontal cells and amacrine cells utilizing γ-aminobutyric acid (GABA) as their primary neurotransmitter. I would like to leave the reader with the image that each bipolar cell type possesses a unique cohort of GABAergic amacrine cell feedback and feedforward connections; that the *apparent* morphological diversity of GABAergic amacrine cells is comprehensible in the idea that many of the variously stratified and arborized GABAergic amacrine cells are merely surround devices for different sets of bipolar cells; that the formal operations of these GABAergic amacrine cells are similar and simply replicated across the sublayers of the inner plexiform layer.

I will restrict this discussion of circuitry to "fast" synaptic processes (Iversen, 1984): Processing where the photoreceptors are viewed as a 2-dimensional sensor array upon which successive scenes of a structurally rich, moving world are imaged; where this array is the input for a system of image operations rapidly executed in parallel on intersecting patches of the sensor matrix to provide a selection of co-transformed scenes. Fast excitation is carried out by photoreceptors and bipolar cells utilizing glutamate as their neurotransmitter (Ehinger et al., 1988; Marc et al.,

1990; Massey, 1990). Most fast inhibition is mediated by GABAergic interneurons and the remainder by glycinergic interneurons (see reviews by Yazulla, 1986; Marc, 1989a). Over 90% of the 50 + types of vertebrate retinal neurons employ glutamate, glycine or GABA as their primary neurotransmitter (e.g., Marc, 1989b) and the interplay of fast conductance changes is the essence of receptive field construction.

This review will discuss (1) visualizing GABAergic neurons; (2) understanding the scope of GABAergic organization throughout the vertebrates; (3) visualizing circuitry; (4) the organization of common microcircuits; and (5) general principles of GABAergic control throughout the retina. I should also warn the reader of my biases towards simple ideas, though that can lead to situations where I discount notions that may later prove to be correct and powerful. I will try to be explicit regarding those points.

**Visualization of GABAergic neurons**

The first step in describing GABAergic circuits is to provide compelling evidence that GABAergic neurons themselves can be characterized with high functional and structural fidelity. The past dozen years of research in the anatomy and biochemistry of retinal GABAergic neurons has involved considerable technical refinement, culminating in rather convincing matches of the components of GABAergic synaptic function. There are three main cell biological mechanisms underlying the rapidity, sustainability and potency of GABAergic neurotransmission: (1) The abilities of neurons to synthesize and mobilize GABA for release; (2) The precise and rapid control of extracellular neurotransmitter levels by potent pre-synaptic neurotransmitter/$Na^+$ symporters; and (3) The mediation of rapid post-synaptic conductance or synaptic efficacy changes by specific GABA receptors. Each of these features can theoretically be associated with visualization techniques. Synthetic and degradative enzymes, the neurotransmitter itself and some of the receptor types (see Brecha, Chapter 1) can be localized by immunocytochemistry. The clearance mechanisms can be documented by autoradiography.

*GABAergic neurons can be visualized with immunoglobulins directed against glutamic acid decarboxylase (GAD)*

Current evidence supports the view that the retina closely mimics the rest of the central nervous system in neurotransmitter synthesis and maintenance of neurotransmitter levels required to sustain synaptic transmission. Data from my laboratory suggest that retinal cells using amino acids as neurotransmitters possess intracellular neurotransmitter concentrations in the 1–10 mM range (Marc et al., 1990; Marc and Basinger, 1991), and that GABAergic cells in particular contain 1–5 mM cytosolic GABA. Obata (1976) reported that cerebellar Purkinje cells maintained an intracellular GABA concentration of about 6 mM.

However, GABA is not a naturally occurring amino acid in non-neural animal tissues (except perhaps pancreatic beta cells; see Solimena et al., 1990) and its selective concentration in neural structures has made it possible to purify the enzymes associated with its synthesis and degradation. The neuronal synthesis of GABA is performed by L-glutamic acid decarboxylase (GAD, EC 4.1.1.15), a pyridoxal phosphate requiring enzyme that apparently exists in two soluble forms: a 59 kDa and a 62–63 kDa form, possibly functional as dimers (Gottlieb et al., 1986; Kaufman et al., 1986; Legay et al., 1987; review by Martin, 1987). This is important for immunocytochemistry in that some antisera have been shown to recognize both forms (Kaufman et al., 1986) but few antisera used in retinal immunocytochemistry have been so tested. Thus GAD isoforms and species variations may strongly influence some immunocytochemical outcomes. The equilibrium constant for GAD favors GABA synthesis and the $K_m$ of brain GAD for glutamate is about 0.45–0.7 mM (Wu, 1976; Spink et al., 1985). This corresponds nicely to the estimated average level of glutamate in GABAergic cells, about 0.3–0.7 mM (Marc et al., 1990; Marc and Basinger, 1991). Moreover, the reverse inhibition of GAD by high GABA levels shows an apparent $K_m$ of about 16 mM (Porter and Martin, 1984), consistent with the apparent 1–5 mM levels reported for horizontal and amacrine cells (Marc and Basinger, 1991). The back reaction should be negligible under normal cellular conditions.

The immunocytochemical localization of GAD in retina has been studied extensively and, for the most part, the conclusions have been consistent across laboratories. One of the very first observations of GAD immunoreactivity (Barber and Saito, 1976) revealed the inner plexiform layer of the rat retina filled with immunoreactive strata. An excellent review of GAD immunocytochemistry was provided by Yazulla (1986), so it is possible to summarize some major points. (1) All vertebrate retinas contain a large contingent of GAD immunoreactive amacrine cells, and they appear to be highly stratified neurons (e.g., Vaughn et al., 1981; Brandon, 1985; Mariani and Caserta, 1986; Yazulla, 1986). (2) Few adult mammalian retinas have displayed convincing GAD immunoreactivity in horizontal cells. In fact, most mammalian preparations have been decidedly GAD immunonegative in the horizontal cell layer (see Brandon, 1985). (3) Most non-mammalian vertebrates have shown the presence of abundant GAD immunoreactive horizontal cells. This points out a significant phylogenetic demarcation in retinal organization that will be elaborated below. Importantly, the correspondence between other labels for GABAergic function (GABA content, GABA symport) have been high, though not an identity in some cases. The general patterns of GAD immunoreactivity in several non-mammalian retinas are shown in Fig. 1. I will revisit some of these data when discussing levels of labeling correspondence below.

*GABAergic neurons can be visualized with immunoglobulins directed against γ-aminobutyric acid conjugates*

The detection of GABAergic neurons with immunoglobulins (IgGs) directed against GABA-glutaraldehyde-protein constructs is now a routine method in many labs (e.g., Storm-Mathisen et al., 1983; Studholme and Yazulla, 1988; Wässle and Chun, 1989; Marc et al., 1990). Anti-GABA IgGs are commercially available and their antigenic specificities easily verifiable (Matute and Streit, 1986; Otterson, 1987; Nabors et al., 1988; Marc et al., 1990). In fact, it is even possible to verify, by immunocytochemistry, that a cell contains an immunoreactivity *kinetically* indistinguishable from a model GABA antigen (Marc et al., 1990; Marc and Basinger, 1991). Electron microscopic immunocytochemistry with anti-GABA IgGs and detection by gold granules coated with linking IgGs is compatible with strong glutaraldehyde fixation and varying degrees of osmication (e.g., Studholme and Yazulla, 1988; Koontz and Hendrickson, 1990). The resolution is far superior to uptake autoradiography, but even so, immunogold procedures suffer from the same "pointillist" statistical requirements as autoradiography: establishment of signal-to-noise criteria, and definition of labelling regime (i.e., in low-density Poisson-like labeling, how many false negatives will appear?). Detection with the horseradish peroxidase (HRP)-diaminobenzidine (DAB) product provides good spatial resolution, moderate signal detectability but may obscure many structural features, notably pre-synaptic specializations. In my laboratory, W.-L. Liu and I have used an overlay technique with digital registration: 100 nm sections are serially processed for high resolution electron microscopy and light microscopic GABA immunoreactivity with silver-intensified immunogold visualization. The pairs of images are digitally registered and overlaid, literally painting a high-signal-to-noise GABA image with a signal reliability of nearly 1.0 on the electron microscopic image. This provides rapid, reliable assignment of thousands of optimally viewed

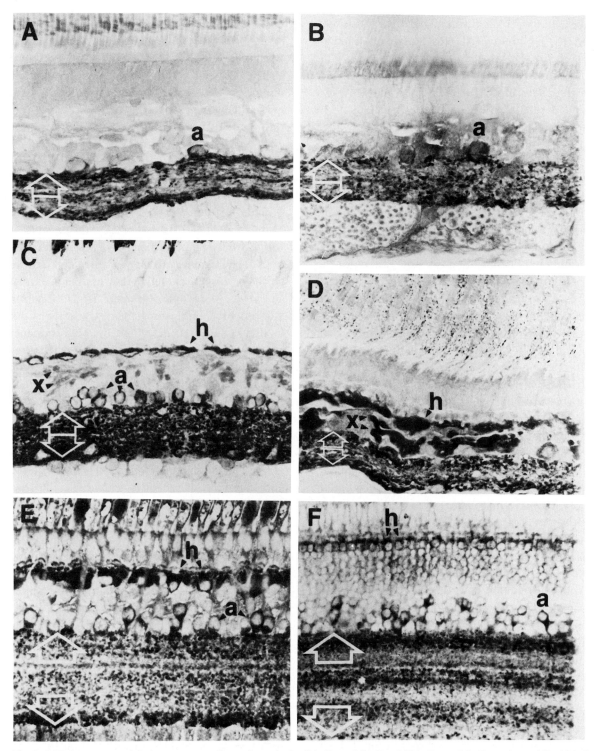

Fig. 1. GAD immunoreactivity in non-mammalian retinas. A, dogfish; B, ratfish; C, goldfish; D, catfish; E, turtle; and F, chick. In all cases the inner plexiform layer is delineated by a white, double-headed arrow. a, immunoreactive amacrine cell bodies; h, immunoreactive horizontal cell bodies; x, immunoreactive horizontal cell axons. A–F, 5 μm sections. Reprinted by permission from Brandon (1985) *Brain Res.*, 334: 286–295.

synaptic processes without grain counts or electron microscopic immunocytochemistry. Its limitations are the inability to resolve the smallest processes and the need for computational resources. In concert with these other methods, however, it provides one more powerful tactic to trace GABAergic circuitry (see Fig. 7).

GABA immunoreactivity has been mapped to many vertebrate retinas (see Phylogenetics), but the general patterns of organization in non-mammalians/ectotherms are easily demonstrated (Fig. 2). In general, a clear population of GABA immunoreactive horizontal cells can be seen in most species (tiger salamander, goldfish and pigeon shown). In addition, the inner plexiform layer is a virtually unbroken field of GABA immunoreactivity and labeled somas are found in both the amacrine and ganglion cell layers, indicating the presence of GABAergic conventional and displaced amacrine cells at least. The GABAergic innervation of the inner plexiform layer is often so dense that it is difficult to resolve the many sublayers that are present. Extensive discussion of stratification concepts for GABAergic systems has been published elsewhere (Marc, 1986; Hurd and Eldred, 1991; Koontz and Hendrickson, 1990). The general impression is that many types of highly stratified GABAergic amacrine cells are stacked through the entire inner plexiform layer. My view is that most of these cells are involved in similar, generic forms of microcircuits for every type of bipolar cell and that the entire population is not so complex after all.

There has been a report of both GABA and GAD immunoreactivity in primate cones (Nishimura et al., 1985) and in a specific subset of lizard cones (Engbretson et al., 1988). However, many workers have reported mammalian cones in general and primate cones in particular (Hendrickson et al., 1985; Mariani and Caserta, 1986) to be clearly GAD immunonegative. Furthermore, all primate cones are strongly glutamate immunoreactive and GABA immunonegative (Marc, unpublished data). From both a physiological and immunochemical view, the conclusions of

Nishimura et al. (1985) must be considered incorrect and their results due to uncompensated cross-reactivities. The issues surrounding lizard cones are as yet unresolved, but the carefulness of that study gives some confidence that a subset of GABAergic photoreceptors could exist in some lacertilians.

*GABAergic neurons can be visualized by autoradiography of high affinity symport of [$^3$H]GABA or GABA analogues*

The first successful marker for GABAergic neurons in an ectotherm retina was light microscopic autoradiography of [$^3$H]GABA uptake (e.g., Voaden et al., 1974; frog). These results revealed three important features that are now obviously common to most non-mammalians: (1) Some horizontal cells and (2) some amacrine cells were strongly labeled by [$^3$H]GABA incubations; (3) Unlike mammalian retinas, most ectotherms lacked Müller's cell uptake of GABA. This latter feature has been extremely fortunate for circuitry analysis since viewing of GABAergic synaptology in bony non-mammalians is largely unobscured by spatial buffering effects (but see below). Similar experiments in goldfish retina (Lam and Steinman, 1971) were augmented by the observations that GAD activity was high in fractions of dissociated goldfish retinal cells enriched for horizontal cells (Lam, 1975). Subsequent immunocytochemical work has convincingly shown that [$^3$H]GABA accumulating goldfish H1 horizontal cells are also GAD immunoreactive (Lam et al., 1979; Yazulla, 1985; Fig. 1). Moreover, goldfish H1 horizontal cells are also GABA immunoreactive (Yazulla, 1986; Ball and Brandon, 1988; Marc et al., 1990; Fig. 2). There are similar correlative data for other species (see Phylogenetics). The concordance of various markers of GABAergic function in ectotherm horizontal cells is almost an identity. Some differences still appear, such as Brandon's (1985) finding that shark horizontal cells are GAD immunonegative and the result from Brunken et al., 1984 that they are GAD immunoreactive. The discrepancy is not easily resolved, but it is proper

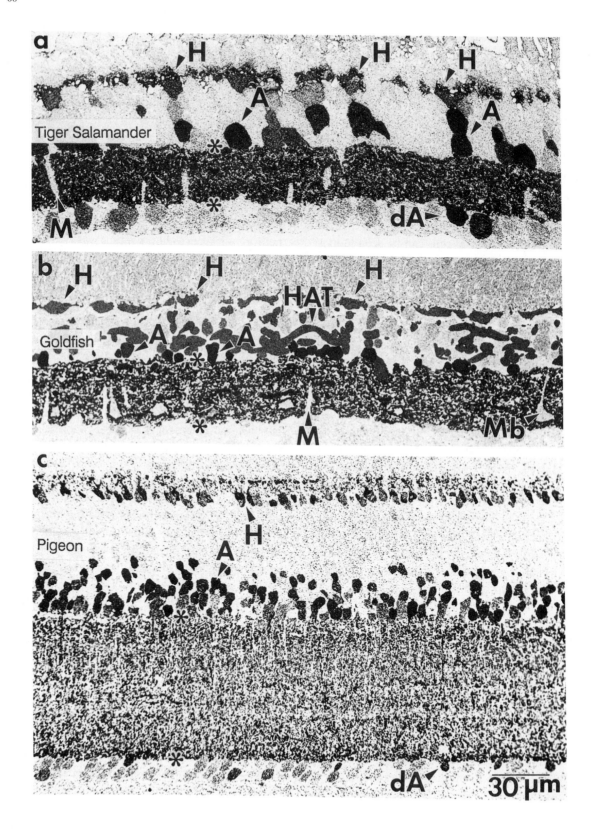

to note the large phylogenetic separation of chondrichthyans from the sources of GAD antigen (which were different in the two cases) and consider the possibility that GAD isoforms undetectable by some anti-GAD IgGs are expressed as possible causes for the difference.

Things have not been so simple for the amacrine cell populations. Initially, the correspondence between GAD immunocytochemistry (Zucker et al., 1984), [³H]GABA uptake (Marc et al., 1978) in amacrine cells and GABA receptor localization (see Yazulla, 1986) in goldfish retina was quite unsatisfactory. The basic flaw in all these studies was an underappreciation of the potency of high affinity GABA symporters (Marc, 1989b and unpublished data; Fig. 3). In effect, the goldfish and other ectotherm retinas possess a strong laminar spatial buffering of extracellular GABA levels due to (1) the horizontal cell layer and (2) the massive accretion of GABAergic synapses throughout the entire inner plexiform layer as is evident from GABA immunoreactivity. Thus exogenously applied [³H]GABA (1–5 $\mu$M) has little opportunity to penetrate very far before it is fully cleared. Under conventional incubation conditions, only H1 horizontal cells and an apparent single population of pyriform amacrine cells arborizing in sublayer 5 of the inner plexiform layer are visible by autoradiography. Tactics that override these barriers, such as (1) retinal slices (Marc, 1986 and unpublished data), (2) long incubations (Marc, 1986) or (3) intravitreal injections (Ball and Brandon, 1986), (4) substrates for which the GABA symporter has lower affinity ([³H] muscimol: Ball and Brandon, 1986; [³H]isuguvacine: Yazulla, 1986; $\delta$-[³H]aminolevulinic acid: Marc, unpublished data), and (5) suppression of

the $K_m$ (Na⁺ depletion: Yazulla and Kleinschmidt, 1983; competitive inhibition by nipecotic acid or unlabeled GABA, Marc, 1986; Marc, 1989b, Muller and Marc, 1990 and unpublished data; Fig. 3) all demonstrate GABA uptake is distributed throughout the inner plexiform layer and that there are actually many GABAergic cells in the amacrine cell layer and the ganglion cell layer. As techniques matured, the levels of correspondence among GAD immunocytochemistry, GABA immunocytochemistry and GABA uptake autoradiography improved (Ball and Brandon, 1986; Yazulla et al., 1986; Ball, 1987; Marc, 1989b) until today it is difficult to document the existence of a GABAergic cell population in the goldfish retina that does not possess both GABA symport and immunoreactivity. The matches are quite good in other species, though the correspondence between GAD and GABA immunoreactivity is not quite an identity in some species (Hurd and Eldred, 1991). The reasons for this are likely complex. Once again, GAD isoforms may not be antigens for all anti-GAD IgGs. But since there are usually more GABA immunoreactive than GAD immunoreactive cells (e.g., Hurd and Eldred, 1990), other phenomena may be involved, assuming that all of the true GAD-containing cells have been effectively marked. One possibility is the potential occurrence of heterologous gap junctions between GABAergic and non-GABAergic amacrine cells, which might lead to some cross labeling (cf. Yazulla and Yang, 1988). Thus a GABA immunoreactive cell might actually be glycinergic, only coupled to a GABAergic cell, and thus GAD immunonegative. It has also been proposed that some cells could accumulate enough GABA from

Fig. 2. GABA immunoreactivity in three non-mammalian retinas: tiger salamander, goldfish and pigeon all displayed at the same scale. Each exhibits a distinctive row of GABA immunoreactive horizontal cells (H), numerous immunoreactive amacrine cells (A) and a few displaced amacrine cells (dA). Note the complete absence of immunoreactivity in Müller's cell processes (M). The inner plexiform layer is bracketed by asterisks and is immunoreactive throughout. Goldfish horizontal cells also display GABA immunoreactive axon terminals (HAT). Bipolar cell terminals such as the ON center cell labeled Mb are immunonegative. Cell Mb is also displayed in Fig. 7. All specimens were processed by the silver intensified immunogold method (Marc et al., 1990). The tiger salamander and pigeon sections were 500 nm thick and the goldfish section was 100 nm thick.

the extracellular space to become GABA immunoreactive. My bias is that such accumulation is kinetically untenable, but evidence for either view has not been convincingly marshalled. In any event, the degrees of correspondence among markers in the goldfish have increased to 92–97%

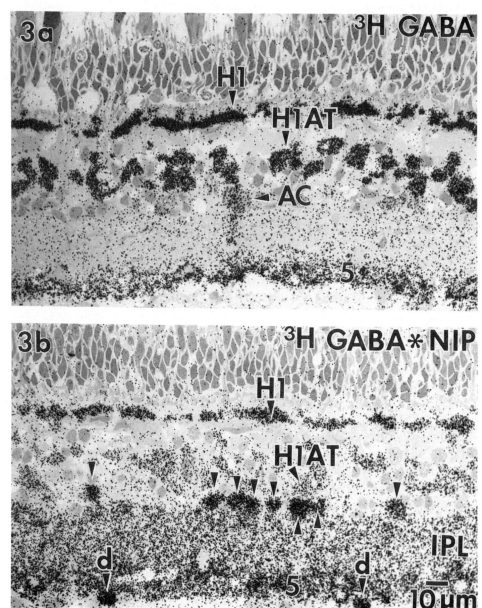

Fig. 3. Spatial buffering of [³H]GABA uptake in the goldfish retina analyzed by light microscopic autoradiography of 500 nm thick sections. (a) A section from a retina incubated 10 minutes in 1 μM [³H]GABA and processed according to Marc et al. (1978), revealing typical labeling of H1 horizontal cells (H1) and their axon terminals (H1AT), a pyriform amacrine cell (AC) destined for sublayer 5 which is dense with label; 14 day exposure. (b) A section from a retina incubated as in (a) but with the addition of 1 mM nipecotic acid. After a 35 day exposure, which roughly equates horizontal cell soma labeling, a massive increase in the number of labeled amacrine cell somas occurs (arrowheads), as well as the appearance of displaced amacrine cells (d) which we now know to be the goldfish equivalent of the starburst amacrine cell (see text). The inner plexiform layer is also much more heavily labeled, indicating the breakdown of the spatial buffer by competitive inhibition.

(Marc, 1989b). For all practical purposes, GAD immunoreactivity, GABA immunoreactivity or [$^3$H]GABA or GABA analogue uptake autoradiography may be employed at the light microscopic or electron microscopic level interchangeably in the goldfish, with high confidence that *bona fide* GABAergic neurons are being marked. This may not be true in all species, but the degree of correspondence is extremely high in most systems that have been carefully examined.

The choice of marker and mode of detection is consequential for ultrastructural visualization. Exploiting the GABA symporter for electron microscopic autoradiography requires either accepting the limited sampling allowed by spatial buffering (Marc et al., 1978; Muller and Marc, 1990) or using conditions to reduce the effects of spatial GABA buffering such as [$^3$H]muscimol uptake (Yazulla and Brecha, 1980) or competitive inhibition with nipecotic acid (Marc, 1989b; Muller and Marc, 1990; Figs. 3,8). The positive attributes of uptake experiments is that they are possible in virtually all species, the reagents are commercially available in high purity, and the technique is compatible with the highest quality ultrastructural preservation, HRP marked neuronal processes (Muller and Marc, 1990) and Golgi impregnation (Pourcho and Goebel, 1983; Kalloniatis and Marc, 1990b). The disadvantages are the technical risks, long signal integration time, low data density and inherent spatial limits of autoradiography. Nevertheless, outstanding morphological documentation has been achieved with autoradiographic methods in many species (e.g., Freed, Chapter 6).

## Phylogenetics

Why do we bother to provide separate descriptions of ectotherm circuitries? There are three striking differences between mammals and *most* non-mammalians. First, the mammalian retina exhibits strong segregation of rod and cone pathways into separate cellular channels whose final common path is realized in the distribution of rod bipolar cell outputs to the glycinergic AII amacrine cell, thence via non-rectifying gap junctions to depolarizing cone bipolar cells and sign-inverting glycinergic synapses onto hyperpolarizing bipolar cells, and finally from the bipolar cells to ganglion cells (Ramon y Cajal, 1893; Famiglietti and Kolb, 1975; Kolb and Nelson, 1983; Dacheux and Raviola, 1986; Strettoi et al., 1990). Conversely, many non-mammalians possess mixed bipolar cells which contact both rods and cones (e.g., Ramon y Cajal, 1893; Stell, 1967; Scholes, 1975; Ishida et al., 1980). Thus no specialized inner plexiform layer circuitry is required to achieve rod-cone convergence into a final common path in ectotherm vertebrates. A second dramatic feature is that almost all non-mammalian vertebrates possess GABAergic horizontal cells and almost all non-mammalian retinal Müller's cells lack a GABA symporter. Third, most non-mammalians possess pleomorphic cones. That is, virtually every spectral class of cones in non-mammalians possesses a strongly differentiated morphology (see review by Marc, 1982); such differentiations can even be made within a spectral class and bespeak connective segregations, the functions of which remain undefined. In contrast, the spectral classes of mammalian cones are monomorphic: essentially identical but for some very subtle variations (Ahnelt et al., 1987). These differences alone, among others, demand a careful separate evaluation of non-mammalian organization before we can safely generalize features of GABAergic circuitry across taxa. This spectrum of differences in retinal organization allows a clear segregation of vertebrate retinas into three types (Marc, 1989c): Type 1, the cartilaginous ectotherms (Cyclostomata; Chondrichthyes); Type 2, the bony non-mammalians composed of the osseous ectotherms (Osteichthyes, Amphibia, Reptilia) and the one non-mammalian endothermic class (Aves); Type 3, the mammalians. A final detail is that, while avians are endotherms and not ectotherms, their retinas are explicitly ectotherm in design.

TABLE 1

Patterns of GABA markers in the vertebrate retina

| Taxon | MC Symport | HC Symport | HC GABA IR | HC GAD IR |
|---|---|---|---|---|
| **Class Cyclostomata** | | | | |
| *Myxinus* sp. (hagfish) | ♦ | ◇ | ♦ | |
| *Ichthyomyzon* sp. (brook lamprey) | ♦ | ◇ | ♦ | |
| *Petromyzon marinus* (lamprey) | | | ♦, a | |
| **Class Chondrichthyes** | | | | |
| *Dasyatis sabina* (ray) | ♦ | ◇ | | |
| *Hydrolagus collei* (ratfish) | ♦ | ◇ | ♦ | |
| *Raja* spp. (skates) | ♦, b | ◇, b | ♦, c | ♦, d |
| *Squalas acanthias* (shark) | ♦ | ◇ | ♦ | ♦, e |
| *Mustelus canis* (shark) | | | | ♦, f |
| **Class Osteichthyes** | | | | |
| *Protopterus* sp. (lungfish) | ◇ | ♦ | ♦ | |
| *Calamoichthyes* sp. (reedfish) | ◇ | ♦ | ♦ | |
| *Polypterus palmas* (bichir) | ◇ | ♦ | ♦ | |
| *Lepisosteus osseus* (gar) | ◇ | ♦ | ♦ | |
| *Carassius auratus* (goldfish) | ◇, g | ♦, g | ♦, h | ♦, i |
| *Carassius carassius* (carp) | ◇ | ♦ | ♦ | ♦ |
| *Ictalurus punctatus* (catfish) | ◇, j | ♦, j | ♦ | ♦, k |
| *Micropterus* sp. (bass) | ◇ | ♦ | ♦ | |
| *Lepomis* sp. (sunfish) | ◇ | ♦ | ♦ | |
| *Lumpenis saggita* (snakefish) | ◇ | ♦ | ♦ | |
| *Porichthyes notatum* (midshipman) | ◇ | ♦ | ♦ | |
| *Cymatogaster aggregata* (shiner perch) | ◇ | ♦ | ♦ | |
| *Betta splendens* (betta) | ◇ | ♦ | ♦ | |
| Δ *Mormyrus* sp. | ♦ | ◇ | ◇ | |
| **Class Amphibia** | | | | |
| *Rana* spp. (frogs) | ◇, l | ♦, l | ♦, m | ♦, n |
| *Xenopus laevis* (clawed frog) | ◇, o | ♦, o | ♦ | |
| *Bufo marinus* (toad) | ◇ | ♦ | ♦ | |
| *Necturus maculosus* (mud puppy) | ◇, p | ♦, p | ♦, q | ♦, r |
| *Ambystoma tigrinum* (tiger salamander) | ◇, s | ♦, s | ♦, t | |
| *Amphiuma means* (congo eel) | ◇ | ♦ | ♦ | |
| (Golden newt) | ◇ | ♦ | ♦ | |
| *Triturus alpestris* (salamander) | | | ♦, u | |
| *Salamandra salamandra* (salamander) | | | ♦, u | |
| *Pleurodeles waltli* (salamander) | | | ♦, u | |
| Δ *Ichthyophis kohtaoensis* (gymnophionid) | | | ◇ | |
| **Class Reptilia** | | | | |
| *Pseudemys scripta elegans* (turtle) | ◇, b | ♦, b | ♦, v | ♦, w |
| *Anolis carolinensis* (anolis) | ◇ | ♦ | ♦ | |
| *Xantusia vigilis* (night lizard) | | | ♦, x | ♦, x |
| Δ *Thamnophis sirtalis* (garter snake) | ♦ | ◇ | ◇ | |
| Δ *Lampropeltis* sp. (King snake) | ♦ | ◇ | ◇ | |
| **Class Aves** | | | | |
| *Gallus domesticus* (chicken) | ◇, y | ♦, y | ♦, q | ♦, k |
| *Columbia livia* (pigeon) | ◇, z | ♦, z | ♦, c | ♦, aa |

TABLE 1 (continued)

| Taxon | MC Symport | HC Symport | HC GABA IR | HC GAD IR |
|---|---|---|---|---|
| **Class Mammalia** | | | | |
| *Setonix brachurya* (wallaby) | | | ◇ | |
| *Rattus norvegicus* (rat) | ♦, bb | ◇, bb | ◇, cc | ◇, dd |
| *Mus musculus* (mouse) | ♦ | ◇ | ◇ | ◇, ee |
| *Oryctolagus cuniculus* (rabbit) | ♦, ff | ◇, ff | ◇, gg | ◇, hh |
| *Sus scrofa* (pig) | | | | ◇, k |
| *Odocoileus* sp. (American deer) | | | ◇ | |
| *Cavia porcellus* (guinea pig) | ♦, ii | ◇, ii | | |
| *Capra hircus* (goat) | ♦, ii | ◇, ii | | |
| Δ *Papio* (baboon) | ♦, jj | ◇, jj | ♦, ◇, kk | ♦, ◇, ll |
| *Saimiri sciureus* (squirrel monkey) | ♦ | ◇ | ◇ | ◇, mm |
| *Homo sapiens* (human) | ♦ | ◇ | ◇, kk | ◇, nn |
| Δ *Macaca* spp. (macaques) | ♦ | ◇ | ♦, ◇, oo | ◇, pp |
| Δ *Felis catus* (cat) | ♦, qq | ◇, qq | ♦, ◇, rr | ♦, ◇, ss |
| Δ *Canis domesticus* (dog) | ♦ | ◇ | ♦ | |
| Δ *Mustela furo* (ferret) | ♦ | ◇ | ♦ | |

Symbols: ♦, symport or immunoreactivity present; ◇, symport or immunoreactivity absent; Δ, species with anomalous labeling relative to Class; letter, representative references; no letter, Marc, unpublished data.

Reference list (RM - Marc, unpublished data): a - Rubinson et al., 1989, 1990. b - Lam, 1976; RM. c - Agardh et al., 1987b; RM. d - Agardh et al., 1987b; Brandon, 1985; Brunken et al., 1986. e - Brandon, 1985; Brunken et al., 1986. f - Brunken et al., 1986. g - Lam and Steinman, 1971; Marc et al., 1978; Yazulla, 1983. h - Mosinger et al., 1986; Yazulla, 1986; Ball, 1987; Marc, 1989b; Marc et al., 1990. i - Lam et al., 1979; Yazulla, 1986; Brandon, 1985; Ball and Brandon, 1986; Yazulla et al., 1986; RM. j - Lam et al., 1978; RM. k -Brandon, 1985. l - Voaden et al., 1974; RM. m - Mosinger et al., 1986; Agardh et al., 1987b; Marc et al., 1990. n - Brandon et al., 1980; Brandon, 1985. o - Hollyfield et al., 1979; Smiley and Basinger, 1990; RM. p - Pourcho et al., 1984; Yazulla, 1986; RM. q - Mosinger et al., 1986; RM. r - Yazulla, 1986. s - Watt et al., 1987; Wu, 1986; RM. t - Yang and Yazulla, 1988; RM. u - Glaesner et al., 1988. v - Mosinger et al., 1986; Hurd and Eldred, 1989; RM. w -Yazulla, 1986; Hurd and Eldred, 1989. x - Engbretson et al., 1988. y - Marshall and Voaden, 1974b; Yazulla and Brecha, 1980; Yazulla, 1986; RM. z - Marshall and Voaden, 1974b; Marc, 1986. aa - Agardh et al., 1987b. bb - Neal and Iversen, 1972; Marshall and Voaden, 1974a; RM. cc - Mosinger et al., 1986; Neal and Iversen, 1972; Marshall and Voaden, 1974a; RM. cc - Mosinger et al., 1986; Neal et al., 1989; RM. dd - Vaughn et al., 1981; Wu et al., 1986. ee - Brandon, 1985; Schnitzer and Russoff 1984; ff - Ehinger, 1970; Marshall and Voaden, 1975; Redburn and Madtes, 1986; RM. gg - Mosinger et al., 1986; Agardh et al., 1987b; RM. hh - Brandon et al., 1979; Brandon, 1985; Yazulla, 1986; Agardh et al., 1987b. ii - Marshall and Voaden, 1975. jj - Marshall and Voaden, 1975; RM. kk - Agardh et al., 1987a; RM. ll - Agardh et al., 1987a. mm - Brecha, 1983. nn - Agardh et al., 1987b; Sarthy and Fu, 1989b - in situ hybridization. oo - Hendrickson et al., 1985; Mosinger et al., 1986; Agardh et al., 1987b; Grünert and Wässle, 1990; Kalloniatis and Marc, unpublished. pp - Hendrickson et al., 1985; Brandon, 1985; Mariani and Caserta, 1986. qq - Marshall and Voaden, 1975; Pourcho, 1980; Nakamura et al., 1980; RM. rr - Wässle and Chun, 1989; Ehinger et al., 1991; RM. ss - Brandon, 1985; Sarthy and Fu, 1989a - in situ hybridization.

*Virtually all non-mammalians possess GABAergic horizontal cells*

When autoradiography for [³H]GABA uptake, or immunocytochemistry for GABA or GAD immunoreactivity is applied to a variety of retinas, almost every type 1 and 2 vertebrate displays evidence of GABAergic horizontal cells (Table 1). The exceptions are themselves instructive. It is not possible to show that the horizontal cells of Cyclostomes (lampreys and hagfishes) or Chondrichthyes (sharks, rays, skates and chimaeras) have GABA symporters (Marc, unpublished data) simply because they are encased in Müller's cells which exhibit potent GABA symport (Lam, 1976; Ripps and Witkovsky, 1985; Marc, unpublished data). When immunocytochemical techniques are applied, however, these vertebrates can easily be shown to possess horizontal cells which are immunoreactive for GAD and/or GABA (Brunken et al., 1984; Rubinson et al., 1989, 1990; Marc, unpublished data). Thus it seems that GABAergic horizontal cells are the norm across most non-mammalian vertebrates.

There are, however, some type 2 vertebrates that lack GABA immunoreactive horizontal cells and GABA symport by horizontal cells: The snakes (O. Ophidia), the caeacelian amphibians (O. Gymnophiona) and some teleost fishes such as the genus Moryrops, a weakly electric fish. The latter two beasts inhabit scotopic niches and apparently lack cones. The former, the snakes, are cone rich but have retinas considered as re-derived from an ancestral rod format (see Crescitelli, 1972) and it is thought that they have experienced an obligate fossorial, and hence scotopic, phase. In any case, I posit that the loss of ancestral cone systems led to the loss of cone driven GABAergic horizontal cells. Further discussion of this topic is inappropriate here. The important point is that most non-mammalians have rich GABAergic horizontal cell networks.

The absence of glial GABA symporters in most non-mammalians is a powerful benefit to circuitry analysis but also raises another point. In type 1 and 3 vertebrates, the glia form a considerable barrier between neuronal GABA symporters deep in the outer plexiform and inner plexiform layers and the substrate, GABA. As this was first observed by Neal and Iversen (1972) in rat retina, how do we know that the purported absence of GABA uptake by most mammalian horizontal cells (even those presumed to be GABAergic by virtue of GABA immunoreactivity, e.g., Wässle and Chun,1990) is not due to strong glial barriers? The neuronal GABA symporters of mammalian amacrine cells can transport [$^3$H]muscimol (which glia cannot), yet cat horizontal cells still remain unlabeled (Wässle and Chun, 1989). Does this mean these cells lack a GABA symporter? Such a conclusion is still tenuous since horizontal cells in non-mammalians clearly show less potent uptake of muscimol than do amacrine cells (e.g., Yazulla and Brecha, 1980). In fact, avian GABAergic horizontal cells have excellent GABA uptake but seem unable to effectively transport either muscimol or isoguvacine (Yazulla and Brecha, 1980; Yazulla, 1986) even though avian GABAergic amacrine cells can transport all three substrates. Thus [$^3$H]muscimol uptake must still be considered a weak test for the presence or absence of a horizontal cell GABA symporter.

*Many amacrine cells in all vertebrates are GABAergic*

Every vertebrate examined by immunocytochemical or autoradiographic means displays a large contingent of GABAergic amacrine cells. Although the detailed forms of most of them remain to be determined, we do have a good sense of the general types of neurons included in this cohort from some species. It is fairly well established that pyriform shaped amacrine cells that stratify in sublayer 5 of the goldfish inner plexiform layer are GABAergic (Marc et al., 1978; Ball and Brandon, 1986; Yazulla et al., 1986). Many other species of teleost fishes (i.e., those listed in Table 1) show a similar or identical cohort of cells. Both autoradiographic and immunocytochemical techniques reveal that GABAergic amacrine cell systems in most species examined so far, especially avians and reptiles, display strong stratification patterns in the inner plexiform layer (e.g., Marc, 1986; Yazulla, 1986; Hurd and Eldred, 1990). This implies that many varieties of GABAergic amacrine cells have input-output operations tightly constrained to certain regions of the neuropil, probably tightly coupled to the laminar distributions of bipolar cell terminals (Marc, 1986).

Of course our real interests in amacrine cell populations are the forms and distributions of individual types of GABAergic amacrine cells, and it turns out that this is the arena in which neurotransmitter colocalization and other markers have been most useful. It is beyond the scope of this review to detail all the possible GABAergic populations in vertebrate retinas. But as an example, it is now quite clear that serotonin-accumulating neurons in the goldfish (Marc et al.,

1988a) are GABAergic (Ball and Tutton, 1990; Marc, unpublished data). This then identifies two subsets of GABAergic neurons: (1) the serotoninergic S1 cells which arborize primarily in sublayer 1 of the inner plexiform layer and are pre-and post-synaptic to off-center bipolar cells; and (2) the more populous serotonin accumulating S2 amacrine cells which terminate in sublayer 3. Since serotonin accumulating neurons in the rabbit retina are also GABAergic (Wässle and Chun, 1988; Sandell and Masland, 1989; Massey et al., 1991), it would not be surprising to discover that all serotonin-labeled amacrine cells in all vertebrates were GABAergic amacrine cells. Moreover, it seems that cholinergic neurons in most retinas will also be GABAergic. The starburst amacrine cells of the rabbit retina are cholinergic/GABAergic cells whose morphologies are well known (Brecha et al., 1988; Vaney and Young, 1988). Similarly, we have shown that the choline acetyltransferase immunoreactive amacrine cells of the goldfish retina co-localize [³H]-GABA uptake and GABA immunoreactivity (Li and Marc, unpublished data) and a subset is also starburst in morphology (Arnold and Marc, unpublished data). In goldfish, at least, all the GABAergic neurons in the ganglion cell layer are displaced GABAergic amacrine cells (Ball and St. Denis, 1986; Marc et al., 1990) and all are probably cholinergic as well (Li and Marc, unpublished data). It is also plausible that many peptidergic neurons will turn out to be GABAergic, as has been demonstrated in Watt and his colleagues (e.g., Watt et al., 1987). If so, yet another type of GABAergic amacrine cell may be one of the tachykinin (substance P) immunoreactive cells described by Yazulla et al. (1985) as being monostratified near sublayer 3 and receiving extensive bipolar cell input. This would be consistent with a theme to be elaborated in this review, that GABAergic amacrine cells are lateral elements receiving their prime inputs from bipolar cells in a manner virtually identical to the horizontal cell network of the outer plexiform layer (see Wu, Chapter 5).

The estimates of the fraction of the amacrine cell layer comprised by GABAergic amacrine cells varies somewhat from species to species and is particularly hard to estimate in those animals with extremely thick amacrine cell layers, such as avians and anuran amphibians. In the goldfish, it appears that roughly 50% of the somas in the amacrine cell layer are GABAergic and about 30–35% are glycinergic. The remainder must be composed of Müller's cells somas, some cone bipolar cells (see Marc et al., 1990), and displaced ganglion cells. In all vertebrates, a large fraction of all somas in the amacrine cell layer derive from GABAergic amacrine cells.

## The anatomy of synaptic transmission

### Conventional synapses are the primary sites of GABAergic transmission

The essence of ultrastructural analyses of circuitry is the synapse and its morphological signatures: pre-synaptic vesicle accumulations, pre-synaptic cytosolic/intracellular membrane face specializations, increased membrane electron opacity, occasional periodic extracellular electron opacities in the synaptic cleft, post-synaptic electron opaque specializations. We presume we may unravel the circuitries of GABAergic neurons based on patterns of conventional synaptic contact. This is not necessarily a foregone conclusion since these synapses may, for some reason, not reflect *bona fide* sites of GABAergic transmission or may not be the only sites. (1) There is evidence that some GABAergic neurons can release GABA by a $Ca^{2+}$-independent mechanism (Schwartz, 1982; Ayoub and Lam, 1984; Schwartz, 1987; Fig. 4a), (2) it has been difficult to document $Ca^{2+}$-dependent GABA release from mammalian amacrine cells in general (e.g., O'Malley and Masland, 1989) and (3) colocalization of neurotransmitter substances raises the query of which neurotransmitter is actually loaded in the vesicles we observe.

I believe we can be confident that neurons containing appropriate GABA markers (uptake or immunoreactivity) communicate via conventional synapses characterized by pre-synaptic accumulations of small, clear vesicles. First, evoked release of pre-loaded GABAergic amacrine cells in the goldfish retina is almost totally $Ca^{2+}$-dependent (Fig. 4b, Ayoub and Lam, 1984). Second, an aspect of synaptic function which receives little attention but remains pivotal is the vesicle loading process. As far as is known, all vesicles mediating synaptic transmission of small molecules such as monamines or amino acids are loaded by ligand/proton antiporters. Glutamate, GABA and glycine antiporters have been kinetically characterized (e.g., Fischer-Bovenkerk et al., 1988; Maycox et al., 1988; Kish et al., 1989). Each is extremely stereospecific and, in fact, there are no known competitive inhibitors of the GABA antiporter. This is important for a very subtle reason. Muscimol, a potent $GABA_A$ receptor agonist, is also a specific but weak substrate for some neuronal but not glial GABA symporters (Yazulla, 1986). GABAergic amacrine cells can be loaded with [$^3$H]muscimol. Models of non-vesicular GABA release are strongly consistent with the view that the GABA/$Na^+$ symporter is responsible for the voltage dependent efflux (Ayoub and Lam, 1984; Yazulla, 1986; Schwartz, 1987). If so, [$^3$H]muscimol should be easy to release from the rabbit retina, if GABAergic amacrine cells release GABA through a $Ca^{2+}$-independent path. However, the same photic, ionic and pharmacologic stimuli which can evoke massive [$^3$H]acetylcholine release in rabbit retina (Linn and Massey, 1991; Linn et al., 1991) are without effect on [$^3$H]muscimol loaded cells (Linn and Massey, personal communication). Why is this so? The answer seems quite simple: No [$^3$H]muscimol was available to any physiological release mechanism. Even 100 $\mu$M muscimol is without effect on the GABA vesicle antiporter

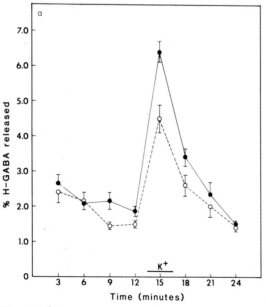

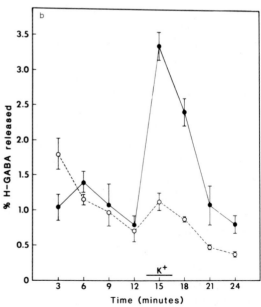

Fig. 4. $Ca^{2+}$ dependence of GABA release from horizontal and amacrine cells in intact goldfish retinas. (a) [$^3$H]GABA was incorporated into horizontal cells by incubation under dim red light illumination. The release profile was elicited by incubations in physiological ($Ca^{2+}$-containing, continuous line) and $Ca^{2+}$-free (dashed line) saline solutions, with 60 mM $K^+$ added for a three minute period to depolarize the cells. Nipecotic acid was added throughout to inhibit GABA uptake. The values are means ± SE of means of a minimum of twelve experiments. (b) A preferential incorporation of [$^3$H]GABA into amacrine cells was accomplished by injection of the label into goldfish eyes, followed by incubation in darkness. The retinas were then used in release experiments as described for horizontal cells. Note the strong dependence of evoked release on the presence of $Ca^{2+}$ for amacrine cells and only a partial dependence for horizontal cells. Reprinted by permission from Ayoub and Lam (1984) *J. Physiol. (London)*, 355: 191–214.

and muscimol cannot enter the vesicular release compartment (Kish et al., 1989). Though starburst amacrine cells have robust muscimol uptake (Massey et al., 1991), they clearly cannot release it. This implies that GABAergic amacrine cells do not use $Ca^{2+}$-independent release as their prime mode of synaptic communication and is a critical concept because the vesicular release model is the underpinning of structural connectivity data. Finally, and very importantly, the distributions of GABA receptors, whether mapped anatomically (see Brecha, Chapter 1) or physiologically (Ishida, Chapter 2; Slaughter and Pan, Chapter 3; Wu, Chapter 5) strongly affirm the view that the very synapses we see in the electron microscope are sites of GABAergic transmission.

### GABAergic horizontal cells utilize both conventional synapses and symporters for GABAergic transmission

It is quite evident that non-mammalian horizontal cells constitute a special case worthy of our attention because there is evidence that they do indeed exploit the transport capacities of the GABA symporter to release GABA in the outer plexiform layer. The GABAergic horizontal cells of the goldfish retina release endogenous GABA by both $Ca^{2+}$-dependent and $Ca^{2+}$-independent processes (Ayoub and Lam, 1985). We now know the somas, proximal dendrites and axon terminals of teleost horizontal cells contain beautiful conventional synapses (Marc and Liu, 1984; Marshak and Dowling, 1987; review by Sakai and Naka, 1988). However, the prime site of GABAergic horizontal cell action seems to be photoreceptor feedback (Murakami et al., 1982; Kaneko and Tachibana, 1986a,b; Wu, 1986; Wu, Chapter 5) even though conventional horizontal cell → cone synapses are absent in most species. The $Ca^{2+}$-independent release of GABA from ectotherm horizontal cells is well documented (Schwartz, 1982; Yazulla and Kleinschmidt, 1983; Ayoub and Lam, 1984, 1985; review by Yazulla, 1986; Schwartz, 1987; Fig. 4a) and by extension, many of us suspect that the process is mediated by GABA sym-

porter molecules aggregated into the tips of the horizontal cell dendrites as they invaginate deeply into the cone pedicle. Since immunochemical probes for at least one neuronal GABA symporter are available (Radian et al., 1990), it may be possible to directly test this hypothesis. A provocative approach, albeit indirect, has been the histochemical localization of p-nitrophenyl-phosphatase activity in goldfish retina, which can be used to map membrane sites of presumed $Na^+$-$K^+$ ATPase accumulations (Yazulla and Studholme, 1987). Among many structures, horizontal cell dendrites in cone pedicles stood out in possessing clear accumulations of reaction product, implying that there is some selective concentration of ATPase activity in those processes and a dearth of reaction product apposed to known sites of vesicular GABAergic transmission in the inner plexiform layer. In any case, the connectivity of GABAergic horizontal cells is clear in spite of not being able to visualize the actual site of synaptic transmission. Furthermore, we can exploit the anatomy of conventional synaptic architecture in horizontal cells as well as amacrine cells when considering connectivities with neurons other than photoreceptors.

### Microcircuits

I use the term *microcircuits* in the sense expressed by Shepherd and Koch (1990): That level of synaptic organization that is the most local in nature and a subset of the next stage, dendritic integration. As I discuss the various microcircuits known in ectotherm retinas, I will focus heavily on my own preferred animal, the goldfish. Moreover I will employ modifications of some common terminology to denote kinds of microcircuits (Table 2). GABA is clearly associated with the generic process of lateral inhibition in the vertebrate retina but different formal paths should be defined. First, *feedback* and *feedforward* should be differentiated in biological and engineering terms (Shepherd and Koch, 1990). *Feedback* is the process where a portion of the output signal of a stage in a serial chain (e.g., photoreceptor or bipolar cell output) is part of the input to the *same stage* (e.g., path 1 in Fig. 10). *Feedforward* is the process where a portion of the output signal of a given stage in a serial chain is part of the input to the next element in the chain (path 2, Fig. 10). Since GABAergic mechanisms, regardless of the receptor mechanism underlying their operations, are virtually always sign-inverting or attenuating in their effects (see discussion on this point by Slaughter and Pan, Chapter 3), all references to feedforward and feedback will imply *negative* feedforward and *negative* feedback. These two neural processes are roughly equivalent to negative feedback and negative feedforward in amplifier design in that feedback involves adding the inverted signal to the input signal prior to the gain step (i.e., the synapse), whereas feedforward adds it after the gain step. This dichotomy is important and retinal synaptology follows many of the same operating rules as elec-

tronic devices (Naka, 1977): i.e., many retinal neurons exhibit operating characteristics diagnostic of feedback processes. With certain mathematical constraints, negative feedback has the capacity to improve the signal reliability, increase the signal-to-noise ratio, broaden the bandwidth, speed the impulse response and enhance the stability (see Marmarelis and Marmarelis, 1977) of a given stage in a retinal circuit. Thus we might expect feedback to be a dominant feature of retinal processing. Yet there is also an inherently spatial dimension that can be recoded as other stimulus qualities such as color, and that dimension is not necessarily mediated exclusively by feedback synapses. Clearly, negative feedforward from one stage to the next, after the gain step (the synapse), can mediate a wide range of spatial, temporal and spectral differentiations. Feedforward will not enhance stability much nor improve signal-to-noise ratio, but it will allow strong signal segregation of parallel input stages to a

TABLE 2

Typographic notation for synaptic transfer

| **Forms of synaptic transfer** | |
| --- | --- |
| Sign-conserving synapse | > |
| Sign-inverting synapse | ≫ |
| Electrical synapse | = |

**Cell notation**

| AC | amacrine cell |
| --- | --- |
| BC | bipolar cell |
| C | cone |
| GC | ganglion cell |
| HC | horizontal cell |
| IPC | interplexiform cell |
| R | rod |
| GABA | GABAergic |
| gly | glycinergic |
| Ser | serotoninergic |

**Examples of synaptic chains**

Excitatory path: BC > GC
Inhibitory path: AC ≫ GC
Reciprocal feedback: BC > ≪ AC
Homologous lateral feedback: BC1 > AC ≫ BC2; BC1 & BC2 same cell type
Heterologous lateral feedback: BCa > AC ≫ BCb; BCa & BCb different cell types
Near feedforward: BC1 > AC1 ≫ GC1; BC1 > GC1
Far feedforward: BC1 > AC1 ≫ GC2; BC1 not > GC2

target without corrupting the input stage. Thus there are different operational consequences to employing feedback or feedforward for a given transfer process.

Though are only two basic forms of inhibitory microcircuits, feedforward and feedback, their implementations may be strongly discriminated in terms of the types and spatial relationships of the cells involved (Table 2; Fig. 10). Table 2 lists some symbols and notations I will use in the remaining text. For example, we may wish to distinguish among (1) feedback paths that involve only two cells in the classical recurrent sense (Shepherd and Koch, 1990), (2) feedback paths from a bipolar cell through a GABAergic amacrine cell to neighboring bipolar cell of the *same* type, and (3) feedback paths from a bipolar cell through a GABAergic amacrine cell to a bipolar cell of a *different* type. Such sequences are labeled (1) reciprocal, (2) homologous lateral and (3) heterologous lateral feedback respectively (Table 2). Furthermore, feedforward connections can involve the same direct chain (near feedforward) or a totally separate vertical chain (far feedforward). I will also equate the common terminology of excitatory with sign-conserving and inhibitory with sign-inverting, depending on whether discussion emphasizes synaptic physiology or circuitry. The following text shows how these types of GABAergic circuits are implemented in the goldfish retina.

*GABAergic horizontal cells synapse on interplexiform cells and some bipolar cells*

The roles of GABAergic horizontal cells in their contributions to the surround properties of cones have been thoroughly discussed in Chapter 5 (Wu) and I will not recapitulate that story here. My intent is to describe GABAergic circuitry in the goldfish retina through the anatomically observable feature of conventional synapses. One well known target of GABAergic horizontal cells is the glycinergic interplexiform cell of the goldfish retina (Marc and Lam, 1981; Marc and Liu, 1984; Kalloniatis and Marc, 1990b; Yazulla and

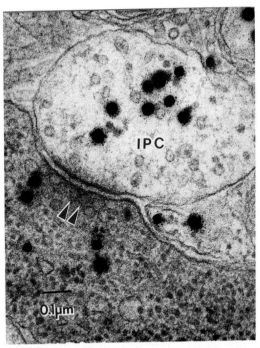

Fig. 5. A synapse between the soma of a GABAergic goldfish horizontal cell and a glycinergic interplexiform cell dendrite; electron microscope autoradiography of [$^3$H]glycine uptake in the goldfish retina. A large conventional synapse with an aggregate of clear vesicles is marked by double arrowheads. Reprinted by permission from Marc and Liu (1984) *Nature*, 311: 266–269.

Studholme, 1990). The glycinergic interplexiform cell sends 2–4 primary dendrites towards the outer plexiform layer where they arborize as a fine plexus of varicosities over a 200 $\mu$m diameter field. The varicosities lie on the distal surfaces of H1 horizontal cell somas and receive direct conventional somatodendritic synapses (Fig. 5; Marc and Liu, 1984). The spatial integration of the glycinergic interplexiform cell is thus quite large, especially considering the addition of horizontal cell coupling to the receptive field. We also know that the targets of the glycinergic interplexiform cells must be either GABAergic amacrine cells or ganglion cells (Marc and Lam, 1981; Muller and Marc, 1990; Fig. 10). We conceive of two minimum length synaptic chains: (1) C > H1 HC ≫ Gly IPC ≫ GABA AC ≫ OFF GC; (2) C > H1 HC ≫ Gly IPC ≫ ON GC. The former chain is net sign-inverting and the latter sign-conserving. We believe these paths may allow certain vertical chains to rapidly reset sensitivity according to the average illumination of the retina (Kalloniatis and Marc, 1990b), a process once thought to be the role of horizontal cells but probably beyond their spatial capabilities.

Marshak and Dowling (1987) also report observing synapses from horizontal cell axon terminals, most of which are GABAergic, onto bipolar cell somas and the processes of both putative glycinergic and dopaminergic interplexiform cells. Van Haesendonck et al. (1991) have similarly observed horizontal cell axon terminal synapses onto tyrosine hydroxylase immunoreactive profiles in the inner nuclear layer, suggesting direct GABAergic input to dopamine interplexiform cell dendrites. Under scotopic conditions, where light driven retinal responses are mediated by rods and not cones, the cone-driven GABAergic horizontal cells should be strongly depolarized and thus tonically release GABA onto dopaminergic interplexiform cell processes, presumably inhibiting dopamine release. This would imply that net dopamine release should be augmented under light-adapted conditions.

The inputs to bipolar cell somas and proximal dendrites are a little more problematic. Unless they occur with sufficient frequency, it is difficult to see how they could much impact a bipolar cell receptive field in the face of powerful horizontal cell feedback to photoreceptors and amacrine cell feedback to the bipolar cell terminals themselves (see below). Also, a direct input from a GABAergic horizontal cell to an ON center bipolar cell would seem to generate the wrong form of surround. Neither the importances nor the mechanisms involved in these unusual circuits have been clarified (see Wu, Chapter 5).

Likewise Sakai and Naka have (1988) documented conventional synapses made by catfish cone horizontal cells, also known to be GABAergic (Lam et al., 1978). In this species it seems that direct synapses onto cone telodendria are frequent and may mediate photoreceptor feedback

in addition to symport. There are also horizontal cell axon terminal outputs to amacrine cell somas and some amacrine cell processes in distal inner plexiform layer. The meanings of these contacts are not clear since we have no sense of their frequencies. It is doubtful that a single horizontal cell axon terminal synapse onto an amacrine cell soma could much influence the amacrine cell's dendritic input-output characteristics.

*GABAergic amacrine cells engage in disynaptic feedback and feedforward inhibitory circuits*

As noted previously, there are many GABAergic amacrine cells in all retinas and it is easy to document some basic forms of connectivity and infer some others. First, from the tremendous frequency of observed contacts, it seems that most types of GABAergic amacrine cells receive direct bipolar cell input, although a truly *intera-macrine* GABAergic cell would easily escape detection. In any case, a dominant form of input to goldfish GABAergic amacrine cells is from bipolar cell ribbons (Marc et al., 1978; Studholme and Yazulla, 1988; Marc, 1989a; Muller and Marc, 1990; Figs. 6,7) and we assume that all such input is sign-conserving (Naka, 1977). More importantly, these GABAergic profiles make abundant synapses on bipolar cells located at the same level of the inner plexiform layer in (1) the reciprocal mode (Marc, 1989b; Muller and Marc, 1990; Figs. 6,7) and (2) in the homologous feedback mode since all Mb (ON center) bipolar cell terminals in sublayer 5 of the inner plexiform layer receive extensive synaptic input around their proximal portions from a single class of pyriform GABAergic amacrine cell (Marc et al., 1978) and overall synaptic input from GABAergic amacrine cells outnumbers reciprocal synapses by about 5:1 (Marc, 1989a). Some of this input is likely to be heterologous lateral feedback when the chromatically heterogeneous nature of the Mb bipolar cell population is taken into account (Ishida et al., 1980) but this has not been established.

Near feedforward synapses are more difficult to document, but the whole feedforward class of inputs to ganglion cells is strongly evidenced in the goldfish retina (Muller and Marc, 1990; Figs. 7,8). The minimum path expected for the concatenation of massive ribbon input to GABAergic amacrine cells and massive GABAergic input to ganglion cell dendrites is obviously $BC > AC \gg GC$. This is consistent with typical models of ganglion cell receptive field organization (see Wu, Chapter 5) and the presence of GABA receptors on goldfish ganglion cells (see Ishida, Chapter 2). Figure 7 illustrates an immunocytochemical overlay procedure for viewing GABAergic feedback and feedforward connections. Four serial 100 nm

sections were cut: the first was processed for light microscopic immunocytochemistry to detect GABA with silver intensified immunogold visualization (Fig. 7a; Marc et al., 1990), and the following 3 were processed for conventional electron microscopy. Section 2 was digitally captured and precision aligned with the appropriate portion of Fig. 7a to produce the overlay Fig. 7b. This identifies 5 GABAergic and 2 non-GABAergic profiles surrounding a type Mb bipolar cell terminal (Fig. 7c,d). Amacrine cell profile 1 makes a clear reciprocal feedback synapse and profile 2 makes a both a reciprocal feedback to the bipolar

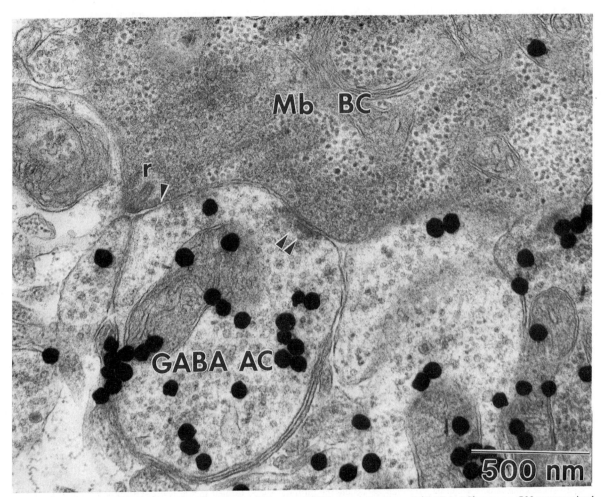

Fig. 6. Reciprocal feedback synapse (double arrowhead) from a GABAergic amacrine cell (GABA AC) onto an ON center mixed rod-cone bipolar cell terminal (Mb BC). The ribbon (r) input is indicated by a single arrowhead. Electron microscope autoradiography of [³H]GABA uptake.

cell and a near feedforward connection to a ganglion cell dendrite (GC2). Profile 4 makes a feedback and feedforward synapse, but it is not known where its input derives. It is likely that, since only the GABAergic pyriform amacrine cells of sublayer 5 innervate this part of the bipolar cell, that some neighboring GABAergic profiles arise from a single amacrine cell and are effectively reciprocal in their function. This connectivity can be found at every level of the inner plexiform layer, including Ma, Mb and cone bipolar cells (Marc, 1989a; Muller and Marc, 1990; Marc, unpublished data). It appears that all reciprocal feedback synapses on bipolar cells may be GABAergic. An apparent exception, the BC > ≪ Ser AC path of serotoninergic S1 amacrine cells (Marc et al., 1988b), is complicated by the fact that those cells are also GABAergic. The domination of feedback to bipolar cells by GABAergic amacrine cells is a general feature of all vertebrate circuitry (Vaughn et al., 1981; Pourcho and Goebel, 1983; Mariani and Caserta, 1986; see Freed, Chapter 6).

*All bipolar cells receive massive GABAergic amacrine cell input at their axon terminals*

A corollary to the involvement of GABAergic amacrine cells in most or all feedback and feedforward paths from bipolar cells is that nearly all of the amacrine cell input to bipolar cells at every level of the inner plexiform layer is GABAergic (Yazulla et al., 1987; Studholme and Yazulla, 1988; Marc, 1989b; Yazulla, 1989; Muller and Marc, 1990). All types of bipolar cell terminals are typically encased in a nest of GABAergic synapses at the electron microscopic level (e.g., Figs. 6,7) and virtually every bipolar cell in every species of vertebrate is ensheathed in GABA immunoreactivity. There should be little doubt that GABA is the prime inhibitory mechanism for bipolar cell control, consistent with the physiological evidence of potent GABA-activated conductances on bipolar cells (e.g., Kondo and Toyoda, 1983; Tachibana and Kaneko, 1987; Wu, Chapter 5). Glycinergic contacts on bipolar cells have been noted previously but are extremely rare (Marc and Lam, 1981; Studholme and Yazulla, 1988; Muller and Marc, 1990) and perhaps physiologically negligible.

*Most and perhaps all ganglion cells receive GABAergic amacrine cell input*

It has long been known that both GABA and glycine seemed to have potent and direct effects on ganglion cells (e.g., Negishi et al., 1978; Frumkes et al., 1981; Ishida, Chapter 2). Anatomically, it is difficult to be certain that one is observing true ganglion cell dendrites in the neu-

Fig. 7. Overlay mapping of light microscopic immunocytochemistry for GABA with serial electron microscopic visualization of synapses. A 100 nm thick section of goldfish inner plexiform layer (same as shown in Fig. 2) was processed for GABA immunoreactivity using silver intensified immunogold visualization (Marc et al., 1990). Serial sections were processed for conventional electron microscopy and the neighbor to the light microscope section digitally aligned and overlaid (Marc et al., 1990). (a) The full width of the goldfish inner plexiform layer showing GABA immunoreactivity throughout, a labeled amacrine cell (AC) and the immunonegative terminal of a type Mb bipolar cell (Mb). The locations of five amacrine cell terminals are indicated. Note in particular the butterfly shape formed by terminals 1 and 2. (b) The digital overlay. GABAergic profiles are dark hatched shapes (1–5) bordering the bipolar cell terminal (Mb BC). The heavy white line is the exact tracing of the bipolar cell border from the electron micrograph. The image corruption is due to the very high degree of processing required to match a light and electron microscopic image. Two unlabeled ganglion cell profiles abut the bipolar cell terminal (GC1, GC2). The position of one synaptic ribbon (r1) and a smooth endoplasmic reticulum cistern (*) are marked. (c) The first of two serial conventional electron microscopic images where each structure can be identified, especially the butterfly shape formed by the two GABAergic terminals (1 and 2). Both ganglion cells are post-synaptic to ribbons, as are amacrine cells 1 and 2 (r1, amacrine cell 1 and GC1, etc.) which also make reciprocal synapses onto the bipolar cell. Profile 4 makes both feedback and feedforward synapses, the latter to an extremely small process marked by a single arrowhead. (d) A serial view of the feedforward synapse from amacrine cell profile 2 to GC2.

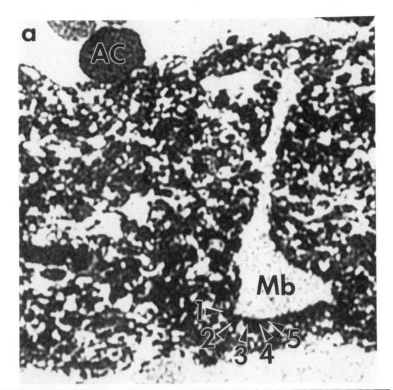

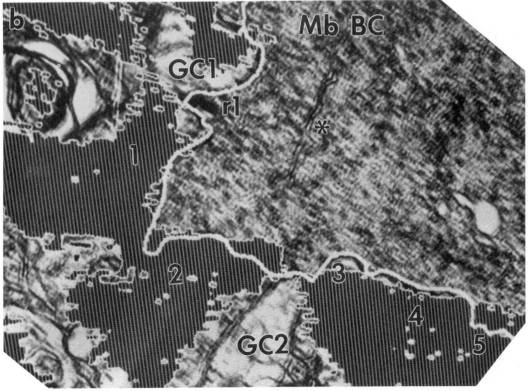

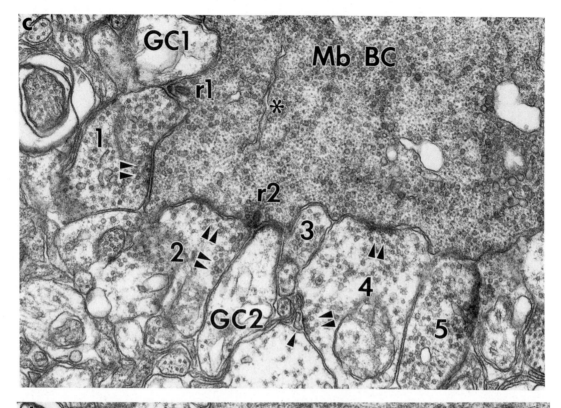

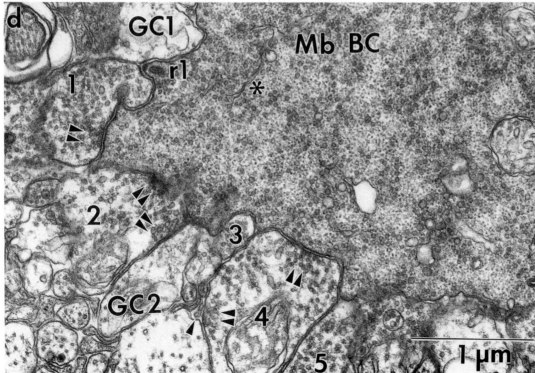

Fig. 7 (continued).

ropil of the inner plexiform layer. By using horseradish-peroxidase backfilling of ganglion cells combined with electron microscopic autoradiography of [³H]GABA and [³H]glycine uptake, it is evident that many and perhaps all varieties of goldfish ganglion cells receive direct GABAergic amacrine cell inputs (Muller and Marc, 1990). Both large caliber and very small (< 100 nm diameter) ganglion cell dendrites can be the targets of amacrine cell input. One particularly interesting type of GABAergic amacrine cell is a large bistratified cell (Marc et al., 1989b and unpublished data) similar in morphology to the large transient amacrine cells of fishes first reported by Murakami and Shimoda (1975) and

later shown to be coupled by gap junctions (Naka and Christensen, 1981; Teranishi et al., 1984). Processes characteristic of such cells receive direct input from bipolar cells, *never* make reciprocal feedback synapses and are directly presynaptic to ganglion cell dendrites (Marc et al., 1988b; Muller and Marc, 1990; Marc, unpublished data; Fig. 8). This is consistent with the model of transient amacrine cell/ganglion cell circuitry proposed by Werblin (1972) for the mud puppy retina and elaborated more fully in ionic substitution and pharmacological studies (Miller and Dacheux, 1976; Slaughter and Miller, 1981; Slaughter and Miller, 1983). This particular circuit, BC > transient AC ≫ transient GC exempli-

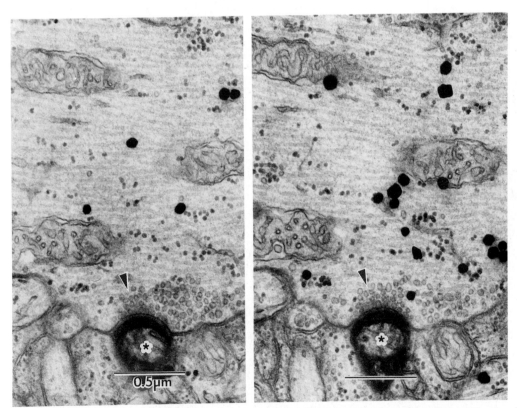

Fig. 8. A double label study of GABAergic amacrine cell inputs onto HRP-labeled ganglion cell dendrites. A pair of serial sections of GABAergic input (arrowhead) onto a ganglion cell dendrite near L70 (about sublayer 4) of the goldfish inner plexiform layer. The amacrine cell is probably a transient cell (see text). Reprinted by permission from Muller and Marc (1990) *J. Comp. Neurol.*, 291: 281–304.

fies the importance of the feedforward format. While it is crucial to mediate powerful surround inhibition for moving signals in the periphery, it is also critical that the bipolar cell stage remain uncorrupted by such a bandpassed surround signal. By extension, certain forms of color coding in

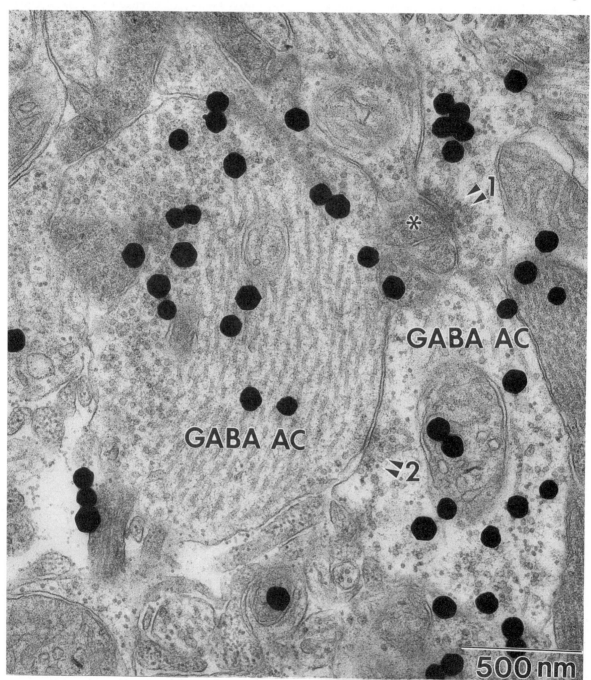

Fig. 9. A GABA AC > GABA AC synapse from mid-inner plexiform layer. Electron microscope autoradiography of [³H]GABA uptake with nipecotic acid coincubation (see text). One GABAergic amacrine cell dendrite makes two synapses, one onto a small unlabeled process (1) and the second onto a large, vesicle-rich GABAergic amacrine cell (2).

ganglion cell surrounds might indeed be mediated by feedforward instead of feedback designs. Such circuitry remains undiscovered.

*Disinhibitory circuits are present in the inner plexiform layer*

There is another common pattern of goldfish GABAergic microcircuitry: inhibitory concatenation through GABA AC ≫ GABA AC, GABA AC ≫ Gly AC, Gly AC ≫ GABA AC or Gly IPC ≫ GABA AC synapses. First, GABA AC ≫ GABA AC synapses have been observed frequently in the inner plexiform layer (Zucker et al., 1984; Muller and Marc, 1990 and unpublished data; Fig. 9) and likely represent disinhibitory connections between two different BC > GABA AC ≫ GC chains at the level of the amacrine cells, perhaps to mediate a process like double color opponency. Moreover, it is obvious that much if not all of the direct input to glycinergic amacrine cells must come from GABAergic amacrine cells since they are not driven by bipolar cells (Marc and Lam, 1981; Marc, 1989b; Yazulla, 1989; Muller and Marc, 1990). How this would ultimately shape glycinergic amacrine cell responses is not known. Conversely, non-GABAergic amacrine cell synapses are clearly made onto GABAergic profiles in the inner plexiform layer and two *minimum* chains are possible: (1) BC > GABA AC ≫ Gly AC ≫ GABA AC ≫ GC (net sign-inverting between the bipolar cell and ganglion cell) and (2) Gly IPC ≫ GABA AC > GC (discussed previously). The actual strengths and consequences of such connections cannot assessed by mere anatomy, but they could logically allow the center and surround balance of a single variety of coded vertical chain to be controlled by more than one kind of surround signal, analogous to the chain we have proposed for glycinergic interplexiform cell operations (Kalloniatis and Marc, 1990b). The remarkable current injection studies of Naka (1977 and following years) have shown at least two kinds of paths from amacrine cells to ganglion cells. For example, the path from sustained ON amacrine cells (probably GABAergic amacrine cells with direct ON bipolar cell input) to sustained ON ganglion cells is sign-inverting and probably monosynaptic. However, the current-driven path from sustained OFF amacrine cells to ON ganglion cells is sign-conserving. Since sustained OFF amacrine cells are almost certainly GABAergic, the most conservative interpretation is that this phenomenon represents the path: OFF BC > OFF GABA AC ≫ ON GABA AC ≫ ON GC. The meanings of such connections for ganglion cell function are certainly not apparent but, as mentioned, can be easily be justified by the need to construct complex ganglion cell surrounds.

## Summary of circuits, concepts and consequences

*Most synapses in the inner plexiform layer are GABAergic*

Autoradiographic or immunocytochemical images illustrate the richness of GABAergic profiles in the inner plexiform layer (e.g., Figs. 2,3b,7). Though we have not counted GABAergic synapses, the fractional volume of the inner plexiform layer comprised of GABAergic profiles is simple to assay with digital imaging (Marc et al., 1990). Applied to Fig. 2, GABAergic amacrine cell processes make up 87% of the inner plexiform layer in tiger salamander, 72% in goldfish and 74% in pigeon. And when we recall that the remaining volume must be partitioned among bipolar cells, ganglion cells, Müller's cells, dopaminergic interplexiform cells and glycinergic amacrine cells, the numerical dominance of GABAergic innervation seems unquestionable. Other than the important role it plays in spatial organization, it is also evident that inhibitory synapses have much lower gain than excitatory synapses if only because excitatory events can activate regenerative mechanisms in ganglion cells. If the relative GABAergic input to a bipolar cell terminal is a measure of the inhibition required to balance the potency of the bipolar cell output (akin to a stable DC level in an operational amplifier), the 5 to 1 dominance of GABAergic amacrine cell inputs to ribbon outputs (Marc, 1989b) is perhaps not very surprising. Finally, these values are similar to the determination by Koontz and Hendrickson (1990) that 70% of the amacrine cell profiles in the macaque were GABA immunoreactive.

*GABAergic horizontal cells and amacrine cells are the primary receptive field surround components of bipolar cell and ganglion cells*

The summary view of circuitry we now have for GABAergic neurons in the goldfish in particular and perhaps ectotherms in general (except for the glycinergic interplexiform cell) is presented in Fig. 10. Both ON and OFF center channels can be seen to be identical in construction past the photoreceptor synapse in terms of their relationships to the $C > BC > GC$ chain.

Even though there is now evidence for some form of direct sign-conserving path between GABAergic horizontal cells and bipolar cells (see Wu, Chapter 5) it remains likely that the strongest inhibitory path for horizontal cells to bipolar cells is via feedback to photoreceptors, primarily due to the large gain of the cone to bipolar cell synapse. Amacrine cells constitute an anatomically strong GABAergic input to bipolar cells both through reciprocal feedback (Fig. 10, path 1) and homologous/heterologous lateral feedback. Thus it would seem that the entire surround of the bipolar cell could be under direct GABAergic control. It is intriguing that bipolar cell surrounds are only completely abolished in salamander in the presence of both $GABA_A$ and $GABA_B$ blockade (see Hare and Owen, 1990; Slaughter and Pan, Chapter 3; Wu, Chapter 5). But an

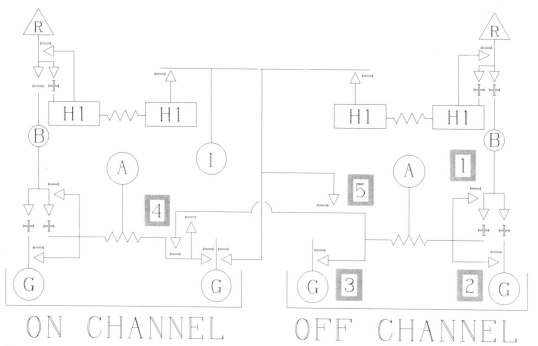

Fig. 10. A summary of GABAergic connections in the goldfish retina for both ON and OFF channels: sign conserving synapses ( + ); sign inverting synapses ( − ); resistor symbols indicate electrotonic coupling. The surround pathways to both types of red cone (R) > bipolar cell (B) > ganglion cell (G) chains from GABAergic horizontal (H) and (A) amacrine cells are identical in form. This figure deletes lamination rules associated with ON and OFF connectivities. Specific types of synaptic interactions include reciprocal feedback (1), near feedforward (2), far feedforward (3), GABA-GABA concatenation (4) and Gly-GABA concatenation (5). The proposed connections of glycinergic interplexiform cells (I) are taken from Kalloniatis and Marc (1990b). This system of connections generates antagonistic surrounds (paths 1,2,3) with the opportunity for other surround pathways to influence center-surround balance (4,5).

additional point is that horizontal cells are unlikely to be the sole or even the dominant determinants of bipolar cell surround features. The massive amacrine cell innervation cannot be ignored.

In a parallel fashion, though feedback to bipolar cells must influence the construction of ganglion cell surrounds, lateral surround inputs from extensive near feedforward (Fig. 10, path 2) and far feedforward (Fig. 10, path 3) must be considered as well. We do not yet know the relative numbers of inhibitory inputs and their dendritic placements, but these will be critical data for modeling receptive fields, especially since the bipolar cell → ganglion cell synapse is also likely to be a high gain step. The presence of concatenated GABAergic synapses in particular (Fig. 10, path 4) and glycine-GABA pairings may mediate disinhibition between various types of vertical chains and certainly can account for most of the patterns of signal transfer observed in current injection experiments. No specific receptive field functions have yet been convincingly attributed to concatenated inhibition. Finally, a particularly rich inhibitory path is exemplified by the flow of signals through the glycinergic interplexiform cell path to presumed GABAergic amacrine cells in the inner plexiform layer. If this is a valid pathway, it not only emphasizes the diversity of circuits possible with just a few "kinds" of inhibitory elements, but it also poses a pharmacological challenge. If this is indeed one parallel surround path, the application of strychnine would actually disinhibit the final GABAergic amacrine cell and change the center-surround balance without really blocking the surround in general. Moreover, since glycinergic amacrine cells are often final inputs in some chain to ganglion cells yet must receive their direct inputs from GABAergic amacrine cells, which also may have direct paths to the same ganglion cell dendrites, blockade with neither glycine nor GABA analogues alone would adequately dissect surround properties. The rules of circuitry need not make physiological analysis easy and the dearth of definitive

ganglion cell receptive field pharmacology using GABA agonists and antagonists is perhaps a testament to the need for combining structural data with (1) physiology and pharmacology from reduced models such as isolated cells (e.g., Ishida, Chapter 2) and the retinal slice preparation (Wu, Chapter 5) to aid in interpreting some of the data from intact retinal preparations. The advent of different $GABA_A$ receptor types with the potential for different conductance properties (Brecha, Chapter 1) and the distinctive and potent actions of $GABA_B$ receptors (Slaughter and Pan, Chapter 3) demonstrates that GABAergic circuitry involves a rich array of inhibitory devices for biological information processing.

## References

Agardh, E., Ehinger, B. and Wu, J.-Y. (1987a) GABA and GAD-like immunoreactivity in the primate retina. *Histochemistry*, 86: 485–490.

Agardh, E., Bruun, A., Ehinger, B., Ekstrom, P., van Veen, T. and Wu, J.-Y. (1987b) Gamma-aminobutyric acid- and glutamic acid decarboxylase-immunoreactive neurons in the retina of different vertebrates. *J. Comp. Neurol.*, 258: 622–630.

Ahnelt, P.K., Kolb, H. and Pflug, R. (1987) Identification of a subtype of cone photoreceptor, likely to be blue sensitive in the human retina. *J. Comp. Neurol.*, 255: 18–34.

Ayoub, G.S. and Lam, D.M.K. (1984) The release of γ-aminobutyric acid from horizontal cells of the goldfish (*Carassius auratus*) retina. *J. Physiol. (London)*, 355: 191–214.

Ayoub, G.S. and Lam, D.M.K. (1985) The content and release of endogenous GABA in isolated horizontal cells of the goldfish retina. *Vision Res.*, 25: 1187–1193.

Ball, A.K. (1987) Immunocytochemical and autoradiographic localization of GABAergic neurons in the goldfish retina. *J. Comp. Neurol.*, 255: 317–325.

Ball, A.K. and Brandon, C. (1986) Localization of [$^3$H]-GABA, -muscimol and -glycine in goldfish retinas stained for glutamate decarboxylase. *J. Neurosci.*, 6: 1621–1627.

Ball, A. and St. Denis, J. (1986) Displaced GABAergic amacrine cells in the ganglion cell layer of the goldfish retina. *Invest. Ophthal. Vis. Sci. Suppl.*, 27: 332.

Ball, A.K. and Tutton, D.A. (1990) Contacts between 'S1' amacrine cells and 'I1' interplexiform cells in the goldfish retina. *Invest. Ophthal. Vis. Sci. Suppl.*, 31: 333.

Barber, R. and Saito, K. (1976) Light microscopic visualization of GAD and GABA-T in immunocytochemical preparations of rodent CNS. In: E. Roberts, T.N. Chase and D.B. Tower (Eds.), *GABA in Nervous System Function*, Raven Press, NY, pp. 113–132.

Brandon, C. (1985) Retinal GABA neurons: localization in vertebrate species using an antiserum to rabbit brain glutamate decarboxylase. *Brain Res.*, 334: 286–295.

Brandon, C., Lam, D.M.K. and Wu, J.-Y. (1979) The gamma-aminobutyric acid system in the rabbit retina: localization by immunocytochemistry and autoradiography. *Proc. Natl. Acad. Sci. USA*, 76: 3557–3561.

Brandon, C., Lam, D.M.K. and Wu, J.-Y. (1980) Immunocytochemical localization of GABA neurons in the rabbit and frog retina. *Brain Res. Bull.*, 5 (Suppl 2): 21–29.

Brecha, N.C. (1983) Retinal transmitters: Histochemical and biochemical studies. In: P. Emson (Ed.), *Chemical Neuroanatomy*, Raven Press, New York, pp. 85–129.

Brecha, N.C., Johnson, D., Piechl, L. and Wässle, H. (1988) Cholinergic amacrine cells of the rabbit retina contain glutamate decarboxylase and γ-aminobutyric acid immunoreactivity. *Proc. Natl. Acad. Sci. USA*, 85: 6187–6191.

Brunken, W.J., Witkovsky, P. and Karten, H.J. (1984) Retinal neurochemistry of three elasmobranch species: An immunohistochemical approach. *J. Comp. Neurol.*, 243: 1–12.

Chun, M.H. and Wässle, H.(1989) GABA-like immunoreactivity in the cat retina: Electron microscopy. *J. Comp. Neurol.*, 279: 55–67.

Crescitelli, F. (1972) The visual cells and visual pigments of the vertebrate eye. In: H.J.A. Dartnall (Ed.) *Photochemistry of Vision. Handbook of Sensory Physiology* VII/1. Springer-Verlag, Berlin, pp. 245–363.

Dacheux, R. and Raviola, E. (1986) The rod pathway in the rabbit retina: A depolarizing bipolar and amacrine cell. *J. Neurosci.*, 6: 331–345.

Ehinger, B. (1970) Autoradiographic identification of rabbit retinal neurons that take up GABA. *Experientia (Basel)*, 26: 1063.

Ehinger, B., Narfström, K., Nilsson, S.E. and van Veen, T. (1991) photoreceptor degeneration and loss of immunoreactive GABA in the Abyssinian cat retina. *Exp. Eye Res.*, 52: 17–25.

Ehinger, B., O.P. Ottersen, J. Storm-Mathisen and J.E. Dowling (1988) Bipolar cells in the turtle retina are strongly immunoreactive for glutamate. *Proc. Nat. Acad. Sci. USA.*, 85:8321–8325

Engbretson, G., Anderson K.J. and Wu, J.-Y. (1988) GABA as a potential transmitter in lizard photoreceptors: immunocytochemical and biochemical evidence. *J. Comp. Neurol.*, 278: 461–471.

Famiglietti, E.V. Jr. and Kolb, H. (1975) A bistratified amacrine cell and synaptic circuitry in the inner plexiform layer of the retina. *Brain Res.*, 84: 293–300.

Fischer-Bovenkerk, C., Kish, P.E. and Veda, T. (1988) ATP-dependent glutamate uptake into synaptic vescicles from cerebellar mutant mice. *J. Neurochem.*, 42: 1054–1059.

Frumkes, T.E., Miller, R.F., Slaughter, M. And Dacheux, R. (1981) Physiological and pharmacological basis of GABA and glycine actions on neurons of the mudpuppy retina. III. Amacrine-mediated inhibitory influences on ganglion cell receptive field organization. *J. Neurophysiol.*, 45: 783–805.

Ishida, A.T., W.K. Stell and D.O. Lightfoot (1980) Rod and cone inputs to bipolar cells in goldfish retina. *J. Comp. Neurol.*, 191: 315–335.

Glaesner, G., Himstedt, W., Weiler, R. and Matute, C. (1988) Putative neurotransmitter in the retinae of three urodele species (*Triturus alpestris, Salamandra salamandra, Pleurodeles waltli*). *Cell Tissue Res.*, 252: 317–328.

Gottlieb, D.I., Chang, Y.C. and Schwob, J.E. (1986) Monoclonal antibodies to glutamic acid decarboxylase. *Proc. Natl. Acad. Sci. USA*, 83: 8808–8812.

Grünert, U. and Wässle, H. (1990) GABA-like immunoreactivity in the macaque monkey retina: A light and electron microscopic study. *J. Comp. Neurol.*, 297: 509–524.

Hare, W.A. and Owen, W.G. (1990) Spatial organization of the bipolar cell's receptive field in the retina of the tiger salamander. *J. Physiol. (London)*, 421: 223–245.

Hendrickson, A., Ryan, M., Noble, B. and Wu, J.-Y. (1985) Colocalization of ($^3$H) muscimol and antisera to GABA and glutamic acid decarboxylase within the same neurons in monkey retina. *Brain Res.*, 348: 391–395.

Hollyfield, J.G., Rayborn, M.E., Sarthy, P.V. and Lam, D.M.K. (1979) The emergence, localization and maturation of neurotransmitter systems during development of the retina in *Xenopus laevis*. I. γ-Aminobutyric acid. *J. Comp. Neurol.*, 188: 587–598.

Hurd II, L.B. and Eldred, W.D. (1989) Localization of GABA- and GAD-like immunoreactivity in the turtle retina. *Visual Neurosci.* 3: 9–20.

Ishida, A.T. (1989) GABA-activated currents in ganglion cells isolated from goldfish retina. In: R. Weiler and N.N. Osborne (Eds.), *Neurobiology of the Inner Retina, NATO ASI Series, Vol. H31a*, Springer-Verlag, Berlin, pp. 350–361.

Ishida, A.T. and Cohen, B.N. (1988) GABA-activated whole cell currents in isolated retinal ganglion cells. *J. Neurophysiol.*, 60: 381–396.

Ishida, A.T., Stell, W.K. and Lightfoot, D.O. (1980) Rod and cone inputs to bipolar cells in the goldfish retina. *J. Comp. Neurol.* 191: 315–335.

Iversen, L.L. (1984) Amino acids and peptides: fast and slow chemical signals in the nervous system? *Proc. Roy. Soc. London B*, 221: 245–260.

Kalloniatis, M. and R.E. Marc (1990a) Golgi impregnated bipolar cells of the goldfish retina. *Invest. Ophthal. Vis. Sci. Suppl.*, 30: 1019.

Kalloniatis, M. and R.E. Marc (1990b) Interplexiform cells of the goldfish retina. *J. Comp. Neurol.*, 297: 340–358.

Kaneko, A. and Tachibana, M. (1986a) Effects of γ-aminobutyric acid on isolated cone photoreceptors of the turtle retina. *J. Physiol. (London)*, 373: 443–461.

Kaneko, A. and Tachibana, M. (1986b) Blocking effects of cobalt and related ions on the γ-aminobutyric acid-induced current in turtle retinal cones. *J. Physiol. (London)*, 373: 463–479.

Kaufman, D.L., McGinnis J.F., Krieger, N.R. and Tobin, A.J. (1986) Brain glutamate decarboxylase cloned in kgt-11:

Fusion protein produces γ-aminobutyric acid. *Science*, 232: 1138–1140.

Kish, P.E., Fischer-Bovenkerk, C. and Ueda, T. (1989) Active transport of γ-aminobutyric acid and glycine into synaptic vesicles. *Proc. Natl. Acad. Sci. USA*, 86: 3877–3881.

Kolb, H. and Nelson, R. (1983) Rod pathways in the retina of the cat. *Vision Res.*, 23: 301–312.

Kondo, H. and Toyoda, J.-I. (1983) GABA and glycine effects on the bipolar cells of the carp retina. *Vision Res*,. 23: 1259–1264.

Koontz, M.A. and Hendrickson, A.E. (1990) Distribution of GABA-immunoreactive amacrine cell synapses in the inner plexiform layer of the macaque monkey retina. *Visual Neurosci.* 5: 17–28.

Lam, D.M.K. (1975) Biosynthesis of γ-aminobutyric acid by isolated axons of cone horizontal cell in the goldfish retina. *Nature*, 254: 345–347

Lam, D.M.K. (1976) Synaptic chemistry of identified cells in the vertebrate retina. *Cold Spring Harbor Symp. Quant. Biol.*, 40: 571–579.

Lam, D.M.K. and Steinman, L.E. (1971) The uptake of (γ-[3]H)aminobutyric acid in the goldfish retina. *Proc. Natl. Acad. Sci. USA* 68: 2777–2781.

Lam, D.M.K., Lasater, E. and Naka, K.-I. (1978) γ-Aminobutyric acid: A neurotransmitter candidate for cone horizontal cells of the catfish retina. *Proc. Natl. Acad. Sci. USA*, 75: 6310–6313.

Lam, D.M.K., Su, Y.Y.T., Swain, L., Marc, R.E., Brandon, C. and Wu, J.-Y. (1979b) Immunocytochemical localization of L-glutamic acid decarboxylase in the goldfish retina. *Nature*, 278: 565–567.

Legay, F., Henry, S., Tappaz, M. (1987) Evidence for two distinct forms of native glutamic acid decarboxylase in rat brain soluble extract: an immunoblotting study. *J. Neurochem.*, 48: 1022–1026.

Linn, D.L. and Massey, S.C. (1991) Acetylcholine release from the rabbit retina mediated by NMDA receptors. *J. Neurosci.*, 11: 123–133.

Linn, D.L., Blazynski, C., Redburn, D.A. and Massey, S.C. (1991) Acetylcholine release from the rabbit retina mediated by kainate receptors. *J. Neurosci.*, 11: 111–122..

Marc, R.E. (1982) Chromatic organization of the retina. In: D. McDevitt (Ed.), *Cellular Aspects of the Eye*, Academic Press, NY, pp. 435–473.

Marc R.E. (1986) Neurochemical stratification in the inner plexiform layer of the vertebrate retina. *Vision Res.*, 26: 223–238.

Marc, R.E. (1989a) The role of glycine in the mammalian retina. In: N. Osborne and G. Chader (Eds.) *Progress in Retinal Research*, Vol. 8, pp. 67–107., Pergamon Press, NY.

Marc, R.E. (1989b) The anatomy of multiple GABAergic and glycinergic pathways in the inner plexiform layer of the goldfish retina. In: R. Weiler and N.N. Osborne (Eds.), *Neurobiology of the Inner Retina, NATO ASI Series, Vol. H31a*, Springer-Verlag, Berlin, pp 53–64.

Marc, R. (1989c) Evolution of retinal circuits. In: J. Erber, R. Menzel, H.-J. Pfluger, D. Todt (Eds.), *Neural Mechanisms of Behavior, Proceedings of the 2nd International Congress of Neuroethology*, Thieme Medical Publishers, Inc., N.Y., pp. 146–147.

Marc, R.E. and Basinger, S.F. (1991) Glutamate, glutamine, aspartate, GABA and taurine levels in neurons, glia and vascular cells of the goldfish retina. *Invest. Ophthalmol. Vis. Sci. Suppl.*, 32: 1188.

Marc, R.E. and Lam, D.M.K. (1981) Glycinergic pathways in the goldfish retina. *J. Neurosci.*, 1: 152–165.

Marc, R.E. and Liu, W.-L.S. (1984) Horizontal cell synapses onto glycine-accumulating interplexiform cells. *Nature*, 311: 266–269.

Marc, R.E. and Sperling, H.G. (1976a) Color receptor identities of goldfish cones. *Science*, 191: 487–489.

Marc, R.E. and Sperling, H.G. (1976b) The chromatic organization of the goldfish cone mosaic. *Vision Res.*, 16: 1211–1224.

Marc, R.E., W.-L.S. Liu and J.F. Muller (1988b) Gap junctions in the inner plexiform layer of the goldfish retina. *Vision Res.*, 28: 9–24.

Marc, R.E., W.-L.S. Liu, K. Scholz and J.F. Muller (1988a) Serotonergic pathways in the goldfish retina. *J. Neuroscience.*, 8: 3427–3450.

Marc, R.E., Stell, W.K., Bok, D. and Lam, D.M.K. (1978) GABA-ergic pathways in the goldfish retina. *J. Comp. Neurol.*, 182: 221–246.

Marc, R.E., Liu, W.-L.S., Kalloniatis, M., Raiguel, S.F. and Van Haesendonck, E. (1990) Patterns of glutamate immunoreactivity in the goldfish retina. *J. Neurosci.*, 10: 4006–4034.

Mariani, A.P. and Caserta, M.T. (1986) Electron microscopy of glutamate-decarboxylase immunoreactivity in the inner plexiform layer of the rhesus monkey retina. *J. Neurocytol.*, 15: 645–655.

Marmarelis, P.Z. and Marmarelis, V.Z. (1978) *Analysis of Physiological Systems: The White-Noise Approach*. Plenum Press, NY, 487 pp.

Marshak, D.W. and Dowling, J.E. (1987) Synapses of cone horizontal cell axons in goldfish retina. *J. Comp. Neurol.*, 291: 281–304.

Marshall, J. and Voaden, M.J. (1974a) An investigation of the cells incorporating [3]H-GABA and [3]H-glycine in the isolated retina of the rat. *Exp. Eye. Res.*, 18: 367–370.

Marshall, J. and Voaden, M.J. (1974b) An autoradiographic study of the cells accumulating [3]H gamma-aminobutyric acid in the isolated retinas of pigeons and chickens. *Invest. Ophthalmol.*, 13: 602–607.

Marshall, J. and Voaden, M.J. (1975) Autoradiographic identification of cells accumulating [[3]H] γ-aminobutyric acid in mammalian retinae: A species comparison. *Vision Res.*, 15: 459–461.

Martin, D.L. (1987) Regulatory properties of brain glutamate decarboxylase. *Cellular and Molecular Neurobiology*, 7: 237–253.

Massey, S.C. (1990) Cell types using glutamate as a neurotransmitter in the vertebrate retina. In: N.N. Osborne and G. Chader (Eds.), *Progress in Retinal Research*, Vol. 9, Pergamon, London, pp. 399–425.

Massey, S.C., Blankenship, K. and Mills, S.L. (1991) Cholinergic amacrine cells in rabbit retina accumulate muscimol. *Visual Neurosci.*, 6: 113–117.

Massey, S.C., Mills, S.L. and Marc, R.E. (1991) Localization of indoleamine uptake and GABA markers in the rabbit retina. *Invest. Ophthalmol. Vis. Sci. Suppl.*, 32: 993.

Matthews, W.D. and Wickelgren, W.O. (1979) Glycine, GABA and synaptic inhibition of reticulospinal neurons of lamprey. *J. Physiol. (London)*, 293: 393–415.

Matute, C. and Streit, P. (1986) Monoclonal antibodies demonstrating GABA-like immunoreactivity. *Histochemistry* 86: 147–157.

Maycox, P.R., Deckworth T., Hell, J.W. and John, R. (1988) Glutamate uptake by brain synaptic vesicles. *J. Biol. Chem.*, 263: 15423–15428.

Miller, R.F. and Dacheux, R.F. (1976) Synaptic organization and ionic basis of on and off channels in mudpuppy retina. III. A model of ganglion cell receptive field organization based on chloride free experiments. *J. Gen. Physiol.*, 67: 679–690.

Mosinger, J.L, Yazulla, S. and Studholme, K.M. (1986) GABA-like immunoreactivity in the vertebrate retina: A species comparison. *Exp. Eye Res.*, 42: 631–644.

Muller, J.F. and Marc,, R.E. (1990) GABA-ergic and glycinergic pathways in the inner plexiform layer of the goldfish retina. *J. Comp. Neurol.*, 291: 281–304.

Murakami, M. and Shimoda, Y. (1975) Identification of amacrine and ganglion cells in the carp retina. *J. Physiol. London.*, 264: 801–818.

Murakami, M., Shimoda, Y., Nakatani, K., Miyachi, E.-I. and Watanabe, S.-I. (1982) GABA-mediated negative feedback from horizontal cells to cones in carp retina. Jpn. J. Physiol., 32: 9110926.

Nabors, L.B., Songu-Mize, E. and Mize, R.R. (1988) Quantitative immunocytochemistry using an image analyzer. II. Concentration standards for transmitter immunocytochemistry. *J. Neurosci. Methods*, 26: 25–34.

Naka, K.-I. (1977) Functional organization of catfish retina. *J. Neurophysiol.*, 40: 26–43.

Naka, K.-I. and Christensen, B. (1981) Direct electrical connections between transient amacrine cells in the catfish retina. *Science*, 214: 462–464.

Nakamura, Y., McGuire, B.A. and Sterling, P. (1980) Interplexiform cell in cat retina: identification by uptake of gamma-($^3$H)-aminobutyric acid and serial reconstruction. *Proc. nat. Acad. Sci. USA*, 77: 658–661.

Neal, M.J. and Iversen, L.L. (1972) Autoradiographic localization of $^3$H GABA in the rat retina. *Nature, New Biol.*, 235: 217–218.

Neal, M.J., Cunningham, J.R., Shah, M.A. and Yazulla, S. (1989) Immunocytochemical evidence that vigibatrin in rats causes GABA accumulation in glial cells of the retina. *Neurosci. Lett.*, 98: 29–32.

Negishi, K., Kato, K., Teranishi, T. and Laufer, M. (1978) Dual actions of some amino acids on spike discharges in the carp retina. *Brain Res.*, 148: 67–84.

Nishimura, Y., Schwartz, M.L. and Rakic, P. (1986) GABA and GAD immunoreactivity of photoreceptor terminals in primate retina. *Nature*, 320: 753–756.

Obata, K. (1976) Association of GABA with cerebellar Purkinje cells: Single cell analysis. In: E. Roberts, T.N. Chase and D.B. Tower (Eds.), *GABA in Nervous System Function*, Raven Press, NY, pp. 7–56.

O'Malley, D.M. and Masland, R.H. (1989) Co-release of acetylcholine and $\gamma$-aminobutyric acid by a retinal neuron. *Proc. Natl. Acad. Sci. USA*, 86: 3414–3418.

Ottersen, O.P. (1987) Postembedding light- and electron microscopic immunocytochemistry of amino acids: description of a new model system allowing identical conditions of specificity testing and tissue processing. *Exp. Brain Res.*, 69: 167–174.

Porter, T.G. and Martin, D.L. (1984) Evidence for feedback regulation of glutamic acid decarboxylase by $\gamma$-aminobutyric acid. *J. Neurochem.* 43: 1464–1467.

Pourcho, R.G. (1980) Uptake of $^3$H-glycine and $^3$H-GABA by amacrine cells in the cat retina. *Brain Res.*, 198: 333–346.

Pourcho, R.G. and Goebel, D.J. (1983) Neuronal subpopulations in cat retina which accumulate the GABA agonist [$^3$H]muscimol: A combined Golgi and autoradiographic study. *J. Comp. Neurol.*, 219: 25–35.

Pourcho, R.G., Goebel, D.J. and McReynolds, J.S. (1984) autoradiographic studies of [$^3$H]-glycine, [$^3$H]-GABA and [$^3$H]-muscimol uptake in the mudpuppy retina. *Exp. Eye Res.* 39: 69–81.

Radian, R., Ottersen, O.P., Storm-Mathisen, J., Castel, M. and Kanner, B.I. (1990) Immunocytochemical localization of the GABA transporter in rat brain. *J. Neurosci.*, 10: 1319–1330.

Ramon y Cajal, S. (1893) Les retine des vertebres. *La Cellule*, 9: 17–257.

Ratliff, F. (1971) The logic of the retina. In: M. Marois (Ed.), *From Theoretical Physics to Biology*, Proceedings of the Third International Conference. S. Karger, Basel, pp. 328–373.

Redburn, D.A. and Madtes Jr., P. (1986) Postnatal development of $^3$H-GABA-accumulating cells in rabbit retina. *J. Comp. Neurol.*, 243: 41–57.

Ripps, H. and Witkovsky, P. (1985) Neuron-glia interaction in brain and retina. In: N.N. Osborne and G.J. Chader (Eds.), *Progress in Retinal Research*, Vol. 4., Pergamon Press, Oxford, pp. 181–219.

Rubinson, K., K. Studholme and S. Yazulla (1989) Immunocytochemical distinction between inner and outer horizontal cells in the lamprey retina. *Soc. Neurosci. Abstr.*, 15: 1209.

Rubinson, K., K. Studholme and S. Yazulla (1990) Horizontal cells in the developing lamprey retina. *Invest. Ophthal. Vis. Sci. Suppl.*, 31: 159.

Sakai, H.M. and Naka, K.-I. (1988) Neuron network in catfish retina: 1967–1987. In: N. Osborne and G. Chader (Eds.), *Progress in Retinal Research*, Vol. 7, Pergamon Press, Oxford, pp. 149–208.

Sandell, J.H. and Masland, R.H. (1989) Shape and distribution of an unusual retinal neuron. *J. Comp. Neurol.*, 280: 489–497.

Sarthy, P.V. and Fu, M. (1989a) Localization of glutamic acid decarboxylase mRNA in monkey and human retina by in situ hybridization. *J. Comp. Neurol.*, 288: 691–697.

Sarthy, P.V. and Fu, M. (1989b) Localization of glutamic acid decarboxylase mRNA in cat retinal horizontal cells by in situ hybridization. *J. Comp. Neurol.*, 288: 593–600.

Schnitzer, J. and Russoff, A. (1984) Horizontal cells of the mouse retina contain glutamic acid decarboxylase-like immunoreactivity during early developmental stages. *J. Neurosci.*, 4: 2948–2955.

Scholes, J.H. (1975) Colour receptors and their synaptic connexions in the retina of a cyprinid fish. *Phil. Trans. R. Soc. London*, 270B: 61–118.

Schwartz, E.A. (1982) Calcium-independent release of GABA from isolated horizontal cells of the toad retina. *J. Physiol. (London)* 323: 211–227.

Schwartz, E.A. (1987) Depolarization without calcium can release γ-aminobutyric acid from a retinal neuron. *Science*, 238: 350–354.

Shepherd, G.M. and Koch, C. (1990) Introduction to synaptic circuits. In: G.M. Shepherd (Ed.), *The Synaptic Organization of the Brain*, Oxford University Press, NY, pp. 3–31.

Slaughter, M.M. and Miller, R.F. (1981) 2-Amino-4-phosphonobutyric acid: A new pharmacological tool for retina research. *Science*, 211: 182–184.

Slaughter, M.M. and Miller, R.F. (1983) An excitatory amino acid antagonist blocks cone input to sign-conserving second-order retinal neurons. *Science*, 219: 1230–1232.

Smiley, J.F. and Basinger, S.F. (1990) Glycine stimulates calcium-independent release of ³H-GABA from isolated retinas of *Xenopus laevis*. *Visual Neurosci.*, 4: 337–348.

Solimena, M., Folli, F., Aparisi, R., Pozza, G. and De Camilli, P. (1990) Autoantibodies to GABA-ergic neurons and pancreatic beta cells in Stiff-Man syndrome. *New Engl. J. Med.*, 322: 1555–1560.

Spink, D.C., Parter, T.G., Wu, S.J. and Martin, D.L. (1985) Characterization of three kinetically distinct forms of glutamate decarboxylase from pig brain. *Biochem. J.*, 231: 695–703.

Stell, W.K. (1967) The structure and relationships of horizontal cells and photoreceptor-bipolar synaptic complexes in the goldfish retina. *Am. J. Anat.*, 121: 401–424.

Stell, W.K. and Hárosi, F.I. (1976) Cone structure and visual pigment content in the retina of the goldfish, *Carassius auratus*. *Vision Res.* 16: 647–657.

Storm-Mathisen, J., Leknes, A.K., Bore, A.T., Vaaland, J.L., Edminson, P., Huang, F.M.S. and Otterson, O.P. (1983) First visualization of glutamate and GABA in neurons by immunocytochemistry. *Nature*, 301: 517–520.

Studholme, K.M. and Yazulla, S. (1988) Localization of GABA and glycine in goldfish retina by electron microscopic postembedding immunocytochemistry: improved visualization of synaptic structures with LR white resin. *J. Neurocytol.*, 17: 859–870.

Strettoi, E., Dacheux, R.F. and Raviola, E. (1990) Synaptic connections of rod bipolar cells in the inner plexiform layer of the rabbit retina. *J. Comp. Neurol.*, 295: 449–466.

Tachibana, M. and Kaneko, A. (1987) Gamma-aminobutyric acid exerts a local inhibitory on the axon terminal of bipolar cells: Evidence for negative feedback from amacrine cells. *Proc. Natl. Acad. Sci. USA*, 84: 3501–3505.

Teranishi, R., Negishi, K. and Kato, S. (1984) Dye coupling between amacrine cells in carp retina. *Neurosci. Lett.*, 51: 73–78.

Van Haesendonck, E. and Missotten, L. (1984) Synaptic contacts between bipolar and photoreceptor cells in the retina of *Callionymus lyra* L. *J. Comp. Neurol.*, 223: 387–399.

Van Haesendonck, E., Marc, R.E. and Missotten, L. (1991) Electron microscopic immunocytochemistry of the dopaminergic interplexiform cell arborization in the outer plexiform layer of the goldfish retina. *Invest. Ophthalmol. Vis. Sci. Suppl.*, 32: 1260.

Vaney, D.I. and Young, H.M. (1988) GABA-like immunoreactivity in cholinergic amacrine cells of the rabbit retina. *Brain Res.*, 438: 369–373.

Vaughn, J.E., Famiglietti, E.V. Jr., Barber, R.P., Saito, K., Roberts, E. and Ribak, C. (1981) GABAergic amacrine cells in rat retina: Immunocytochemical identification and synaptic connectivity. *J. Comp. Neurol.*, 197: 113–127.

Voaden, M.J., Marshall, J. and Murani, N. (1974) The uptake of (³H) gamma-aminobutyric acid and (³H) glycine by the isolated retina of the frog. *Brain Res.*, 67: 115–132.

Walls, G.L. (1942) *The Vertebrate Eye and Its Adaptive Radiation*. Cranbrook Institute of Science, Bloomfield Hills, MI, USA.

Watt, C.B., Li, T., Lam, D.M.K., and Wu, S.M. (1987) Interactions between enkephalin and γ-aminobutyric acid in the larval tiger salamander retina. *J. Physiol. (London)* 280: 449–470.

Werblin, F. (1972) Lateral interactions at the inner plexiform layer of vertebrate retina: Antagonistic responses to change. *Science*, 175: 1008–1010.

Wu, J.-Y. (1976) Purification, characterization and kinetic studies of GAD and GABA-T from mouse brain. In: E. Roberts, T.N. Chase and D.B. Tower (Eds.), *GABA in Nervous System Function* Raven Press, NY, pp. 7–56.

Wu, J.-Y., Denner, L.A., Wei, S.C., Lin C.-T., Song, G.-X., Xu, Y.F., Liu, J.W. and Lin, H.S. (1986) Production and characterization of polyclonal and monoclonal antibodies to rat brain L-glutamate decarboxylase. *Brain Res.*, 373: 1–14.

Wu, S.M. (1986) Effects of gamma-aminobutyric acid on cones and bipolar cells of the tiger salamander retina. *Brain Res.*, 365: 70–77.

Wässle, H. and Chun, M.H. (1988) Dopaminergic and indoleamine-accumulating amacrine cells express GABA-like immunoreactivity in the cat retina. *J. Neurosci.*, 8: 3383–3394.

Wässle, H. and Chun, M.H. (1989) GABA-like immunoreactivity in the cat retina: light microscopy. *J. Comp. Neurol.*, 279: 43–54.

Yang, C.Y. and Yazulla, S. (1988) Localization of putative GABAergic neurons in the larval tiger salamander by immunocytochemical and autoradiographical methods. *J. Comp. Neurol.*, 272: 343–357.

Yazulla, S. (1983) Stimulation of GABA release from retinal horizontal cells by potassium and acidic amino acid agonists. *Brain Res.*, 275: 61–74.

92

Yazulla, S. (1986) GABAergic mechanisms in retina. In: N. Osborne and J. Chader (Eds.), *Progress in Retinal Research, Vol. 5.*, Pergamon Press, NY, pp. 1–52.

Yazulla, S. (1989) Transmitter-specific synaptic contacts involving mixed rod-cone bipolar cell terminals in goldfish retina. In: R. Weiler and N.N. Osborne (Eds.), *Neurobiology of the Inner Retina, NATO ASI Series, Vol. H31a*, Springer-Verlag, Berlin, pp. 91–102.

Yazulla, S. and Brecha, N.C. (1980) Binding and uptake of the GABA analogue, $^3$H-muscimol, in the retinas of goldfish and chick. *Invest. Ophthalmol.*, 19: 1415–1426.

Yazulla, S. and Kleinschmidt, J. (1983) Carrier mediated release of GABA from retinal horizontal cells. *Brain Res.*, 263: 63–75.

Yazulla, S. and Studholme, K.M. (1987) Ultracytochemical distribution of ouabain-sensitive, $K^+$-dependent, p-nitrophenylphosphatase in the synaptic layers of goldfish retina. *J. Comp. Neurol.*, 261–74–84.

Yazulla, S. and Studholme, K.M. (1990) Multiple subtypes of glycine-immunoreactive neurons in the goldfish retina: Single and double-label studies. *Visual Neurosci.*, 4: 299–309..

Yazulla, S. and Yang, C.-Y. (1988) Colocalization of GABA and glycine immunoreactivities in a subset of retinal neurons in the tiger salamander. *Neurosci. Lett.*, 95: 37–41.

Yazulla, S., Studholme, K. and Wu, J.-Y. (1986) Comparative distribution of $^3$H-GABA uptake and GAD immunoreactivity in goldfish retinal amacrine cells: A double label analysis. *J. Comp. Neurol.*, 244: 149–162.

Yazulla, S., Studholme, K. and Wu, J.-Y. (1987) GABAergic input to the synaptic terminals of mb$_1$ bipolar cells in the goldfish retina. *Brain Res.*, 411: 400–405.

Yazulla, S., Studholme, K. and Zucker, C.L. (1985) Synaptic organization of Substance P-like immunoreactive amacrine cells in goldfish retina. *J. Comp. Neurol.*, 231: 232–238.

Zucker, C.L., Yazulla, S. and Wu, J.-Y. (1984) Non-correspondence of $^3$H-GABA uptake and GAD localization in goldfish amacrine cells. *Brain Res.*, 298: 154–158.

R.R. Mize, R.E. Marc and A.M. Sillito (Eds.)
Progress in Brain Research, Vol. 90

CHAPTER 5

# Functional organization of GABAergic circuitry in ectotherm retinas

Samuel M. Wu

*Cullen Eye Institute, Baylor College of Medicine, Houston, TX 77030, USA*

## Introduction

In the vertebrate retina, photoreceptors trans-duce light into electrical signals that are transmit-ted to retinal ganglion cells, the output neurons of the retina, along two pathways. The central pathway consists of photoreceptor-bipolar cell and bipolar cell-ganglion cell synapses whereas the lateral pathway consists of the input and output synapses of horizontal cells and amacrine cells, the lateral interneurons of the retina. The central and lateral pathways are responsible for mediat-ing the center-surround antagonistic receptive fields of retinal bipolar cells and ganglion cells. Such receptive fields are believed to be the basic alphabet for encoding spatial information in the visual system (Hubel and Wiesel, 1961, 1962). The neurotransmitter used by synapses in the central pathway is probably glutamate, which, except in one synapse, exerts excitatory (or sign-preserving) actions on postsynaptic neurons (Copenhagen and Jahr, 1988; Slaughter and Miller, 1981, 1983a,b; Nawy and Jahr, 1990; Yang and Wu, 1990). The neurotransmitters used by synapses in the lateral pathway are mainly in-hibitory (sign-inverting), which include gamma-aminobutyric acid (GABA), glycine and in some species dopamine and serotonin (Marc et al., 1978; Marc, 1985; Ehinger and Dowling, 1987). The main function of these inhibitory neurotrans-mitters is to provide antagonistic surround inputs

to bipolar cells and ganglion cells. Additionally, these neurotransmitters may be used to modulate various functions of retinal neurons.

The best studied neurotransmitter in the lat-eral synaptic pathway is GABA. At least in ec-totherms, GABA is used by subpopulations of horizontal cells and amacrine cells as their neuro-transmitter, and it exerts postsynaptic actions on cones, bipolar cells and ganglion cells. In this chapter, I shall review some of the studies con-cerning GABAergic synapses in ectotherm reti-nas. These studies not only help us understand how GABAergic synapses work, but also provide important information on how lateral synapses in general (GABAergic or not) function and how the center-surround antagonistic receptive fields are formed in the retina.

Figure 1 depicts the major synaptic connec-tions between various cell types in the retina. The left portion shows the synaptic organization of the on- or depolarizing bipolar cell (DBC)-path-way whereas the right portion shows the off- or hyperpolarizing bipolar cell (HBC)-pathway. Ma-jor GABAergic synapses are marked by numbers in Fig. 1: (1) feedback synapses from HC to cones; (2) feedforward synapses from HC to bipo-lar cells; (3) feedback synapses from amacrine cell to bipolar cell terminals; (4) feedforward synapses from amacrine cells to ganglion cells; (5) amacrine-amacrine cell synapses. In addition to these five types of GABAergic synapses, GABA

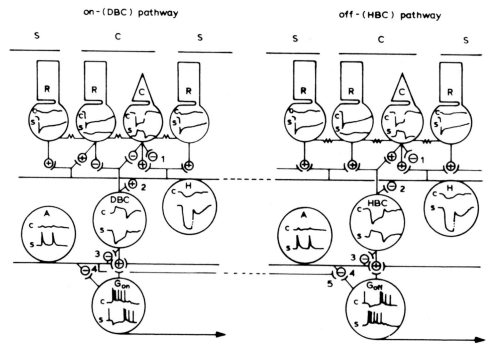

Fig. 1. Summary diagram of major synaptic connections of the on-(DBC) pathway (left) and off-(HBC) pathway (right). Voltage responses to center (C) and surround (S) light stimuli are shown in each cell. R, rod; C, cone; DBC, depolarizing bipolar cell; HBC, hyperpolarizing bipolar cell; H, horizontal cell; A, amacrine cell; $G_{on}$, on ganglion cell; $G_{off}$, off ganglion cell; (⤳) electrical synapse; (+), sign-preserving chemical synapse; (−), sign-inverting chemical synapses. Synapses marked 1–5 are possible GABAergic synapses which are described in the text.

receptors may exist in synapses between photoreceptors and HCs in some vertebrate species (Yang and Wu, 1989b). In the following sections, I shall describe mechanisms and functions of the five GABAergic synapses shown in Fig. 1. Moreover, the modulatory actions of GABA on retinal neurons will also be discussed.

## GABAergic synapses in the outer retina

In the ectotherm retina, GABA is used by populations of horizontal cells (HCs) as their neurotransmitter (see Marc, Chapter 4). HC outputs are probably mediated by the HC-cone feedback synapse and the HC-bipolar cell feedforward synapse (Fig. 1). In this section, I shall focus on two ectotherms, the tiger salamander (Class Amphibian) and the teleost fish (Class Osteichthyes), with emphasis on the basic synaptic mechanisms in the former, and the circuitry mediating color

information processing in the latter. Immunocytochemical localization of GABA in the tiger salamander and teleost fish retinas are given in Chapter 4 of this volume.

### Feedback synapses between HCs and cones

Figure 2A shows the effects of bicuculline, a $GABA_A$ antagonist, on the feedback depolarizing signals in cones of the tiger salamander. The left traces are the simultaneous light responses of a cone whose outer segment is truncated (i.e., broken off to eliminate the masking effect of phototocurrent on the feedback light response) and a HC. Detailed description of the truncated cone preparation is given elsewhere (Wu, 1991). In the presence of 100 $\mu$M bicuculline (right traces), the feedback response in cones is suppressed whereas the HC response (the presynaptic response to the feedback response) is unaffected. This result is consistent with the notion that salamander HCs use GABA as their neurotransmitter and the HC-cone feedback synapse is probably a sign-inverting chemical synapse mediated by $GABA_A$ receptors. Certain studies have indicated that GABA receptors other than bicuculline-sensitive $GABA_A$ forms mediate HC to cone feedback (O'Hare and Owen, 1990; Slaughter and Pan, Chapter 3). However, on balance, the results of Wu (1991) and others strongly favor the involvement of $GABA_A$ receptors in HC-cone feedback synapse.

Figure 2B shows the feedback depolarizing signal in cones reverses near the membrane voltage polarized by $-0.1$ nA of current injection. The input resistance of the cones is about 250 $M\Omega$ and the reversal potential ($E_s$) of the feedback synapse in cones is estimated to be about

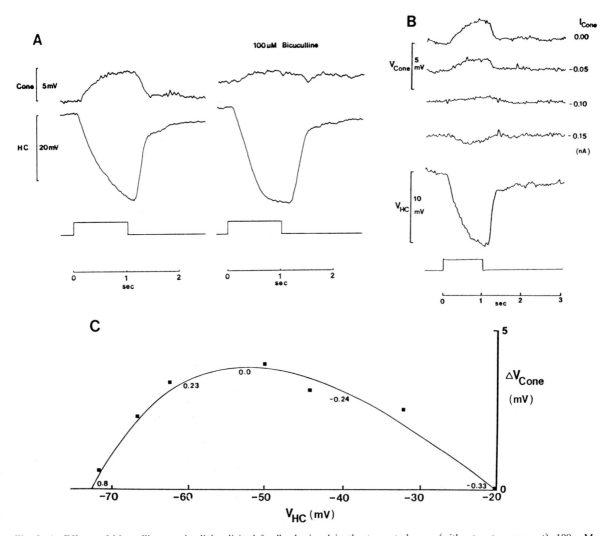

Fig. 2. A. Effects of bicuculline on the light-elicited feedback signal in the truncated cone (without outer segment). 100 $\mu$M bicuculline suppressed the feedback signal in cone but exert little effect on the simultaneously recorded HC. This result suggests that the feedback synapse from HCs to cones is probably mediated by $GABA_A$ receptors. B. Effects of membrane hyperpolarization on the feedback signals in the truncated cone. The depolarizing feedback signal reversed at about $V_{cone} = -67$ mV $[V_{rest} + I_c R_c = -40$ mV $+ (-0.11$ nA)(250 $M\Omega$)]. C. Input-output relation of the HC cone feedback synapse for light-evoked responses. The curve is bell-shaped with slope gains ($-0.33$ to $+0.8$) marked at various HC voltages (from Wu, 1991).

−67 mV (Wu, 1991). Based on this observation, one can conclude that the light-evoked feedback signals in cones are controlled by two factors: (1) the magnitude of GABA-mediated postsynaptic conductance decrease *increases* as brighter light gives rise a larger HC hyperpolarization; and (2) the driving force $(V - E_s)$ of the postsynaptic current *decreases* as brighter light hyperpolarizes the cones closer to the reversal potential of the feedback synapse. These two factors exert opposite effects on the postsynaptic responses and thus result in a bell-shaped input-output relation for the light-evoked feedback signals (Fig. 2C). The slope gain of the feedback synapse is negative at low light intensities (small HC responses) and positive at high light intensities (large HC responses). The maximum feedback signal in cones is observed when $V_{HC}$ is hyperpolarized to approximately −52 mV (slope gain is zero).

In the teleost fish, the feedback circuitry from HCs to cones is more complex. There are three spectral classes of cones and three types of cone-driven HCs which exhibit different response patterns to stimuli of various wavelengths. The synaptic contacts of the cone-HC cascade in the goldfish retina are shown in Fig. 3A (Stell and Lightfoot, 1975). The H1 HCs (L-type) receive sign-preserving synaptic inputs primarily from red-sensitive cones (R-cones) and they feedback (via presumably sign-inverting synapses, like the salamander feedback synapse) to all three types of cones (R-cones, G-cones and B-cones). The H2 HCs (biphasic C-type) receive sign-preserving inputs from G-cones which consist of responses derived from the G-cone photocurrent and from the H1 HCs through the feedback synapse. This synaptic arrangement results in hyperpolarizing responses to short-wavelength stimuli and depolarizing responses to long-wavelength stimuli in H2 HCs. The H3 (triphasic C-type) HCs receive sign-preserving input from B-cones which consist of responses derived from B-cone photocurrent and from the H1 and H2 HCs through feedback synapses. This arrangement gives rise to hyperpolarizing responses to long- and short- wavelength

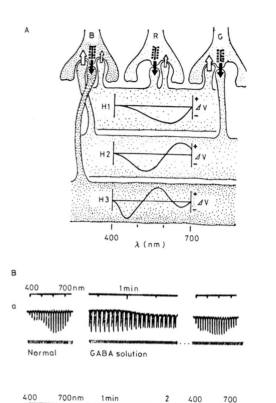

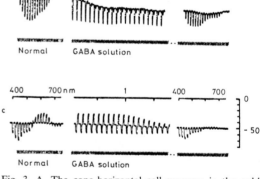

Fig. 3. A. The cone-horizontal cell synapses in the goldfish retina. B, R and G are blue-, red- and green-sensitive cones; H1, H2 and H3 are monophasic (L-type), biphasic (C-type) and triphasic (C-type) HCs, respectively. Solid arrows are sign preserving synapses, whereas open arrows are sign-inverting synapses (from Stell and Lightfoot, 1975). B. Effects of GABA on the monophasic (a), biphasic (b) and triphasic (c) HCs in the carp retina (from Murakami et al, 1982a,b).

stimuli and depolarizing responses to medium-wavelength stimuli (Fig. 3A).

Autoradiographic and immuncytochemical evidence has shown that H1 HCs in the teleost fish probably use GABA as the neurotransmitter (see Marc, Chapter 4). Murakami and co-workers (Murakami et al., 1982a,b) therefore examined the effects of GABA on the H1, H2 and H3 HCs in the carp retina. Figure 3B shows that application of GABA selectively suppresses the depolarizing responses of H2 HCs to long-wavelength stimuli, and the responses of H3 HCs to medium- and long-wavelength stimuli. Their findings are consistent with Stell's model (Fig. 3A) which predicts that application of GABA saturates all feedback synapses from H1 HCs and thus leaves the H2 and H3 HC responses solely mediated by the G-cone and B-cone photocurrents, respectively. A problem in this argument is that H2 HCs appear not to be GABAergic, the depolarizing responses to medium-wavelength in H3 HCs should persist in the presence of GABA. One possible explanation of the absence of H3 depolarizing responses in GABA is that the GABAergic feedback synapse from H1 to B-cones may interact with the non-GABAergic feedback synapse from H2 to B-cones. An alternative explanation is that the H2 neurotransmitter is GABA-like, thus application of GABA blocks the H2-H3 synapse.

*Feedforward synapses between horizontal cells and bipolar cells*

It has been more than twenty years since chemical synapses between HCs and bipolar cells were observed anatomically (Dowling and Werblin, 1969). Nevertheless, direct demonstration of signal transmission across these synapses has been difficult, because it is hard to distinguish between the HC-cone-bipolar feedback signal and the HC-bipolar feedforward signal (Naka, 1972). Recently, by selectively blocking the photoreceptor-DBC synapses with L-AP4, Yang and Wu have been able to demonstrate a sustained hyperpolarizing response in DBCs in the tiger salamander retina. This sustained hyperpolarizing response in the presence of L-AP4 is probably mediated by the HC-DBC feedforward synapse and analysis of

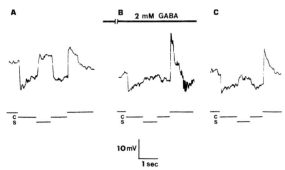

Fig. 4. Effects of 2 mM GABA on the center (C) and surround (S) responses of the HBC. The surround response is selectively suppressed, indicative of the involvement of GABAergic HCs and/or amacrine cells in mediating the surround responses of bipolar cells (from Wu, 1986).

this and the feedback responses suggests that the feedforward synapse contributes about one-quarter to one-third of the surround responses of the DBCs (Yang and Wu, 1991). At the present time, there are no compounds which can selectively block the photoreceptor-HBC synapses without affecting the HC responses. Therefore it is not yet possible to demonstrate signal transmission across the HC-HBC feedforward synapse, although there is no reason to believe that the lateral synaptic arrangements in DBC and HBC are different.

Figure 4 shows the effect of GABA on HBCs in the tiger salamander retina. Application of 2 mM GABA suppresses the surround response without affecting the center response. The surround response partially recovers after GABA removal. This result is consistent with the notion that GABAergic HCs in the tiger salamander retina are responsible for mediating the surround responses in bipolar cells. If the surround response of the HBC is mediated by both the feedback and feedforward synapses, this result also implies that both synapses are probably GABAergic.

In the fish retina, evidence of GABA actions on HC-bipolar cell feedforward synapses is sparse. Iontophoretic application of GABA in the outer retina elicits little response in bipolar cells (Kondo and Toyoda, 1983). Similar results are obtained from isolated fish bipolar cells while GABA is applied to the dendritic or somatic regions (Tachibana and Kaneko, 1987). These results suggest that the GABAergic H1 HCs in the fish retina probably do not make feedforward synapses on bipolar cells.

## GABAergic synapses in the inner retina

In most vertebrate species, several subpopulations of amacrine cells (ACs) use GABA as their neurotransmitter (see Marc, Chapter 4, and Freed, Chapter 6). These GABAergic amacrine cells make synapses on bipolar cell axon termi-

nals, other amacrine cells and ganglion cells in the inner plexiform layer.

*Feedback synapses between GABAergic amacrine cells and bipolar cells*

Anatomical evidence has revealed that in most vertebrate retinas, amacrine cells make chemical synapses on bipolar cell axon terminals (Dowling and Werblin, 1969; Wong-Riley, 1974). In the goldfish, several types of amacrine cells make GABAergic synapses onto bipolar cell terminals (Marc et al., 1978; Marc, 1989). Iontophoretic application of GABA in the inner plexiform layer

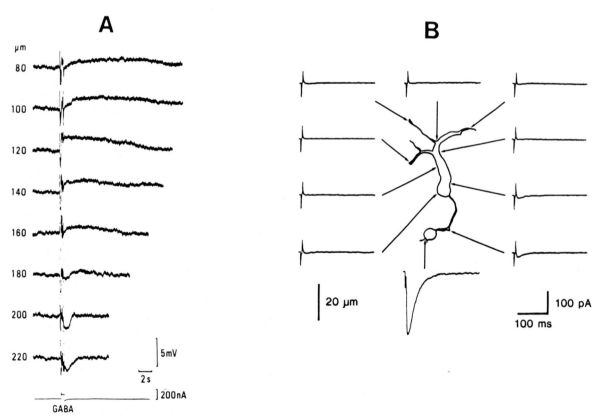

Fig. 5. A. Responses of a DBC in the carp retina to GABA applied at various retinal depths (from the photoreceptor side, marked by numbers, in $\mu$m, on the left of each trace (from Hondo and Toyoda, 1983). B. GABA-induced responses recorded from a solitary bipolar cell of the goldfish. GABA was applied iontophoretically to various parts of the cell clamped at −66 mV. The largest current was observed when GABA was applied to the axon terminal region of the bipolar cell (from Tachibana and Kaneko, 1987).

elicit large responses in bipolar cells (Fig. 5A), and isolated fish bipolar cells exhibit high GABA sensitivity near the axon terminal region (Fig. 5B). These results strongly suggest that GABAergic amacrine cells exert feedback actions on bipolar cell terminals in the teleost retina.

In the tiger salamander, the slow narrow-field amacrine cells probably use GABA. Maguire et al. (1989a,b) have shown that application of baclofen, a $GABA_B$ receptor agonist, reduces the L-type calcium current in bipolar cell axon terminals and makes the bipolar cell output more transient, through the action of a G-protein (Fig. 6, see also Slaughter and Pan, Chapter 3). This baclofen-induced reduction of calcium current is probably involved in modulating glutamate release from bipolar cell terminals to amacrine cells and ganglion cells.

*Feedforward synapses from amacrine cells to ganglion cells*

GABAergic inputs in retinal ganglion cells have been intensively studied in the mudpuppy retina by Frumkes et al. (1981). These authors suggest that the on-type, off-type and on-off type ganglion cell receive inhibitory inputs from GABAergic amacrine cells which may be either on-off amacrine cells or sustained on amacrine cells. A summary of their work is given in Fig. 7. GABAergic amacrine cells appear to primarily inhibit the on ganglion cells but not the off cells, in the catfish and skate (Lasater and Lam, 1984; Cohen, 1985), but the consequences of GABA uptake in the inner plexiform layer may complicate these conclusions (see Marc, Chapter 4). The GABAergic amacrine-ganglion cell synapses, along with the GABAergic amacrine-bipolar cell synapses, form a network of lateral connections in the inner plexiform layer that are responsible for mediating the antagonistic surround responses of retinal ganglion cells. It is also noteworthy that 87% of the isolated goldfish ganglion cells recorded by Ishida and Cohen (1988) exhib-

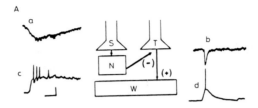

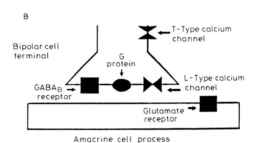

Fig. 6. A. Scheme for interactions mediating change detection. *Vertical arrows* represent glutamate pathways; *diagonal arrow* indicates a GABA pathway. The slow narrow field amacrine cell (N) receives excitatory input (a) from a slow bipolar cell terminal (S). The output of this cell (c) in turn feeds back to a separate class of transient bipolar terminals (T), truncating release from this terminal via a $GABA_B$ receptor. (The slow amacrine cell also inhibits the fast wide field amacrine cell (W) directly via a $GABA_A$ receptor.) The traces represent inferred signals in this pathway. a. Inferred output of the sustained bipolar terminal recorded as the excitatory synaptic current in the narrow field amacrine cell. b. Inferred output of the transient or fast bipolar terminal recorded as the excitatory current in the wide field amacrine cell. c. Output of the narrow field amacrine cell recorded under current clamp. This is a steadily spiking signal. d. Output of the wide field amacrine cell recorded under current clamp, showing single-spike activity (from Maguire et al., 1989a). B. Circuitry for the $GABA_B$ modulatory pathway that blocks an excitatory input to a class of amacrine cell. A GABA input from a separate class of GABAergic, narrow field, sustained amacrine cells impinges upon the $GABA_B$ receptors at the bipolar-amacrine cell synapse. The $GABA_B$ receptors act by way of G proteins to down-regulate L-type calcium currents at the terminals. The T-type calcium channels are located at other sites, including the soma and/or dendrites and are not modulated by the $GABA_B$ pathway (from Maguire et al., 1989b).

ited GABA activated currents and that goldfish off ganglion cells have GABAergic synapses on their dendrites (Muller and Marc, 1990).

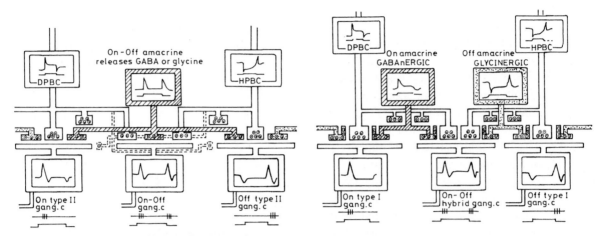

Fig. 7. A model of the GABAergic and glycinergic pathways in the mudpuppy inner retina (updated by R.F. Miller from Figs. 14 and 15 of Frumkes et al., 1981).

*Amacrine-amacrine cell synapses*

Anatomical evidence has shown that numerous chemical synapses are formed between amacrine cells in the vertebrate retina. Some of these synapses are serial and some are reciprocal (Dowling, 1987). In the tiger salamander, application of GABA elicits a postsynaptic response in the transient wide-field amacrine cells through

perhaps $GABA_A$ receptors. The reversal potential is about $-60$ mV, indicative of the involvement of chloride conductance (Maguire et al., 1989b).

## Modulatory roles of GABA in the retina

In addition to the neurotransmitter actions described in the previous sections, GABA appears

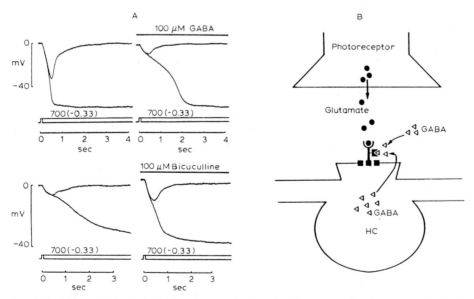

Fig. 8. A. Effects of GABA and bicuculline on horizontal cell response rise time (HCRRT). B. Summary diagram illustrating possible mechanisms of GABA-mediated modulation of the HCRRT (from Yang and Wu, 1989b).

to act like a neuromodulator in some synapses in the ectotherm retinas. The neurotransmitter actions of GABA are fast, short-lasting and probably directly involved in gating of postsynaptic chloride channels. The neuromodulatory actions, on the other hand, are usually slow, long-lasting and probably involved in long-term modification of synaptic efficacy and/or kinetics. Figure 8A shows that effects of GABA and bicuculline on the horizontal cell response rise time (HCRRT) in the tiger salamander retina. Under dark-adapted conditions, the HCRRT is slow, with a time-to-peak of about 3 s, and under light-adapted conditions, the HCRRT becomes much faster (time-to-peak ~ 0.8 s). This adaptation-induced change in HCRRT can be mimicked by application of GABA or bicuculline (Yang and Wu, 1989b). Application of 100 $\mu$M GABA mimics dark-adaptation and 100 $\mu$M of bicuculline mimics light-adaptation. Since HCs are the primary neurons in the outer retina that contain GABA, it is possible that GABA is released continuously in darkness from HCs and it self-regulates (slows down the kinetics) the postsynaptic receptor-channel complexes in the HC membrane. Under light-adapted conditions, HCs are hyperpolarized and thus the rate of GABA released is reduced. HCRRT becomes faster. This can also be achieved by bicuculline, which antagonises the self-regulating action of GABA. A summary diagram illustrating the possible mechanisms underlying the modulation of HCRRT by GABA is given in Fig. 8B.

## Functions of GABAergic synapses in the retina

GABA is one of the major inhibitory neurotransmitters in the vertebrate retina and at least in ectotherms, it is involved in every type of lateral synapse in both plexiform layers. By analyzing the functions of GABAergic synapses, we may not only understand how GABA mediates visual information processing, but also gain considerable insights of how lateral inhibitory synapses in retina

function in general. There are at least six functions of GABAergic synapses in the retina:

### (a) GABAergic synapses set up negative feedback systems for the photoreceptor-bipolar-ganglion cell pathway

Evidence described in this article indicates that at least some of the HC-cone and AC-bipolar cell feedback synapses are GABAergic and sign-inverting. These synapses constitute negative feedback circuits in the photoreceptor-bipolar and bipolar-ganglion cell synapses. Based on the principles of system analysis, negative feedback improves the reliability, signal-to-noise ratio, response band width and stability of the forward signals (Marmarelis and Marmarelis, 1978). In the retina, the photoreceptor-bipolar-ganglion cell synapses constitute the direct and express route for signal transmission between the photoreceptors and the brain, the GABAergic negative feedback synapses help to secure the performance and accuracy of signal transfer in this pathway.

### (b) GABAergic feedback synapses modulate dynamic range of retinal neurons

In the vertebrate retina, different types of neurons operate within different light intensity (dynamic) ranges. The dynamic range for photoreceptors and horizontal cells, for example, are much wider than those of the bipolar cells and ganglion cells (Werblin, 1972). Since photoreceptor-bipolar synaptic transmission is limited within a window of the photoreceptor voltage (Belgum and Copenhagen, 1987; Wu 1988b), a tonic negative feedback signal can shift the dynamic range of bipolar cells towards the right in the intensity axis (Fig. 9). Physiologically, when a steady background illumination tonically activates the feedback synapses between HCs and cones, the operating range of the bipolar cells shift to the right so that a brighter light stimulus is required to generate a given bipolar cell response. This type of feedback-mediated reset in light sensitivity may

102

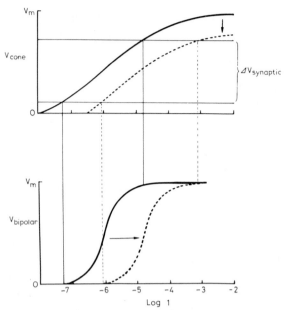

Fig. 9. *V*-log *I* curves for a cone *(upper portion)* and a bipolar cell *(lower portion)* are plotted as solid lines when no background illumination is present. The two horizontal lines in the upper plot indicate the voltage window for cone-to-bipolar cell synaptic transmission. Dashed curves are the *V*-log *I* plots for the cone and bipolar cell in the presence of background illumination. The amplitude of cone responses is reduced by sign-inverting feedback signals from the horizontal cells. The *V*-log *I* curve of bipolar cell is shifted to the right. The arrows indicate the transition from darkness to bright background illumination (from Wu, 1988a).

also occur in the inner retina, and possibly through the whole visual pathway.

## (c) GABAergic synapses mediate color opponency in retinal neurons

As described above, GABAergic synapses between the H1 HCs and cones are responsible for mediating the depolarizing responses of the H2 and perhaps the H3 HCs to red lights. These synapses provide an example of how color opponency may work. In several vertebrate species, color-coded bipolar cells, amacrine cells and ganglion cells have been observed, and each of these cells are at least partially innervated by GABAergic interneurons (Kaneko, 1973). It is likely that GABA, along with other inhibitory neurotransmitters, is involved in providing the necessary

sign inversion in establishing color opponency in the retina.

## (d) GABAergic synapses mediate surround responses in the retina

It has been proposed for over twenty years that antagonistic surround responses in retinal bipolar cells and ganglion cells are mediated by lateral interneurons, the HCs and ACs, which send signals laterally in the outer and inner plexiform layers. Results described in this chapter show that the actions of GABAergic interneurons in ectotherm retinas are consistent with this notion. When light falls onto the surround regions of the bipolar or ganglion cell receptive fields, it polarizes the HCs and ACs. These HC and AC polarizations result in responses in bipolar and ganglion cells of the opposite polarity to the responses elicited by center illuminations. Some of these polarity inversions, as described in the previous sections, are mediated by GABAergic mechanisms, GABA may act on chloride channels through $GABA_A$ receptors or on second-messenger system through $GABA_B$ receptors. As evident from the tiger salamander cones, when polarity inversion is mediated by chloride channels, the value of the chloride equilibrium potential (see Ishida, Chapter 2) becomes strategically very important in determining the strength of the signal inversion: under conditions while the membrane potential ($V_m$) is above $E_{Cl}$, sign-inversion occurs with increasing strength as ($V_m - E_{Cl}$) is larger. GABAergic synapses may fail to give rise to polarity inversion (or antagonistic surround) under conditions while $V_m$ is close to or below $E_{Cl}$ (also see the discussion of shunting and hyperpolarizing inhibition, Slaughter and Pan, Chapter 3).

## (e) GABAergic synapses mediates movement detection in the retina

Movement detecting ganglion cells have been observed in many vertebrate retinas and Barlow and Levick (1965) proposed that they are mediated by movement-detecting subunits (MDS).

Based on the results obtained from the tiger salamander retina, Werblin and co-workers have shown that the MDS probably involves amacrine cells and bipolar cell axon terminals, and GABA plays a key role in this circuitry (Fig. 10). According to this scheme, the narrow field sustained GABAergic amacrine cells feedback to bipolar cell terminals and make the bipolar cell output transient. Consequently, the wide-field amacrine cells and some ganglion cells exhibit transient responses at the onset and cessation of the light stimuli. The transient wide-field amacrine cells (W cells) send inhibitory signals to ganglion cells with a delay compared with the bipolar cell inputs. When the speed of movement of a visual object matches the product of the lateral distance between W-cells and ganglion cells and the delay, inhibition cancels excitation in ganglion cells. A scheme showing how directional sensitivity of retinal ganglion may occur is given in Fig. 10B. In this case W-cell inhibition needs to be unidirectional, and thus movement of a visual object in one direction (null direction) is inhibited by the W-cells whereas movements in other directions are not.

*(f) GABA mediates synaptic plasticity and visual adaptation*

Results described in this chapter also suggest that, in darkness, when the extracellular concentration of GABA is high, it slows down the HCRRT. This modulatory action of GABA occurs probably in the postsynaptic membrane in HCs, because the GABA does not alter response kinetics in either the photoreceptors or bipolar cells which share the same synapses with the HCs (Yang and Wu, 1989a). Horizontal cells exert inhibitory actions on bipolar cells that send output signals to the inner retina. Under dark-adapted conditions, the HC responses are slow, and the amplitudes of the responses to short light steps are small. This may result in a slower or smaller inhibition on the bipolar cell responses. Under light-adapted conditions (after prolonged light exposure), HC responses become faster, and the responses to short light steps become larger. This results in a faster and stronger inhibition on the bipolar cell responses. Consequently, the bipolar cell responses are more transient under light-adapted conditions. The differences in response waveform of outer retinal neurons under

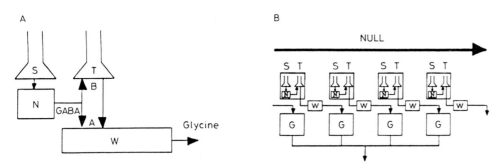

Fig. 10. A. Change-detecting subunit. The sustained-responding bipolar cell terminal (S) provides excitatory synaptic input to the narrow-field sustained amacrine cell (N). The narrow-field amacrine cell feeds back to the transient bipolar cell terminal (T) at GABA$_B$ receptor to truncate the sustained signal arriving via its axon. (There is also a narrow-field feed-forward GABA$_A$ input to the wide-field amacrine cell, presumed to originate from the narrow-field amacrine cell.) The output from this terminal, in turn, drives the wide-field amacrine cell (W) that augments the transient input by generating a single spike, and it propagates this signal laterally. B. Implementing the movement-detecting subunit in the Barlow-Levick model. The movement-detecting subunit (MDS) shown in the upper series of boxes is composed of the OFF responding, change-detecting subunit with the same circuitry, as shown in A. A complementary set of interactions, from the on-system, should also be included in the complete MDS. This MDS drives the lateral inhibitory element, W, the wide-field amacrine cell that propagates in the null direction and feeds forward to the ganglion cell dendrites via a glycinergic synapse. The lower boxes (G) represent the dendrites of a single ganglion cell that integrates the activity from a local population of subunits (from Werblin et al., 1988).

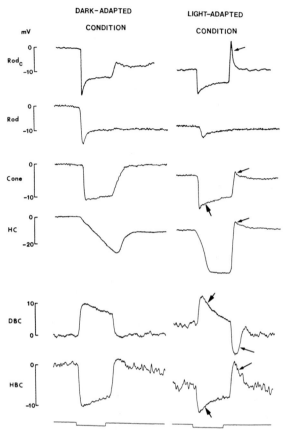

Fig. 11. Light responses of (from top to bottom) a rod$_c$, a rod, a cone, an HC, a DBC and an HBC to a 1 s, 700 nm light step under dark-adapted conditions (left column) and in the presence of background illumination (right column). Note the response rise time of the HC is much slower under dark-adapted conditions. The on-transient responses of the cone, DBC and HBC (thick arrows), and the off-transient responses of the rod$_c$, cone, HC, DBC and HBC (thin arrows) are more pronounced under light-adapted conditions (from Frumkes and Wu, 1990).

dition to acting like a classical neurotransmitter (e.g., open chloride channels in cones and bipolar cells), GABA also acts like a neuromodulator (e.g., slows down the HCRRT, acts on G-proteins). This dual role of GABA in retina and perhaps in the brain warrants attention and further investigation.

## Acknowledgements

This work was supported by grants from National Institutes of Health (EY04446), the Retina Research Foundation (Houston), and Research to Prevent Blindness, Inc.

## References

Attwell, D., Borges, S., Wu, S.M. and Wilson, M. (1987) Signal clipping by the rod output synapse. *Nature*, 382: 522–524.

Bader, C.R., Bertrand, D. and Schwartz, E.A. (1982) Voltage-activated and calcium-activated currents studied in solitary rod inner segments from the salamander retina. *J. Physiol.*, 331: 253–284.

Barlow, H.B. and Levick, W.R. (1965) The mechanisms of directionally selective units in rabbit's retina. *J. Physiol.*, 178: 477–504.

Baylor, D.A., Fuortes, M.G.F. and O'Bryan, P.M. (1971) Receptive fields of single cones in the retina of the turtle. *J. Physiol.*, 24: 265–294.

Belgum, J.H. and Copenhagen, D.R. (1988) Synaptic transfer of rod signals to horizontal and bipolar cells in the retina of the toad. *J. Physiol.*, 396: 225–245.

Cohen, J.L. (1985) Effects of glycine and GABA on ganglion cells of the retina of the skate *Raja crinacca. Brain Res.*, 332: 169–173.

Copenhagen, D.R. and Jahr, C.E. (1988) Release of excitatory amino acids from turtle photoreceptors detected with NMDA receptor-rich membrane patch. *Invest. Ophthalmol. Visual Sci. (Suppl.)*, 29: 223.

Dowling, J.E., Werblin F. (1969) Organization of the retina of the mudpuppy, *Necturus maculosus*. I. Synaptic structure. *J. Neurophysiol.*, 32: 315–388.

Dowling, J.E. (1987) *The Retina, an Approachable Part of the Brain.* Harvard University Press.

Ehinger, B. and Dowling, J.E. (1987) Retinal neurocircuitry and transmission. In: *Handbook of Chemical Neuroanatomy* Vol. 5, A. Bjorklund, T. Hokfelt and L.W. Swanson (Eds.), Ch. IV. pp. 389–446. Elsevier.

Frumkes, T.E., Miller, R.F., Slaughter, M. and Dacheux, R.F. (1981) Physiological and pharmacological basis of GABA and glycine action on neurons of mudpuppy retina. III. Amacrine-mediated inhibitory influences on ganglion cell

dark- and light-adapted conditions are given in Fig. 11. It is probably economical, if not advantageous, for the retina to transmit only transient signals than to transmit constant information under light-adapted conditions.

In summary, GABAergic synapses in ectotherm retinas appear to be involved in several vital functions. These include spatial and temporal resolution of visual images as well as adaptation-induced changes in synaptic efficacy. In ad-

receptive-field organization: a model. *J. Neurophysiol.*, 45: 783–804.

Frumkes, T.E. and Wu, S.M. (1990) Independent influences of rod-adaptation upon cone-mediated responses to light onset and offset in distal retinal neurons. *J. Neurophysiol.*, 64: 1043–1054.

Hubel, D.H., Wiesel, T.N. (1961) Integrative action in the cat's lateral geniculate body. *J. Physiol.*, 155: 385–398.

Hubel, D.H., Wiesel, T.N. (1962) Receptive fields, binocular interaction and functional architecture in the cat's visual cortex. *J. Physiol.*, 160: 106–154.

Ishida, A.T. and Cohen, B.N. (1988) GABA-activated whole cell currents in isolated retinal ganglion cells. *J. Neurophysiol.*, 60: 381–396.

Kondo, H. and Toyoda, J.-I. (1983) GABA and glycine effects of the bipolar cells of the carp retina. *Vision Res.*, 23: 1259–1264.

Kaneko, A. (1973) Receptive field organization of bipolar and amacrine cells in the goldfish retina. *J. Physiol.*, 235: 133–153.

Lasater, E.M. and Lam, D.M.K. (1984) The identification and some functions of GABAergic neurons in the distal catfish retina. *Vision Res.*, 24: 497–506.

Maguire, G.W., Lukasiewicz, P.D. and Werblin, R. (1989a) Amacrine cell interactions underlying the response to change in the tiger salamander retina. *J. Neurosci.*, 9: 726–735.

Maguire, G.W., Maple, B.R., Lukasiewicz, P.D. and Werblin, F. (1989b) Calcium channel currents of bipolar cell axon terminals are modulated via $GABA_B$ receptors. *Proc. Natl. Acad. Sci. USA*, 86: 10144–10147.

Marc, R.E., Stell, W.K., Bok, D., Lam, D.M.K. (1978) GABAergic pathways in the goldfish retina. *J. Comp. Neurol.*, 182: 221–246.

Marc, R.E. (1985) The role of glycine in retinal circuitry. In: Morgan W.H. (Ed.), *Retinal Transmitters and Modulators: Models for the Brain. Vol. I*, CRC Press, Boca Raton, FL, pp. 119–158.

Marc, R.E. (1989) The anatomy of multiple GABAergic and glycinergic pathways in the inner plexiform layer of the goldfish retina. In: *Neurobiology of the inner retina*. Weiler R, Osborne NN, (Eds.), Berlin, Springer,. pp. 53–64.

Marmarelis, P.Z. and Marmarelis, V.Z. (1978) *Analysis of physiological systems, the white-noise approach*. Plenum Press, New York.

Muller, J.F. and Marc, R.E. (1990) GABAergic and glycinergic pathway in the inner plexiform layer of the goldfish retina. *J. Comp. Neurol.*, 291: 281–304.

Murakami, M., Shimoda, Y., Nakatani, K., Miyachi, E., Watanabe, S. (1982b) GABA-mediated negative feedback and color opponency in carp retina. *Jpn. J. Physiol.*, 32: 927–935.

Murakami, M., Shimoda Y., Nakatani, K., Miyachi, E., Watanabe, S. (1982a) GABA-mediated negative feedback from horizontal cells to cones in carp retina. *Jpn. J. Physiol.*, 32: 911–926.

Naka, K.I. (1972) The horizontal cells. *Vision Res.*, 22: 653–660.

Nawy, S. and Jahr, C.E. (1990) Suppression by glutamate of cGMP-activated conductance in retinal bipolar cells. *Nature*, 346: 269–271.

O'Hare, W.A. and Owen, W.G. (1990) Spatial organization of the bipolar cells receptive fields in the retina of the tiger salamander. *J. Physiol.*, 421: 223–245.

Slaughter, M.M. and Miller, R.F. (1981) 2-Amino-4-phosphonobutyric acid: a new pharmacological tool for retina research. *Science*, 211: 182–185.

Slaughter, M.M. and Miller, R.F. (1983a) An excitatory amino-acid antagonists blocks cone input to sigh-conserving second-order retinal neurons. *Science*, 219: 1230–1232.

Slaughter, M.M. and Miller, R.F. (1983b) Bipolar cells in the mudpuppy retina use an excitatory amino-acid neurotransmitter. *Nature*, 303: 537–538.

Stell, W.K., Lightfoot, D.O. (1975) Color-specific interconnections of cones and horizontal cells in the retina of the goldfish. *J. Comp. Neurol.*, 159: 473–502.

Tachibana M. and Kaneko A. (1987) $\gamma$-Aminobutyric acid exerts a local inhibitory action on the axon terminal of bipolar cells: Evidence for negative feedback from amacrine cells. *Proc. Natl. Acad. Sci. USA*, 84: 3501–3505.

Werblin, F.S. (1972) Lateral interactions at inner plexiform layer of the vertebrate retina: antagonistic responses to change. *Science*, 175: 1008–1010.

Werblin, F.S. and Dowling, J.E. (1969) Organization of the retina of the mudpuppy. *Necturus maculosus*. II. Intracellular recording. *J. Neurophysiol.*, 32: 339–355.

Werblin, F.S., Maguire, G., Lukasiewicz, P., Eliasof, S. and Wu, S.M. (1988) Neural interactions mediating the detection of motion in the retina of the tiger salamander. *Vis. Neurosci.*, 1: 317–329.

Wong-Riley, M.T.T. (1974) Synaptic organization of the inner plexiform layer in the retina of the tiger salamander. *J. Neurocytol.*, 3: 1–33.

Wu, S.M. (1986) Effects of gamma-aminobutyric acid on cones and bipolar cells of the tiger salamander retina. *Brain Res.*, 365: 70–77.

Wu, S.M. (1988a) Electrical interactions between the neuronal cells of the retina: encoding of visual images in the vertebrate retina. In: M. Tso (Ed.), *Retinal Disease: Biomedical Foundations and Clinical Management*. Lippincott, PA, pp. 112–121.

Wu, S.M. (1988b) Synaptic transmission from photoreceptors to second-order retinal neurons. In: D.M.K. Lam (Ed.) *Proceedings of the Retinal Research Foundation Symposium*. Portfolio Publishing Co., Inc., The Woodlands, TX, pp. 128–140.

Wu, S.M. (1991) Input-output relations of the feedback synapse between horizontal cells and cones in the tiger salamander retina. *J. Neurophysiol.*, 65: 1197–1206.

Yang, X.L. and Wu, S.M. (1989a) Effects of background illumination on horizontal cell responses in tiger salamander retina. *J. Neurosci.*, 9: 815–826.

Yang, X.L. and Wu, S.M. (1989b) Effects of prolonged light

exposure, gamma-aminobutyric acid and glycine on the HC responses in the tiger salamander retina. *J. Neurophysiol.*, 61: 1025–1035.

Yang, X.L. and Wu, S.M. (1990) Effects of CNQX, APB, PDA, and kynurenate on horizontal cells of the tiger salamander retina. *Visual Neurosci.*, 3: 207–212.

Yang, X.L. and Wu, S.M. (1991) Feedforward lateral inhibition in retinal bipolar cells: input-output relation of the horizontal cell-depolarizing bipolar cell synapse. *Proc. Natl. Acad. Sci. USA*, 88: 3310–3313.

R.R. Mize, R.E. Marc and A.M. Sillito (Eds.)
Progress in Brain Research, Vol. 90

CHAPTER 6

# GABAergic circuits in the mammalian retina

Michael A. Freed

*Building 36, Room 2C02, National Institutes of Health, Bethesda, MD 20892, USA*

## Introduction

The evidence that GABA ($\gamma$-aminobutyric acid) is a neurotransmitter within the mammalian retina has been reviewed before (Enna and Karbon, 1986; Yazulla, 1986): there is an uptake carrier with a high affinity for GABA (Goodchild and Neal, 1973; Starr and Voaden, 1972); both flash-ing lights and high $K^+$ release GABA (Bauer, 1978; Lam et al., 1980); there are GABA recep-tors (Enna and Snyder, 1976); the retina contains GABA and its synthetic enzyme glutamic acid decarboxylase (GAD) (Graham, 1972; Kuriyama et al., 1968). These findings are compelling but do not implicate particular neuronal types to be GABAergic. Thus, they will not be discussed

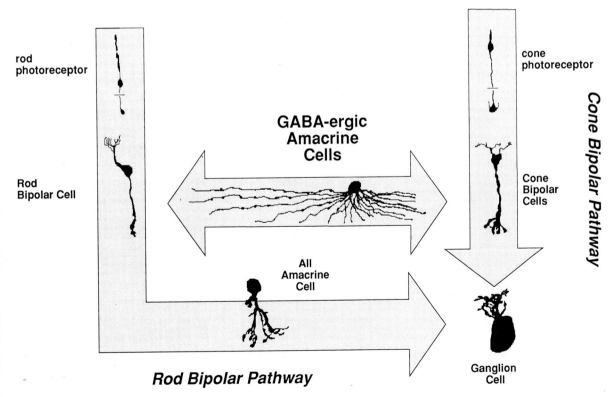

Fig. 1. The rod bipolar and cone bipolar pathways.

further here. This chapter will focus on specific GABAergic retinal neurons and discuss their role in the retinal circuitry of eutherian mammals.

Many distinct types of interneuron convey the visual scene, transduced by the rods and cones, to the ganglion cells (Ramón Y Cajal, 1972). The cat retina has been estimated to contain 33 types of interneuron and 23 types of ganglion cell (Kolb et al., 1981). These interneurons form two major pathways, the rod bipolar pathway and the cone bipolar pathway (Kolb and Famiglietti, 1974; Sterling et al., 1988). This arrangement may be common to mammals (Dacheux and Raviola, 1986; Müller, 1989; Vaughn et al., 1981; Voigt and Wässle, 1987). The pathways begin in the outer plexiform layer (see Fig. 1). Here, rods and cones contact separate bipolar cell types, the rod and cone bipolar cells. The rod and cone bipolar cells lead to the inner plexiform layer, where both pathways ultimately converge upon the same ganglion cells. The rod pathway is less direct, however, since it includes an intermediate amacrine cell, the AII amacrine cell. Rod and cone signals also intermingle due to gap junctions between rod and cones. As would be expected from the sensitivity of rods to dim light, the rod bipolar pathway functions under conditions of low illumination and the cone bipolar pathway functions under conditions of high illumination (Kolb and Famiglietti, 1974; Smith et al., 1986).

This chapter's theme is that GABAergic circuits modify signals running through both rod and cone bipolar pathways. These modifying circuits, in keeping with their name, are often circular chains of neurons, as distinct from the linear bipolar pathways, and therefore seem to mediate feedback. Another function of these modifying circuits can be understood in the context that, since each neuronal type is repeated across the retina, rod and cone bipolar pathways represent many parallel routes: the modifying circuits convey information laterally between these parallel routes. One modifying circuit cell is the horizontal cell, which interacts with rods, cones and bipolar cells in some manner not fully under-

stood. In mammals, there are at least 2 types of horizontal cell (Ramón Y Cajal, 1972). There is equivocal evidence that both types of horizontal cell are GABAergic. Another modifying circuit cell is the amacrine cell, which interacts with bipolar cells, ganglion cells and other amacrine cells. There is good evidence that specific types of amacrine cells are GABAergic. A third kind of modifying neuron, the interplexiform cell, receives synapses from amacrine cells in the inner plexiform layer and synapses upon bipolar cell dendrites in the outer plexiform layer, constituting a longer feedback loop. In mammals, there is good evidence that 2 types of interplexiform cell are GABAergic.

## Specific types of GABAergic neurons

Putative GABAergic neurons have been located by several methods: Autoradiography of tritiated GABA or its tritiated analogues (isoguvacine, diaminobutyric acid, muscimol), after these substances are accumulated by neurons, shows grains over somas and processes. To use this method, neurons with high-affinity uptake, which show many autoradiographic grains, must be distinguished from those neurons with low-affinity uptake, which show few grains. A second method, immunohistochemistry, locates endogenous GABA. Immunohistochemistry also locates GAD the enzyme that synthesizes GABA from glutamate. Since immunohistochemistry may recognize molecules that share epitopes with GABA or GAD, the qualifications GABA-like immunoreactivity or GAD-like immunoreactivity are used (GABA-IR or GAD-IR). This means that cells without GAD or GABA may be recognized. On the other hand, immunohistochemistry may fail to recognize cells with GAD, since an antibody may not recognize all isoforms of this enzyme. A third method, in situ hybridization, confirms the presence of GAD: DNA and RNA probes show the transcription of the GAD gene in neurons (Sarthy and Fu, 1989a,b). A fourth method preloads GABA-accumulating cells with

[$^3$H]GABA, stimulates them with light to release [$^3$H]GABA, and then uses autoradiography to demonstrate the resulting depletion of [$^3$H]GABA from the cells (O'Malley and Masland, 1989).

Given the variety methods for identifying putative GABAergic neurons, it is natural to ask to what extent these methods identify the same neurons. Comparing the results of GAD and GABA immunohistochemistry, virtually all amacrine cells that show GAD-IR also show GABA-IR (Hendrickson et al., 1985; Mosinger and Yazulla, 1987). This is expected and may only indicate that cells use GAD to synthesize GABA. Reversing this comparison, about 87% of amacrine cells that show GABA-IR also show GAD-IR (Mosinger and Yazulla, 1987). This may mean that some cells take up GABA but do not synthesize it. This is confirmed by comparing the results of GAD immunohistochemistry and the uptake of the GABA analogues [$^3$H]GABA and [$^3$H]muscimol: only about 71–78% of analogue-accumulating cells show GAD-IR (Hendrickson et al., 1985; Mosinger and Yazulla, 1985).

These results indicate that the population with GAD-IR is smaller than either GABA-accumulating or GABA-containing populations. So there is good, but not perfect, agreement between the various methods in mammals. Given that the agreement is not perfect, none of these methods are infallible markers for GABAergic cells. Yet, all these methods provide evidence that cells have GABA available for release. Thus, a reasonable approach to identifying GABAergic neurons is to consider the evidence for each cell type in turn.

*Horizontal cells*

The evidence for GABAergic horizontal cells in adult eutherian mammals is equivocal. This is in contrast to the good evidence for GABAergic horizontal cells in lower vertebrates (see Wu, Chapter 5, and Marc, Chapter 4). Some studies of mammals report GABA-IR and GAD-IR in horizontal cells (Bolz and McGuire, 1985; Grünert and Wässle, 1990; Osborne et al., 1986; Pourcho

and Owczarzak, 1989; Wässle and Chun, 1989). Yet, other studies report no specific staining (Agardh et al., 1987; Brandon, 1985; Hendrickson et al., 1985; Mosinger et al., 1986). In those studies that report immunostaining, horizontal cells of both types stain, but stain less intensely than amacrine cells. The results of in situ hybridization vary too: they show horizontal cells transcribe the GAD gene in cat, but not primate (Sarthy and Fu, 1989a,b). Even for the same investigator and the same animal, horizontal cell staining is sporadic, occurring in some sections and not in others (Grünert and Wässle, 1990; Mosinger and Yazulla, 1987). The cause of sporadic staining, and even reported differences between animals, may be sampling error: A study of monkey that paid attention to retinal position showed that central horizontal cells stain while peripheral horizontal cells do not (Grünert and Wässle, 1990).

Other evidence fails to support GABAergic horizontal cells. If horizontal cells release GABA within the photoreceptor invagination, the site where it interacts with the photoreceptor and the bipolar cell, then one of these cell types must take up GABA to clear it from the invagination. Yet, no such uptake is observed (Brandon et al., 1979; Freed et al., 1983; Hendrickson et al., 1985; Pourcho, 1980; Wässle and Chun, 1989). Thus, a cautious approach to evidence would indicate that the case for mammalian GABAergic horizontal cells is unproven. Yet, it would be surprising that a basic part of the retinal circuit should function so differently in mammals versus other orders of vertebrate, or in the central versus the peripheral retina.

*Amacrine cells*

In cat and rabbit, putative GABAergic amacrine cells make up about 25–40% of amacrine cells in the inner nuclear layer (Freed et al., 1983; Mosinger and Yazulla, 1985; Pourcho, 1981; Wässle and Chun, 1989), and most of the amacrine cells in the ganglion cell layer (Brecha et al., 1988; Wässle et al., 1989). The same approximate portion of amacrine cells accumulates GABA, accumulates muscimol, contains GABA-IR and contains GAD-IR. The immunostaining of amacrine cells is reproducible and intense. Amacrine cells also contain messenger RNA for GAD (Sarthy and Fu, 1989a,b). The only other transmitter implicated for so many amacrine cells (about 40%) is glycine (Pourcho, 1980), indicating that GABA is a major amacrine transmitter of the mammalian retina.

Using autoradiography of either [$^3$H]muscimol or [$^3$H]GABA, specific types of putative GABAergic amacrine cells have been studied most extensively in the cat. Initially, Pourcho (1980, 1981) divided the somas of GABA-accumulating amacrine cells into 5 classes denoted A(GABA$_1$) to A(GABA$_5$). Next, to find the partial morphology of GABA-accumulating amacrine cells, my collaborators and I (Freed et al., 1983) reconstructed amacrine cells and divided them into 4 classes denoted type 1 to type 4 (see Fig. 2). Finally, Pourcho and Goebel (1983) developed a clever technique to show the complete morphology of muscimol-accumulating amacrine cells: Golgi staining combined with autoradiography of [$^3$H]muscimol accumulations. This technique allowed Pourcho and Goebel to identify muscimol-accumulating amacrine cells according to Kolb et al.'s (1981) classification scheme, denoted A1-A22.

For the cat, the classification of GABA-accumulating amacrine cells (including interplexiform cells) indicates at least 7 of a total of perhaps 22 amacrine cell types. Each type has been described in some detail. This detail allows the identification of specific types of putative GABAergic amacrine cell in studies of synaptic connections, light responses, and pharmacology, and so will be summarized here. These specific types are also schematized in Fig. 3. In the following summary, the direction "up" will be synonymous with "toward the outside of the eye" and "down" with "towards the inside of the eye", the standard orientation of retinal micrographs. Also, the reader needs to know that the top third

of the inner plexiform layer is called sublamina $a$, while the bottom two thirds is called sublamina $b$. All measures are of diameters.

A2 = A(GABA$_2$) = type 2. The A2 amacrine accumulates muscimol and has been identified with the GABA-accumulating A(GABA$_2$) and type 2 (Freed et al., 1983; Pourcho, 1980; Pourcho and Goebel, 1983). The soma is medium-sized (9–10 $\mu$m) and contains an electron-lucent cytoplasm. The soma is round on top, but flat on the bottom. The nuclear surface is either invaginated or smooth. Medium caliber (0.8 $\mu$m) primary processes extend from the edge of the soma bottom and a stouter primary process stems from its middle. All processes ramify within sublamina $a$. The A2 amacrine has a narrow (90–100 $\mu$m) dendritic field (Kolb et al., 1981; Pourcho and Goebel, 1983).

A10 = A(GABA$_1$). The A10 accumulates muscimol and has been identified with the GABA-accumulating A(GABA$_1$) (Pourcho and Goebel, 1983). This type has with a medium-sized soma (9–11 $\mu$m) and a pale cytoplasm. The A10 ramifies broadly within S2-S4 and has a small (100–200 $\mu$m) dendritic field (Kolb et al., 1981; Pourcho and Goebel, 1983).

A13 = A(GABA$_3$) = type 1. The A13 accumulates muscimol and has been identified with the GABA-accumulating A(GABA$_3$) and type 1 (Freed et al., 1983; Pourcho, 1980; Pourcho and Goebel, 1983). The soma is large (12–15 $\mu$m) and contains an electron-dense cytoplasm filled with copious endoplasmic reticulum. The soma is round on top but flat on the bottom, like the carapace of a crab. The nuclear surface is smooth. From the edges of the soma bottom stem medium (0.6 $\mu$m) primary processes which ramify within sublamina $a$. Narrower (0.4 $\mu$m) processes stem from the edges of the soma bottom and from the medium processes and descend vertically into sublamina $b$. Processes that stem from the middle of the soma bottom are absent. The A13 has a

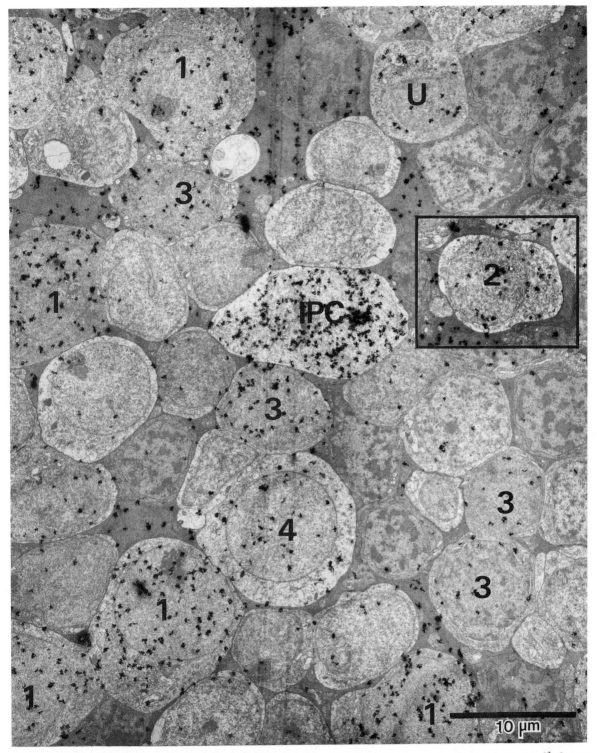

Fig. 2. Electron microscopic autoradiograph of tangential section through amacrine somas. Grains, indicating [³H]GABA accumulate intensely over one type of interplexiform cell (IPC) and less intensely over four types of GABA-accumulating amacrine cells (1 = A13, A17; 2 = A2; 3 = type 3; 4 = A18; U = unclassified; from Freed et al., 1983).

small dendritic field (< 200 μm; Kolb et al., 1981; Nelson and Kolb, 1985; Pourcho and Goebel, 1983).

A17 = A(GABA₃) = type 1. The A17 accumulates muscimol and, like the A13, has been identified with the GABA-accumulating A(GABA₃) and type 1 (Freed et al., 1983; Pourcho, 1980; Pourcho and Goebel, 1983). The soma is medium-sized (9–13 μm; Nelson and Kolb, 1985) with an electron-dense cytoplasm, much endoplasmic reticulum, and a flattened bottom. The nuclear surface is smooth. From the edges of the soma bottom stem medium diameter (0.6 μm) primary processes. Narrower (0.1 μm), varicose, dendrites branch from the primary processes and descend gradually to the bottom of the inner plexiform layer. The A17 has a wide dendritic field (500–1200 μm; Nelson and Kolb, 1985).

A19. Originally, I identified my type 4 with the A19, but this may be mistaken. Recently, it has been shown that the A18 interplexiform cell contains GABA-IR (see below; Wässle and Chun, 1988). The A18 has the largest soma of any cell in the amacrine layer (15–17 μm); this is how my type 4 and Pourcho's A(GABA₄) were described,

indicating that they may be identical with the A18, not the A19.

The A19 accumulates muscimol (Pourcho and Goebel, 1983). The soma is large (12–15 μm), and lies either in the inner nuclear or ganglion cell layer (Freed et al., 1990). Thick (0.5–2.0 μm) straight processes radiate from the soma and ramify in sublamina *a*. The dendritic arbor is wide (500 μm). Like other amacrine cells (Dacey, 1988), the A19 has long, very thin (< 0.2 μm), processes that extend some distance (800 μm) from the dendritic field. These thin processes may be axons (Freed et al., 1990).

A(GABA₅) = type 3. The Golgi classification of this GABA- and muscimol-accumulating amacrine cell is unknown. Yet, it has been observed by both myself and R. Pourcho in electron micrographs. A small soma (8 μm) has very electron-dense cytoplasm (Freed et al., 1983; Pourcho, 1980; Pourcho and Goebel, 1983). Empty vacuoles appear in cytoplasm; this is perhaps an artifact. The nuclear surface is invaginated or smooth. A very thick extension of soma descends into the inner plexiform layer, suggesting that this amacrine cell's processes extends deep into the inner plexiform layer and ramify in sublamina *b*.

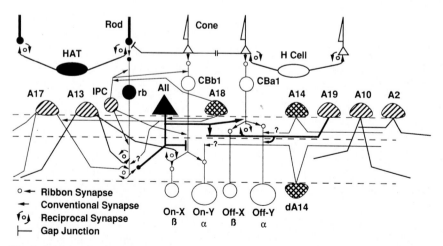

Fig. 3. GABAergic circuits in the cat retina. All putative GABAergic neurons are cross-hatched. Colocalization of GABA with another transmitter is indicated with double-hatching. IPC, interplexiform cell; rb, rod bipolar cell; H cell, horizontal cell; HAT, horizontal cell axon terminal; CB, cone bipolar cell; A, amacrine cell; dA, displaced amacrine cell; X, Y, ganglion cells.

## Interplexiform cells

An interplexiform cell is distinguished from other amacrine cells by thin but extensive processes which ramify in the outer plexiform layer. Mammalian interplexiform cells commonly are of two types. Originally, investigators thought these two types to be GABAergic and dopaminergic (Dowling and Ehinger, 1978; Dowling et al., 1980; Nakamura et al., 1980; Ryan and Hendrickson, 1987; Wulle and Schnitzer, 1989). Recently, however, there is evidence the dopaminergic neurons may also be GABAergic (see below). In any case, the two types of interplexiform cell can be distinguished by their morphology.

In cat, the non-dopaminergic type of interplexiform cell type makes up about 2% of the GABA- and muscimol-accumulating neurons in the amacrine cell layer (Nakamura et al., 1980). It accumulates more GABA and muscimol than amacrine cells (see Fig. 2). The interplexiform cell also contains GABA-IR (Chun and Wässle, 1989; Grünert and Wässle, 1990; Pourcho and Owczarzak, 1989; Ryan and Hendrickson, 1987; Wässle and Chun, 1989). The medium-sized soma (10–12 $\mu$m) is oval and appears placed on end. The soma contains an electron lucent cytoplasm. Medium diameter primary processes extend into the inner plexiform layer and diffusely stratify throughout this layer. Thin (0.3–0.4 $\mu$m) processes extend upward from the apex of the soma, or from the inner plexiform layer processes, and ramify in the outer plexiform layer. The dendritic field in either plexiform layer is small (about 200 $\mu$m; Pourcho and Goebel, 1983).

## Colocalization with other transmitters

Cholinergic, dopaminergic, and putative indoleaminergic types of amacrine cell may also be GABAergic. For 2 types of cholinergic and 1 type of dopaminergic amacrine cell, the case for GABAergic transmission is either as compelling, or almost as compelling, as can be made for any amacrine cell. Some of the indoleamine-accumulating types, putatively serotonergic, prove to be identical with putative GABAergic types already described (A17, A19). The evidence that these indoleamine-accumulating types are GABAergic is better than the evidence they are serotonergic.

## Cholinergic amacrine cells

GABA-IR, GAD-IR and accumulations of [$^3$H]GABA and [$^3$H]muscimol have been found in starburst-shaped amacrine cells of rabbit, cat, and rat (Brecha et al., 1988; Chun et al., 1988; Kosaka et al., 1988; Mariani and Hersh, 1988; Massey et al., 1991; O'Malley and Masland, 1989; Vaney and Young, 1988). The evidence that starburst amacrine cells are cholinergic is good: they immuno-stain for choline acetyltransferase, accumulate choline with a high affinity, and release acetylcholine. Since there is strong evidence that acetylcholine (ACh) is a retinal transmitter (reviewed by Neal, 1983), the colocalization of GABA and ACh shows the coexistence of two functional transmitters in the same cell.

Cholinergic amacrine cells are similar in several mammals (Masland and Mills, 1979; Pourcho and Osman, 1986; Voigt, 1986). There are two types, one in the inner nuclear layer where most amacrine cells lie, which ramifies in sublamina $a$, and another displaced to the ganglion cell layer, which ramifies in sublamina $b$. Cholinergic amacrine cells form the majority of displaced amacrine cells in rabbit and cat; this is presumably the basis for the observation that most displaced amacrine cells stain for GAD-IR (Brecha et al., 1988; Wässle et al., 1989). In cat, the cholinergic amacrine cells are identified as the A14 and dA14 (Pourcho and Osman, 1986).

The cholinergic cells release both GABA and ACh, but under different conditions. Flashing lights or moving bars cause them to release ACh, but not GABA (Friedman and Redburn, 1990; Masland and Livingston, 1976; O'Malley and Masland, 1989). Depolarization with high potassium cause them to release both ACh and GABA. The resulting depletion of GABA from the cholinergic cell has been directly visualized using autoradiography. O'Malley and Masland (1989) have found that the release of ACh from the retina is calcium dependent, but that the release of GABA is not. This suggests that ACh is released in vesicles, but that GABA is released by other means. GABA may be released by the same carrier responsible for GABA uptake, made to run in reverse by depolarization. Such a reversal of the carrier may be a mode of synaptic transmission in fish horizontal cells, where it is independent of both extracellular and intracellular $Ca^{2+}$ (Schwartz, 1987). Yet, under the conditions of O'Malley and Masland's study, it is difficult to ascribe the apparent carrier-mediated release to the cholinergic amacrine cells specifically, since numerous glial cell, known to have GABA carriers, would also release GABA. Also, in this same study, an intracellular stores of calcium can not be excluded as a possible source of calcium for vesicular release (for an alternative to carrier-mediated release see Marc, Chapter 4).

Given the coexistence of GABA and ACh in the starburst amacrine cells, it is particularly interesting that GABA suppresses the light-evoked release of ACh (Masland and Livingston, 1976). $GABA_A$ receptors may mediate this suppression, since it is blocked by $GABA_A$ antagonists. $GABA_B$ receptors may be involved in an enhancement of ACh release, since baclofen, a $GABA_B$ agonist, causes release of ACh independent of light (Friedman and Redburn, 1990). It has been suggested that starburst cells inhibit their own release of ACh, either directly through autoreceptors (Brecha et al., 1988), or indirectly through a loop of intermediary interneurons. Indeed, this intermediary neuron may be a bipolar cell that synapses upon the cholinergic amacrine cell because blocking glutaminergic bipolar synapses with 6–7-dinitroquinoxaline-2,3-dione also blocks the effects of $GABA_A$ antagonists on ACh release (Linn and Massey, 1991).

Some investigators have suggested the utility of two transmitters in one cell (Masland et al., 1989; Vaney et al., 1989). These suggestions are too complex to describe here. Given the inability

of light to cause a measurable release of GABA, a less complex, but more disappointing, explanation is that cholinergic cells are not GABAergic, but simply GABA-receptive; they clear GABA from the synapse by accumulating it. Yet, this explanation is hard to accept since the cholinergic cells show just as many indications of being GABAergic, including GAD-IR, as any amacrine cell type discussed so far.

### Dopaminergic amacrine cells

In cat, the dopaminergic amacrine cell, A18, which shows tyrosine-hydroxylase like immunoreactivity (TH-IR), often shows GABA-IR. This neuron, however, does not show high-affinity uptake of muscimol, but requires concentrations in excess of those required by other cell types (Wässle and Chun, 1988). A similar colocalization of TH-IR with GABA-IR and GAD-IR has also been found in rat retina (Kosaka et al., 1987). This colocalization implies that two functional transmitters exist in the same cell, since there is good evidence that dopamine is a retinal transmitter (reviewed by Kamp, 1985; Massey and Redburn, 1987).

All mammals examined possess dopaminergic retinal neurons and these neurons are remarkably similar: their somas are large (up to 20 $\mu$m) compared to other cells in the inner nuclear layer and their dendrites ramify at the border at the very top of the inner plexiform layer (Dacey, 1988; Mitrofanis and Finay, 1990; Nguyen-Legros et al., 1981; Nguyen-Legros et al., 1984; Oyster et al., 1985; Törk and Stone, 1979). These dendrites form rings that encircle and contact the stout primary processes of the AII amacrine cell (Pourcho, 1982; Voigt and Wässle, 1987). In addition to dendrites, dopaminergic cells have thin, axon-like processes, which dip toward the bottom of the inner plexiform layer and then back up again to the top (Kolb et al., 1990).

Some, but not all, dopaminergic neurons have been demonstrated to direct a process toward the outer plexiform layer. Since this process is the defining characteristic of an interplexiform cell, its sporadic appearance creates uncertainty whether retinal dopaminergic neurons in a given mammal are all interplexiform cells, or whether they vary between amacrine and interplexiform types. Yet, a thin upward-directed process could be easily missed. Since the morphology of dopaminergic neurons is otherwise uniform, and variability is uncharacteristic of retinal cell types, (see Sterling, 1983 for review), the dopaminergic neuron may be a single type of interplexiform cell (but see Oyster et al., 1985). This suggests that mammals have two kinds of interplexiform cells: one that is GABAergic only, another that is both dopaminergic and GABAergic.

*Indoleamine-accumulating cells*

Holmgren-Taylor (Ehinger and Holmgren, 1979; Holmgren-Taylor, 1982) reported that most (75%) of the amacrine varicosities in a reciprocal synaptic relationship to the rod bipolar cell are indoleamine-accumulating. She identified varicosities by injecting 5,6-dihydroxytryptamine (5,6-DHT) into the vitreous and observing the toxic effects of accumulating this indoleamine. These effects include swollen mitochondria and increased electron density of membranes (Dowling and Ehinger, 1978). My collaborators and I (Freed et al., 1987) reported that more than 90% of these same reciprocal amacrine varicosities are GABA-accumulating. At the time, these findings appeared mutually contradictory, suggesting either GABAergic or serotoninergic reciprocal amacrine cells.

This contradiction was resolved recently by a demonstration that the same amacrine cell types accumulate both GABA and indoleamines (Osborne and Beaton, 1986; Wässle and Chun, 1988). Indeed, the indoleamine-accumulating population of amacrine cells seems to be a subset of the putative GABAergic population: in cat, more than 70% of cells with GAD-IR also accumulate serotonin (Wässle and Chun, 1988). In rabbit, about 20% of cells with GABA-IR also accumulate serotonin and the indoleamine 5,7-dihydroxytryptamine (5,7-DHT; Osborne and

Beaton, 1986). There are few, if any, amacrine cells that are members of the indoleamine-accumulating population only.

The types of putative GABAergic neurons that accumulate indoleamines has been found by a new technique: Cells are made fluorescent by accumulating indoleamines and then injected with lucifer dye to show their morphology (Tauchi and Masland, 1984). In cat, after dye injection, two GABAergic types were found to accumulating the indoleamine 5,6-DHT: the A17 and the A19 (Wässle et al., 1987).

In rabbit, after dye injection, 3 cell types are found to accumulate the indoleamine 5,7-DHT: types S1, S2 and S3. Although detailed study of specific GABA-ergic cell types has not been published in rabbit, it can be inferred that these 3 types are putative GABAergic cells. Types S1 and S2 resemble the A17 and A13 amacrine cells in cat because they stratify diffusely and their dendrites descend toward the bottom of the inner plexiform layer (Sandell and Masland, 1986; Vaney, 1986). The S1 and S2 resemble the A17 and A13 in another way: they are reciprocal to the rod bipolar cell (Sandell et al., 1989). Furthermore, it can be inferred that S1 and S2 are GABA-immunoreactive. About 75–80% of indoleamine-accumulating amacrine cells in rabbit are GABA-immunoreactive (Osborne and Beaton, 1986; Wässle and Chun, 1988). Since this is a greater portion of indoleamine-accumulating cells than are of type S1 (Vaney, 1986), this implies that both S1 and S2 are putative GABAergic neurons (Wässle and Chun, 1988). The third indoleamine-accumulating type in rabbit (S3) is an interplexiform cell, that occurs infrequently across the retina and accumulates GABA (Sandell and Masland, 1986, 1989). Thus rabbit, like other mammals, has a putative GABAergic interplexiform cell type.

Before putative GABAergic types can be accepted as serotonergic, there are certain criteria worth considering. One of these is that they show high affinity uptake of indoleamines. In cat, this criteria is not met (Wässle and Chun, 1988). Only the A20 amacrine cell, not thought to be GABAergic or to provide varicosities reciprocal to the rod bipolar cell, accumulates indoleamines when the isolated retina is bathed in concentrations of 5,6-DHT approximate to the $K_m$ for high-affinity uptake (Osborne, 1980; Thomas and Redburn, 1979). Other cell types, including putative GABAergic amacrine cells, require concentrations 100 times in excess of this to accumulate indoleamines by low-affinity uptake.

Holmgren-Taylor studied amacrine varicosities reciprocal to the rod bipolar cell after intravitreal injection of 5,6-DHT. It is hard to determine exactly what concentrations in the cat retina these injections produced, but it is possible to infer that they were sufficient for low-affinity uptake. A small amount of 5,6-DHT (20 g) injected into the vitreous labels the high-affinity A20 intensely, but the A22 and the A19 only faintly (Wässle and Chun, 1988). None of these 3 types are known to be reciprocal to the rod bipolar cell. Twice this amount of 5,6-DHT labels the A17, which is reciprocal to the rod bipolar cell. Presumably this larger amount of 5,6-DHT causes nonspecific labeling of the A17, as high concentrations do in the bath, since this amount also labels the Y ganglion cell, not thought to be either GABAergic or indoleamine-accumulating. To label the reciprocal varicosities, Holmgren-Taylor injected even more (50 $\mu$g) of 5,6-DHT into the vitreous, an amount sufficient for low-affinity uptake. Additionally, she chose to study regions of retina where the labeling, and thus the concentration of 5,6-DHT, were highest. The evidence indicates that amacrine varicosities reciprocal to the rod bipolar cell suffered toxic effects because of their low-affinity uptake of indoleamines.

Another criteria for serotonergic transmission is that the candidate neuron contains sufficient quantities of endogenous serotonin. Although there are no established minimum criteria for quantity, the evidence suggests that a putative GABAergic neuron contains much less serotonin than GABA. A more than 1000-fold disparity between the total amounts of serotonin and

GABA in the retina supports this idea ($\sim 1 \times 10^{-10}$ versus $4 \times 10^{-7}$ M per gram wet weight; Ehinger et al., 1981; Kuriyama et al., 1968; Mitchell and Redburn, 1985; Osborne et al., 1982). A parsimonious amount of serotonin is also borne out by immunohistochemical studies of eutherian mammals: these studies fail to detect any endogenous serotonin in neurons (for prototherians, see Young and Vaney, 1990). Immunohistochemical studies of serotonin must raise serotonin levels artificially to detect it (Ehinger et al., 1981). In contrast, GABA is easily localized in amacrine cells without artificial increases. The levels of synthetic enzymes indicate the same disparity: a study of tryptophan hydroxylase (Florén and Hansson, 1980), the enzyme that synthesizes serotonin, reports no detectable levels. A study of tryptophan hydrolase-like immunoreactivity in guinea pig (Osborne et al., 1989) located a small number of unidentified amacrine cells. In contrast, GAD-IR has been repeatedly demonstrated and localized in many amacrine cells.

In general, the evidence for any sort of serotonergic transmission in the mammalian retina is contradictory. There is some doubt whether high potassium releases serotonin (Nowak et al., 1985; but see Osborne, 1980; Thomas and Redburn, 1979). Two studies (Blazynski et al., 1985; Osborne et al., 1989) show serotonin elevates cAMP levels, but another study (Florén and Hansson, 1980) reports no such effect. It has been suggested that other indoleamines might be the natural transmitter, but these also may be present at very low levels (Florén, 1979; Osborne et al., 1982).

In support of serotonergic neurotransmission, there is evidence that serotonin and its antagonists reduce the firing of retinal ganglion cells. Thier and Wässle (1984) observed the effects of serotonin and its antagonist 5-methoxy-$N$,$N$-dimethyltryptamine on 22 cat retinal ganglion cells. They found a decrease in spontaneous rate. When the light-evoked response was referenced to the spontaneous rate (see below), they found no change in light-evoked responses from 20 cells. For 2 cells, the antagonist suppressed a response, but that this was accompanied by "a reduction in the amplitude of the extracellularly recorded spike". This reduction of spike amplitude suggests a hyperpolarizing shunt of the membrane resistance which may reduce firing during the stimulus and at other times. The reduction in firing may occur because shunting reduces, in an ohmic fashion, voltages that cause spontaneous and light-evoked firing. In this case, light-evoked and spontaneous firing would be reduced by some common ratio. Reduction of both light-evoked responses (not referenced to spontaneous rate) and spontaneous firing by serotoninergic antagonists have also been reported in rabbit (Brunken and Daw, 1986, 1988a,b). So, in both cat and rabbit, ganglion cells may be directly sensitive to serotonin and related drugs.

In summary, both rabbit and cat have two types of diffuse putative GABAergic amacrine cells whose terminal processes run along the bottom of the inner plexiform layer and contact rod bipolar cells and at least one type of putative GABAergic interplexiform cell. These cell types may contain only small amounts of serotonin. Why GABAergic amacrine cells accumulate indoleamines is not clear.

**GABA-receptive cell types**

Recently a $GABA_A$ receptor has been isolated and monoclonal antibodies made against it. This allows immunocytochemical staining for the receptor, and identification of presumed GABA-receptive neurons in primates. Unfortunately, the identify of specific neuronal types has not been published, only the identity of general cell classes: the antibodies stain amacrine and ganglion cell somas, but not photoreceptors or horizontal cells (Hughes et al., 1989; Mariani et al., 1987; Richards et al., 1987; see Brecha, Chapter 1). There may be, however, other types of stained neuron. Inspection of one illustration shows a stained neuron (Fig. 4 of Hughes et al., 1989) which resem-

bles a starburst amacrine cell. Inspection of many illustrations suggests that bipolar cells may be labeled too: stained somas, in the middle of the inner nuclear layer, show a thick stalk which descends into the inner plexiform layer, but no ascending stalk. To me, this descending stalk looks like the axon of a bipolar cell. Perhaps bipolar cell axons stain but their dendritic terminals do not. Large ganglion cell somas and dendrites are stained which are probably of the parasol type, thought to correspond to the Y cells of cat.

Whole-cell and patch-clamp recordings of the rat and mouse show $GABA_A$ receptors on identified rod bipolar cells and untyped ganglion cells (Lipton, 1989; Tauck et al., 1988; Karschin and Wässle, 1990; Suzuki et al., 1990; Yeh et al., 1990). On these cells, GABA receptors gate a channel selective to chloride, and are blocked by the $GABA_A$ antagonist bicuculline. There is no evidence of $GABA_B$ receptors: In mammals, baclofen has no effect on bipolar cell channels, and ganglion cell channels exhibit only typical $GABA_A$ conductances. These conductances are resistant to cytosolic dilution by patch electrodes ("washout"), and thus provide no evidence for the second messengers typical of $GABA_B$ receptors (Lipton, 1989). Since $GABA_A$ immunostaining seems to outline bipolar cell axons and somas, but not dendritic terminals, it is interesting that the rod bipolar axons and somas are sensitive to puffs of GABA, but the dendritic terminals are not (Karschin and Wässle, 1990; Suzuki et al., 1990; but see Yeh et al., 1990).

To summarize: the results of both patch clamping and receptor immunohistochemistry indicate that amacrine cells, bipolar cells, and ganglion cells, possess $GABA_A$ receptors. These cell classes are known to be postsynaptic to GABAergic amacrine cells in the inner plexiform layer (see below). Specific types of GABA-receptive neurons may include cholinergic amacrine cells, the rod bipolar cell and the Y-type ganglion cell. The sites of horizontal cell interaction, the bipolar dendrites and receptors, do not appear to possess these receptors, another indication of the uncertain role of GABA in the outer plexiform layer.

## Circuits

Figure 3 is a circuit diagram for GABAergic circuits in the cat retina including all the putative GABAergic and GABA-receptive types discussed above. Its construction is based on electron microscopic sections of Golgi- or horseradish peroxidase-stained cells, as well as serial section reconstruction (Freed and Sterling, 1988; Kolb and Nelson, 1985; McGuire et al., 1986; Nelson and Kolb, 1984, 1985; Kolb et al., 1990). Like most circuit diagrams, it is uninformative unless one traces particular circuits through the various components. There is not room in this chapter to trace and discuss all circuits. The horizontal cell's synaptic interaction with the photoreceptor can be omitted since it seems similar in mammal and cold-blooded vertebrate, and the GABAergic nature of this interaction is better documented in cold-blooded vertebrates. The interactions of GABAergic amacrine cells and the cone bipolar pathway are important but will be left for a future publication (A19 cell, Freed, Kolb and Nelson, in preparation). This section of the chapter will focus on amacrine cells synaptically associated with the rod bipolar cell. Before it does, some general comments about GABAergic circuits are necessary

The circuit diagram of Fig. 3 lacks an important dimension. It does not specify how many individuals of each type are synaptically associated. Neither does it specify the related information about the number, distribution, and source of GABAergic synapses on each GABA-receptive cell type. At this point such information is very sketchy. Instead, a survey of GABAergic synapses has been accomplished by adapting, to the electron microscope, immunohistochemical methods for locating GAD-IR and GABA-IR (Chun and Wässle, 1989; Grünert and Wässle, 1990; Koontz and Hendrickson, 1990; Mariani and Caserta,

1986; Vaughn et al., 1981). Immunolabeled, presumably GABAergic, amacrine synapses are spread throughout the depth of the inner plexiform layer, in contrast to the laminar distributions of GAD-IR in light microscopic studies (Brandon, 1985). Apparently, GABAergic amacrine processes ramify in discrete lamina but this does not indicate the distribution of their synapses. The distribution of $GABA_A$ receptors in the inner plexiform layer is also laminated, so the distribution of GABAergic synapses is not identical to the distribution of GABA-receptive processes either (Hughes et al., 1989; Mariani et al., 1987; Richards et al., 1987).

Five studies of central retina have identified the processes *post*synaptic to GABAergic amacrine synapses as either bipolar cell, ganglion cell, or amacrine cell. Three studies of cat, rat and macaque are in agreement: at about half of GABAergic synapses, the postsynaptic processes are rod and cone bipolar cells (Chun and Wässle, 1989; Koontz and Hendrickson, 1990; Vaughn et al., 1981). The remaining GABAergic synapses are presynaptic to ganglion cells and amacrine cells with about equal frequency. Although two studies (Grünert and Wässle, 1990; Mariani and Caserta, 1986) differ on proportions or are not directly comparable, all studies agree that a substantial output from GABAergic amacrine cells is to bipolar cells.

Identification of processes *pre*synaptic to GABAergic amacrine cells has been made also. Rod and cone bipolar cells are an important input to GABAergic amacrine cells: more than half (51–88%) of the synapses upon GABAergic amacrines come from bipolar cells, with the remainder from amacrine cells (Chun and Wässle, 1989; Grünert and Wässle, 1990; Koontz and Hendrickson, 1990; Mariani and Caserta, 1986).

The GABAergic amacrine cells specialize in feedback synapses. Rod and cone bipolar cells contact amacrine cell varicosities at a dyad (Dowling and Boycott, 1976); at this site two processes are postsynaptic to the bipolar cell: the amacrine cell and one other cell. This other cell may be either a ganglion cell or another amacrine cell. A reciprocal synapse occurs when the amacrine cell process returns a synapse back upon the same bipolar cell. Chun and Wässle (1989) found that about 40% of the bipolar cell input to the GABAergic amacrine cell is reciprocated. Many reciprocal synapses are missed in single sections, so probably the proportion of reciprocal input to the GABAergic amacrine is much higher. Koontz and Hendrison (1990) have stated that all reciprocal amacrine synapses upon bipolar cells they could find were GABAergic.

The GABAergic amacrine cells in mammals are somewhat clannish: most (60–100%) amacrine inputs to GABAergic amacrine cells are from other GABAergic amacrine cells (Chun and Wässle, 1989; Grünert and Wässle, 1990; Vaughn et al., 1981). This may be due to the frequency of GABAergic processes in the inner plexiform layer, which causes GABAergic amacrine processes to encounter one another often. That GABAergic amacrine processes are frequent is hinted at: 70% of amacrine synapses are GABA-ergic (Koontz and Hendrickson, 1990). In addition, it is interesting, but of uncertain import, that GABAergic amacrine cells seem to have many more (3–5 ×) outputs than inputs (Chun and Wässle, 1989; Grünert and Wässle, 1990; Vaughn et al., 1981).

It may be possible to infer from these surveys the proportion of GABAergic synapses upon a retinal cell type. For example, there is a concentration of GABAergic amacrine synapses upon ganglion cells at the top of sublamina *b*, where the primate correlate of the On-Y cell ramifies. It would be, however, preferable to directly observe the pattern of GABAergic synapses upon an individual cell of identified type. If, for example, all GABAergic synapses are close to the Y cell's soma, this would have important nonlinear effects on its light response (Koch et al., 1982). Thus, it would be worth summarizing the pattern of GABAergic synapses upon an identified neuron. My collaborators and I (Freed et al., 1987) have found the pattern of GABAergic input upon

the rod bipolar cell. Many other investigators have contributed to an understanding of the rod bipolar cell-GABAergic amacrine circuit, making it one of the better characterized GABAergic circuits in mammal.

### The rod bipolar-reciprocal amacrine circuit

My collaborators and I (Smith et al., 1986) have concluded that gap junctions between photoreceptors are "closed" under conditions of extreme darkness, leaving the rod bipolar pathway the only operating pathway to the ganglion cells. A computer simulation of the large rod-cone network indicated the utility of closing the gap junctions: to keep small currents, caused by single quanta, from being diluted in the network. This makes the structure of the rod bipolar axon terminal particularly interesting as a final common path for signals. As can be seen in the circuit diagrams (Figs. 1 and 3), signals going down the rod pathway must go through the rod bipolar axon terminal → AII amacrine synapse. At virtually every such synapse, an amacrine varicosity is positioned that makes a reciprocal synapse back upon the rod bipolar cell (Kolb, 1979; McGuire et al., 1984; Strettoi et al., 1990). Thus, this reciprocal amacrine influences virtually all signals to the ganglion cells in the dark. Our study showed that almost all (> 90%) of the reciprocal amacrines are GABA-accumulating, indicating that GABA-ergic feedback is important to the rod bipolar pathway in mammals. A similar preponderance of GABAergic feedback upon rod bipolar cells in goldfish is discussed in Chapter 4 of this volume.

Figure 4, taken from our study, shows four rod bipolar axon terminals reconstructed from serial electron microscope sections (parts A–D). Each reconstruction is a series of profiles traced from the sections and stacked one upon the other to give a three-dimensional view of the entire axon terminal. In addition, all of the processes either presynaptic or postsynaptic to the axon terminal were reconstructed; these are represented in the figure by their largest profiles. Each rod bipolar axon terminal is represented three times to allow

120

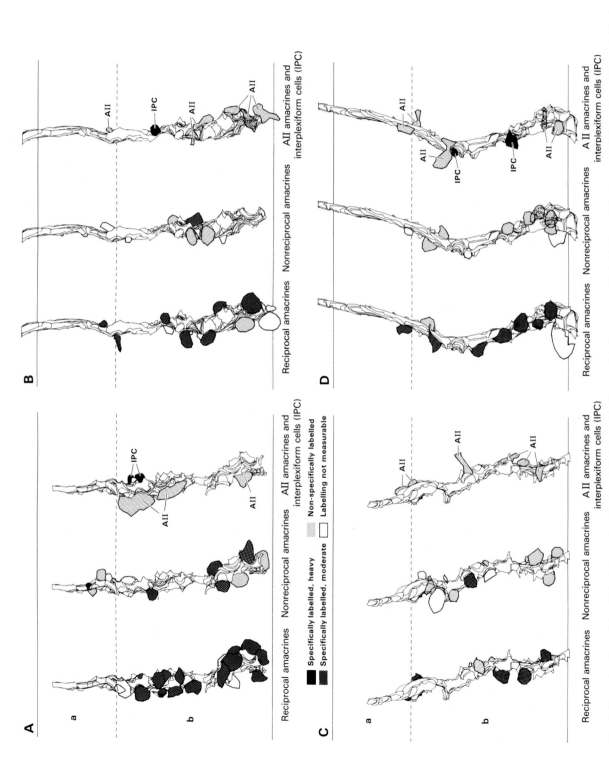

Fig. 4. Reconstruction of 4 rod bipolar axon terminals and their synaptically associated processes. Each bipolar cell is represented three times. For each bipolar cell: left panel, distribution of reciprocal amacrine processes; middle panel, non-reciprocal amacrine processes; right panel, AII and interplexiform cell processes (from Freed et al., 1987).

all of the processes to be represented without obscuring the axon terminal. Thus, each axon terminal is literally covered with synaptically-interacting processes.

Every section of the series used to reconstruct the rod bipolars was also prepared for autoradiography to show the location of [$^3$H]GABA after it was injected into the vitreous. We counted the grains over all the profile of all of these processes, measured their areas, and calculated the density of grains. Ninety percent of the reciprocal amacrine varicosities, and 100% of interplexiform varicosities, showed specific accumulations of grains. In addition, there are non-reciprocal amacrine varicosities, of uncertain origin, which are only presynaptic to the rod bipolar, not postsynaptic. Forty percent of non-reciprocal varicosities had specific accumulations. Specific accumulations did not lie over processes of the rod bipolar cell or the AII amacrine cell.

We knew that the autoradiographic grains represented [$^3$H]GABA, since chromatography showed that over 90% of radioactivity in the retina was due to [$^3$H]GABA. In addition, we checked the distribution of grain densities among processes: this distribution was bimodal, as would result from cells with high- and low-affinity uptake. Thus, specific accumulations of grains over neurons are due to high-affinity uptake, indicating the reciprocal amacrines are probably almost all GABAergic. In confirmation, amacrine varicosities reciprocal to the rod bipolar have been found to contain GABA-IR and GAD-IR (Chun and Wässle, 1989; Pourcho and Owczarzak, 1989; Vaughn et al., 1981). Also, the putative GABAergic types A17, A13, S1, and S2 have been shown to contribute reciprocal synapses to the rod bipolar cell. Other amacrine types, not known to be GABAergic, contribute reciprocal varicosities upon the rod bipolar cell, but our results suggest that they contribute less than 10% of these varicosities.

The very structure of the rod bipolar cell output implies massive GABAergic feedback. To determine whether this feedback is positive or negative one needs to known the light-evoked responses of all participants in the dyad. So far, the recorded responses are all to a step function (a flash of light). Intracellular recording and staining of the AII amacrine cell shows a depolarization to the onset of the step which decays with time (a transient response; Dacheux and Raviola, 1986; Nelson and Kolb, 1983). Recording from the A17 and its analogue in rabbit (S1) shows a depolarizing to the onset of the step, but with little decay (a sustained response; Nelson and Kolb, 1985; Raviola and Dacheux, 1987). Surprisingly, the A13 response is of opposite polarity: a sustained hyperpolarization.

Since all of these amacrine cells, AII, A13, and A17, are postsynaptic at the dyad, the opposite polarity of the A13 is unexpected. Different inputs may cause these different responses: the A17 receives predominant rod bipolar input (with occasional input from the A18), while the A13 receives input from cone bipolar cells in addition (see circuit diagram, Fig. 3). It is possible, therefore, that the response recorded at the A13 soma reflects this additional input, and the A13 varicosities at the rod bipolar dyad might be electrically isolated from the soma (Ellias and Stevens, 1980). In this case, the response polarity of all the reciprocal varicosities, would be depolarizing, like the A17 response.

The few intracellular recordings from rod bipolar cells published so far disagree as to whether its response is hyperpolarizing or depolarizing (Dacheux and Raviola, 1986; Nelson et al., 1976). The reason for this disagreement is that the rod bipolar cell soma is extremely difficult to record from in situ, since it is small and lies interstitial in the retina. To improve recording conditions, rod bipolar cells have been isolated from the rat retina, placed in a dish, and patch electrodes used to make whole-cell recordings (Karschin and Wässle, 1990; Yamashita and Wässle, 1990). The response to light was eliminated by this isolation, of course. Instead, the natural transmitter of the rod photoreceptors, glutamate, and its agonist 2-amino-4-phosphonobutyric acid (APB), were puffed onto the rod bipolar cell. It was reasoned that these puffs should have the opposite effect to light, since light curtails photoreceptor release of transmitter. APB was found to close channels with a reversal potential positive to the rod bipolar cell's potential in the dark. This indicated that light, having the opposite effect, opened these channels and depolarized the cell.

Since the rod bipolar cell seems to depolarize to light, it can be inferred that input upon the AII and A17 amacrine cell from the rod bipolar cell is sign conserving. It can also be inferred that the return synapses of the reciprocal amacrine are sign inverting: upon depolarization the reciprocal amacrine releases GABA, which increases chloride conductance in the rod bipolar cell. Presumably, the chloride reversal potential is negative to the rod bipolar dark potential and an increase in chloride conductance causes a hyperpolarization. This all adds up to negative feedback at the dyad.

In light of the evidence presented for negative feedback, it is somewhat disappointing that its effects are not obvious in the responses of the intact retina so far recorded. The transient response of the AII cell might indicate feedback, but is probably not a result of the reciprocal synapse: Neither the A17 cell or the rod bipolar cell is transient. Yet, the A17 is postsynaptic at the same synapses as the AII cell. Therefore, the AII transient response may be due to its intrinsic properties, and not due to the reciprocal synapse (Werblin, 1977). The A17 and AII cells have a quicker response (less rise time) at the onset of the step than the rod bipolar cell, which may indicate feedback, since it shows increased gain and high frequency response. Unfortunately, the responses recorded so far are not definitive, since their characteristics could be approximated by either positive or negative feedback, depending on the frequency response and gain of the elements in the feedback loop. For example, a response to high frequency can be enhanced by either negative feedback with low pass character-

istics, or positive feedback with high pass characteristics. Thus, it is clear that, despite much data about a very simple GABAergic circuit, the rod bipolar dyad is still only vaguely understood.

## Effects of GABA-antagonists on circuitry

Extracellular and intracellular records of ganglion cells in situ show complex effects of $GABA_A$ antagonists. Unfortunately, the reported effects of these antagonists, even for the same cell type in the same animal, often disagree. Each study stresses a different division of four ganglion cell types (On-X, On-Y, Off-X, Off-Y). Caldwell and Daw (1978) separate X and Y cells, and report that picrotoxin alters the center-surround balance of Y but not X cells. Ikeda and Sheardown (1983) separate On and Off cells, claiming that bicuculline blocks inhibition in On but not Off cells. Saito (1981,1983) reports that bicuculline alters center-surround balance in On-Y, but not in Off-Y, On-X or Off-X cells. Bolz et al. (1985) claim that all four types of ganglion cell are affected by bicuculline.

Differences among these studies may be due to differences in the route of drug application: some studies perfuse drugs into the retinal circulation or into the bath surrounding an isolated retina. Other studies iontophorese drugs into a more limited volume of the retina. More important, investigators differ in their interpretation and description of post stimulus time histograms. Figure 5 simulates a post stimulus time histogram of a ganglion cell response before and during a drug application. There are two incorrect interpretations of this histogram. One investigator, noting that the spike frequency during light-On is greater with the drug than without, might conclude that the effect of the drug is to increase the On-excitation. Another investigator, noting that the complete inhibition of firing at light-Off has become a partial inhibition, might conclude that the effect of the drug is to block the Off-inhibition. In fact, Fig. 5 was constructed by raising the firing rate at all times during the histogram by the

A

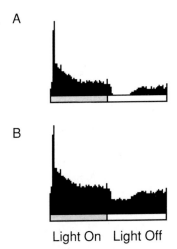

B

Light On    Light Off

Fig. 5. Simulation of ganglion cell response to light before (A) and during (B) a drug that raises the spontaneous rate of firing. See text for explanation.

same amount. Thus, the responses at light-On and light-Off have not changed at all, if response is defined as the difference between the firing during the stimulus and the spontaneous rate. This illustrates the need for a non-zero rate of firing, both spontaneous and during inhibition, to serve as a reference for the response *. Since GABA$_A$-antagonists increase the spontaneous rate of On-center cells, and have variable effects on the spontaneous rate of Off-center cells (Bolz et al., 1985; Saito, 1983), this criterion is applied

to the following summary of GABA$_A$ antagonist effects on ganglion cell responses. The GABA$_A$ antagonists used are bicuculline and picrotoxin.

*On ganglion cell responses*

On-Y cells, under mesopic and scotopic conditions, show a differential effect of GABA$_A$ antagonists on center and surround, since the surround response (surround-On, surround-Off) is reduced more than the center responses (Caldwell and Daw, 1978; Kirby and Enroth-Cugell, 1976; Saito, 1981, 1983). The center response is reduced very little. Examination of records from most studies indicates a common effect of these antagonists: The initial transient of the center excitatory response (center-On) commonly decays faster, leaving this transient more distinct from the subsequent sustained portion of the excitatory response (Fig. 2 of Kirby and Enroth-Cugell, 1976; Fig. 2 of Saito, 1983; Fig. 5 of Bolz et al., 1985).

For On-X cells, under mesopic conditions, when spontaneous rate is allowed for, there is little evidence that GABA$_A$ antagonists have any large effect on their light responses, including any differential effect on center and surround (Bolz et al., 1985; Caldwell and Daw, 1978; Ikeda and Sheardown, 1983; Kirby and Enroth-Cugell, 1976; Saito, 1981, 1983).

*Off ganglion cell responses*

For 14 Off-Y cells, under the mesopic conditions adaptation, GABA$_A$ antagonists had no differential effect on center and surround amplitudes (Saito, 1981; Saito, 1983). Kirby and Enroth-Cugell (Kirby and Enroth-Cugell, 1976) reported a differential effect, that the surround response decreased more than the center, but this was based on an unspecified number of Off-Y cells. The inhibitory responses (center-On, surround-Off) are reduced. The initial transients of excitatory responses (center-Off, surround-On) are often increased in amplitude and commonly decay more quickly (Fig. 5. of Caldwell and Daw, 1978; Fig. 4 of Saito, 1983; Fig. 8 of Bolz et al., 1985).

---

* In an analysis of circuitry, the voltage responses of a cell are important, since they reflect synaptic inputs. Firing frequency, an easily measured quantity, is only an epiphenomenom of voltage change: If membrane voltage is above the threshold for firing, firing frequency is proportional to membrane voltage (Fourtes, 1959; personal observations). The frequency of spontaneous firing sums with the frequency of light-evoked firing because the voltages that cause firing sum at the spike generating site. This indicates the need to subtract the spontaneous firing frequency from the light-evoked firing frequency to derive a response. For this derivation to be valid, the spontaneous frequency must be above zero, otherwise the voltage of the cell is below threshold for firing and so indeterminate. Similarly, firing frequency during an inhibitory response must be above zero, or else the true voltage change of the inhibitory response is indeterminate.

For Off-X cell, under mesopic conditions, GABA$_A$ antagonists have little differential effect on center and surround (Bolz et al., 1985; Caldwell and Daw, 1978; Kirby and Enroth-Cugell, n rabbit, after dye in1976; Saito, 1981; Saito, 1983). The center size is not affected (Bolz et al., 1985). The inhibitory responses (center-On, surround-Off) are reduced. The amplitudes of excitatory responses (center-Off, surround-On) are little affected but, at least in cat, their initial transients decay more quickly (Fig. 1 of Ikeda and Sheardown, 1983; Fig. 4 of Saito, 1983; Fig. 7 of Bolz et al., 1985).

*X versus Y cells*

For Y cells, the effect of GABA$_A$ antagonists depends on conditions of adaptation. Under photopic or high mesopic conditions the center and surround responses of On- and Off-Y cells are affected very little by GABA$_A$ antagonists (Frishman and Linsenmeier, 1982; Kirby and Schweitzer-Tong, 1981a). Under conditions of scotopic to high mesopic adaptation, GABA$_A$ antagonists reduce the center size of of On-center but increase the center size of Off-Y cells (Kirby and Schweitzer-Tong, 1981a,b).

Unlike X cells, Y cell's receptive fields have complex, nonlinear, components laid over the center and surround. Hockstein and Shapley have introduced the concept of nonlinear subunits, which are multiple domains, smaller than the center or surround, and distributed throughout the receptive field (Hochstein and Shapley, 1976). Under photopic conditions, picrotoxin reduces the sensitivity of these nonlinear subunits (Frishman and Linsenmeier, 1982).

A moving pattern outside the surround alters the response of Y cell, but not X cells. This response to a moving pattern is blocked by picrotoxin (Caldwell and Daw, 1978; Frishman and Linsenmeier, 1982).

*Other ganglion cell types*

In addition to the X and Y cells, both cat and rabbit have ganglion cells with more complex

receptive fields, the W cells. Unlike X and Y cells, W cells are excited most by certain directions of movement, speeds of movement and orientations. Picrotoxin, under mesopic conditions, eliminates these characteristics, simplifying the receptive fields to a center-surround structure like that of X and Y cells (Caldwell et al., 1978). For example, one W cell type has a center-surround receptive field like the Y cell; unlike the Y cell, this cell type is selective for high speeds of movement. Picrotoxin causes this cell type to respond to both high and low speeds of movement, as a Y cell does. Another W cell type is orientation selective. Picrotoxin causes this cell type to lose orientation selectivity, simplifying the receptive field to a center-surround structure

**Discussion**

The most general statement that can be made about GABA$_A$ antagonists is that they modify the center-surround structure of X and Y receptive fields, but never abolish the center or surround completely (Caldwell and Daw, 1978). In the case of On-X, Off-X, and Off-Y cells, bicuculline has little effect on center-surround balance.

The weak effects of GABA$_A$ antagonists on center-surround structure provide no evidence for GABAergic horizontal cells. Horizontal cells, through their reciprocal interaction with photoreceptors and bipolar cells, are thought to create a center-surround structure in rod and cone bipolar cells (Mangel and Miller, 1987). Rod and cone bipolar pathways convey this center-surround structure to ganglion cells. Even if horizontal cells are not the sole origin of ganglion cell surrounds, the resistance of On-X cell responses to GABA$_A$ drugs seems to indicate that a GABAergic horizontal cell does not contribute to any ganglion cell responses, since On-X ganglion cells share with all ganglion cells the same horizontal cell input.

It could be argued, in favor of GABAergic horizontal cells in mammals, that the site of horizontal cell synaptic interactions, the photoreceptor invagination, is protected from drugs. Yet, another drug of similar size, APB, is able to reach this site and block On-center bipolar cells. As would be expected, blocking the On-bipolar cell pathways (rod, cone $\rightarrow$ CBb$_1$ $\rightarrow$ On ganglion cell) abolishes the center response, and presumably the surround response, of On-center ganglion cells. Also, it might be that the horizontal cell is presynaptic at GABA$_B$ receptors and thus not blocked by GABA$_A$ antagonists; this possibility has not been investigated in mammals. In salamander, there is some suggestion that horizontal cells are presynaptic at both GABA$_A$ and GABA$_B$ receptors, since drugs specific to each receptor have little effect on bipolar cell surrounds (Miller et al., 1981; Slaughter and Bai, 1989; see Slaughter and Pan, Chapter 3; see Wu, Chapter 5), but a combination of $\delta$-aminovaleric acid and picrotoxin, which may block both receptor types, has been shown to eliminate bipolar cell surrounds (Hare and Owen, 1990). No report exists of this combination's affect on the mammalian retina. Thus, the histological and physiological evidence in mammal for GABAergic horizontal cells is equivocal, but all means of gathering such evidence have not been tried.

Comparison of the circuit diagram with the reported effects of GABA$_A$ antagonists rules out sites better than it indicates them. The On-Y response is affected by GABA$_A$ antagonists, while the On-X response is not. This rules out as a site of drug action any common inputs to the On-X and On-Y cells. The CBb$_1$ bipolar cell is such a common input. Indeed, it is the predominant bipolar cell input to both ganglion cell types, and is known to have a center-surround receptive field (Freed and Sterling, 1988; McGuire et al., 1986; Nelson and Kolb, 1983). It is unclear why the A13 amacrine, which contacts cone bipolar cells, is not a site of drug action: perhaps these inputs to the CBb1 are rare. This leaves direct GABAergic input to the On-Y cell to mediate GABA$_A$ effects, perhaps from the dA14 and other GABAergic amacrine cells. These GABAergic inputs may contribute to the On-Y surround. The

sensitivity of On-Y cells to antagonists is consistent with the evidence for concentrated GABAergic input upon their dendrites.

The Off-X and Off-Y cell also share a common, predominant, bipolar cell input from CBa$_1$ (Nelson et al., 1989). Presumably, the effects of GABA antagonists common to both Off-X and Off-Y are due to this common input. These common effects are the reduction of inhibition, and the enhancement of transients. The receptive fields of both Off-X and Off-Y cells are known to reflect a greater variety of influences than On-X and On-Y cells, and include both excitatory and inhibitory inputs (Belgum et al., 1987; Chen and Linsenmeier, 1989a; Chen and Linsenmeier, 1989b). It may be that GABAergic amacrine cells contribute to the inhibitory responses of Off ganglion cells.

The complex receptive field features that distinguish Y and W cells from X cells appear to originate in amacrine cells. Amacrine cells contribute a greater proportion of input to the Y cells and W cells than to the X cells (Kolb, 1979). To date, however, most amacrine cells presynaptic to Y and W cells have not been typed. An exception is the GABA-accumulating type A19, known to contact the Off-Y cell. The A19 has a receptive field and an On-Off response with many similarities to the nonlinear subunits of the Y cells and thus may be the cause of them (Freed et al., 1990). GABAergic amacrine cells contribute to the complex feature of W cells too, such as orientation, speed and direction selectivities. In both Y and W cell, complex features appear to overlay the basic center-surround receptive field structure contributed by the bipolar pathways. Again, GABAergic amacrines modify, but do not create, this structure.

Most of the pharmacological studies discussed above were done under conditions of illumination too bright to favor the rod bipolar pathway. However, the circuit diagram indicates reciprocal GABAergic synapses upon cone bipolar cells as well as rod bipolar cells. Thus, given the ubiquity of GABAergic feedback on both rod and cone bipolar pathways, and assuming that all such synapses operate alike, some pervasive sign of GABAergic feedback should appear in the pharmacological studies. Indeed, apparent in the summary presented here is a common effect of $GABA_A$ antagonists, which is to accentuate the transient excitatory responses and make them even more transient. This common effect does point to some sort of feedback. Unfortunately, this common effect is no more indicative of negative feedback than positive feedback, since, as discussed, the frequency response of the feedback loop is unknown.

The enhancement of transients by GABA analogues also occurs in mudpuppy. In this animal, baclofen, a $GABA_B$ agonist, as well as bicuculline, the $GABA_A$ antagonist make sustained ganglion responses more transient and increases the amplitude of transients in transient amacrine and ganglion cells (Bai and Slaughter, 1989; Frumkes et al., 1981; Slaughter and Bai, 1989). In some transient neurons, these effects appear to have a simple electrogenic basis. In other transient neurons this transient enhancement appears to be an emergent property of retinal circuitry, (e.g., reciprocal synapses?) and so is not well understood.

It might appear odd that bicuculline, a $GABA_A$ antagonist, mimics baclofen, a $GABA_B$ agonist, but such a equivalency is suggested by results in mudpuppy. Here, bicuculline blocks $GABA_A$ receptors, but leaves $GABA_B$ receptors alone. In this circumstance, GABA binds solely to $GABA_B$ receptors, and has an effect indistinguishable from that of baclofen (Slaughter and Bai, 1989). Although, in mammals, bipolar cells and ganglion cells don't seem to have $GABA_B$ receptors, amacrine cells may have both $GABA_A$ and $GABA_B$ receptors, as they do in mudpuppy (Maguire et al., 1989). Thus, in mammals, bicuculline may block $GABA_A$ receptors, leaving tonically released GABA to act like baclofen. Such an equivalence between bicuculline and baclofen is suggested by a recent study of cat: baclofen, like

bicuculline, makes ganglion cell responses more transient (Ikeda et al., 1990).

## Conclusion

The structure of the rod bipolar cell dyad synapse, with its putative reciprocal GABAergic amacrine, is well characterized, and recently some success at isolating its constituent neurons has been made. Yet, these results do not serve to explain the photic responses of constituent neurons when they sit in the intact retina, or the pharmacological effects of GABA drugs on the intact retina. It may be that the retina, as simple as it is, has too many GABAergic sites for drug action to be understood from the circuit diagram. Perhaps individual circuits must be removed from the retina to be understood. Recently, it has been possible to grow bipolar cell synapses in culture (Gleason and Wilson, 1989). GABAergic amacrine cells can also be grown in culture (Akagawa and Barnstable, 1986). Future studies may combine bipolar and amacrine cells in culture to reconstitute the GABAergic feedback circuit. Methods of recording from retinal slices have been developed which include low-noise electrodes and better visual control of the targeted cell (Werblin, 1977). Such methods provide easier access to the retinal interior. Adapted to the mammalian retina, these methods will aid investigation of GABAergic circuits there. The identification of GABAergic amacrine cell types, as reviewed here, will confer an advantage to future studies of GABA circuits. There are 10 putative GABAergic amacrine cells in cat (7 GABA-accumulating + 2 cholinergic + 1 dopaminergic). It will be interesting to see the variety of roles they play in retinal circuitry.

## References

Agardh, E., Bruun, A., Ehinger, B., Ekström, van Veen, T. and Wu, J.-Y. (1987) Gamma-aminobutyric acid-and glutamic acid decarboxylase-immunoreactive neurons in the retina of different vertebrates. *J. Comp. Neurol.*, 258: 622–630.

Akagawa, K. and Barnstable, C.J. (1986) Identification and characterization of cell types in monolayer cultures of rat retina using monoclonal antibodies. *Brain Res.*, 383: 110–20.

Bai, S.-H. and Slaughter, M.M. (1989) Effects of baclofen on transient neurons in the mudpuppy retina: electrogenic and network actions. *J. Neurophysiol.*, 61: 382–390.

Bauer, B. (1978) Photic release of radioactivity from rabbit retina reloaded with [$^3$H]GABA. *Acta Ophthalmol.*, 56: 277–283.

Belgum, J.H., Dvorak, D.R., McReynolds, J.S. and Miyachi, E. (1987) Push-pull effect of surround illumination on excitatory and inhibitory inputs to mudpuppy retinal ganglion cells. *J. Physiol. (London)*, 388: 233–43.

Blazynski, C., Ferrendelli, J.A. and Cohen, A.I. (1985) indoleamine-sensitive adenylate cyclase in rabbit retina: Characterization and distribution. *J. Neurochem.*, 45: 440–447.

Bolz, J., Frumkes, T., Voigt, T. and Wässle, H. (1985) Action and localization of gamma-aminobutyric acid in the cat retina. *J. Physiol. (London)*, 362: 369–93.

Bolz, J. and McGuire, B. (1985) GABA-like immunoreactivity in horizontal cells of the cat retina. *Soc. Neurosci. Abstr.*, 11: 1215.

Brandon, C. (1985) Retinal GABA neurons: localization in vertebrate species using an antiserum to rabbit brain glutamate decarboxylase. *Brain Res.*, 344: 286–95.

Brandon, C., Lam, D.M. and Wu, J.Y. (1979) The gamma-aminobutyric acid system in rabbit retina: localization by immunocytochemistry and autoradiography. *Proc. Natl. Acad. Sci. USA*, 76: 3557–61.

Brecha, N., Johnson, D., Peichl, L. and Wässle, H. (1988) Cholinergic amacrine cells of the rabbit retina contain glutamate decarboxylase and gamma-aminobutyric acid immunoreactivity. *Proc. Natl. Acad. Sci. USA*, 85: 6187–91.

Brunken, W.J. and Daw, N.W. (1986) 5-HT$_2$ antagonists reduce ON-responses in the rabbit retina. *Brain Res.*, 384: 161–5.

Brunken, W.J. and Daw, N.W. (1988a) The effects of serotonin agonists and antagonists on the response properties of complex ganglion cells in the rabbit's retina. *Vis. Neurosci.*, 1: 181–188.

Brunken, W.J. and Daw, N.W. (1988b) Neuropharmacological analysis of the role of indoleamine-accumulating amacrine cells in the rabbit retina. *Vis. Neurosci.*, 1: 275–285.

Caldwell, J.H. and Daw, N.W. (1978) Effects of picrotoxin and strychnine on rabbit retinal ganglion cells: changes in centre surround receptive fields. *J. Physiol. (London)*, 276: 299–310.

Caldwell, J.H., Daw, N.W. and Wyatt, H.J. (1978) Effects of picrotoxin and strychnine on rabbit retinal ganglion cells: lateral interactions for cells with more complex receptive fields. *J. Physiol. (London)*, 276: 277–98.

Chen, E.P.C. and Linsenmeier, R.A. (1989a) Centre components of cone-driven retinal ganglion cells - differential sensitivity to 2-amino-4-phosphonobutyric acid. *J. Physiol. (London)*, 419: 77–93.

Chen, E.P.C. and Linsenmeier, R.A. (1989b) Effects of 2-amino-4-phosphonobutyric acid on responsivity and spatial summation of X cells in the cat retina. *J. Physiol. (London)*, 419: 59–75.

Chun, M.H. and Wässle, H. (1989) GABA-like immunoreactivity in the cat retina: Electron microscopy. *J. Comp. Neurol.*, 279: 55–67.

Chun, M.H., Wässle, H. and Brecha, N. (1988) Colocalization of [$^3$H]muscimol uptake and choline acetyltransferase immunoreactivity in amacrine cells of the cat retina. *Neurosci. Lett.*, 94: 259–63.

Dacey, D.M. (1988) Dopamine-accumulating retinal neurons revealed by in vitro fluorescence display a unique morphology. *Science*, 240: 1196–8.

Dacheux, R.F. and Raviola, E. (1986) The rod bipolar pathway in the rabbit retina; a depolarizing bipolar and amacrine cell. *J. Neurosci.*, 6: 331–345.

Dowling, J.E. and Boycott, B.B. (1976) Organization of the primate retina: Electron microscopy. *Proc. R. Soc. London Biol.*, 166: 80–111.

Dowling, J.E. and Ehinger, B. (1978) Synaptic organization of the dopaminergic neurons in the rabbit retina. *J. Comp. Neurol.*, 180: 203–220.

Dowling, J.E., Ehinger, B. and Floren, I. (1980) Fluorescence and electron microscopical observations on the amine-accumulating neurons of the Cebus monkey retina. *J. Comp. Neurol.*, 192: 665–85.

Ehinger, B., Hansson, C. and Tornqvist, K. (1981) 5-Hydroxytryptamine in the retina of some mammals. *Exp. Eye Res.*, 33: 663–672.

Ehinger, B. and Holmgren, I. (1979) Electron microscopy of the indoleamine-accumulating neurons in the retina of the rabbit. *Cell Tissue Res.*, 197: 175–94.

Ellias, S.A. and Stevens, J.K. (1980) The dendritic varicosity: a mechanism for electrically isolating the dendrites of cat retinal amacrine cells? *Brain Res.*, 196: 365–72.

Enna, S.J. and Karbon, E.W. (1986) GABA Receptors: An Overview. In: R.W. Olsen and J.C. Venter (Eds.), *Benzodiazepine / GABA Receptors and Chloride Channels: Structural and Functional Properties*, Vol. 5, Alan R. Liss, New York, pp. 41–56.

Enna, S.J. and Snyder, H. (1976) Gamma-aminobutyric acid (GABA) receptor binding in mammalian retina. *Brain Res.*, 115: 174–179.

Fourtes, M.G.F. (1959) Initiation of impulses in visual cells of Limulus. *J. Physiol. (London)*, 148: 14–28.

Florén, I. (1979) Arguments against 5-Hydroxytryptamine in the rabbit retina. *J. Neural Trans.*, 46: 1–15.

Florén, I. and Hansson, C. (1980) Investigations into whether 5-hydroxytryptamine is a neurotransmitter in the retina of rabbit and chicken. *Ophthalmol. Vis. Sci.*, 19: 117–125.

Freed, M., Smith, R. and Sterling, P. (1987) Rod bipolar array in the cat retina: pattern of input from rods and GABA-accumulating amacrine cells. *J. Comp. Neurol.*, 266: 445–455.

Freed, M.A., Nakamura, Y. and Sterling, P. (1983) Four types of amacrine in the cat retina that accumulate GABA. *J. Comp. Neurol.*, 219: 295–304.

Freed, M.A., Nelson, R., Pflug, R. and Kolb, H. (1990) On-Off amacrine cell in cat retina has multiple axon-like processes. *Invest. Ophthal. Vis. Science (Suppl.)*, 31: 114–115.

Freed, M.A. and Sterling, P. (1988) The ON-alpha ganglion cell of the cat retina and its presynaptic cell types. *J. Neurosci.*, 8: 2303–20.

Friedman, D.L. and Redburn, D.A. (1990) Evidence for functionally distinct subclasses of γ-aminobutyric acid receptors in rabbit retina. *J. Neurochem.*, 55: 1189–1199.

Frishman, L.J. and Linsenmeier, R.A. (1982) Effects of picrotoxin and strychnine on non-linear responses of Y-type cat retinal ganglion cells. *J. Physiol. (London)*, 324: 347–363.

Frumkes, T.E., Miller, R.F., Slaughter, M. and Dacheux, R.F. (1981) Physiological and pharmacological basis of GABA and glycine action on neurons of mudpuppy retina. III. Amacrine-mediated inhibitory influences on ganglion cell receptive-field organization: a model. *J. Neurophysiol.*, 45: 783–804.

Gleason, E. and Wilson, M. (1989) Development of synapses between chick retinal neurons in dispersed culture. *J. Comp. Neurol.*, 287: 213–224.

Goodchild, M. and Neal, M.J. (1973) The uptake of [$^3$H]γ-aminobutryric acid by the retina. *Br. J. Pharmacol.*, 47: 529–542.

Graham, L.T. (1972) Intraretinal distribution of GABA content and GAD activity. *Brain Res.*, 36: 476–479.

Grünert, U. and Wässle, H. (1990) GABA-like immunoreactivity in the Macaque monkey retina: a light and electron microscopic study. *J. Comp. Neurol.*, 297: 509–524.

Hare, W.A. and Owen, W.G. (1990) Spatial organization of the bipolar cell's receptive field in the retina of the tiger salamander. *J. Physiol. (London)*, 421: 223–245.

Hendrickson, A., Marianne, R., Noble, B. and Wu, J.-Y. (1985) Colocalization of [$^3$H]muscimol and antisera to GABA and glutamic acid decarboxylase within the same neurons in monkey retina. *Brain. Res.*, 348: 391–396.

Hochstein, S. and Shapley, R.M. (1976) Linear and nonlinear spatial subunits in Y cat retinal ganglion cells. *J. Physiol. (London)*, 262: 265–284.

Holmgren-Taylor, I. (1982) Electron microscopical observations on the indoleamine-accumulating neurons and their synaptic connections in the retina of the cat. *J. Comp. Neurol.*, 208: 144–56.

Hughes, T.E., Carey, R.G., J., V., deBlas, A.L. and Karten, H.J. (1989) Immunohistochemical localization of GABA$_A$ receptors in the retina of the new world primate *Saimiri sciureus*. *Vis. Neurosci*, 2: 565–581.

Ikeda, H. and Sheardown, M.J. (1983) Transmitters mediating inhibition of ganglion cells in the cat retina: iontophoretic studies in vivo. *Neuroscience*, 8: 837–853.

Ikeda, H., Hankins, M.W. and Kay, C.D. (1990) Actions of baclofen and phaclofen upon On-ganglion and Off-ganglion cells in the cat retina. *Eur. J. Pharm.*, 190: 1–9.

Kamp, C. (1985) The dopaminergic system in retina. In: W.W. Morgan (Eds.), *Retinal Transmitters and Modulators: Models for the Brain*. CRC, Boca Raton, FL, pp. 1–32.

Karschin, A. and Wässle, H. (1990) Voltage- and transmitter-gated currents in isolated rod bipolar cells of rat retina. *J. Neurophysiol.*, 63: 860–876.

Kirby, A.W. and Enroth-Cugell, C. (1976) The involvement of gamma-aminobutyric acid in the organization of the cat retinal ganglion cell receptive fields. *J. Gen. Physiol.*, 68: 465–484.

Kirby, A.W. and Schweitzer-Tong, D.E. (1981a) GABA-antagonists alter spatial summation in receptive field centres of rod- but not cone-drive cat retinal ganglion Y-cells. *J. Physiol. (London)*, 320: 303–8.

Kirby, A.W. and Schweitzer-Tong, D.E. (1981b) GABA-antagonists and spatial summation in Y-type cat retinal ganglion cells. *J. Physiol. (London)*, 312: 335–344.

Koch, C., Poggio, T. and Torre, V. (1982) Retinal ganglion cells: A functional interpretation of dendritic morphology. *Phil. Trans. Soc. London B*, 298: 227–264.

Kolb, H. (1979) The inner plexiform layer in the retina of the cat: electron microscopic observations. *J. Neurocytol.*, 8: 295–329.

Kolb, H., Cuenca, N., Wang, H.H. and Dekorver, L. (1990) The synaptic organization of the dopaminergic amacrine cell in the cat retina. *J. Neurocytol.*, 19: 343–366.

Kolb, H. and Famiglietti, E.V. (1974) Rod and cone pathways in the inner plexiform layer of cat retina. *Science*, 186: 47–49.

Kolb, H. and Nelson, R. (1985) Functional neurocircuitry of amacrine cells in the cat retina. In: A. Gallego and P. Gouras (Eds.), *Neurocircuitry of the Retina, A Cajal Memorial*. Elsevier, Amsterdam, pp.

Kolb, H., Nelson, R. and Mariani, A. (1981) Amacrine cells, bipolar cells and ganglion cells of the cat retina: a Golgi study. *Vision. Res.*, 21: 1081–1114.

Koontz, M.A. and Hendrickson, A.E. (1990) Distribution of GABA-Immunoreactive amacrine cell synapses in the inner plexiform layer of macaque monkey retina. *Vis. Neurosci.*, 5: 17–28.

Kosaka, T., Kosaka, K., Hataguchi, Y., Nagatsu, I., Wu, J.-Y., Ottersen, O.P., Storm-Mathisen, J. and Hama, K. (1987) Catecholaminergic neurons containing GABA-like and/or glutamic acid decarboxylase-like immunoreactivity in various brain regions of the rat. *Exp. Brain Res.*, 66: 191–210.

Kosaka, T., Tauchi, M. and Dahl, J.L. (1988) Cholinergic neurons containing GABA-like and/or glutamic acid decarboxylase-like immunoreactivities in various brain regions of the rat. *Exp. Brain Res.*, 70: 605–17.

Kuriyama, K., Sisken, B., Haber, B. and Roberts, E. (1968) The γ-aminobutyric acid system in rabbit retina. *Brain Res.*, 9: 165–168.

Lam, D.M.-K., Fung, S.-C. and Kong, U.-C. (1980) Postnatal development of GABA-ergic neurons in the rabbit retina. *J. Comp. Neurol.*, 193: 89–102.

Lipton, S. (1989) GABA-activated single channel currents in outside-out membrane patches from rat retinal ganglion cells. *Vis. Neurosci.*, 3: 275–279.

Linn, D.M. and Massey, S.C. (1991) GABA inhibits ACh

release from the rabbit retina: a direct effect of bipolar cell feedback? *Soc. Neurosci. Abstr.*, 16: 713

Mangel, S.C. and Miller, R.F. (1987) Horizontal cells contribute to the receptive field surround of ganglion cells in the rabbit retina. *Brain Res.*, 414: 182–186.

Maguire, G., Lukasiewicz, P. and Werblin, F. (1989) Amacrine cell interactions underlying the response to change in the tiger salamander retina. *J. Neurosci.*, 9: 726–735.

Mariani, A.P. and Caserta, M.T. (1986) Electron microscopy of glutamate decarboxylase (GAD) immunoreactivity in the inner plexiform layer of the rhesus monkey retina. *J. Neurocytol.*, 15: 645–655.

Mariani, A.P., Cosenza-Murphy, D. and Barker, J.L. (1987) GABAergic synapses and benzodiazepine receptors are not identically distributed in the primate retina. *Brain. Res.*, 415: 153–157.

Mariani, A.P. and Hersh, L.B. (1988) Synaptic organization of cholinergic amacrine cells in the rhesus monkey retina. *J. Comp. Neurol.*, 267: 269–280.

Masland, R.H., Cassidy, C. and O'Malley, D.M. (1989) The release of acetylcholine and GABA by neurons of the rabbit retina. In: R. Weiler and N.N. Osborne (Eds.), *Neurobiology of the Inner Retina*, Vol. 31, Springer-Verlag, Berlin, pp. 15–26.

Masland, R.H. and Livingston, C.J. (1976) Effect of stimulation with light on the synthesis and release of acetylcholine by an isolated mammalian retina. *J. Neurophysiol.*, 39: 1210–1219.

Masland, R.H. and Mills, J.W. (1979) Autoradiographic identification of acetylcholine in the rabbit retina. *J. Cell Biol.*, 83: 159–78.

Massey, S.C. and Redburn, D.A. (1987) Transmitter circuits in the vertebrate retina. *Prog. Neurobiol.*, 28: 55–96.

Massey, S.C. Blankenship, K. and Mills, S.L. (1991) Cholinergic amacrine cells in the rabbit retina accumulate muscimol. *Visual Neurosci.*, 6: 113–117

McGuire, B.A., Stevens, J.K. and Sterling, P. (1984) Microcircuitry of bipolar cells in cat retina. *J. Neurosci.*, 4: 2920–38.

McGuire, B.A., Stevens, J.K. and Sterling, P. (1986) Microcircuitry of beta ganglion cells in cat retina. *J. Neurosci.*, 6: 907–918.

Miller, R.F., Frumkes, T.E., Slaughter, M. and Dacheux, R.F. (1981) Physiological and pharmacological basis of GABA and glycine action on neurons of mudpuppy retina. I. Receptors, horizontal cells, bipolars and G-cells. *J. Neurophysiol.*, 45: 743–763.

Mitchell, C.K. and Redburn, D.A. (1985) Analysis of pre- and postsynaptic factors of the serotonin system in rabbit retina. *J. Cell. Biol.*, 100: 64–73.

Mitrofanis, J. and Finay, B.L. (1990) Developmental changes in the distribution of retinal catecholaminergic neurons in hamster and gerbils. *J. Comp. Neurol.*, 292: 480–494.

Mosinger, J.L. and Yazulla, S. (1985) Colocalization of GAD-like immunoreactivity and [³H]GABA uptake in amacrine cells of rabbit retina. *J. Comp. Neurol.*, 240: 396–406.

Mosinger, J.L. and Yazulla, S. (1987) Double-label analysis of GAD- and GABA-like immunoreactivity in the rabbit retina. *Vision Res.*, 27: 23–30.

Mosinger, J.L., Yazulla, S. and Studholme, K.M. (1986) GABA-like immunoreactivity in the vertebrate retina: A species comparison. *Exp. Eye Res.*, 42: 631–644.

Müller, B. (1989) Demonstration of neurons in the presumed rod pathway of the tree shrew retina. *J. Comp. Neurol.*, 282: 581–594.

Nakamura, Y., McGuire, B.A. and Sterling, P. (1980) Interplexiform cell in cat retina: identification by uptake of γ-[³H]aminobutyric acid and serial reconstruction. *Proc. Natl. Acad. Sci. USA*, 77: 658–61.

Neal, M.J. (1983) Cholinergic mechanisms in the vertebrate retina. In: N. Osborne and G. Chader (Eds.), *Progress in Retinal Research*, Vol. 2, Pergamon Press, Oxford, pp. 191–212.

Nelson, R. and Kolb, H. (1983) Synaptic patterns and response properties of bipolar and ganglion cells in the cat retina. *Vision Res.*, 23: 1183–95.

Nelson, R. and Kolb, H. (1984) Amacrine cells in scotopic vision. *Ophthalmic. Res.*, 16: 21–6.

Nelson, R. and Kolb, H. (1985) A17: A broad-field amacrine cell in the rod system of the cat retina. *J. Neurophysiol.*, 54: 592–614.

Nelson, R., Kolb, H., Chandler, N. and DeKorver, L. (1989) Neural-circuitry of Off-alpha and Off-beta ganglion cells in cat retina. *Invest. Ophthalmol. Vis. Sci. (Suppl.)*, 30: 69.

Nelson, R., Kolb, H., Famiglietti, E.V. and Gouras, P. (1976) Neural responses in the rod and cone systems of the cat retina: intracellular records and procion stains. *Invest. Ophthalmol.*, 15: 946–953.

Nguyen-Legros, J., Berger, B., Vigny, A. and Alvarez, C. (1981) TH-like immunoreactive interplexiform cells in the rat retina. *Neurosci. Lett.*, 27: 255–259.

Nguyen-Legros, J., Botter, C., Phuc, L.H., Vigny, A. and Gay, M. (1984) Morphology of primate's dopaminergic amacrine cells as revealed by TH-like immunoreactivity on retinal flat-mounts. *Brain Res.*, 295: 145–153.

Nowak, J.Z., Szyc, H. and Nawrocki, J. (1985) Does 5-HT play a neurotransmitter role in mammalian retina? Studies on uptake and potassium-stimulated release of ¹⁴C-GABA and ¹⁴C-GABA from bovine and rabbit retina slices. *Pol. J. Pharmacol. Pharm.*, 37: 57–68.

O'Malley, D.M. and Masland, R.H. (1989) Co-release of acetylcholine and gamma-aminobutyric acid by a retinal neuron. *Proc. Natl. Acad. Sci. USA*, 86: 3414–8.

Osborne, N. (1980) In vitro experiments on the metabolism, uptake and release of 5-hydroxytryptamine in bovine retina. *Brain Res.*, 184: 283–297.

Osborne, N.N., Barnett, N.L., Ghazi, H., Calas, A. and Maitre, M. (1989) Studies on the localization of serotonergic neurones and the types of serotonin receptors in the mammalian retina. In: R. Weiler and N.N. Osborne (Eds.), *Neurobiology of the Inner Retina*, Vol. 31, Springer-Verlag, Berlin, pp.

Osborne, N.N. and Beaton, D.W. (1986) Direct histochemical localisation of 5,7-dihydroxytryptamine and the uptake of serotonin by a subpopulation of GABA neurones in the rabbit retina. *Brain Res.*, 382: 158–62.

Osborne, N.N., Nesselhut, T., Nicholas, D.A., Patel, S. and

Cuello, A.C. (1982) Serotonin-containing neurons in vertebrate retinas. *J. Neurochem.*, 39: 1519–1528.

Osborne, N.N., Patel, S., Beaton, D.W. and Neuhoff, V. (1986) GABA neurones in retinas of different species and their postnatal development in situ and in culture in the rabbit retina. *Cell Tissue Res.*, 243: 117–23.

Oyster, C.W., Takahashi, E.S., Cilluffo, M. and Brecha, N.C. (1985) Morphology and distribution of tyrosine hydroxylase-like immunoreactive neurons in the cat retina. *Proc. Natl. Acad. Sci. USA*, 82: 6335–9.

Pourcho, R.G. (1980) Uptake of [$^3$H]glycine and [$^3$H]GABA by amacrine cells in the cat retina. *Brain Res.*, 198: 33–46.

Pourcho, R.G. (1981) Autoradiographic localization of [$^3$H]muscimol in the cat retina. *Brain Res.*, 215: 187–99.

Pourcho, R.G. (1982) Dopaminergic amacrine cells in the cat retina. *Brain Res.*, 252: 101–9.

Pourcho, R.G. and Goebel, D.J. (1983) Neuronal subpopulations in cat retina which accumulate the GABA agonist, ($^3$H)muscimol: a combined Golgi and autoradiographic study. *J. Comp. Neurol.*, 219: 25–35.

Pourcho, R.G. and Osman, K. (1986) Cytochemical identification of cholinergic amacrine cells in cat retina. *J. Comp. Neurol.*, 247: 497–504.

Pourcho, R.G. and Owczarzak (1989) Distribution of GABA immunoreactivity in the cat retina: A light- and electron-microscopic study. *Vis. Neurosci.*, 2: 425–435.

Raviola, E. and Dacheux, R.F. (1987) Excitatory dyad synapse in rabbit retina. *Proc. Natl. Acad. Sci. USA*, 84: 7324–7328.

Richards, J.G., Schoch, P., Häring, P., Takacs, B. and Möhler, H. (1987) Resolving GABA$_A$/Benzodiazepine receptors: Cellular and subcellular localization in the CNS with monoclonal antibodies. *J. Neurosci.*, 7: 1866–1886.

Ryan, M.K. and Hendrickson, A.E. (1987) Interplexiform cells in macaque monkey retina. *Exp. Eye Res.*, 45: 57–66.

Saito, H. (1981) The effects of strychnine and bicuculline on the responses of X- and Y-cells of the isolated eye-cup preparation of the cat. *Brain Res.*, 212: 243–8.

Saito, H. (1983) Pharmacological and morphological differences between X- and Y-type ganglion cells in the cat's retina. *Vision Res.*, 23: 1299–308.

Sandell, J.H., Masland, R.H., Raviola, E. and Dacheux, R.F. (1989) Connections of indoleamine-accumulating cells in the rabbit retina. *J. Comp. Neurol.*, 283: 303–313.,

Sandell, J.S. and Masland, R.H. (1986) A system of indoleamine-accumulating neurons in the cat retina. *J. Neurosci.*, 6: 331–3347.

Sarthy, P. and Fu, M. (1989a) Localization of L-glutamic acid decarboxylase messenger RNA in cat retinal horizontal cells by in situ hybridization. *J. Comp. Neurol.*, 288: 593–600.

Sarthy, P. and Fu, M. (1989b) Localization of L-glutamic acid decarboxylase messenger RNA in monkey and human retina by in situ hybridization. *J. Comp. Neurol.*, 288: 691–697.

Schwartz, E.A. (1987) Depolarization without calcium can release γ-aminobutyric acid from a retinal neuron. *Science*, 238: 350–5.

Slaughter, M.M. and Bai, S.-H. (1989) Differential effects of baclofen on sustained and transient cells in the mudpuppy retina. *J. Neurophysiol.*, 61: 374–381.

Smith, R.G., Freed, M.A. and Sterling, P. (1986) Microcircuitry of the dark-adapted cat retina: functional architecture of the rod-cone network. *J. Neurosci.*, 6: 3505–3517.

Starr, M.S. and Voaden, M.J. (1972) The uptake of ($^{14}$C)-γ-aminobutyric acid by isolated retina of the rat. *Vision Res.*, 12: 549–557.

Sterling, P. (1983) Microcircuitry of the cat retina. *Ann. Rev. Neurosci.*, 6: 149–85.

Sterling, P., Freed, M.A. and Smith, R.G. (1988) Architecture of rod and cone circuits to the On-beta ganglion cell. *J. Neurosci.*, 8: 623–42.

Strettoi, E., Dacheux, R.F. and Raviola, E. (1990) Synaptic connections of rod bipolar cells in the inner plexiform layer of the rabbit retina. *J. Comp. Neurol.*, 295: 449–466.

Suzuki, S., Tachibana, M. and Kaneko, A. (1990) Effects of glycine and GABA on isolated bipolar cells of the mouse retina. *J. Physiol.*, 421: 645–662.

Tauchi, M. and Masland, R.H. (1984) The shape and arrangement of the cholinergic neurons in the rabbit retina. *Proc. R. Soc. London B*, 223: 101–119.

Tauck, D.L., Frosch, M.P. and Lipton, S.A. (1988) Characterization of GABA- and glycine-induced currents of solitary rodent retinal ganglion cells in culture. *Neuroscience*, 27: 193–203.

Thier, P. and Wässle, H. (1984) Indoleamine-mediated reciprocal modulation of on-centre and off-centre ganglion cell activity in the retina of the cat. *J. Physiol. (London)*, 351: 613–30.

Thomas, T.N. and Redburn, D.A. (1979) 5-hydroxytryptamine: a neurotransmitter of bovine retina. *Exp. Eye Res.*, 28: 55–61.

Törk, I. and Stone, J. (1979) Morphology of catecholamine-containing amacrine cells in the cat's retina, as seen in retinal whole mounts. *Brain Res.*, 169: 261–73.

Vaney, D.I. (1986) Morphological identification of serotonin-accumulating neurons in the living retina. *Science*, 233: 444–6.

Vaney, D.I., Collin, S.P. and Young, H.M. (1989) Dendritic relationships between cholinergic amacrine cells and direction-selective retinal ganglion cells. In: R. Weiler and N.N. Osborne (Eds.), *Neurobiology of the Inner Retina*, Vol. 31, Springer-Verlag, Berlin, pp. 158–168.

Vaney, D.I. and Young, H.M. (1988) GABA-like immunoreactivity in cholinergic amacrine cells of the rabbit retina. *Brain Res.*, 438: 369–373.

Vaughn, J.E., Famiglietti, E.V. Jr. et al. (1981) GABAergic amacrine cells in rat retina: immunocytochemical identification and synaptic connectivity. *J. Comp. Neurol.*, 197: 113–27.

Voigt, T. (1986) Cholinergic amacrine cells in the rat retina. *J. Comp. Neurol.*, 248: 19–35.

Voigt, T. and Wässle, H. (1987) Dopaminergic innervation of AII amacrine cells in mammalian retina. *J. Neurosci.*, 7: 4115–4128.

Wässle, H. and Chun, M.H. (1988) Dopaminergic and indoleamine-accumulating amacrine cells express GABA-like immunoreactivity in the cat retina. *J. Neurosci.*, 8: 3383–3394.

Wässle, H. and Chun, M.H. (1989) GABA-like immunoreactivity in the cat retina: light microscopy. *J. Comp. Neurol.*, 279: 43–54.

Wässle, H., Grünert, U., Rohrenbeck, J. and Boycott, B.B. (1989) Cortical magnification factor and the ganglion cell density of the primate retina. *Nature*, 341: 643–646.

Wässle, H., Voigt, T. and Patel, B. (1987) Morphological and Immunocytochemical identification of indoleamine-accumulating neurons in the cat retina. *J. Neurosci.*, 7: 1574–1585.

Werblin, F.S. (1977) Regenerative amacrine cell depolarization and formation of on-off ganglion cell response. *J. Physiol. (London)*, 264: 767–85.

Wulle, I. and Schnitzer, J. (1989) Distribution and morphology of tyrosine hydroxylase-immunoreactive neurons in the developing mouse retina. *Dev. Brain Res.*, 48: 59–72.

Yamashita, M. and Wässle, H. (1990) Responses of dissociated rod bipolar cells of the rat retina to 2-amino-4-phosphonobutyric acid (APB). *Soc. Neurosci. Abstr.*, 16: 712.

Yazulla, S. (1986) GABAergic mechanisms in the retina. *Prog. Ret. Res.*, 5: 1–52.

Yeh, H.H., Lee, M.B. and Cheun, J.E. (1990) Properties of GABA-activated whole-cell currents in bipolar cells of the rat retina. *Vis. Neurosci.*, 4: 349–357.

Young, H.M. and Vaney, D.I. (1990) The retinae of prototherian mammals possess neuronal types that are characteristic of non-mammalian retinae. *Vis. Neurosci.*, 5: 61–66.

R.R. Mize, R.E. Marc and A.M. Sillito (Eds.)
Progress in Brain Research, Vol. 90

CHAPTER 7

# Development of GABAergic neurons in the mammalian retina

## Dianna A. Redburn

*Department of Neurobiology and Anatomy, The University of Texas Medical School, P.O. Box 20708, Houston, TX 77225, USA*

## Introduction

GABAergic systems in the mammalian retina have been localized within many anatomically distinct and functionally diverse subclasses of amacrine cells (Ehinger, 1970; Brandon et al., 1979; Nakamura et al., 1980; Freed et al., 1983; Kolb and Nelson, 1984; Koontz and Hendrickson, 1990). Some populations of GABAergic amacrine cells have a dense distribution and limited retinal coverage consistent with a role for GABAergic transmission in shaping details of the visual image. Functional studies support this type of role for GABA in local feedback and feedforward circuits, for example the picrotoxin sensitive responses of directionally sensitive ganglion cells (Ariel and Daw, 1982). Other subclasses of GABAergic interneurons are sparsely distributed across the retina and have extensive retinal coverage. Examples include subclasses of amacrine cells in which GABA is co-localized with neuroactive peptides (Brecha, 1983; Stell et al., 1984; Lam et al., 1985). GABAergic interplexiform cells with widely distributed axon terminals in the outer retina (Nakamura et al., 1980; Mosinger et al., 1986; Mosinger and Yazulla, 1987), also fit in this latter category whose function is described as neuromodulatory. These cells could be responsible for contributing to a widespread and tonic inhibition by GABA in the retina. Finally, it is possible that GABA may also be a transmitter of another type of interneuron, the horizontal cell (Osborne et al., 1986; Mosinger and Yazulla, 1987), and of small subclasses of ganglion and bipolar cells in mammals (Mosinger and Yazulla, 1987; Yu et al., 1987; Wässle and Chun, 1989; Grünert and Wässle, 1990).

The anatomical and functional diversity of GABAergic cells in retina precludes simple schemes for describing how GABA circuitry is arranged in the adult (cf. Wu, Chapter 5; Marc Chapter 4; Freed, Chapter 6) and provides an even greater challenge in discerning how that circuitry might be established during development. It is from this perspective that the topic of this chapter has been approached. In reviewing these data, it should be kept in mind that many experimental approaches described herein do not permit detailed analyses of individual GABAergic cell types, but rather document overall changes in the levels of GABAergic markers that give a general view of GABA "tone" during inner plexiform layer development. In most cases, it has not been possible to follow, in a straightforward and direct manner, the appearance and maturation of a functionally distinct subclass of GABAergic amacrine cell.

In addition to the limitations caused by complexity in adult circuitry, another complication further confounds interpretations drawn from developmental studies of GABAergic neurons in retina: Neonatal GABAergic systems are even more complex than in the adult (Schnitzer and Rusoff, 1984; Osborne et al., 1986; Redburn and Madtes, 1986; Finlay and Sengelaub, 1989). GABAergic markers appear early in prenatal development and are localized in larger numbers and more diverse types of cells than in the adult. Thus it appears that postnatal maturation of the GABA system involves a process of selective pruning rather than simple addition. The developmental *decrease* in anatomical diversity may also be reflected in a decrease in functional diversity since functions other than synaptic transmission have been ascribed to GABA early in development (see below). Even if the immature system is different in cellular form and function from that seen in the adult, it seems unlikely that immature characteristics end abruptly and have no relationship to adult systems. Understanding the developing system may provide critical insights regarding the dominant inhibitory influence of GABA in the adult retina.

### Development of the mammalian retina

In order to examine the development of GABAergic retinal neurons, it is necessary to review the maturational processes responsible for overall retinal development. (For an excellent review, see Finlay and Sengelaub, 1989.) Most of the information regarding mammalian development is based on rodent models (Cajal, 1893, 1929; Polyak, 1941; Sidman, 1961; Hinds and Hinds, 1974, 1978, 1983), although similar information exists for primate retina as well (Polyak, 1941; Duke-Elder and Cook, 1963; Mann, 1969). Initially the retina evaginates from the neural tube to form a primitive optic vesicle. A layer of pseudostratified epithelial cells lines the walls of the vesicle and serves as a precursor of the neural retina (Hinds and Ruffett, 1971). These ventricular cells are multipotential, with a single retinal progenitor cell capable of giving rise to diverse cell types (Turner and Cepko, 1987). Prior to the onset of neurogenesis, processes from each ventricular cell span the entire thickness of the retina

and form junctional contacts with basement membranes at both the outer and the inner retinal surfaces (Whitley and Young, 1986; Sheffield and Fischhman, 1970). Mitotic division occurs after ventricular cells release their attachments at the vitreal surface, allowing their cell bodies to move near the outer surface of the retina and assume a more rounded shape (Sauer, 1935). The daughter cells then undergo DNA replication while re-establishing their fusiform shape and sending processes to contact the vitreal surface. It has been suggested that this polarized morphology, in particular the presence of a process extending to the vitreal surface, is necessary for maintaining proliferative potential. The only differentiated cells to retain contacts with the vitreal surface are the Müller cells, and they also retain their mitotic activity (in response to injury) in adult animals (Reh, 1989). In addition, experimental removal of the basement membrane which these processes normally contact has been shown to induce premature differentiation of all germinal cells (Reh et al., 1987; Reh and Radke, 1988). Therefore, it is possible that the failure to re-establish contact with this surface after cytokinesis is a first step toward initiating neuronal differentiation. According to this model, each neuroblastic cell making contact with the vitreal surface would repeat the proliferative cycle, alternating between a fusiform and a rounded cell shape, analogous to the interkinetic migration along radial glia observed in the developing brain (Rakic, 1982). Although some authors refer to the presence of radial glia within retina (Schnitzer, 1988), there is little direct evidence for a separate population of these cells which are distinct from ventricular cells. Some authors speculate that given the relatively short distance through which retinal cells are required to migrate, radial glia may not be necessary to provide guidance (Polley et al., 1989). Rather, other factors may provide cues for migration and subsequent differentiation.

Differentiation of cell types in the retina follows a specific temporal sequence which has been divided into three phases. Based on [$^3$H]thymidine studies (Sidman, 1961; Carter-Dawson and LaVail, 1979; Johns et al., 1979; Polley et al., 1986; Zimmerman et al., 1988), several different classes of retinal cells, called cohorts, appear to have concurrent periods of neurogenesis. Based on studies in cat and rabbit, the first cohort differentiates prenatally and consists of ganglion cells, type A horizontal cells and cones. The second cohort consisting of Müller cells, type B horizontal cells and bipolar cells differentiates postnatally. Amacrine cells are considered as a separate, highly diverse cohort with some cells differentiating prenatally and others postnatally. No information is currently available on neurogenesis of interplexiform cells, although our recent data (Messersmith and Redburn, 1991) suggests that at least some differentiate prenatally.

Synaptogenesis within the two plexiform layers of the retina generally peaks in the perinatal period of non-primate mammals (Blanks et al., 1974; McArdle et al., 1977; Carter-Dawson and LaVail, 1979; Maslim and Stone, 1986; Redburn and Madtes, 1986). The first synapses of the outer plexiform layer are formed between cones and type A horizontal cells. Type B horizontal cells make contact with rods and cones somewhat later. In the inner plexiform layer, the first synapses to be observed are those from amacrine cells which project to other amacrines and to ganglion cell dendrites. Bipolar cells are among the last cells to mature. Thus, second order neurons in the visual pathway which connect outer to inner retina, may represent the final connection added to complete the primary visual pathway in retina. Based on these findings, it has been suggested that the two plexiform layers must develop independently of each other (Maslim and Stone, 1986). However, there is at least one exception to this theory. A limited population of interplexiform cells have been observed at birth (Messersmith and Redburn, 1991), with processes projecting to both plexiform layers. Thus some interaction between the two developing layers may occur.

Functional maturation of the retina has been most extensively studied in rabbit where light responses in ganglion cells are first recorded at 8 days after birth (Masland, 1977; Dacheux and Miller, 1981a,b). The first functional synapses appear to be the receptor-to-bipolar and bipolar-to-third order neuronal connections, namely the so-called vertical pathway. Surround influences involving interneuron pathways mature more slowly.

## Development of GABAergic systems

A variety of markers have been used to monitor the appearance of GABAergic transmission during development. Uptake and release of [$^3$H]-GABA or [$^3$H]muscimol, immunocytochemical localization of GABA or its synthesizing enzyme, GAD, and electrophysiological analysis of GABA-mimetic compounds have all been reported. One of the major conclusions drawn from these studies is that the GABA system is among the first neurotransmitter systems expressed in retinal development. Fung et al. (1982) report that uptake of [$^3$H]GABA by cells in the amacrine and ganglion cell layers is first observed autoradiographically on embryonic day 22 in rabbit retina whereas uptake of [$^3$H]glycine and [$^3$H]-dopamine by amacrine cells is first seen on embryonic day 25 and 27, respectively. Schnitzer and Rusoff (1984) report GAD immunoreactive cells in mouse retina as early as embryonic day 17.

Early, prenatal expression of GABAergic markers is also seen in other parts of brain. Studies using autoradiographic localization of [$^3$H]GABA uptake (Chronwall and Wolff, 1980), immunocytochemical localization of antibodies to GAD (Wolff et al. 1984), and antibodies to GABA itself (Lauder et al., 1986), have demonstrated that the GABA system is expressed very early relative to other transmitter systems in developing rat brain. First observed with GABA antibodies at embryonic day 13, a broad network of fibers within the marginal zone, subplate, and intermediate zones also express [$^3$H]GABA uptake and GAD immunolabeling by E18.

Our own studies on the postnatal development of rabbit retina have also shown that GABAergic systems are well-developed before birth. A large and diverse group of retinal cells is labeled either by autoradiographic localization of [$^3$H]GABA or immunocytochemical staining with GABA antisera (Redburn and Madtes, 1986; Keith and Redburn, 1987; Redburn and Keith, 1987; Messersmith and Redburn, 1991). Although we have not utilized double-label analyses, corresponding groups of cells are stained with both labels. A summary of our observations follows.

*Cells in the amacrine and ganglion cell layers*

At birth, two substrata of cell bodies within the amacrine cell layer are labeled with [$^3$H]-GABA and GABA-antisera. The proximal sublamina contains a high density of labeled cells with large, oval-shaped cell bodies. From immunocytochemical studies, we estimate that approximately 30% of the cells in this layer are labeled. The second, more distal sublamina is much less distinct and generally contains fewer labeled cells which are pyramidal in shape.

Greater than 80% of all cell bodies in the ganglion cell layer are labeled both by autoradiography and immunocytochemistry, as are elements of the nerve fiber layer. Analysis of autoradiograms at the EM level confirm that labeling is associated with fiber bundles and not surrounding elements. Cells of both large and small diameter are labeled, thus we assume that at birth both displaced amacrine cells and ganglion cells contain endogenous GABA and have a GABA uptake system.

*Inner plexiform layer*

Retinas from neonatal animals show intense labeling of elements in the inner plexiform layer. In well oriented sections, a distinct bilaminar pattern is observed, roughly corresponding to the position of sublamina 2 and 4 in the adult retina. Each immunofluorescent layer appears as a con-

tinuous band with a relatively uniform thickness of approximately 6 $\mu$m. The labeling pattern appears to result from the highly restricted branching of a limited number of large-diameter neurites, caused in part by their exclusion from the central one-third of the inner plexiform layer. Labeled processes do not appear to cross this zone of exclusion. Thus, it appears that cells in the ganglion and amacrine cell layers contribute fibers to the proximal and distal sublaminae respectively.

*Interplexiform cells*

In the middle region of the developing inner nuclear layer, an additional group of cells with morphological characteristics of interplexiform cells are intensely labeled with GABA antisera. A single descending process projects from the cell body and joins the inner plexiform layer where it becomes indistinguishable from other labeled processes there. A single ascending process projects to the developing outer plexiform layer where it branches abruptly, forming a very extensive, thinly branched but widely distributed dendritic arborization of more than 100 $\mu$m. These cells represent a rather small population and it is perhaps for this and other technical reasons that we are unable to convincingly demonstrate uptake of [$^3$H]GABA into this cell type autoradiographically.

As stated above, it has long been held that the two plexiform layers develop more or less independently of each other, only to be linked at later stages of retinal development by bipolar processes (Blanks et. al., 1974; McArdle et al., 1977; Maslim and Stone, 1986). However, our data clearly demonstrate that the inner and outer plexiform layers are linked at birth by processes from interplexiform cells.

*Type A horiozontal cells*

Every mature cell in the neonatal horizontal cell layer is labeled by [$^3$H]GABA uptake and by GABA antisera. However, labeling with both markers is less intense than in other cells described above. These cells appear to form a distinct population first characterized as type A horizontal cells by Cajal (1883). Schnitzer and Rusoff (1984) report staining of mouse prenatal type A horizontal cells with GAD antibodies. The cell bodies are large, pale staining and semilunar in shape with a highly regular cell-to-cell spacing of approximately 30 $\mu$m. Thick processes project horizontally from the soma and are the first recognizable element to define the position of the developing outer plexiform layer.

## Changes in GABAergic markers during postnatal development

During postnatal development of the rabbit retina, there is a significant decrease in the number and distribution of labeled cell bodies. Up to postnatal day five, all type A horizontal cells, most cells in the amacrine and ganglion cell layers and a small population of interplexiform cells are labeled. By postnatal day 5 and beyond, labeling intensity declines in cell bodies and processes of horizontal cells. In mouse retina, GAD immunoreactivity is uniformly expressed by the entire prenatal population of type A horizontal cells and yet is absent in the adult. Since our own studies as well as [³H]thymidine studies by others suggest that there is no massive cell death or replacement of type A horizontal cells during this period, we assume that the loss of endogenous levels of GABA and of the ability to take up GABA represents a down-regulation of this transmitter phenotype during postnatal maturation of the type A horizontal cell.

We are less certain about the fate of GABA immunoreactive interplexiform cells during development. Labeled interplexiform cells are rarely observed in our preparations from adult rabbit. Mosinger et al. (1986) report a small population of interplexiform cells in adult rabbit which are labeled with GABA antisera. The fact that we have not observed labeled interplexiform cells in retinas of 20 day old rabbits could be due to the fact that the cell population is very limited in size.

The major change seen in the inner retina during postnatal development is a decrease in the number of immunocytochemically labeled cells in both amacrine and ganglion cell layers. We estimate that by postnatal day 20, the frequency of labeling in both amacrine and ganglion cell layers decreases by more than 50%, perhaps due to GABAergic cell death, change in transmitter phenotype, and/or dilution by postnatal development of non-GABAergic amacrine and displaced amacrine cells as well as by overall retinal growth. The average volume of the remaining labeled somata increases by roughly one third along with a shift to a more spherical cell shape.

Müller cells are not generally considered to be GABAergic since it appears that under normal circumstances they do not release GABA. However, in the adult mammalian retina, they do have an active uptake system for GABA and metabolic enzymes, i.e., GABA transaminase, which rapidly metabolize any GABA that has been internalized (Ehinger, 1970). Thus, while Müller cells treated with GABA transaminase inhibitors may artificially contain internal stores of GABA and may be induced to release it when depolarized by elevated levels of potassium, it is unlikely that this occurrence is important in normal retinal function. Nevertheless, the rate of removal of GABA by uptake and metabolism of Müller cells clearly influences the level of extracellular GABA. In this way the Müller cell is thought to play an important role in GABAergic transmission. Our studies show no accumulation of [³H]GABA in Müller cells until approximately 5 days after birth. It is interesting to note that prior to the onset of Müller cell maturation, only neurons, specifically those with relatively mature morphology have GABA uptake sites. Neither ventricular cells nor neuroblastic cells accumulate GABA. Thus it may well be that in neonatal retina, GABA "tone" is relatively high because of the lack of metabolic activity in Müller cells.

The lack of glial uptake early in development may simply reflect the fact that, in rabbit, Müller cells first become post-mitotic at a later time

(Reichenbach and Reichelt, 1986). Similar results were obtained with [$^3$H]thymidine studies in cat retina (Polley et al., 1986, 1989). However, based on the distribution of glial markers such as glial fibrillary acidic protein, vimentin, galactocerebroside and others, Schnitzer (1988) suggests that some Müller cells are present in rabbit retina at birth and that staining increases in the early postnatal period. Our own [$^3$H]thymidine studies in rabbit retina clearly show that many Müller cells undergo mitotic division postnatally. Resolution of these conflicting results might be achieved in future experiments which could combine [$^3$H]thymidine autoradiography with vimentin immunocytochemistry. It does seem certain, however, that regardless of the birthdate of Müller cells, robust glial uptake of GABA is not expressed until the fifth postnatal day.

It is our general observation that the appearance of [$^3$H]GABA accumulation in Müller cells in the retina marks the division between two distinct phases of retinal development. Prior to this time only cells of the first cohort are mature. The outer plexiform layer is composed of the GABAergic type A horizontal cell and its pre/postsynaptic partner, the cone photoreceptor pedicle. The density of GABA immunoreactive cell bodies in both the amacrine and ganglion cell layers reaches its peak. The inner and outer plexiform layers are linked by a sparse population of GABA containing interplexiform cells.

Around postnatal day 5, a second phase in retinal development begins with the appearance of the second cohort of maturing cells which includes Müller cells, bipolar cells, rod cells and type B horizontal cells. At this time, GABAergic markers in type A horizontal cells begin to decline, as do the numbers of GABA immunoreactive cells in the amacrine and ganglion cell layer. At this time, uptake of GABA in Müller cells begins to predominate over neuronal uptake. If this period represents a pruning cycle for the GABA system, then the final complement of adult GABAergic cells might be established at this time. Final synaptic maturation occurs during a third, perhaps more prolonged phase. It may be that neurons initiate synapses only after their numbers have stabilized. Evidence for this suggestion is supported by data from Horsburgh and Sefton (1987) showing that such is probably the case for amacrine and bipolar cells in the rat retina.

Our results described above are in general agreement with work from other laboratories yet there are specific differences regarding horizontal cell development which merit discussion. The central point of disagreement is the degree to which the endogenous pool of GABA (as measured by immunoreactivity) is down-regulated in horizontal cells during development. Our results suggest that GABA levels are decreased dramatically. We have found only a single example of a GABA immunoreactive cell in the outer plexiform layer in rabbits 20 days of age or older. Certain other investigators likewise report no GAD labeling of type A horizontal cells in the adult rabbit retina (Brandon et al., 1979; Brandon, 1985). In contrast, Osborne et al. (1986) report consistent staining of type A horizontal cells with GABA antisera in rabbit retina as late as postnatal day 8 and some staining in the adult. These authors do not mention the presence of interplexiform cells and it is possible that some of the labeled processes they show in the outer plexiform layer in adult rabbit are associated with this cell type rather than horizontal cells. On the other hand, Mosinger and Yazulla (1987) report that on occasion, they have also observed GABA and GAD immunoreactivity in type A horizontal cells in the adult rabbit. In these instances, co-localization of the two labels was unequivocally associated with horizontal cell bodies and their processes. It was clearly distinct from staining seen in interplexiform cells. Because of the sporadic nature of the staining, these authors could not determine with confidence if the inconsistent staining pattern was due to regional localization. Nevertheless, since all horizontal cells are strongly labeled by GABA antisera at birth, it does appear there is at least some degree of down-regulation of endogenous pools of GABA. Furthermore, horizontal cells take up [³H]GABA early in development but fail to do so in the adult. Thus there is considerable evidence for the overall down-regulation of the GABAergic system in rabbit type A horizontal cells although uncertainties remain about sporadic instances of immunocytochemical labeling in the adult.

An additional complexity has recently been recognized, namely that the GABA system in the outer retina may not be similar in all mammalian species. There is general agreement among most laboratories, that many type A horizontal cells are convincingly immunoreactive to GABA in the adult cat (Nishimura et al., 1985; Ryan and Henderickson, 1987; Agardh et al., 1987a; Pourcho and Owczarzak, 1989; Wässle and Chun, 1989). Likewise, horizontal cells in the monkey are stained with GABA antisera, but only in central regions of the retina (Grünert and Wässle, 1990). The actual significance of this finding is still uncertain however, since there is unanimous agreement that adult horizontal cells of all mammalian species examined (including rodent, feline and primate), do not accumulate [³H]GABA (Redburn and Madtes, 1986; Yazulla, 1986; Grünert and Wässle, 1990). Similarly, electrophysiological analyses show no evidence of GABAergic transmission in the outer plexiform layer of the adult rabbit retina (Massey, S., personal communication) or any other mammalian species of which we are aware. Non-mammalian vertebrates have subpopulations of mature horizontal cells which are immunoreactive to GABA and GAD but, in contrast to mammalian horizontal cells, they take up [³H]GABA and they have well-documented inhibitory effects on both photoreceptors and bipolar cells (Yazulla, 1986; see Wu, Chapter 5; Marc, Chapter 4).

To summarize, we suggest that populations of neonatal horizontal cells are capable of uptake, storage and release of [³H]GABA. They also contain endogenous levels of GABA and GAD. During development it appears that this GABAergic system declines. Uptake capability is lost,

although in some mammalian species such as monkey and cat, endogenous stores of GABA may be retained to a larger extent (perhaps in certain regions) in the adult than is the case in other species such as rabbit or mouse. Unlike the non-mammalian vertebrates, there is no evidence for a functional role for GABA in the outer retina of the adult mammalian retina.

*Biochemical analyses of GABAergic development*

In addition to the morphological studies described above, biochemical analyses of various aspects of the GABA system have also been reported. In general, these results show that the total number of uptake sites, the level of GAD activity, the amount of stimulated release of [³H]GABA (Lam et al., 1980; Fung et al., 1982) and receptor sites for GABA (Redburn and Mitchell, 1981; Madtes and Redburn, 1982), all remain at a fairly low but measurable level until a few days after birth. A large increase is observed postnatally until adult levels are reached. In many cases, adult levels are generally reached around the time of eye opening. While these studies provide information regarding overall GABA tone in the developing retina, it is clear that diverse GABAergic cell types may express different rates of maturation. Results are further confounded by cell death and/or down-regulation in some populations during the neonatal period. It may be, however, that these later increases in GABAergic markers are associated with synaptogenesis in those cells which constitute the mature GABAergic circuitry.

Electrophysiological studies in kittens suggest that functional GABAergic organization does not mature until 11–12 weeks of age (Ikeda and Robbins, 1985). At 7–8 weeks, kittens exhibit immature responses characterized as having low selectivity to inhibitory transmitters (namely GABA vs glycine), low sensitivity to exogenously applied GABA agonists, and high sensitivity to GABA antagonists. Although the cellular or molecular mechanisms responsible for maturation of these GABA receptor responses are unknown, it is interesting to note that similar characteristics are observed in both the immature neuromuscular junction and sympathetic ganglia.

Changes in receptor localization and composition have also been seen during this developmental period in kittens (Robbins and Ikeda, 1989). At early stages, low levels of $GABA_A$ receptors linked to benzodiazepine regulatory sites are present on both ON and OFF retinal ganglion cells. During maturation, GABAergic transmission in the ON pathway is increased (more benzodiazepine-linked GABA receptors and more GABA released); whereas in the OFF pathway, GABAergic transmission is decreased (fewer GABA receptors with no benzodiazepine coupling and less GABA released). The development of other aspects of GABAergic function in mammalian retina, including inhibition of acetylcholine and dopamine release, and establishment of receptive fields in directionally sensitive ganglion cells, has not been examined.

*The role of GABA in development*

Given the early expression of GABAergic systems in neonatal retina and its subsequent decline, it is of interest to determine if there is special significance to the early appearance of GABA and if it reflects a special role for GABA in developmental processes. Some such role might be reasonably suggested based simply on its presence and the current model of development as a process which proceeds under the direction of a balanced mixture of positive and negative signals. The alternative would be for the GABA transmitter system to be held silent for an extended period after it is first expressed. This alternative is made less likely by the finding that exogenously applied GABA does exert trophic influences on a variety of developing neuronal tissues. Addition of GABA to the culture medium enhances neurite outgrowth in primary cultures of embryonic chick brain and retina (Spoerri, 1988), and in neuroblastoma tumor cell lines (Spoerri and Wolff, 1981). Similar effects are seen after exposure of rat superior cervical ganglion to GABA

(Wolff et al., 1978). Mattson and Kater (1989) have also shown that, in cultures of identified cells from *Helisoma*, neurotransmitters such as GABA hyperpolarize growth cones, thus maintaining them in the state required for continued growth. In primary cultures of rat cerebellum, GABA was found to enhance neurite outgrowth and, in addition, to induce the formation of low-affinity GABA receptors (Hansen et al., 1984). The relationship between these two effects is unclear. However, it is possible that they both reflect growth of processes bearing GABA receptors.

We have found that blocking GABA uptake in neonatal rabbit retina with intraoculation injections of nipecotic acid (and presumably increasing extracellular levels of endogenous GABA) also leads to increases in low-affinity GABA receptors (Madtes and Redburn, 1983). Thus, it appears that developing neuronal tissue from a variety of sources, including retina, is capable of responding to exogenous GABA as well as to pharmacologically induced increases in endogenous GABA. These effects are consistent with a role for GABA as a trophic substance which stimulates or sustains outgrowth of processes from developing neurons. However, these findings do not specifically answer the question of whether or not endogenous GABA has a significant influence on retinal development under normal conditions, or how identified cell types might be specifically influenced.

We have chosen to address these issues by focusing on the role of the GABAergic horizontal cell in the postnatal development of specific elements of the outer plexiform layer. This choice was based on various characteristics of this region of the retina and the specific cell types involved.

The outer retina in the neonatal rabbit is immature at birth and undergoes an intense period of differentiation, maturation and synaptogenesis within the first five postnatal days (McArdle et al., 1977). At birth the only cells in the outer retina which have established mature morphological characteristics are the type A horizontal cells.

They are also the only cells in the outer retina to express GABAergic properties. Cells in the second cohort of neurogenesis (rods, type B horizontal cells, bipolar cells and some amacrine cells and Müller cells) continue to undergo mitosis and interkinetic migration during this period. Migrating cells which will eventually reside in the inner nuclear layer must pass through the horizontal cell layer composed of large, closely spaced somata and a dense network of broad processes.

Initially rod and cone axons follow the same vertical path as other migrating cells; however their growth stops along a common horizontal plane in register with horizontal cell processes. Because cones become postmitotic and mature earlier than rods, their terminals are the first to invade the outer plexiform layer. At postnatal day five, the ratio of cone-to-rod terminals is very high, with cone pedicles forming a regular array of pre/postsynaptic contacts with horizontal cells

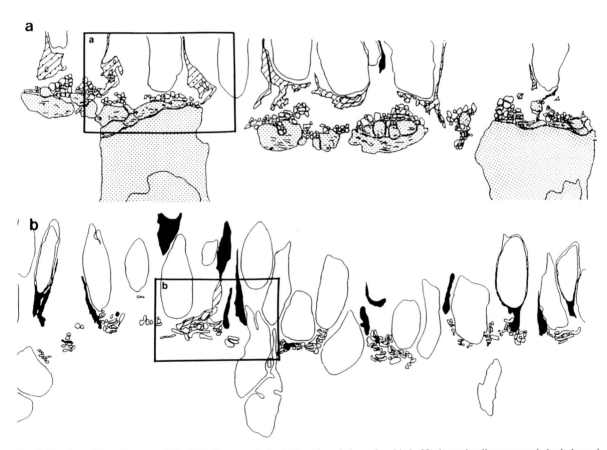

Fig. 1. Tracing of the elements of the OPL from control rabbit retina, 5 days after birth. Horizontal cell processes (stippled area) form a contiguous lateral layer upon which clusters of small processes (open area) may rest. A regular array of cone terminals (cross-hatched areas) appear along the outermost border of the developing OPL. Rod terminals (black area) are rarely seen at this stage in development. Boxed area indicates borders for Fig. 2a. (b) Tracing of elements of the OPL from newborn rabbit retina 5 days after kainic acid administration. Horizontal cells and their processes are absent. Photoreceptors and neuroblastic cell bodies are separated from cells in the inner retina by a thin, irregular layer. Clusters of small processes (open area) within the layer tend to be fewer in number and have larger diameters than controls (a). They commonly appear in horizontal stacks. In contrast to controls, rod terminals (black areas) predominate and cone terminals (cross-hatched area) are rarely present. Boxed area indicates borders for Fig. 2b. (Reprinted with permission from Messersmith and Redburn, 1990, Pergamon Press, Inc.)

(see Figs. 1 and 2). Rod spherules are added several days later, forming a slightly more distal layer and eventually outnumbering cone terminals by many fold (Fernald, 1989).

Two characteristics of these horizontal cells are of particular interest. First, they assume their mature position early in development and thus appear to be the first component of the outer plexiform layer to be expressed. Second, their position establishes the location of the developing outer plexiform layer. Growing fibers entering the layer appear first in patches and then as a continuous layer which remains closely associated with the flattened, distal surfaces of the horizontal cell processes. Postnatal growth of the outer plexiform layer is restricted to this area, and results in the trilaminar arrangement seen in the adult, with horizontal cell processes comprising the innermost border, photoreceptor terminals forming the outermost border, and many other smaller diameter processes, presumably from bipolar cells and other types of horizontal cells, filling in the middle layer.

Both of these properties of horizontal cells are similar to those described for pioneer or pathfinder cells in other parts of the CNS: namely, they grow to a target area and, once there, begin to attract later growing fibers (Weiss, 1941). Examples include pathfinding axons in the retina of *Daphnia* (Lopresti et al., 1973) and pioneer neurons in the developing innervation of rat diaphragm (Bennett and Pettigrew, 1974). Reviews by Edwards (1982) and Goodman (1982) also provide strong evidence for pioneer cells from their own work in the insect nervous system. In embryonic rat brain, pioneer cells send cortical afferents to invade the telencephalic vesicle, providing guidance for subsequent ingrowth of fibers and also providing a stimulus for the beginning of neuronal differentiation in this region (Lauder et al., 1986). It is of particular interest to note that this pioneer system has been shown to be GABAergic.

The GABAergic nature of the neonatal horizontal cell suggests that the emerging outer plexiform layer may exist in a GABA-rich environment which theoretically could maintain developing GABA-receptive cells (such as cones) in a hyperpolarized state. The structural barrier provided by the broad horizontal cell processes, and the trophic effects of GABA on growth cones (Mattson and Kater, 1989), are two possible factors which could influence the growth of photoreceptor terminals and other processes in the region of the outer plexiform layer. We have attempted to address these possibilities by exploiting the fact that horizontal cells possess kainic acid receptors. After lesioning GABAergic horizontal cells at birth with kainic acid, we were able to examine the development of the outer plexiform layer in the absence of horizontal cells (Messersmith and Redburn, 1990).

*Acute effects of kainic acid on retinal morphology*

We examined rabbit retinas 3 h after an intraocular injection of kainic acid on the day of birth. Kainic acid was found to be toxic to a variety of cells in the inner retina, but highly specific in its toxicity to horizontal cells in the outer retina. The entire complement of horizontal cells was swollen and thus they appeared to behave as a single homogeneous population. Photoreceptors were insensitive to kainic acid. Cone and rod terminals were normal in appearance; synaptic vesicles and synaptic ribbons remained intact. Immature cells showed no morphological response to kainic acid, suggesting that immature cells do not possess kainic acid receptors.

Twenty-four hours after the kainic acid injection, no cells with excitotoxic swelling or necrosis were observed. There was no evidence for recovery of the kainic acid sensitive cells and the entire population of type A horizontal cells was absent. Likewise, the normal complement of cells in the amacrine and ganglion cell layers was diminished, suggesting that necrotic cells had been removed and not replaced. With the loss of horizontal cells, the position of the outer plexiform layer was no longer discernible and neuroblastic cells occupied the majority of the outer retina, extend-

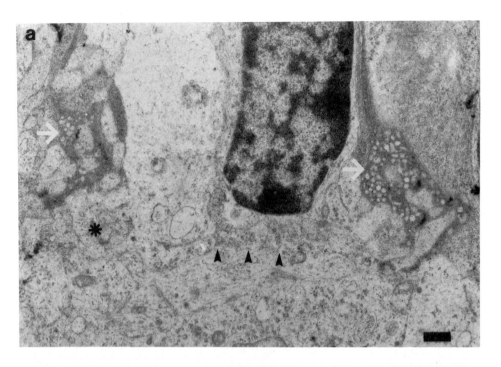

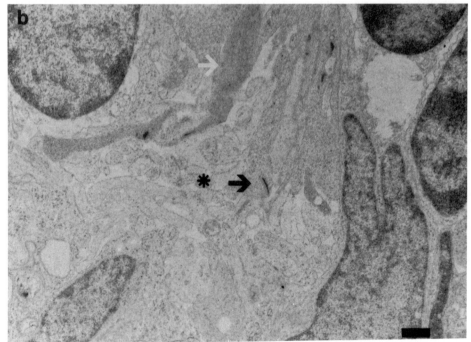

Fig. 2. (a) Selected electron micrograph from OPL tracing (Fig. 1a), control rabbit retina postnatal day 5. Two cone photoreceptor terminals with the characteristics of darkly stained cytoplasm and multiple synaptic ribbons (white arrows) are aligned along the distal border of the OPL. In close apposition to these terminals are clusters of small processes (asterisk). The small processes rest upon the large lateral neurites (black arrowheads) of the horizontal cells. Bar = 0.8 μm. (b) Selected electron micrograph from OPL tracing (Fig. 1b), newborn rabbit retina 5 days after kainic administration. The majority of the photoreceptor terminals present in these retinas possess rod characteristics; they have lightly stained cytoplasm, small round (spherule) endings and a single synaptic ribbon (black arrow). This is in contrast to the darkly stained cytoplasm and multiple ribbons (white arrow) characteristic of the cone terminals seen infrequently in treated retinas. The clusters of small processes (asterisk) are loosely arranged between the photoreceptor terminals and uniquely shaped nuclei. Bar = 0.7 μm. (Reprinted with permission from Messersmith and Redburn, 1990, Pergamon Press, Inc.)

ing from the distal surface through the discontinuous amacrine cell layer.

### Development after kainic acid treatment

Five days after the horizontal cells were lesioned, a distinct but somewhat altered outer plexiform layer was observed even in the absence of horizontal cells (see Figs. 1 and 2). The inner and outer nuclear layers were separated by groups of small processes, horizontally arranged within the outer plexiform layer, and by rod terminals which were generally restricted to their normal position along the outer border. The presence of these elements after treatment negates the hypothesis that the horizontal cell acts simply as a barrier which is necessary and sufficient to establish the boundary between inner and outer nuclear layers.

The most pronounced alteration was a dramatic reversal in the rod to cone cell ratio, with rods representing the dominant type of terminal after lesioning. The array of cone terminals normally seen at postnatal day 5 was absent. Thus, it appears that loss of the horizontal cell target was sufficient to disrupt normal development of presynaptic cone terminals. Kainic acid-insensitive targets which apparently were adequate for rod synaptogenesis did not suffice for cones. It is possible that the lack of cone terminals in treated tissues reflect delayed cell death within the cone cell population. We have no morphological evidence which supports this suggestion; however, we have observed a significant number of connecting cilia in the inner nuclear layer, leading us to speculate that the entire cone cell body might be displaced in these tissues. It is possible that, without the horizontal cells, cones continue to migrate past their normal targets and thus appear in the inner nuclear layer. Similar experiments which use kainic acid to lesion the GABAergic cortical subplate neurons early in development, show somewhat comparable results (Ghosh et al., 1990). In the absence of pioneering subplate neurons, axons growing from the lateral geniculate continue to migrate beyond their normal target position.

To determine if the loss of GABA plays any role in the developmental alterations observed after kainic acid lesioning of horizontal cells, the effects of the $GABA_A$ receptor antagonists picrotoxin and bicuculline, and the $GABA_B$ receptor antagonist phaclofen were examined. Intraocular injections were applied on the day of birth, and subsequent development of the outer plexiform layer was assessed on postnatal day 5. None of the antagonists tested caused morphological damage to any cells in the retina; horizontal cells remained intact. However, the $GABA_A$ antagonists altered the cone-to-rod ratio in a manner similar to that seen with kainic acid lesioning. Phaclofen had no observable effect on development.

Based on these results, we suggest that GABAergic type A horizontal cells may have an important influence on the development of the outer plexiform layer. Removal of this influence either by direct lesioning of the cell or by blocking the action of the GABA causes a disruption of postnatal development in a highly specific manner. Cone terminals, which are the normal synaptic partners of the type A horizontal cells, fail to appear in their appropriate position within the outer plexiform layer. It is interesting to note that, in general, the pharmacologically induced disruption did not block the differentiation of rod cells nor the migration of rod terminals to their correct synaptic position. This suggests that growing axons of rods and cones respond to different guidance cues. The presence of $GABA_A$ receptors on cone axons and their absence on rods could offer one possible explanation for this difference. Unfortunately, the distribution of GABA receptors in neonatal rabbit retina has not been examined to date.

In preliminary experiments using cone-specific peanut agglutinin histofluorescence, we have traced the movement of cones after picrotoxin treatment and find that some appear to be displaced to the inner retina (Redburn et al., 1991).

We speculate that the cones may have reached this position because picrotoxin blocked their ability to respond to the guiding influences of GABA in the outer plexiform layer. If the effect of GABA on growing cone terminals is similar to that reported in neurons from other tissue, it might be expected that GABAergic horizontal cells provide a hyperpolarizing milieu in which growth of cone axonal processes would be sustained. The GABA uptake system could function to help restrict the region of influence over which these effects might be expressed. Thus extracellular regions in close proximity to the horizontal cell layer would represent a concentrated source of GABA to keep axonal processes hyperpolarized and thus in a state of active growth. Responsive cells (developing cones with GABA receptors?) might respond to the positive concentration gradient in order to help find their way to the outer plexiform layer. Continued growth beyond the targeted layer would be inhibited because movement away from the GABA-rich region would result in a relatively depolarized state with concomitant cessation of growth. This hypothesis, while highly speculative, is attractive because it is consistent with data from a variety of different experimental approaches. It is also amenable to a number of rather direct tests of its validity, some of which are currently underway.

## References

Agardh, E., Ehinger, B. and Wu, J.Y. (1987) GABA and GAD-like immunoreactivity in the primate retina. *Histochemistry*, 86: 485–490.

Ariel, M. and Daw, N.W. (1982) Pharmacological analysis of directionally sensitive retinal ganglion cells. *J. Physiol.*, 324: 161–185.

Bennett, M.R. and Pettigrew, A.G. (1974) The formation of synapses in striated muscle during development. *J. Physiol. London.*, 241: 515–545.

Blanks, J.C., Adinolfi, A.M. and Lolley, R.N. (1974) Synaptogenesis in the photoreceptor terminal of the mouse retina. *J. Comp. Neurol.*, 156: 81–94.

Brandon, C. (1985) Retinal GABA neurons: Localization in vertebrate species using an antiserum to rabbit brain glutamate decarboxylase. *Brain Res.*, 344: 286–295.

Brandon, C., Lam, D.M.K. and Wu, J.Y. (1979) The γ-aminobutyric acid system in rabbit retina: Localization by immunocytochemistry and autoradiography. *Proc. Natl. Acad. Sci. USA*, 76: 3557–3561.

Brecha, N. (1983) Retinal neurotransmitters: Histochemical and biochemical studies. In P.C. Emson (Ed.), *Chemical Anatomy,* Raven Press, New York, pp. 85–129.

Cajal, S. (1893) *La retines des vertebres.* English translation by D. Maguire and R.W. Rodieck, Appendix 1 In R.W. Rodieck (Ed.), *The Vertebrate Retina, Principles of Structure and Function*, W.H. Freeman, San Francisco, 1973.

Cajal, S. (1929) *Studies on Vertebrate Neurogenesis* (translated by L. Guth), C.C. Thomas, Springfield, Ill., 1960.

Carter-Dawson, L.D. and LaVail, M.M. (1979) Rods and cones in the mouse retina. II. Autoradiographic analysis of cell generation using tritiated thymidine. *J. Comp. Neurol.*, 188: 263–272.

Chronwall, B.M. and Wolff, J.R. (1980) Prenatal and postnatal development of GABA-accumulating cells in the occipital neocortex of rat. *J. Comp. Neurol.*, 190: 187–208.

Chun, M.H. and Wässle, H. (1989) GABA-like immunoreactivity in the cat retina: Electron microscopy. *J. Comp. Neurol.*, 279: 55–67.

Dacheux, R.F. and Miller, R.F. (1981a) An intracellular electrophysiological study of the ontogeny of functional synapses in the rabbit retina. I. Receptors, horizontal, and bipolar cells. *J. Comp. Neurol.*, 198: 307–326.

Dacheux, R.F. and Miller, R.F. (1981b) An intracellular electrophysiological study of the ontogeny of functional synapses in the rabbit retina. II. Amacrine cells. *J. Comp. Neurol.*, 198: 327–334.

Duke-Elder, S. and Cook, C. (1963) Embryology. In: S. Duke-Elder (Ed.), *System of Ophthalmology, Vol. 3, Normal and Abnormal Development*, C.V. Mosby, St. Louis, pp. 11–57 and 81–99.

Edwards, J.S. (1982) Pioneer fibers. In: N. Spitzer (Ed.), *Neuronal Development*, Plenum Press, New York, pp. 255–266.

Ehinger, B. (1970) Autoradiographic identification of rabbit retinal neurons that take up GABA. *Exper. Basel*, 26: 1063.

Fernald, R.D. (1989) Retinal rod neurogenesis. In: B.L. Finlay and D.R. Sengelaub (Eds.), *Development of the Vertebrate Retina*, Plenum Press, New York, pp. 69–86.

Finlay, B.L. and Sengelaub, D.R. (1989) (Eds.), *Development of the Vertebrate Retina*, Plenum Press, New York.

Freed, M.A., Nakamura, Y. and Sterling, P. (1983) Four types of amacrine in the cat retina that accumulate GABA. *J. Comp. Neurol.*, 219: 295–304.

Fung, S.-C., Kong, Y.-C. and Lam, D.M.K. (1982) Prenatal development of GABAergic, glycinergic and dopaminergic neurons in the rabbit retina. *J. Neurosci.*, 2: 1623–1632.

Ghosh, A., Antonini, A., McConnell, S.K. and Shatz, C.J. (1990) Requirement for subplate neurons in the formation of thalamocortical connections. *Nature*, 347: 179–181.

Goodman, C.S. (1982) Embryonic development of identified neurons in the grasshopper. In: N. Spitzer (Ed.), *Neuronal Development*, Plenum Press, New York, pp. 171–211.

146

Grünert, U. and Wässle, H. (1990) GABA-like immunoreactivity in the macaque monkey retina: a light and electron microscopic study. *J. Comp. Neurol.*, 297: 509–524.

Hansen, G.H., Meier, E. and Schousboe, A. (1984) GABA influences the ultrastructure composition of cerebellar granule cells during development in culture. *Int. J. Devl. Neurosci.*, 2: 247–257.

Hinds, J.W. and Hinds, P.L. (1974) Early ganglion cell differentiation in the mouse retina: An electron microscopic analysis utilizing serial sections. *Dev. Biol.*, 37: 381–416.

Hinds, J.W. and Hinds, P.L. (1978) Early development of amacrine cells in the mouse retina: An electron microscopic, serial section analysis. *J. Comp. Neurol.*, 179: 277–300.

Hinds, J.W. and Hinds, P.L. (1983) Development of retinal amacrine cells in the mouse embryo: Evidence for two modes of formation. *J. Comp. Neurol.*, 213: 1–23.

Hinds, J.W. and Ruffett, T.L. (1971) Cell proliferation in the neural tube: An electron microscopic and Golgi analysis in the mouse cerebral vesicle. *Z. Zellforsch.*, 115: 226–264.

Horsburgh, G.W. and Sefton, A.J. (1987) Cellular degeneration and synaptogenesis in the developing retina of the rat. *J. Comp. Neurol.*, 263: 553–566.

Ikeda, H. and Robbins, J. (1985) Postnatal development of GABA- and glycine-mediated inhibition of feline retinal ganglion cells in the area centralis. *Dev. Brain Rev.*, 23: 1–17.

Johns, P., Rusoff, A. and Dubin, M.W. (1979) Postnatal neurogenesis in the kitten retina. *J. Comp. Neurol.*, 187: 545–556.

Keith, M.E. and Redburn, D.A. (1987) GABA-immunoreactivity in the developing rabbit retina. *Invest. Ophthalmol. Vis. Sci. Suppl.*, 28: 349.

Kolb, H. and Nelson, R. (1984) Neuronal architecture of the cat retina. *Prog. Ret. Res.*, 3: 21–60.

Koontz, M.A. and Hendrickson, A.E. (1990) Distribution of GABA immunoreactive amacrine cell synapses in the inner plexiform layer of macaque monkey retina. *Vis. Neurosci.*, 5: 17–28.

Lam, D.M.K., Fung, S.C. and Kong, Y.C. (1980) Postnatal development of GABAergic neurons in the rabbit retina. *J. Comp. Neurol.*, 193: 89–102.

Lam, D.M.K., Li, H.B., Su, T.Y.Y. and Watt, C.B. (1985) The signature hypothesis: Co-localizations of neuroactive substances as anatomical probes for circuitry analyses. *Vision Res.*, 25: 1353–1364.

Lauder, J.M., Han, V.K.M., Henderson, P., Vendoorn, T. and Towle, A.C. (1986) Prenatal ontogeny of the GABAergic system in the rat brain: An immunocytochemical study. *Neuroscience*, 19: 465–493.

Lopresti, V., Macagno, E.R. and Levinthal, C. (1973) Structure and development of neuronal connections in isogenic organisms. Cellular interactions in the development of the optic lamina of Daphnia. *Proc. Natl. Acad. Sci. USA*, 70: 433–437.

Madtes, P.C. Jr. and Redburn, D.A. (1982) [$^3$H]-GABA binding in developing rabbit retina. *Neurochem. Res.*, 7: 495–503.

Madtes, P.C. and Redburn, D.A. (1983) Intraocular injections of nipecotic acid produce a preferential block of neuronal [$^3$H]GABA accumulation in adult rabbit retina. *Invest. Ophthalmol. Vis. Sci.*, 24: 886–892.

McArdle, C.B., Dowling, J.E. and Masland, R.H. (1977) Development of outer segments and synapses in the rabbit retina. *J. Comp. Neurol.*, 175: 253–274.

Mann, I. (1969) *The Development of the Human Eye*, Grune & Stratton, New York.

Masland, R.H. (1977) Maturation of function in the developing rabbit retina. *J. Comp. Neurol.*, 175: 275–286.

Maslim, J., and Stone, J. (1986) Synaptogenesis in the retina of the cat. *Brain Res.*, 373: 35–48.

Mattson, M.P. and Kater, S. (1989) Excitatory and inhibitory neurotransmitters in the generation and degeneration of hippocampal neuroarchitecture. *Brain Res.*, 478: 337–348.

Messersmith, E.K. and Redburn, D.A. (1990) Kainic acid lesioning alters development of the outer plexiform layer in neonatal rabbit retina. *Int. J. Dev. Neurosci.*, 8: 447–461.

Messersmith, E.K. and Redburn, D.A. (1991) γ-Aminobutyric acid immunoreactivity in multiple cell types of the developing rabbit retina. *Vis. Neurosci.*, in press.

Mosinger, J., Yazulla, S. and Studholme, K.M. (1986) GABA-like immunoreactivity in the vertebrate retina: A species comparison. *Exper. Eye Res.*, 42: 631–644.

Mosinger, J and Yazulla, S. (1987) Double-label analysis of GAD-and GABA-like immunoreactivity in the rabbit retina. *Vis. Res.*, 27: 23–30.

Nakamura, Y., McGuire, B.A. and Sterling, P. (1980) Interplexiform cell in cat retina: Identification by uptake of γ-[$^3$H]-aminobutyric acid and serial reconstruction. *Proc. Natl. Acad. Sci. USA*, 77: 658–661.

Nishimura, Y., Schwartz, M.L. and Rakic, P. (1985) Localization of γ-aminobutyric acid and glutamic acid decarboxylase in rhesus monkey. *Brain Res.*, 359: 351–355.

Osborne, N.N., Patel, S., Beaton, D.W. and Neuhoff, V. (1986) GABA neurones in retinas of different species and their postnatal development in situ and in culture in the rabbit retina. *Cell Tissue Res.*, 243: 117–123.

Polley, E.H., Zimmerman, R.P. and Fortney, R.L. (1986) Interaction of a temporal sequence of cell birthdays and a spatial gradient of morphological maturation in the mammalian retina. *Invest. Ophthalmol. Vis. Sci. (Suppl.)*, 27: 326.

Polley, E.H., Zimmerman, R.P. and Fortney, R.L. (1989) Neurogenesis and maturation of cell morphology in the development of the mammalian retina. In: B.L. Finlay and D.R. Sengelaub (Eds.), *Development of the Vertebrate Retina*, Plenum Press, New York, pp. 3–29.

Polyak, S.L. (1941) *The Retina*, University of Chicago Press, Chicago.

Pourcho, R.G. and Owczarzak, M.T. (1989) Distribution of GABA immunoreactivity in the cat retina: A light- and electron-microscopic study. *Vis. Neurosci.*, 2: 425–435.

Rakic, P. (1982) Organizing principles for development of primate cerebral cortex. In: S.C. Scharma (Ed.), *Organizing Principles of Neural Development*, Plenum Press, New York, pp. 21–48.

Redburn, D.A., Blanchard, V. and Messersmith, E.K. (1991) Picrotoxin disrupts development of the cone photoreceptor distribution in rabbit retina. *Invest. Ophthalmol. Vis. Sci. Suppl.*, 32: 925.

Redburn, D.A. and Madtes, P. (1986) Postnatal development of [³H]GABA-accumulating cells in rabbit retina. *J. Comp. Neurol.*, 243: 41–57.

Redburn, D.A. and Mitchell, C.K. (1981) [³H]musicmol binding in synaptosomal fractions from bovine and developing rabbit retina. *J. Neurosci. Res.*, 6: 487–495.

Redburn, D.A. and Keith, M.E. (1987) Developmental alterations in retinal GABAergic neurons. In: D.A. Redburn and A. Schousboe (Eds.), *Neurotrophic Activity of GABA During Development. Neurology and Neurobiology*, Vol. 32, Alan R. Liss, New York, pp. 98–108.

Reh, T.A. (1989) The regulation of neuronal production during retinal neurogenesis. In: B.L. Finlay and D.R. Sengelaub (Eds.), *Development of the Vertebrate Retina*, Plenum Press, New York, pp. 43–67.

Reh, T.A., Nagy, T. and Gretton, H. (1987) Retinal pigmented epithelial cells induced to transdifferentiate to neurons by laminin. *Nature (London)*, 330: 68–71.

Reh, T.A. and Radke, K. (1988) A role for the extracellular matrix in retinal neurogenesis *in vitro*. *Dev Biol.*, 129: 283–293.

Reichenbach, A. and Reichelt, W. (1986) Postnatal development of radial glial (Müller) cells of the rabbit retina. *Neurosci Lett.*, 71: 125–130.

Robbins, J. and Ikeda, H. (1989) Benzodiazepines and the mammalian retina. III. Postnatal development. *Brain Res.*, 479: 334–338.

Sauer, F.C. (1935) Mitosis in the neural tube. *J. Comp. Neurol.*, 62: 377–405.

Schnitzer, J. (1988) Immunocytochemical studies on the development of astrocytes, Müller (glial) cells, and oligodendrocytes in the rabbit retina. *Dev. Brain Res.*, 44: 59–72.

Schnitzer, J. and Rusoff, A.C. (1984) Horizontal cells of the mouse retina contain glutamate acid decarboxylase-like immunoreactivity during early developmental stages. *J. Neurosci.*, 4: 2948–2955.

Sheffield, J.B. and Fischman, D.A. (1970) Intercellular junctions in the developing neural retina of the chick embryo. *Z. Zellforsch.*, 104: 405–418.

Sidman, R.L. (1961) Histogenesis of mouse retina studied with thymidine-³H. In: G.K. Smelser (Ed.), *Structure of the Eye*, Academic Press, New York, pp. 487–492.

Spoerri, P.E. and Wolff, J.R. (1982) Effect of GABA-administration on murine neuroblatoma cells in culture. I. Increased membrane dynamics and formation of specialized contacts. *Cell Tissue Res.*, 218: 567–579.

Spoerri, P.E. (1988) Neurotrophic effects of GABA in cultures of embryonic chick brain and retina. *Synapse*, 2: 11–22.

Stell, W.K., Walker, S.E., Chohan, K.S. and Ball, A.K. (1984) The goldfish nervus terminalis: A luteinizing hormone-releasing hormone and molluscan cardioexcitatory peptide immunoreactive olfacto-retinal pathway. *Proc. Natl. Acad. Sci. USA*, 81: 940–944.

Turner, D.L. and Cepko, C.L. (1987) A common progenitor for neurons and glia persists in rat retina late in development. *Nature (London)*, 328: 131–136.

Wässle, H. and Chun, M.H. (1989) GABA-like immunoreactivity in the cat retina: Light microscopy. *J. Comp. Neurol.*, 279: 43–54.

Weiss, P. (1941) Nerve patterns: Mechanics of nerve growth. *Growth*, 5: 163–203.

Whiteley, H.E. and Young, S. (1986) The external limiting membrane in developing normal and dysplastic canine retina. *Tissue Cell*, 18: 231–239.

Wolff, J.R., Joo, F. and Dames, W. (1978) Plasticity in dendrites shown by continuous GABA administration in superior cervical ganglion of adult rat. *Nature*, 274: 72–74.

Wolff, J.R., Böttcher, H., Zetzsche, T., Oertel, W.H. and Chronwall, B.M. (1984) Development of GABA-ergic neurons in rat visual cortex as identified by glutamate decarboxylase-like immunoreactivity. *Neurosci. Lett.*, 47: 207–212.

Yazulla, S. (1986) GABAergic mechanisms in the retina. In: N. Osborne and G. Chader (Eds.), *Progress in Retinal Research*, Pergamon Press, Oxford, Vol. 5, pp. 1–52.

Yu, B.C.W., Watt, C.B., Lam, D.M.K. and Fry, K.R. (1979b) GABAergic ganglion cells in the rabbit retina. *Brain Res.*, 439: 376–382.

Zimmerman, R.P., Polley, E. and Fortney, R.L. (1988) Cell birthdays and rate of differentiation of ganglion and horizontal cells of the developing cat's retina. *J. Comp. Neurol.*, 274: 77–90.

# SECTION II

# Subcortical visual pathways

R.R. Mize, R.E. Marc and A.M. Sillito (Eds.)
Progress in Brain Research, Vol. 90

CHAPTER 8

# GABA$_A$ and pre- and post-synaptic GABA$_B$ receptor-mediated responses in the lateral geniculate nucleus

Ivan Soltesz and Vincenzo Crunelli *

*Department of Visual Science, Institute of Ophthalmology, Judd Street, London, England, UK*

## Introduction

Although retinal and geniculate receptive fields are quite similar, the anatomical location per se, as well as the chemical diversity of its afferents, suggest that the lateral geniculate nucleus (LGN) is of strategic importance in the processing of visual information (for reviews, see Sherman and Spear, 1982; Sherman and Koch, 1986; Steriade et al., 1990b). $\gamma$-Aminobutyric acid (GABA) plays a key role in the inhibitory control of visual signals in the LGN (Hubel and Wiesel, 1961; Singer and Bedworth, 1973; Dubin and Cleland, 1977; Hale et al., 1982; Lindstrom, 1982; Ahlsen et al., 1985; Lindstrom and Wrobel, 1990) since centre-surround inhibition, long-range inhibition, binocular inhibition and the inhibition responsible for the orientation bias of LGN thalamocortical (TC) cells are all affected by the GABA$_A$ receptor antagonist bicuculline applied in the vicinity of the recorded cells (Sillito and Kemp, 1983; Vidyasagar, 1984; Berardi and Morrone, 1984; Pape and Eysel, 1986; Eysel et al., 1987; Francesconi et al., 1988; Norton et al., 1989, see also Norton and Godwin, Chapter 10, and Sillito,

Chapter 17). In addition to this "classical" inhibitory role mediated by GABA$_A$ receptors, however, GABA also acts on another type of receptors, the GABA$_B$ receptors that are not blocked by bicuculline (Bowery et al., 1980; Bormann, 1988; Bowery et al., 1990).

In this chapter we review the results that have emerged in the last 5 years from the electrophysiological studies concerning the action of GABA in in vitro slices of the ventral and dorsal LGN (vLGN, dLGN) of cats and rats. In particular, the effects of pre- and postsynaptic GABA$_B$ receptor activation are helping us to appreciate the variety of responses that GABA can generate in the visual thalamus. Presynaptic GABA$_B$ receptors exert a negative control on GABA and glutamate release, while the activation of postsynaptic GABA$_B$ receptors present on TC cells evokes a late, long-lasting inhibitory postsynaptic potential (IPSP) that is responsible for a weak inhibition as well as for burst-firing excitation of these cells (Hirsch and Burnod, 1987; Crunelli et al., 1988; Soltesz et al., 1988, 1989b,c; Crunelli and Leresche, 1991).

### The basic circuitry of the dorsal LGN (dLGN) and its GABAergic components

In the cat, visual information from the retina to the visual cortex via the dorsal LGN (dLGN) is

---

* Present address: Department of Physiology, University of Wales, College of Cardiff, Museum Avenue, Cardiff CF1 1SS, Wales, UK.

152

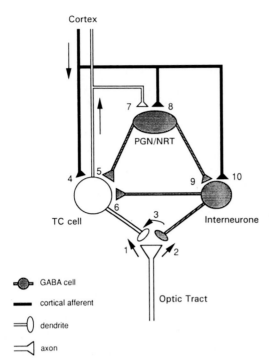

Fig. 1. Schematic drawing of the GABAergic connections in the dLGN. The position of terminals in the drawing does not indicate the exact anatomical location of a synapse but only the existence of a synaptic connection between cells. PGN, perigeniculate nucleus; NRT, nucleus reticularis thalami; TC cell, thalamocortical cell.

carried in three, largely independent and segregated channels, the X, Y and W pathway. TC cells in each of these groups possess many features that are different from those of the other groups, e.g., cell morphology, laminar distribution, synaptic connections and visual response properties (Peters and Palay, 1966; Sherman and Spear, 1982; Friedlander et al., 1981; Wilson et al., 1984; Jones, 1985; Mize et al., 1986; Steriade et al., 1990b). TC cells of all three groups, however, receive their visual information through the terminals of the optic tract fibres and send their axons to cells of the visual cortex (Fig. 1).

Twenty to thirty percent of cells in the A laminae of the dLGN do not project to the visual cortex (i.e., Golgi type II neurones, local circuit cells or interneurones) (Guillery, 1966; Famiglietti and Peters, 1972; Szentagothai, 1973; Lieberman, 1973; Hamori et al., 1974; Parnavelas et al.,

1977; Sterling and Davis, 1980; Jones, 1985) and are immunopositive to glutamic acid decarboxylase and GABA (Fig. 1) (O'Hara et al., 1983; Fitzpatrick et al., 1984; Ottersen and Storm-Mathisen, 1984; Montero and Singer, 1984; Hamos et al., 1985; Montero and Zempel, 1985; Gabbott et al., 1985; Madarasz et al., 1985; Sherman and Friedlander, 1988) (see also Uhlrich and Cucchiaro, Chapter 9). The dendrites of these GABA containing interneurones display a large number of complex appendages, which, together with terminals from the optic tract and the dendrites of X cells, take part in triadic synaptic arrangements within complex glomerular zones. Here, retinal axon terminals make synaptic contacts on both the dendrites of TC cells (synapse 1 in Fig. 1) and the appendages of the interneurone dendrite (synapse 2); the latter, in turn, are presynaptic to TC cell dendrites (synapse 3). Interneurones also have axons (Jones, 1985; Montero, 1987; Steriade et al., 1990b) and thus they can exert their action through conventional, action potential-evoked GABA release (synapse 6) as well as through dendritic operations (synapse 2).

The second major GABAergic input to TC cells originates from neurones of the perigeniculate nucleus (PGN) in the cat and of the visual segment of the nucleus reticularis thalami (NRT) in the rat (Fig. 1) (Houser and Vaughn, 1980; Montero and Scott, 1981; Ide, 1982; Montero and Singer, 1985). Recent evidence in the cat indicates the presence of separate GABAergic projections from the PGN and the NRT to the dLGN (Cucchiaro et al., 1990; see Uhlrich and Cucchiaro, Chapter 9). The PGN/NRT cells receive inputs from corticofugal afferents (synapse 8 in Fig. 1) and from axon collaterals of TC cells (synapse 7). The axons of PGN/NRT cells, in turn, make synapses on dLGN TC cells (synapse 5).

An important feature of the GABAergic connections in the dLGN is the presence of GABA-GABA synapses between dLGN interneurones (not shown in Fig. 1) (Jones, 1985; Montero and Singer, 1985). In the cat, GABA-GABA synapses are also formed between PGN cells and dLGN interneurones (synapse 9; Fig. 1) (Montero and Singer, 1985; Montero, 1986), though the presence of NRT to dLGN interneurones synapses in the rat has so far proved elusive (Montero and Scott, 1981). Other extrathalamic sources of GABA, for example from the pretectum, have also been reported (Bickford et al., 1990) (see Uhlrich and Cucchiaro, Chapter 9).

It is also worth noting that, in addition to morphological differences, dLGN interneurones also differ from TC cells and from the GABAergic PGN/NRT cells in their passive and active membrane properties. Thus, dLGN interneurones have a higher input resistance than TC cells, a relatively linear voltage-current relationship and they are not electrically compact (Jahnsen and Llinas, 1984; Deschenes et al., 1984; Crunelli et al., 1987a,d; Bloomfield et al., 1987; McCormick and Pape, 1988; Spreafico et al., 1988; Bloomfield and Sherman, 1989). As far as the active membrane properties are concerned, the major differences reported so far are the lack of low threshold $Ca^{2+}$ potentials in the interneurones (but not in PGN/NRT cells, see Mulle et al., 1985; Avanzini et al., 1989) and of the slow, mixed $Na^+/K^+$ inward rectifying current, $I_h$ (McCormick and Pape, 1988, 1990; Leresche et al., 1990, 1991; Soltesz et al., 1991).

## Localization of $GABA_A$ and $GABA_B$ binding sites in the LGN

Autoradiographic and immunocytochemical studies have revealed relatively high densities of both $GABA_A$ (Palacios et al., 1981; Schoch et al., 1985; Richards et al., 1987; De Blas et al., 1988; Vitorica et al., 1988) and $GABA_B$ binding sites in the dLGN (Bowery et al., 1987; Chu et al., 1990). In the rat, the ratio of $GABA_A$ and $GABA_B$ binding sites seems to be around 3:1 and probably reflects differences in receptor affinity (i.e., GABA binds with 3–4 times higher affinity to $GABA_A$ than to $GABA_B$ receptors) and/or in receptor number (Chu et al., 1990). Bowery et al.

(1987), however, reported a similar density of $GABA_A$ and $GABA_B$ binding sites in the thalamus, with the dLGN having a concentration of $GABA_B$ binding sites higher than the vLGN and among the highest in the brain.

Using a monoclonal antibody raised against the $\alpha$ subunit of the $GABA_A$/benzodiazepine receptor/$Cl^-$ channel complex, a recent immunocytochemical study at the light and electron microscope level has revealed differences in the distribution of this antigen between the various classes of neurones in the cat dLGN (Soltesz et al., 1990). The strongest immunoreactivity is found on the somatic plasma membrane and in the endoplasmic reticulum of the GABA-negative neurones (i.e., TC cells) that have the smallest soma area and cellular laminated bodies, which are likely to be a feature of X cells (LeVay and Fester, 1977). The second strongest immunoreactive cell group has large somata, is GABA-negative and contains no cellular laminated bodies. Immunoreactivity in these cells is strong on the plasma membrane of the soma and dendrites, but is scant or absent intracellularly. GABA-positive cells (i.e., local circuit cells, interneurones) show weak intracellular immunoreactivity and little, if any, immunoreactivity at the somatic and proximal dendritic plasma membrane. The synaptic junctions formed by many boutons establishing symmetrical synapses with dendrites and soma of TC cells are immunopositive, but no immunoreactivity can be detected at the synapses established by the presynaptic dendrites of the interneurones, not even after detergent treatment. These results suggest that interneurones in the cat dLGN do not possess the $\alpha$ subunit of the $GABA_A$ receptor-complex neither on their soma membrane nor on their dendritic appendages. Thus, either $GABA_A$ receptors are absent from the interneurones or, if present, their $\alpha$ subunit is not the one recognized by the monoclonal antibody used in this study (cf. Luddens and Wisden, 1991). Interestingly, immunoreactivity to this $\alpha$ subunit antibody is detected at intra- and extrasynaptic membrane sites, suggesting that GABA may act at both synaptic and non-synaptic sites (Soltesz et al., 1990).

### Effect of postsynaptic GABA$_A$ and GABA$_B$ receptor activation

In vitro, activation of the GABA$_A$ receptors present on TC cells of the rat and cat LGN (by iontophoretically or bath applied GABA) produces a fast, Cl$^-$ dependent hyperpolarization that is associated with a marked decrease in input resistance, is blocked by bicuculline and picrotoxin (a Cl$^-$ channel blocker) and has a reversal potential of $-65$ mV. The hyperpolarization per se and the decrease in input resistance produce a strong inhibition of spontaneous and optic tract-evoked firing (Crunelli et al., 1988; Soltesz et al., 1989c). When the iontophoretic pipette is positioned more than 50 $\mu$m away from the recording electrode and/or when higher iontophoretic currents are used, GABA also evokes a fast depolarization that is blocked by bicuculline and has a reversal potential of $-45$ mV. This GABA$_A$ receptor-mediated depolarization is associated with a marked decrease in input resistance and thus results in a strong inhibition of firing. Often, the bicuculline sensitive hyperpolarization and depolarization can be observed during the same iontophoretic application of GABA, with the former often preceding the latter (Crunelli et al., 1988).

In contrast, selective activation of the GABA$_B$ receptors (by iontophoretically or bath applied baclofen) evokes a slow, K$^+$ dependent hyperpolarization that is associated with a relatively small decrease in input resistance, is blocked by phaclofen (a GABA$_B$ receptor antagonist, Kerr et al., 1987) but not by bicuculline and picrotoxin and has a reversal potential of $-80$ mV. This GABA$_B$ receptor-mediated hyperpolarization is capable of producing some inhibition of spontaneous firing that is not, however, as strong as during GABA$_A$ receptor activation and is extremely dependent on the membrane potential of the cell (see below). Identical results are obtained when selective activation of GABA$_B$ receptors is

achieved by using GABA in the presence of bicuculline and picrotoxin (Hirsch and Burnod, 1987; Crunelli et al., 1988; Soltesz et al., 1988).

It is important to note at this point that the GABA$_A$ receptor-mediated hyperpolarizing/depolarizing effect of iontophoretically and bath applied GABA described above for the in vitro studies occur in the majority of LGN cells, a result similar to the findings in vivo where the spontaneous firing of almost every TC cell in the dLGN (X and Y, on and off centre) is abolished by iontophoretically applied GABA (Sillito and Kemp, 1983; Sillito, personal communication). In view of the differential distribution of the $\alpha$ subunit of the GABA$_A$ receptor in the dLGN (Soltesz et al., 1990), these findings indicate that a different composition of subunits of the GABA$_A$ receptor does not markedly affect its functional properties and/or that the iontophoretic studies carried out in vivo and in vitro have not been sensitive enough to show the subtle differences in potency between different types of GABA$_A$ receptors in dLGN TC cells.

### "Physiological" activation of postsynaptic GABA$_A$ and GABA$_B$ receptors: the early and the late IPSP

Electrical stimulation of the optic tract in vitro evokes a complex sequence of synaptic potentials (Yamamoto, 1974; Kelly et al., 1979; Godfraind and Kelly, 1981) that, between $-55$ and $-65$ mV for instance, consists of a depolarizing potential followed by two hyperpolarizing ones (Fig. 2A, bottom trace) (Hirsch and Burnod, 1987; Crunelli et al., 1988; Soltesz et al., 1988). The depolarizing potential is a monosynaptic excitatory postsynaptic potential (EPSP) that is mediated by an excitatory amino acid (possibly glutamate) acting on $N$-methyl-D-aspartate (NMDA) and non-NMDA receptors (Kemp and Sillito, 1982; Crunelli et al., 1987b; Soltesz et al., 1989a; Sillito et al., 1990; Sharfman et al., 1990).

The two hyperpolarizing potentials represent two IPSPs that can be easily distinguished on the

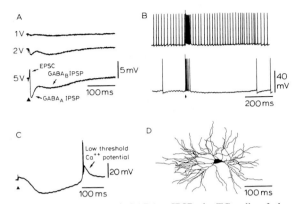

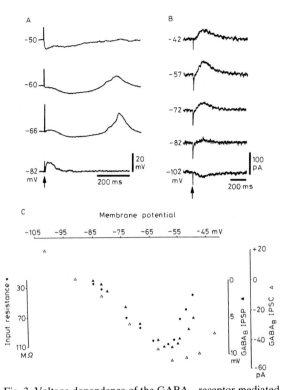

Fig. 2. A. GABA$_A$ and GABA$_B$ IPSPs in TC cells of the dLGN in vitro: intracellular voltage records show the GABA$_A$ and GABA$_B$ IPSPs evoked in a TC cell of the rat dLGN by electrical stimulation of the optic tract (arrow head) (membrane potential, $-60$ mV). Using low intensities of stimulation (1 and 2 V) both the GABA$_A$ and the GABA$_B$ IPSP are evoked in the absence of a preceding EPSP, while at higher intensities (5 V) the complete sequence of potentials (EPSP, GABA$_A$ and GABA$_B$ IPSPs) is present. The small depolarizing hump present between the GABA$_A$ and the GABA$_B$ IPSPs is similar to the one observed in vivo. B shows intracellular voltage traces recorded with a horseradish peroxidase filled microelectrode from the TC cell shown in D. The GABA$_B$ IPSP evoked by stimulation of the optic tract (arrow) decreases the probability of action potential discharges at $-50$ mV (bottom trace). However, the GABA$_B$ IPSP has no effect on the stronger, repetitive action potential firing observed when the cell is depolarized (by steady dc current injection) to $-35$ mV (top trace). Note that, although present at $-50$ mV, the hyperpolarization associated with the GABA$_B$ IPSP is hardly visible at more depolarized potentials because of its non-linear relationship with the membrane potential (cf. Fig. 3A and C). C. Stimulation of the optic tract (in the presence of bicuculline, 50 $\mu$M) evokes a small EPSP followed by an 18 mV GABA$_B$ IPSP. On return of the membrane potential to its resting level a low-threshold Ca$^{2+}$ potential with a burst of action potentials is generated. D is the camera lucida reconstruction of the horseradish peroxidase filled dLGN cell in lamina A from which the records shown in B were recorded. The A/A$_1$ lamina border is vertical and to the right (for detail, see Soltesz et al., 1989b). Reproduced, with permission, from Crunelli et al. (1988) and from Soltesz et al. (1989b).

Fig. 3. Voltage dependence of the GABA$_B$ receptor mediated IPSP and IPSC. A. Intracellular voltage records show the GABA$_A$ and GABA$_B$ IPSP evoked by stimulation of the optic tract (arrow) and recorded at the four membrane potentials indicated on the left hand side of each trace. The GABA$_A$ IPSP reverses in polarity at around $-65$ mV, while the GABA$_B$ IPSP becomes flat at $-82$ mV. The GABA$_B$ IPSP recorded at $-50$ mV is smaller than that recorded at $-60$ mV. Note that, at membrane potentials negative to $-55$ mV, the hyperpolarization associated with the GABA$_B$ IPSP is capable of activating a low threshold Ca$^{2+}$ potential (TC cell in the cat dLGN recorded in 0.5 mM Mg$^{2+}$ and 3 mM Ca$^{2+}$). B shows the late, GABA$_B$ receptor mediated IPSC evoked by stimulation of the optic tract (arrow) in a TC cell of the cat dLGN clamped at the different membrane potentials indicated. The GABA$_B$ IPSC reverses at around $-87$ mV in this cell. Note the rectification of the IPSC at potential positive to $-57$ mV (top trace). Bicuculline (50 $\mu$M) was present in the perfusate. C. Plot of the amplitude of the GABA$_B$ IPSP (▲), the amplitude of the GABA$_B$ IPSC (△) and input resistance (●) *versus* membrane potential. (The values for GABA$_B$ IPSP and input resistance are from the same TC cell of the rat dLGN, those for the GABA$_B$ IPSC are from the same cell as in B). At membrane potentials outside the range of resting membrane potentials of TC cells in vitro ($-55$ to $-65$ mV), the amplitude of the GABA$_B$ IPSP and IPSC decreases, closely following changes in the input resistance of the cell. A and C: reproduced, with permission, and rearranged from Soltesz et al. (1989b) and Crunelli et al. (1988).

basis of their different electrophysiological and pharmacological properties. The first IPSP is characterized by a short latency to onset (3–4 ms), a short latency to peak and a short duration (30–40 ms) (Fig. 2A). It is associated with a marked decrease in the input resistance of the cell, its amplitude is linearly related to the membrane potential and its reversal potential ($-70$ mV) is sensitive to changes in extra- and intracellular $Cl^-$ concentration. Furthermore, it is reversibly blocked by bicuculline (Fig. 4) and picrotoxin at concentrations that are similarly effective against the fast, $Cl^-$ dependent hyperpolarization evoked by exogenously applied GABA. Thus, the early IPSP represents a $GABA_A$ receptor-mediated IPSP (Fig. 2A) (Hirsch and Burnod, 1987; Crunelli et al., 1988; Soltesz et al., 1989b).

The second IPSP has a relatively longer latency to onset (30–50 ms) and to peak, and a long duration (200–300 ms) (Fig. 2A). It is associated with a smaller decrease in input resistance, its amplitude is not linearly related to membrane potential (cf. Fig. 3A,C) and its reversal potential ($-80$ mV) is sensitive to changes in the extracellular $K^+$, but not $Cl^-$, concentration. In addition, it is reversibly blocked by the $GABA_B$ receptor antagonists phaclofen and 2-OH-saclofen (see Kerr et al., 1987, 1988) at concentrations that are similarly effective against the slow, $K^+$ dependent hyperpolarization evoked by exogenously applied baclofen. Indeed, the late inhibitory postsynaptic current (IPSC) that underlies the $GABA_B$ IPSP is also reversibly blocked by 2-OH-saclofen (Lightowler, Soltesz and Crunelli, unpublished observations). Thus, the late, long-lasting IPSP represents a $GABA_B$ receptor-mediated IPSP (Fig. 2A) (Hirsch and Burnod, 1987; Crunelli et al., 1988; Soltesz et al., 1988, 1989b).

Recently, a "miniature" $GABA_A$ IPSP, that precedes the $GABA_A$ and $GABA_B$ IPSP described above, has been observed in TC cells of the anterior thalamic nuclei in vivo following stimulation of the prethalamic fibers (arising in the mammillary body) but not of the cortical afferents (Paré et al., 1990). As shown in Fig. 5C (arrow head), in some TC cells in the cat dLGN a miniature $GABA_A$ IPSP has been observed following stimulation of the optic tract.

## Origin of the two IPSPs

Both the early, $GABA_A$ receptor-mediated and the late, $GABA_B$ receptor-mediated IPSPs (as well as the miniature $GABA_A$ IPSP) can be evoked by stimulation of the optic tract in rat and cat slices that do not contain the NRT and the PGN (Hirsch and Burnod, 1987; Crunelli et al., 1988; Soltesz et al., 1989b). This finding puts an end to the controversy concerning the lack of intrageniculate inhibition (Sumimoto et al., 1976; Shosaku et al.,1989; Steriade et al., 1990b) and indicates that *GABA released from the dLGN interneurones is capable of generating a miniature, an early and a late IPSP*. Thus, the late, long-lasting depression of visual responsiveness observed in TC cells of the cat and rat dLGN (see Norton and Godwin, Chapter 10) can no longer be ascribed *only* to the recurrent (late) inhibition from the PGN/NRT. Indeed, a series of new questions should now be addressed: are there two groups of interneurones (as it has been suggested in the cat dLGN on the basis of morphological findings, Montero and Zempel, 1985) mediating the $GABA_A$ and the $GABA_B$ IPSP, respectively?; is the $GABA_A$ IPSP generated at the dendro-dendritic synapse (synapse 3 in Fig. 1) and the $GABA_B$ IPSP at the axonal synapse (synapse 6) or vice versa? or, does the suggestion put forward by Paré et al. (1990) for the anterior thalamic nuclei (i.e., that the miniature $GABA_A$ IPSP is generated at the dendro-dendritic synapse and the $GABA_A$ and $GABA_B$ IPSP at the axonal synapse) apply to the dLGN interneurones as well?

It is important to note at this point that the ability of rat and cat dLGN interneurones to generate $GABA_A$ and $GABA_B$ IPSPs does not exclude the possibility that in vivo both types of IPSP can also be evoked by GABA released from PGN/NRT cells (synapse 5 in Fig. 1). Although such evidence is still lacking for the dLGN, experiments in TC cells of the rat ventrobasal nucleus (Sumitomo et al., 1988) and anterior thalamic nuclei (Thomson, 1988, 1990) have shown the presence of $GABA_A$ and $GABA_B$ IPSPs originating from the NRT. Indeed, both PGN/NRT-mediated $GABA_A$ and $GABA_B$ IPSPs may contribute to the "late" inhibition of visual responses

(Ahlsen and Lindstrom, 1982; Eysel et al., 1987; see Norton and Godwin, Chapter 10, and Sillito, Chapter 17) and to the sleep spindles (Steriade et al., 1985, 1990a).

As far as the corticofugal afferents are concerned, in a few TC cells it has been possible to evoke what appeared to be a pure orthodromic response following electrical stimulation of the optic radiation. This response consists of an EPSP followed by a $GABA_A$ and a $GABA_B$ IPSP whose electrophysiological and pharmacological properties were identical to those evoked by stimulation of the optic tract (Soltesz et al., 1989b). Nevertheless, these results cannot be taken as conclusive evidence that direct activation of the interneurones by the corticofugal afferents can generate the two types of IPSPs in TC cells since in these experiments the IPSPs might have been evoked by the GABAergic cells of the PGN.

## X and Y cells in the dLGN display $GABA_A$ and $GABA_B$ IPSPs

The typical EPSP-$GABA_A$ IPSP-$GABA_B$ IPSP sequence of synaptic potentials described in the previous sections is observed in a high proportion of TC cells of the dLGN in vitro (e.g., 70% in the rat dLGN, Crunelli et al., 1988). Three additional observations, however, need to be discussed here with respect to possible differences in the interneurone-mediated GABA IPSPs between TC cell types in the dLGN.

(i) It is a common finding of all the in vitro studies that low intensity of stimulation can evoke $GABA_A$ and $GABA_B$ IPSPs without a preceding EPSP, though a small EPSP can be observed by increasing the intensity and/or duration of stimulation (Fig. 2A) (Hirsch and Burnod, 1987; Crunelli et al., 1988; Soltesz et al., 1989b). Undoubtedly, the amplitude of the optic tract-evoked EPSP is under strict control from the $GABA_A$ IPSP and in some TC cells (Fig. 4B), though not in all (Fig. 4A), bicuculline can unmask a prominent EPSP.

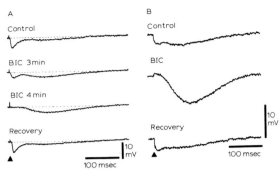

Fig. 4. The effect of bicuculline on the $GABA_A$ and $GABA_B$ IPSP. Intracellular voltage records show that bicuculline applied in the perfusion medium (10 $\mu$M) (A) reversibly abolishes the $GABA_A$ IPSP and increases the amplitude and the duration of the $GABA_B$ IPSP. Iontophoretic application of bicuculline (80 nA, 2 s) (B) from an independently mounted multibarrelled micropipette markedly increased the amplitude of the $GABA_B$ IPSP, but it did not, in this cell, prolong its duration. In both A and B the intensity of stimulation was adjusted so that in the control experiments no EPSP could be evoked, although in B the block of the $GABA_A$ IPSP revealed a clear, though small, EPSP. Membrane potential is $-55$ mV in A and $-60$ mV in B. Reproduced, with permission, from Crunelli et al. (1988).

(ii) In some cells either one of the two IPSPs is evoked by stimulation of the optic tract (e.g., 11% for the $GABA_A$ IPSP and 16% for the $GABA_B$ IPSP in the rat, Crunelli et al., 1988) while the other IPSP is not observed even after changing the intensity, duration, frequency and number of stimuli or, indeed, the position of the stimulating electrode along the optic tract or in the slice itself close to the recording electrode (Hirsh and Burnod, 1987; Crunelli et al., 1988; Soltesz et al., 1988, 1989b). In addition, there are cells that, in control condition, appear to show only $GABA_A$ IPSPs though $GABA_B$ IPSPs become visible in the presence of bicuculline (see below).

(iii) There appears to be a considerable variation in the amplitude of both $GABA_A$ and $GABA_B$ IPSPs between TC cells both in the rat and cat dLGN (Hirsch and Burnod, 1987; Crunelli et al., 1988; Soltesz et al., 1989b; Sharfman et al., 1990).

In an attempt to correlate cell types to the presence of IPSPs, one in vitro study, using intracellular injection of horseradish peroxidase, has shown that TC cells with morphological features similar to X and Y geniculate cells respond with $GABA_B$ IPSPs to optic tract stimulation (Fig. 2D) (Soltesz et al., 1989b). Thus, both cell types have functional $GABA_B$ receptors on their membranes, which, using optimal stimulation parameters and/or in the presence of favourable conditions (e.g., low extracellular $K^+$, bicuculline), can be activated by optic tract stimulation.

In slices, of course, one can never be certain whether the differences in the presence and/or amplitude of any response between cells are indeed attributable to physiological differences or to other variables inherent to this technique (survival of CNS tissue in vitro; level of oxygenation; choice of perfusion medium, etc.; cf. Kerkut and Wheal, 1981; Kelly, 1982; Dingledine, 1984). This problem is of particular importance in studies investigating synaptic potentials, since, in this case, factors such as the angle of cutting of the slice, the position of the recorded cell with respect to the stimulated afferents, different sur-

vival of excitatory and inhibitory synapses have also to be considered.

This notwithstanding, it appears that most of the findings reported for the $GABA_A$ and $GABA_B$ IPSPs in vitro are similar to the situation in vivo. Examples of an early, short-lasting and a late, long-lasting IPSP were observed in TC cells of the dLGN following electrical stimulation of the optic tract/chiasm in vivo (cf. Fig. 4b and c of Burke and Sefton, 1966), though they both appeared to be reversed in polarity by recording with $Cl^-$-filled electrodes. Recent investigations have enlarged and clarified these original findings

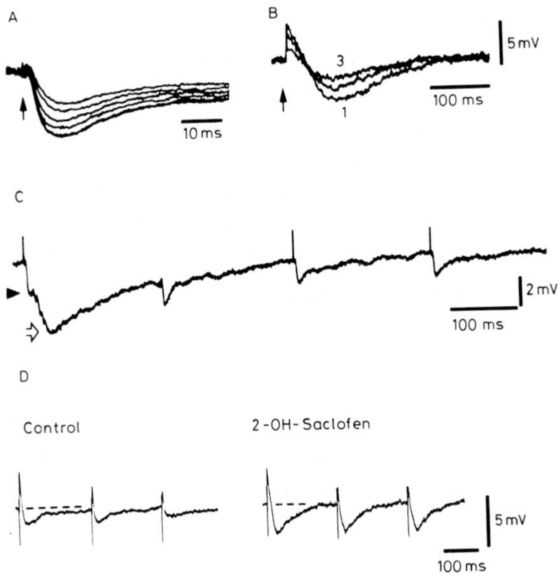

Fig. 5. Frequency-dependent decrease in the amplitude of $GABA_A$ (A, C and D) and $GABA_B$ IPSP (C and B), its blockade by 2-OH-saclofen (D) and the presence of a miniature, $GABA_A$ IPSP in TC cells of the cat dLGN (C). A. Superimposed intracellular voltage records show the decrease in the amplitude of the fifth $GABA_A$ IPSP (in each train) evoked at increasing frequencies of stimulation (from top to bottom, 3, 2, 1, 0.5, 0.35 and 0.25 Hz). Note that no decrease is present at the two lowest frequencies (traces obtained at 0.35 and 0.25 Hz are identical) (membrane potential, $-55$ mV) (arrow marks the time of stimulation). B. Superimposed traces show the decrease in the amplitude of the $GABA_B$ IPSP evoked by stimulation of the optic tract at 2 Hz. The first three responses of the train are shown. Records obtained in the presence of bicuculline (50 $\mu$M) (membrane potential, $-60$ mV) (arrow marks the time of stimulation). Records in A and B were obtained from two TC cells in the rat dLGN. C. Intracellular voltage record from a TC cell in lamina $A_1$ of the cat dLGN shows the response to a 5 Hz train of stimuli. The first stimulus evokes a small, fast $GABA_A$ IPSP (arrow head) (a miniature $GABA_A$ IPSP according to Paré et al., 1990), followed by a $GABA_A$ (open arrow) and a $GABA_B$ IPSP. At the third and fourth stimuli the $GABA_A$ and the $GABA_B$ IPSP are markedly reduced while the amplitude of the miniature $GABA_A$ IPSP is only slightly decreased. The fast upward deflections represent the stimulus artifact (membrane potential, $-51$ mV). D. Intracellular voltage records from a rat dLGN cell show the first three responses obtained by a 5 Hz train of stimuli delivered to the optic tract. In control, the first stimulus evokes a $GABA_A$ and a small $GABA_B$ IPSP. In the second and third stimulus the $GABA_A$ IPSP is progressively decreased in amplitude. In the presence of 2-OH-saclofen (400 $\mu$M), the amplitude of the $GABA_A$ IPSPs has increased and no decrease is present along the train. The fast downward deflections represent the stimulus artifact (membrane potential, $-55$ mV). In A and C, note the absence of an EPSP preceding the IPSPs. A and B reproduced, with permission, from Crunelli et al. (1988).

in the dLGN (Bloomfield and Sherman, 1988; Hu et al., 1989) as well as in other thalamic nuclei following stimulation of the appropriate sensory and/or cortical afferents (Roy et al., 1984; Paré et al., 1990). Although no attempt to characterize the nature of the receptors responsible for these two IPSPs has been carried out in vivo, their electrophysiological properties (e.g., latency to onset and to peak, duration, voltage dependency, reversal potential) strongly indicate that they represent a $GABA_A$ and a $GABA_B$ IPSP similar to those observed in vitro. Indeed, it appears that both $GABA_A$ and $GABA_B$ IPSPs are present in physiologically identified geniculate X and Y cells (Bloomfield and Sherman, 1988) and might therefore contribute to the early and late phase of inhibition observed in these two types of cells during visual stimulation (see Norton and Godwin, Chapter 10, and Sillito, Chapter 17). However, the presence of the PGN in these in vivo experiments has meant that the origin of these two IPSPs could not be unequivocally ascribed to the dLGN interneurones or to the PGN cells (while this has been possible in the in vitro studies, see above).

Other important similarities between the in vivo and in vitro studies include the findings that both the $GABA_A$ and the $GABA_B$ IPSPs can be observed in the absence of a preceding EPSP (Hu et al., 1989; cf. Paré et al., 1990) and that there are variations in the amplitude of the two IPSPs between TC cells (Hu et al., 1989; Paré et al.,1990). Thus, it is possible that in the dLGN there are subpopulations of TC cells with different activation thresholds for the excitatory and inhibitory synapses, and with different activation threshold and/or site of generation for the two types of GABA receptors. In addition, there might also be differences between TC cell types in the distribution of presynaptic $GABA_B$ receptors since recent findings have shown that the miniature $GABA_A$ IPSP shows a smaller frequency-dependent decrease in amplitude than the one of the $GABA_A$ and $GABA_B$ IPSP in vivo (Paré et al., 1990) and in vitro (Fig. 5C) (see below).

These possible differences in the presence and relative size of depolarizing and hyperpolarizing synaptic potentials between TC cells brings us to problem of the presence of lagged and non-lagged cells in the cat dLGN. Though the subject of intense debate, there is anatomical and electrophysiological evidence that a group of X neurones (the lagged X cells) show a relatively more powerful phase of inhibition during the early part of prolonged visual stimulation than other, non-lagged cells (Mastronarde, 1987a,b; Humphrey and Weller, 1988a,b; Hartveit and Heggeland, 1990; Heggeland and Hartveit, 1990). Indeed, the presence of lagged and non-lagged Y cells has also been recently reported (Mastronarde, 1988). The different distribution of $GABA_A$ receptors, the different activation thresholds of EPSP and IPSPs, the voltage sensitivity of the $GABA_B$ IPSP, a likely differential distribution of the miniature $GABA_A$ IPSP and some intrinsic, voltage-dependent conductances of TC cells (e.g., the $I_A$ current, see McCormick, 1990) should all be considered in the interpretation of these in vivo results concerning the existence of lagged and non-lagged cells. Undoubtedly, the availability of new intracellular staining techniques (e.g., biocytin) that allow a better resolution of the morphological details together with a superior quality of intracellular recordings will help to clarify this controversial issue.

### Role of the $GABA_B$ IPSP in TC cells: inhibition and burst-firing excitation

The hyperpolarization of the $GABA_B$ IPSP (and its associated decrease in input resistance) is able to inhibit repetitive action potential firing in TC cells of the dLGN (Fig. 2B). This effect is maximal at potentials close to the in vitro resting membrane potential ($-55$ to $-65$ mV), but is less pronounced and disappears altogether at more depolarized potentials (Hirsch and Burnod, 1987; Crunelli et al., 1988; Soltesz et al., 1989b). As elegantly shown by Connors et al. (1988) in cortical cells, the GABA$_B$ IPSP "would tend to reduce background firing rates and responsiveness to weak excitatory stimuli but leaves responsiveness to strong transient stimuli unimpaired" (see Connors, Chapter 16). Thus, the GABA$_B$ IPSP appears to be more suited to a subtle control of excitability than to the modulation of the receptive field properties of dLGN TC cells.

The non-linear relationship between the amplitude of GABA$_B$ IPSP and the membrane potential (in the voltage region positive to $-55$ mV) is of particular relevance to the voltage dependent inhibition described above, as are the rectifying membrane properties of TC cells (Fig. 3C). Recent experiments indicate that the amplitude of the late GABA$_B$ IPSC (recorded using the single electrode voltage clamp technique) has a maximum at the same membrane potential as the GABA$_B$ IPSP ($-55$ to $-65$ mV) (Fig. 3B and C). At more depolarized potentials the amplitude of the GABA$_B$ IPSC decreases, while in the voltage range $-65$ to $-100$ mV it is voltage independent, i.e., it is linearly related to the membrane potential (Fig. 3B and C) (but cf. Gahwiler and Brown, 1985; Hablitz and Thalmann, 1987). Notwithstanding some of the problems associated with studying synaptic currents with this technique (cf. Johnston and Brown, 1983), these results indicate that the voltage dependency of the GABA$_B$ IPSC, possibly together with the rectifying properties of TC cells, is responsible for the reduction in the amplitude of the GABA$_B$ IPSP (Fig. 3A) and the associated decreases in inhibitory action that are observed at potentials positive to $-55$ mV (Fig. 2B).

Inhibition of firing, however, is not the only effect produced by the late, long-lasting GABA$_B$ IPSP. In fact, as shown in Fig. 2C, a single GABA$_B$ IPSP is capable of evoking a low-threshold Ca$^{2+}$ potential, which in turn, depending on its amplitude, evokes a single or a burst of action potentials (Crunelli et al., 1988; Soltesz et al., 1989b). This sequence of events only occurs in a relatively narrow region of membrane potentials ($-60$ to $-70$ mV) and is mainly due to an

interplay between the GABA$_B$ IPSP and $I_T$ (Crunelli and Leresche, 1991), the Ca$^{2+}$ current responsible for the low threshold Ca$^{2+}$ potentials (Coulter et al., 1989; Crunelli et al., 1989; Hernandez-Cruz and Pape, 1989; Suzuki and Rogawski, 1989). The mechanism underlying the interaction between the GABA$_B$ IPSP and $I_T$ has been recently reviewed in Crunelli and Leresche (1991). Undoubtedly, this "priming" action of GABA$_B$ IPSPs in burst-firing excitation of TC cells is involved in the late (100–150 ms) burst of excitation (and subsequent rhythmic excitation) recorded in dLGN TC cells following electrical stimulation of the optic tract in vivo (cf. Figs. 2d, 3a and c in Burke and Sefton, 1966). Indeed, it may also play a role in the oscillatory activities observed in TC cells during certain stages of sleep (Steriade et al., 1990a) or during the spike and wave discharges of petit mal attacks (Gloor and Fariello, 1988) (though TC cells still retain the ability to produce oscillations even when the receptors for GABA or other neurotransmitters are blocked, see Leresche et al., 1990, 1991; Crunelli and Leresche, 1991). Clearly, to identify the full extent of any possible contribution of GABA$_B$ IPSP-mediated inhibition and/or burst-firing excitation to the processing of visual information in the dLGN we still have to wait for experiments on the effects of selective GABA$_B$ antagonists on visual responses (see Baumfalk and Albus, 1988). A final point of clarification needs to be added here. In the initial study describing the GABA$_B$ IPSP (Crunelli et al., 1988) this synaptic potential was shown to evoke burst-firing excitation only in the presence of bicuculline, since, as explained in the next section, in control condition it was too small to deactivate $I_T$. However, later in vitro "experiments carried out in 3 mM Ca$^{2+}$ and 0.5 mM Mg$^{2+}$, or in 3.25 mM K$^+$, have shown GABA$_B$ IPSPs sufficiently large to generate a low threshold Ca$^{2+}$ potential" (Soltesz et al., 1989) and its associated burst-firing excitation even in the absence of bicuculline (cf. Fig.2A of Soltesz et al., 1989).

## Bicuculline increases the amplitude of the GABA$_B$ IPSP

Our knowledge about the role of GABA mediated inhibition in shaping the visual response properties of TC cells in dLGN comes, to a large extent, from in vivo studies using bicuculline as a selective antagonist of GABA$_A$ receptors (see Norton and Godwin, Chapter 10, and Sillito, Chapter 17). In vitro, however, bicuculline (as well as picrotoxin), applied either iontophoretically or in the perfusion medium, not only blocks GABA$_A$ IPSPs but also markedly increases the amplitude of the GABA$_B$ IPSP (Fig. 4) (Hirsch and Burnod, 1987; Crunelli et al., 1988; Soltesz et al., 1988, 1989b) and IPSC (Lightowler, Soltesz and Crunelli, unpublished observation).

The exact mechanism of this enhancement is still uncertain. It is not due to a loss of selectivity by bicuculline (or picrotoxin) in vitro since, even at concentrations higher than those enhancing the GABA$_B$ IPSP, this substance seems to have no effect on the slow hyperpolarization evoked in TC cells by the selective GABA$_B$ agonist baclofen. Since the latency to onset of the GABA$_B$ IPSP and IPSC is about 30–35 ms, it is unlikely that this effect of bicuculline involves a release of the GABA$_B$ IPSP from a direct "shunting" action of the GABA$_A$ IPSP immediately preceding it. In addition, an interaction between the Cl$^-$ influx associated with GABA$_A$ receptor activation and the second messenger system responsible for the GABA$_B$ IPSP is also unlikely since a similar bicuculline-evoked increase of the GABA$_B$ IPSP can be observed at different extracellular Cl$^-$ concentrations and when recording with KCl filled microelectrodes.

Thus, as in the case of other neurones (Newberry and Nicoll, 1985), the most likely explanations for this effect of bicuculline on the GABA$_B$ IPSPs have, so far, been based upon the local synaptic circuitry in the dLGN.

(i) The simplest one is that in vitro the interneurones responsible for the GABA$_B$ IPSPs (if there are two separate sets of interneurones), or the release site responsible for the GABA$_B$ IPSP (if the same interneurone is responsible for GABA$_A$ and GABA$_B$ IPSPs), are under a *tonic* GABA$_A$ mediated inhibitory control either from other interneurones or from the GABAergic cells of the PGN/NRT. Bicuculline would simply release the interneurones from this inhibition allowing a larger release of GABA and, thus, an enhanced GABA$_B$ IPSP and IPSC (see Fig. 10 of Crunelli et al., 1988). Indeed, the presence of spontaneous IPSPs is a common finding in intracellular recording from TC cells in the cat dLGN in vitro (cf. Fig. 5A of Crunelli et al., 1987c; and Fig. 1B of Sharfman et al., 1990). Though this is not the case in TC cells of the rat dLGN during standard current clamp intracellular recordings, using patch electrodes the majority of rat dLGN cells maintained in thin slices show a baseline current trace covered with spontaneous, bicuculline sensitive IPSC (Leresche and Llano, personal communication).

(ii) In the cat, the lack of immunostaining in dLGN interneurones for a monoclonal antibody raised against the $\alpha$ subunit of the GABA$_A$ receptor (Soltesz et al., 1990) and the likely presence of intrageniculate axon collaterals of TC cells (not shown in Fig. 1) *, has meant that an alternative possibility could also be considered. In the control condition, a TC cell is under GABA$_A$ inhibitory control during the first 30–40 ms (duration of GABA$_A$ IPSPs) immediately after stimulation of the optic tract. In the presence of bicuculline, the interneurones (which in this explanation we consider responsible for both

---

* The presence of intrageniculate axon collaterals of TC cells is still a matter of great controversy (Friedlander et al., 1981; Jones, 1985; Steriade et al., 1990b). Owing to the improved resolution of new intracellular labelling techniques, these intrageniculate axon collaterals of TC cells are being recognized in a relatively higher percentage of cells. Clearly, whether they make synaptic contacts with the interneurones remains to be established.

GABA$_A$ and GABA$_B$ IPSPs) could receive an additional, longer excitation from the axon collateral of this TC cell that could now evoke action potentials for a relatively longer period: this will lead to increased GABA release and enhanced GABA$_B$ IPSP (see Fig. 6B of Soltesz et al., 1989b). Indeed not every TC cell needs to have an intrageniculate axon collateral since each interneurone contacts more than one TC cell.

Whatever the exact mechanism of the bicuculline-induced increase in the amplitude of GABA$_B$ IPSPs, we believe that it is now necessary to re-investigate the action of this GABA$_A$ antagonist in vivo in the presence of a GABA$_B$ antagonist, and thus, to ascertain which, if any, of the effects of bicuculline on the visual response properties of TC cells in the dLGN can be ascribed to a block of GABA$_A$ IPSPs and/or to a concomitant increase in the amplitude of GABA$_B$ IPSPs. In this respect, two points need to be raised. Firstly, due to the non-linear relationship of the GABA$_B$ IPSPs with the membrane potential (Fig. 3) it might be difficult to ascertain the relative contribution of GABA$_A$ and GABA$_B$ receptors from the results of experiments using extracellular single unit recordings. Secondly, one cannot exlude the possibility that in vivo the GABA$_B$ IPSPs are already of a maximum amplitude and, thus, they will not be affected by bicuculline. Finally, a technical consideration: although 2-OH-saclofen might appear to be the GABA$_B$ antagonist of choice because of its higher potency when compared to phaclofen, its action on presynaptic GABA$_B$ receptors (see below) should be considered in the interpretation of the results.

## Are there presynaptic GABA$_B$ receptors in the dLGN?

A wealth of biochemical and electrophysiological experiments suggests that GABA can decrease its own release as well as that of glutamate via presynaptic GABA$_B$ receptors (Bowery et al., 1980; Dolphin and Scott, 1987; Deisz and Prince,

1989; Starke et al., 1989; Bowery et al., 1990; Deisz and Zieglgansberger; 1990; Waldmeier and Baumann, 1990). In dLGN TC cells, both the GABA$_A$ and the GABA$_B$ IPSP show a decline in amplitude with increasing frequencies of stimulation (Fig. 5A, B and C) (Crunelli et al., 1988; Soltesz et al., 1989b). In other neurones, such frequency-dependent decreases in the amplitude of GABA IPSPs have been shown to be due to presynaptic GABA$_B$ receptors (Deisz and Prince, 1989) and, in the light of our preliminary results obtained with 2-OH-saclofen (and discussed below), it is possible that, in the dLGN too, GABA modulates glutamate and GABA release through presynaptic GABA$_B$ receptors.

Firstly, 2-OH-saclofen increases the amplitude of the optic tract-evoked GABA$_A$ IPSP by 10–20% (Fig. 5D). Secondly, and more importantly, 2-OH-saclofen reduces the frequency-dependent decrease in the amplitude of GABA$_A$ IPSPs (Fig 5D). Although a reduction in GABA uptake might contribute to some of these effects of 2-OH-saclofen (cf. Kerr et al., 1988), these results suggest that 2-OH-saclofen blocks presynaptic GABA$_B$ receptors, and this leads to an increase in GABA release. Thus, in addition to interneurone-interneurone and PGN-interneurone synapses, dLGN interneurones might be capable of controlling GABA release by a negative feed-back mechanism through presynaptic GABA$_B$ receptors present on their axon or dendritic terminals. During visual processing in vivo, this negative control of GABA release by presynaptic GABA$_B$ receptors will be of major importance owing to the relatively high firing rate of the retinal afferents. Preliminary observations also indicate that baclofen (in the presence of Ba$^{2+}$ which blocks the postsynaptic, K$^+$ dependent GABA$_B$ receptors) is capable of decreasing the amplitude of the optic tract-evoked EPSP, suggesting that presynaptic GABA$_B$ receptors might be present on the optic nerve terminals. Finally, a pharmacological consideration: phaclofen does not produce any of the effects described above for 2-OH-saclofen, indicating that at concentrations that

abolish the postsynaptic $GABA_B$ response, i.e., 1
mM phaclofen and 400 $\mu$M 2-OH-saclofen, the
latter is more potent than the former on presynaptic $GABA_B$ receptors, at least on those present in the dLGN.

## GABA mediated responses in the rat vLGN: lack of optic tract-evoked $GABA_B$ IPSPs

The retino-receptive lateral geniculate body consists of two main parts, the vLGN and dLGN
(Jones, 1985). The dLGN has its embryonic origins in the dorsal diencephalon, while the vLGN
is derived from the ventral diencephalon, and
these two embryonic structures then fuse to form
the LGN. The vLGN, or an homologous structure, is present in the brains of all vertebrate
species, but, with increasing size and development of the visual cortex, there is a concomitant
reduction in the relative size and probably in the
relative importance of the vLGN. The vLGN
projects to the superior colliculus, and not to the
visual cortex, and its main role has been suggested to be the processing of information regarding light intensity (Legg and Cowey, 1977; Brauer
and Schober, 1982; Taylor, 1986; Taylor and
Lieberman, 1987).

The two main groups of neurones in the rat
vLGN, the projecting cells and the Golgi type II
(non-projecting) interneurones are connected
mainly through dendro-dendritic synapses which
are part of triadic arrangements (Lieberman et
al., 1973; Mounty et al., 1977; Jones, 1985). Glutamic acid decarboxylase- and GABA-like immunoreactivity (Taylor, 1986) as well as $GABA_A$
and $GABA_B$ binding sites are present in the
neuropil of the vLGN (Bowery et al., 1987; Chu
et al., 1990). Unlike the dLGN, however, the
extrageniculate GABAergic afferents to the
vLGN do not originate from the NRT (since no
connection exists between these two nuclei, see
Mackay-Sim et al., 1983; Cosenza amd Moore,
1984) but from the pretectum (Campbell, 1982;
Campbell et al., 1984; Taylor, 1986).

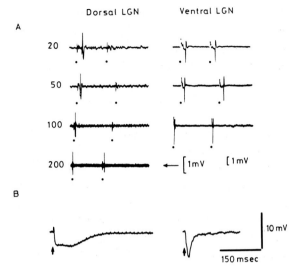

Fig. 6. The effect of double (A) and single (B) shock stimulation of the optic tract recorded extracellularly in vivo (A) and
intracellularly in vitro (B), respectively, from the rat vLGN
and dLGN. A. Extracellular single unit recordings show the
response to suprathreshold conditioning and test shocks to
the optic tract (marked by dots) delivered at the intervals
indicated on the left hand side of each trace. The cell in the
dLGN fails to respond to the test shock at 20, 50 and 100 ms
intervals. The cell in the vLGN responds to the test shock at
all intervals. B. Intracellular voltage traces show the typical
response recorded from a dLGN (left) and a vLGN (right) cell
in vitro following stimulation of the optic tract (arrow). The
dLGN cell showed both a $GABA_A$ and a $GABA_B$ IPSP while
the vLGN cell responded only with a $GABA_A$ IPSP. Reproduced, with permission, from Hale and Sefton (1978) and
from Soltesz et al. (1989c).

In contrast to what has been observed in the
dLGN, extracellular single unit recordings indicate that the majority of vLGN cells do not show
a centre-surround antagonism in their receptive
fields (Fukuda et al., 1977; Hale and Sefton,
1978; Sumimoto et al., 1979). In addition, they
lack a long-lasting post-excitatory inhibition, i.e.,
their probability of firing is suppressed only for a
relatively short period of time following an electrical shock to the optic tract and/or nerve,
whereas a long-lasting (200 ms) decrease in excitability is present in TC cells of the dLGN (Fig.
6A) (Hale and Sefton, 1978). An explanation of
this difference has been that the long-lasting inhibition in the dLGN is mediated by the GABAer-

gic cells of the NRT which are known to innervate the dLGN but not the vLGN. As discussed below, however, an alternative possibility is provided by the in vitro studies showing the inability of optic tract stimulation to activate the $GABA_B$ receptors that are present in the vLGN (Soltesz et al., 1989c).

Similar to what has been observed in the dLGN in vitro, iontophoretically applied GABA evokes both bicuculline sensitive and insensitive hyperpolarizations in the vLGN. This latter response as well as the slow hyperpolarization evoked by baclofen are antagonized by phaclofen, indicating that both $GABA_A$ and $GABA_B$ receptors are present in vLGN neurones (Soltesz et al., 1989c).

In these neurones, however, electrical stimulation of the optic tract evokes only a short latency, short duration IPSP (Fig. 6B) whose electrophysiological and pharmacological properties (including its sensitivity to bicuculline) are similar to the $GABA_A$ IPSP recorded in TC cells of the dLGN. Thus, the IPSP recorded in vLGN neurones is a $GABA_A$ receptor-mediated IPSP. This optic tract evoked $GABA_A$ IPSP of vLGN neurones is never followed by a late, long-lasting IPSP, though, in the same slice, $GABA_B$ receptor mediated IPSPs can be routinely observed in TC cells of the dLGN (Fig. 6B) (Soltesz et al., 1989c). Thus, in vLGN neurones electrical stimulation of the optic tract evokes only $GABA_A$ but not $GABA_B$ receptor mediated IPSPs, though functionally active, phaclofen-sensitive $GABA_B$ receptors are present on these cells. It is conceivable that $GABA_A$ IPSPs represent the physiological basis of the short-lasting inhibition observed in vLGN neurones in vivo, while the lack of optic tract evoked $GABA_B$ IPSPs underlies the lack of long-lasting inhibition (Fig. 6A). Thus, the absence of innervation of the rat vLGN by the NRT may not be the only cause for the lack of long-lasting post-excitatory inhibition in vLGN neurones. As far as the role of $GABA_B$ receptors present on the vLGN cells is concerned, they may represent extrasynaptic receptors or, more likely, they might be activated by other GABA containing afferents, for instance, by those originating in the pretectum.

## Conclusions and outlook

Undoubtedly, the success of understanding the processing of visual information by the cortex depends upon our knowledge of the neuronal integration occurring at subcortical levels of the visual system. Thus, the exploration of the LGN is of particular importance not only because its TC cells form the immediate input to the visual cortex but also because of its suggested role in feeding back to the cortex the output of the cortical processing. Inherent to a highly non-linear neuronal system such as the LGN is the capability to generate a rich repertoire of temporal and spatial activity patterns in its distributed circuits. Clearly, if we are to understand the computations taking place in this nucleus we have to integrate the findings of many disciplines. We are beginning to understand the genetic basis of cellular phenotypes in the LGN (Hendry et al., 1988; Sequier et al., 1988; Hockfield and Sur, 1990) and monoclonal antibodies raised against different subunits of $GABA_A$ (Luddens and Wisden, 1991) (as well as other neurotransmitter) receptors are showing the diversity of receptor subtypes which might underlie the large variety of behaviours observed in LGN neurones. Intracellular recordings in in vitro LGN slices have paved the way in the study of the repertoire of these possible electrical behaviours. As far as GABA is concerned, these investigations have provided conclusive evidence that, following stimulation of the optic tract fibres, GABA released from rat and cat dLGN interneurones can generate $GABA_A$ and $GABA_B$ receptor-mediated IPSPs in TC cells. In addition, they have indicated that presynaptic $GABA_B$ receptors can modulate GABA and glutamate release in the dLGN. It is now necessary to demonstrate which of these GABA-mediated responses are used by the LGN in the processing of visual information.

## Acknowledgments

We are indebted to our colleagues Drs. M. Haby, D. Jassick-Gerschenfeld, N. Leresche, M. Pirchio, C.E. Pollard, S. Lightowler and Miss Z. Emri and K. Tóth who, at different stages, were involved in the work reported in this paper. Supported by grants of the Wellcome Trust to V. Crunelli.

## References

Ahlsen, G. and Lindstrom, S. (1982) Excitation of perigeniculate neurones via axon collaterals of principal cells. *Brain. Res.*, 236: 477–481.

Ahlsen, G., Lindstrom, S. and Lo, F.S. (1985) Interaction between inhibitory pathways to principal cells in the lateral geniculate nucleus of the cat. *Exp. Brain Res.*, 58: 134–143.

Avanzini, G., De Curtis, M., Panzica, F. and Spreafico, R. (1989) Intrinsic properties of nucleus reticularis thalami neurones of the rat studied in vitro. *J. Physiol.*, 416: 111–122.

Baumfalk, U. and Albus, K. (1988) Phaclofen antagonizes baclofen-induced suppression of visually evoked responses in the cat's striate cortex. *Brain Res.*, 463: 398–402.

Berardi, N. and Morrone, M.C. (1984) The role of $\gamma$-aminobutyric acid mediated inhibition in the response properties of cat lateral geniculate nucleus neurons. *J. Physiol.*, 357: 505–523.

Bickford, M.E., Cucchiaro, J.B. and Sherman, S.M. (1990) A GABAergic pretectal projection to the lateral geniculate nucleus in the cat. *Soc. Neurosci.*, 16: 72.9.

Bloomfield, S.A., Hamos, J.E. and Sherman, S.M. (1987) Passive cable properties and morphological correlates of neurons in the lateral geniculate nucleus of the cat. *J. Physiol. (London)*, 383: 653–692.

Bloomfield, S.A. and Sherman, S.M. (1988) Postsynaptic potentials recorded in neurons of the cat's lateral geniculate nucleus following electrical stimulation of the optic chiasm. *J. Neurophysiol.*, 60: 1924–1945.

Bloomfield, S.A. and Sherman, S.M. (1989) Dendritic current flow in relay cells and interneurons of the cat's lateral geniculate nucleus. *Proc. Natl. Acad. Sci. USA*, 86: 3911–3914.

Bormann, J. (1988) Electrophysiology of $GABA_A$ and $GABA_B$ receptor subtypes. *Trends Neurosci.*, 11: 112–116.

Bowery, N.G., Bittiger, H. and Olpe, H.-R. (1990) *$GABA_B$ Receptors in Mammalian Functions*. Wiley, London.

Bowery, N.G., Hill, D.R., Hudson, A.L., Doble, A., Middlemiss, D.N., Shaw, J. and Turnbull, M. (1980) (−)Baclofen decreases neurotransmitter release in the mammalian CNS by an action at a novel GABA receptor. *Nature*, 283:92–94.

Bowery, N.G., Hudson, A.L. and Price, G.W. (1987) $GABA_A$ and $GABA_B$ receptor site distribution in the rat central nervous system. *Neuroscience*, 20: 365–383.

Brauer, K. and Schober, W. (1982) Identification of geniculotectal relay neurons in the rat's ventral lateral geniculate nucleus. *Exp. Brain.Res.*, 45: 84–88.

Burke, W. and Sefton, A.J. (1966) Inhibitory mechanisms in lateral geniculate nucleus of rat. *J. Physiol.*, 187: 231–246.

Campbell, G. (1982) Anatomical studies of the rat pretectum. PhD thesis, University of London.

Campbell, G., Hunt, S.P., Liberman, A.R., Ohara, P.T., Ottersen, O.P., Storm-Mathisen, J. and Wu, J.Y. (1984) Immunohistochemical identification of GAD- and GABA-containing neurones in the olivary pretectal nucleus (OPN) of rat and mouse. *J. Physiol.*, 353: 45P.

Chu, D.C.M., Albin, R.L., Young, A.B. and Penney, J.B. (1990) Distribution and kinetics of $GABA_B$ binding sites in rat central nervous system: A quantitative autoradiographic study. *Neuroscience*, 34: 341–357.

Connors, B.W., Malenka, R.C. and Silva, L.R. (1988) Two inhibitory postsynaptic potentials, and $GABA_A$ and $GABA_B$ mediated responses in neocortex of rat and cat. *J. Physiol. (London)*, 406:443–468.

Cosenza, R.M. and Moore, R.Y. (1984) Afferent connections of the ventral lateral geniculate nucleus in the rat: an HRP study. *Brain Res.*, 310:367–370.

Coulter, D.A., Huguenard, J.R. and Prince, D.A. (1989) Calcium currents in rat thalamocortical relay neurones: kinetic properties of the transient low-threshold current. *J. Physiol.*, 414: 587–604.

Crunelli, V., Kelly, J.S., Leresche, N. and Pirchio, M. (1987a) The ventral and dorsal lateral geniculate nucleus of the rat: intracellular recordings in vitro. *J. Physiol.*, 384: 587–601.

Crunelli, V., Kelly, J.S., Leresche, N. and Pirchio, M. (1987b) On the excitatory post-synaptic potential evoked by stimulation of the optic tract in the rat lateral geniculate nucleus. *J. Physiol.*, 384: 603–618.

Crunelli, V., Leresche, N., Hynd, J.W., Patel, N.M. and Parnavelas, J.G. (1987c) An in vitro preparation of the cat lateral geniculate nucleus. *J. Neurosci. Methods*, 20:211–219.

Crunelli, V., Leresche, N. and Parnavelas, J.G. (1987d) Membrane properties of morphologically identified X and Y cells in the lateral geniculate nucleus of the cat in vitro. *J. Physiol.*, 390: 243–256.

Crunelli, V., Haby, M., Jassik-Gerschenfeld, D., Leresche, N. and Pirchio, M. (1988) $Cl^-$ and $K^+$-dependent inhibitory postsynaptic potentials evoked by interneurones of the rat lateral geniculate nucleus. *J. Physiol.*, 399: 153–176.

Crunelli,V., Lightowler, S. and Pollard, C.E. (1989) A T-type $Ca^{2+}$ current underlies low-threshold $Ca^{2+}$ potentials in cells of the cat and rat lateral geniculate nucleus. *J. Physiol.*, 413: 543–561.

Crunelli, V. and Leresche, N. (1991) A role of $GABA_B$ receptors in excitation and inhibition of thalamocortical cells. *Trends Neurosci.*, 14: 16–21.

Cucchiaro, J.B., Uhlrich, D.J. and Sherman, S.M. (1990) A projection from the thalamic reticular nucleus to the dorsal lateral geniculate nucleus in the cat: a comparison with the perigeniculate projection. *Soc. Neurosci. Abstr.*, 16:72.8.

De Blas, A.L., Vitorica, J. and Friedrich, P. (1988) Localization of the GABA-A receptor in the rat brain with a monoclonal antibody to the 57,000 Mr peptide of the GABA-A receptor/benzodiazepine receptor/Cl⁻ channel complex. *J. Neurosci.*, 8: 602–614.

Deisz, R.A. and Prince, D.A. (1989) Frequency-dependent depression of inhibition in guinea-pig neocortex in vitro by GABA$_B$ receptor feed-back on GABA release. *J. Physiol.*, 412: 513–541

Deisz, R.A. and Zieglgansberger, W. (1990) GABA$_B$ receptors control GABA release of neocortical neurones. In: S. Kalsner and T.C. Westfall (Eds.), *Presynaptic receptors and the question of autoregulation of neurotransmitter release.* NY Acad. Sci., New York.

Deschenes, M., Paradis, M., Roy, J.P. and Steriade, M. (1984) Electrophysiology of neurones of lateral thalamic nuclei in cat: Resting properties and burst discharges. *J. Neurophysiol.*, 51: 1196–1219.

Dingledine, R. (1984) *Brain Slices.* New York, Plenum Press.

Dolphin, A.C. and Scott, R.H. (1987) Calcium channel currents and their inhibition by (−)baclofen in rat sensory neurones: modulation by guanine nucleotides. *J. Physiol.*, 386: 1–17.

Dubin, M.W. and Cleland J.G. (1977) Organization of visual inputs to interneurons of lateral geniculate nucleus of the cat. *J. Neurophysiol.*, 40: 410–427.

Eysel, U.T., Pape, H.-C. and van Schayck, R. (1987) Contributions of inhibitory mechanisms to the shift responses of X and Y cells in the cat lateral geniculate nucleus. *J. Physiol.*, 388: 199–212.

Famiglietti, E.V. and Peters, A. (1972) The synaptic glomerulus and the intrinsic neuron in the dorsal lateral geniculate nucleus of the cat. *J. Comp. Neurol.*, 144: 285–334.

Fitzpatrick, D., Penny, G.R. and Schemechel, D.E. (1984) Glutamic acid decarboxylase-immunoreactive neurons and terminals in the lateral geniculate nucleus of the cat. *J. Neurosci.*, 4: 1809–1829.

Francesconi, W., Müller, C.M. and Singer, W. (1988) Cholinergic mechanisms in the reticular control of transmission in the cat lateral geniculate nucleus. *J. Neurophysiol.*, 59:1690–1718.

Friedlander, M.J., Lin, C.S., Stanford, L.R. and Sherman, S.M. (1981) Morphology of functionally identified neurons in lateral geniculate nucleus of the cat. *J. Neurophysiol.*, 46: 80–129.

Fukuda, Y., Sumimoto, I. and Sugitani, I. (1977) Properties of cells in the ventral part of the rat's lateral geniculate nucleus. *Proc. XXVII IUPS Meeting*, 247.

Gabbott, P.L.A., J. Somogyi, M.G. Stewart and Hamori, J. (1985) GABA-immunoreactive neurons in the rat dorsal lateral geniculate nucleus: light microscopical observations. *Brain Res.*, 346: 171–175.

Gahwiler, B.H. and Brown, D.A. (1985) GABA$_B$-receptor-activated K⁺ current in voltage clamp CA$_3$ pyramidal

cells in hippocampal cultures. *Proc. Natl. Acad. Sci. USA*, 82: 1558–1562.

Gloor, P. and Fariello, R.G. (1988) Generalized epilepsy: some of its cellular mechanisms differ from those of focal epilepsy. *Trends Neurosci.*, 11: 63–68.

Godfraind, J.-M. and Kelly, J.S. (1981) Intracellular recording from thin slices of the lateral geniculate nucleus of rats and cats. In: G.A. Kerkut and H.V. Wheal (Eds.), *Electrophysiology of Isolated Mammalian CNS Preparations*, Academic Press, London, pp. 257–284.

Guillery, R.W. (1966) A study of Golgi preparations from the lateral geniculate nucleus of the adult cat. *J. Comp. Neurol.*, 128:21–50.

Hablitz, J.J. and Thalmann, R.H. (1987) Conductance changes underlying a late synaptic hyperpolarisation in hippocampal CA$_3$ neurons. *J. Neurophysiol.*, 58: 160–171.

Hale, P.T. and Sefton, A.J. (1978) A comparison of the visual and electrical response properties of the cells in the dorsal and ventral lateral geniculate nuclei. *Brain Res.*, 153: 591–595.

Hale, P.T., Sefton, A.J., Baur, L.A. and Cottee, L.J. (1982) Interrelations of rat's thalamic reticular and dorsal lateral geniculate nuclei. *Exp. Brain.Res.*, 45: 217–229.

Hamori, J., Pasik, T., Pasik, P. and Szentagothai, J.H. (1974) Triadic synaptic arrangements and their possible significance in the lateral geniculate nucleus of the monkey. *Brain Res.*, 80: 379–393.

Hamos, J.E., van Horn, S.C., Raczkowski, D., Uhlrich, D.J. and Sherman, S.M. (1985) Synaptic connectivity of a local circuit neuron in lateral geniculate nucleus of the cat. *Nature*, 317: 618–621.

Hartveit, E. and Heggelund, P. (1990) Neurotransmitter receptors mediating excitatory input to the cat lateral geniculate nucleus. II. Non-lagged cells. *J. Neurophysiol.*, 63: 1361–1372.

Heggelund, P. and Hartveit, E. (1990) Neurotransmitter receptors mediating excitatory input to the cat lateral geniculate nucleus. I. Lagged cells. *J. Neurophysiol.*, 63: 1347–1360.

Hendry, S.H.C., Jones, E.G., Hockfield, S. and McKay, R.D.G. (1988) Neuronal populations stained with the monoclonal antibody cat-301 in the mammalian cerebral cortex and thalamus. *J. Neurosci.*, 8: 518–542.

Hernandez-Cruz, A. and Pape, H.-C. (1989) Identification of two calcium currents in acutely dissociated neurons from the lateral geniculate nucleus. *J. Neurophysiol.*, 61: 1270–1283.

Hirsch, J.C. and Burnod, Y. (1987) A synaptically evoked late hyperpolarization in the rat dorsolateral geniculate neurons in vitro. *Neuroscience*, 23: 457–468.

Hockfield, S. and Sur, M. (1990) Monoclonal antibody Cat-301 identifies Y-cells in the dorsal lateral geniculate nucleus of the cat. *J. Comp. Neurol.*, 300:320–330.

Houser, C.R. and Vaughn, J.E. (1980) GABA neurons are the major cell type of the nucleus reticularis thalami. *Brain Res.*, 200: 341–354.

Hu, B., Steriade, M. and Deschenes, M. (1989) The effects of brainstem peribrachial stimulation on reticular thalamic neurons. *Neuroscience*, 31: 1–12.

Hubel, D.H. and Wiesel, T.N. (1961) Integrative action in the cat's lateral geniculate body. *J. Physiol.*, 150: 91–104.

Humphrey, A.L. and Weller, R.E. (1988a) Functionally distinct groups of X-cells in the lateral geniculate nucleus of the cat. *J. Comp. Neurol.*, 268: 429–447.

Humphrey, A.L. and Weller, R.E. (1988b) Structural correlates of functionally distinct X-cells in the lateral geniculate nucleus of the cat. *J. Comp. Neurol.*, 268: 448–468.

Ide, L.S. (1982) The fine structure of the perigeniculate nucleus in the cat. *J. Comp. Neurol.*, 210: 317–334.

Jahnsen, H. and Llinas, R.R. (1984) Electrophysiological properties of guinea-pig thalamic neurones: An in vitro study. *J. Physiol.*, 349: 205–226.

Johnston, D. and Brown, T.H. (1983) Interpretation of voltage-clamp measurements in hippocampal neurons. *J. Neurophysiol.*, 50: 464–486.

Jones, E.G. (1985) *The Thalamus*. New York, Plenum Press.

Kelly, J.S., Godfraind, J.M. and Maruyama, S. (1979) The presence and nature of inhibition in small slices of dorsal lateral geniculate nucleus of rat and cat incubated in vitro. *Brain Res.*, 168: 388–392.

Kelly, J.S. (1982) Intracellular recording from neurones in brain slices in vitro. In: L.L. Iversen, S.D. Iversen and S.M. Snyder (Eds.), *Handbook of Psychopharmacology*, Plenum Press, New York, pp. 95–183.

Kemp, J.A. and Sillito, A.M. (1982) The nature of the excitatory transmitter mediating X and Y cell inputs to the cat dorsal geniculate nucleus. *J. Physiol.*, 323: 377–391.

Kerkut, G.A. and Wheal, H.V. (1981) *Electrophysiology of Isolated Mammalian CNS Preparations*. London, Academic Press.

Kerr, D.I.B., Ong, J., Prager, R.H., Gynther, B.D. and Curtis, D.R. (1987) Phaclofen: a peripheral and central baclofen antagonist. *Brain. Res.*, 405: 150–154.

Kerr, D.I.B., Ong, J., Johnston, G.A.R., Abbenate, J. and Prager, R.H. (1988) 2-Hydroxy-saclofen: an improved antagonist at central and peripheral GABA_B receptors. *Neurosci. Lett.*, 91: 92–96.

Legg, C.R. and Cowey, A. (1977) The role of the ventral lateral geniculate nucleus and posterior thalamus in intensity discrimination in rats. *Brain Res.*, 123:261–273.

Leresche, N., Jassik-Gerschenfeld, D., Haby, M., Soltesz, I. and Crunelli, V. (1990) Pacemaker-like and other types of spontaneous membrane potential oscillations of thalamocortical cells. *Neurosci. Lett.*, 113: 72–77.

Leresche, N., Lightowler, S., Soltesz, I., Jassik-Gerschenfeld, D. and Crunelli, V. (1991) Low frequency oscillatory activities intrinsic to rat and cat thalamocortical cells. *J. Physiol.*, 441: 155–174.

LeVay, S. and Fester, D. (1977) Relay cell classes in the lateral geniculate nucleus of the cat and the effects of visual deprivation. *J. Comp. Neurol.*, 172:563–584.

Lieberman, A.R. (1973) Neurones with presynaptic perikaria and presynaptic dendrites in the rat lateral geniculate nucleus. *Brain Res.*, 59: 35–39.

Lieberman, A.R., Ohara, P.T., Taylor, A.M., Hunt, S.P. and

Wu, J.-Y. (1983) Immunohistochemical studies of glutamatic acid decarboxylase (GAD) in the ventral lateral geniculate nucleus (LGv) and intergeniculate leaflet (IGL) of the lateral geniculate body of the rat. *J. Anat.*, 136: 627P.

Lindstrom, S. (1982) Synaptic organization of inhibitory pathways to principal cells in the lateral geniculate nucleus of the cat. *Brain Res.*, 234: 447–453.

Lindstrom, S. and Wrobel, A. (1990) Private inhibitory systems for the X and Y pathways in the dorsal lateral geniculate nucleus of the cat. *J. Physiol. (London)*, 429:259–281.

Luddens, H. and Wisden, W. (1991) Function and pharmacology of multiple GABA_A receptor subunits. *TIPS*, 12:49–52.

Mackay-Sim, A., Sefton, A.J. and Martin, P.R. (1983) Subcortical projections of lateral geniculate and thalamic reticular nuclei in the hooded rat. *J. Comp. Neurol.*, 213:24–35.

Madarasz, M., Somogyi, Gy., Somogyi, J. and Hamori, J. (1985) Numerical estimation of γ-aminobutyric acid (GABA)-containing neurons in three thalamic nuclei of the cat: direct GABA immunocytochemistry. *Neurosci. Lett.*, 61: 73–78.

Mastronarde, D.M. (1987a) Two classes of single-input X-cells in cat lateral geniculate nucleus. II. Retinal inputs and the generation of receptive-field properties. *J. Neurophysiol.*, 57: 381–413.

Mastronarde, D.M. (1987b) Two classes of single-input X-cells in cat lateral geniculate nucleus. I. Receptive-field properties and classification of cells. *J. Neurophysiol.*, 57: 357–380.

Mastronarde, D.N. (1988) Branching of X and Y functional pathways in cat lateral geniculate nucleus. *Soc. Neurosci.*, 14: 127.6.

McCormick, D.A. (1990) Possible ionic basis for lagged visual responses in cat LGNd relay neurons. *Soc. Neurosci. Abstr.*, 16:72.6.

McCormick, D.A. and Pape, H.-C. (1988) Acetylcholine inhibits identified interneurons in the cat lateral geniculate nucleus. *Nature*, 334: 246–248.

McCormick, D.A. and Pape, H.-C. (1990) Properties of a hyperpolarization-activated cation current and its role in rhythmic oscillation in thalamic relay neurones. *J. Physiol.*, 431: 291–318.

Mize, R.R., Spencer, R.F. and Horner, L.H. (1986) Quantitative comparison of retinal synapses in the dorsal and ventral (parvicellular) C laminae of the cat dorsal lateral geniculate nucleus. *J. Comp. Neurol.*, 248: 57–73.

Montero, V.M. (1987) Ultrastructural identification of synaptic terminals from the axon of type 3 interneurons in the cat lateral geniculate nucleus. *J. Comp. Neurol.*, 264: 268–283.

Montero, V.M. and Scott, G.L. (1981) Synaptic terminals in dorsal lateral geniculate nucleus from neurons of the thalamic reticular nucleus. A light and electron microscope autoradiographic study. *Neuroscience*, 6:2561–2577.

Montero, V.M. and Singer, W. (1984) Ultrastructure and synaptic relations of neural elements containing glutamic acid decarboxylase (GAD) in the perigeniculate nucleus of the cat. *Exp. Brain. Res.*, 56: 115–125.

Montero, V.M. and Singer, W. (1985) Ultrastructure identification of somata and neural processes immunoreactive to antibodies against glutamic decarboxylase (GAD) in the dorsal lateral geniculate nucleus of the cat. *Exp. Brain Res.*, 59: 151–165.

Montero, V.M. and Zempel, J. (1985) Evidence for two types of GABA-containing interneurons in the A-laminae of the cat lateral geniculate nucleus: a double-label HRP and GABA-immunocytochemical study. *Exp. Brain Res.*, 60: 603–609.

Mounty, E.J., Parnavelas, J.G. and Lieberman, A.R. (1977) The neurons and their postnatal development in the ventral lateral geniculate nucleus of the rat. *Anat. Embryol.*, 151: 35–51.

Mulle, C., Steriade, M. and Deschenes, M. (1985) Absence of spindle oscillations in the cat anterior thalamic nuclei. *Brain Res.*, 334: 165–168.

Newberry, N.R. and Nicoll, R.A. (1985) Comparison of the action of baclofen with γ-aminobutiric acid on rat hippocampal pyramidal cells in vitro. *J. Physiol. (London)*, 360:161–185.

Norton, T.T., Holdefer, R.N. and Godwin, D.W. (1989) Effects of bicuculline on receptive field center sensitivity of relay cells in the lateral geniculate nucleus. *Brain Res.*, 488:348–352.

O'Hara, P.T., Lieberman, A.R., Hunt, S.P. and Wu, J.Y. (1983) Neural elements containing glutamic acid decarboxylase (GAD) in the dorsal lateral geniculate nucleus of the rat. Immunohistochemical studies by light and electron microscopy. *Neuroscience*, 8: 189–211.

Ottersen, O.P. and Storm-Mathisen, J. (1984) Glutamate-and-GABA-containing neurons in the mouse and rat brain, as demonstrated with a new immunocytochemical technique. *J. Comp. Neurol.*, 229: 374–392.

Palacios, J.M., Wamsley, J.K. and Kuhar, M.J. (1981) High-affinity GABA receptors: Autoradiographic localization. *Brain Res.*, 222: 285–307.

Pape, H.-C. and Eysel, U.T. (1986) Binocular interactions in the lateral geniculate nucleus of the cat: GABAergic inhibition reduced by dominant afferent activity. *Exp. Brain Res.*, 61: 265–271.

Paré, D., Curró Dossi, R. and Steriade, M. (1990) Genesis of inhibitory postsynaptic potentials (IPSPs) by interneurons in the feline anterior thalamic (AT) nuclei. *Soc. Neurosci. Abstr.*, 16:202.1.

Parnavelas, J.G., Mounty, E.J., Bradford, R. and Lieberman, A.R. (1977) The postnatal development of neurons in the dorsal lateral geniculate nucleus of the rat: a Golgi study. *J. Comp. Neurol.*, 171:481–500.

Peters, A. and Palay, S.L. (1966) The morphology of lamina A and A1 of the dorsal nucleus of the lateral geniculate body of the cat. *J. Anat.*, 100: 451–486.

Richards, J.G., Schoch, P., Haring, P., Takacs, B. and Mohler, H. (1987) Resolving GABA-A/benzodiazepine receptors: cellular and subcellular localization in the CNS with monoclonal antibodies. *J. Neurosci.*, 7: 1866–1886.

Roy, J.P., Clerq, M., Steriade, M. and Deschenes, M. (1984) Electrophysiology of neurons of lateral thalamic nuclei in cat: mechanisms of long-lasting hyperpolarisations. *J. Neurophysiol.*, 51: 1220–1235.

Scharfman, H.E., Lu, S.-M., Guido, W., Adams, P.R. and Sherman, S.M. (1990) N-Methyl-D-aspartate receptors contribute to excitatory postsynaptic potentials of cat lateral geniculate neurons recorded in thalamic slices. *Proc. Natl. Acad. Sci. USA*, 87: 4548–4552.

Schoch, P., Richards, J.G., Haring, P., Takacs, B., Stahli, C., Staehelin, T., Heafely, W. and Mohler, H. (1985) Co-localization of GABA$_A$ receptors and benzodiazepine receptors in the brain shown by monoclonal antibodies. *Nature*, 314: 168:171.

Sequier, J.M., Richards, J.G., Malherbe, P., Price, G.W., Mathews, S. and Mohler, H. (1988) Mapping of brain areas containing RNA homologous to cDNAs encoding the α- and β-subunits of the rat GABA$_A$ γ-aminobutyrate receptor. *Proc. Natl. Acad. Sci.USA*, 85: 7815–7819.

Sherman, S.M. and Friedlander, M.J. (1988) Identification of X versus Y properties for interneurons in the A-laminae of the cat's lateral geniculate nucleus. *Exp. Brain Res.*, 73:384–392.

Sherman, S.M. and Koch, C. (1986) The control of retinogeniculate transmission in the mammalian lateral geniculate nucleus. *Exp. Brain. Res.*, 63: 1–20.

Sherman, S.M. and Spear, P.D. (1982) Organization of visual pathways in normal and visually deprived cats. *Physiol. Rev.*, 62: 738–855.

Shosaku, A., Kayama, Y., Sumitomo, I., Sugitani, M. and Iwama, K. (1989) Analysis of recurrent inhibitory circuit in rat thalamus: Neurophysiology of the thalamic reticular nucleus. *Prog. Neurobiol.*, 32:77–102.

Sillito, A.M. and Kemp, J.A. (1983) The influence of GABAergic inhibitory processes on the receptive field structure of X and Y cells in cat dorsal lateral geniculate nucleus (dLGN). *Brain Res.*, 277: 63–78.

Sillito, A.M., Murphy, P.C., Salt, T.E. and Moody, C.I. (1990) Dependence of retinogeniculate transmission in cat on NMDA receptors. *J. Neurophysiol.*, 63: 347–355.

Singer, W. and Bedworth, N. (1973) Inhibitory interaction between X and Y units in the cat lateral geniculate nucleus. *Brain Res.*, 49: 291–307.

Soltesz, I., Haby, M., Leresche, N. and Crunelli, V. (1988) The GABA$_B$ antagonist phaclofen inhibits the late K$^+$-dependent IPSP in cat and rat thalamic and hippocampal neurones. *Brain Res.*, 448: 351–354.

Soltesz, I., Haby, M., Jassik-Gerschenfeld, D., Leresche, N. and Crunelli, V. (1989a) NMDA and non-NMDA receptors mediate both high and low frequency synaptic potentials in the rat lateral geniculate nucleus. *Soc. Neurosci.*, 15: 516.19.

Soltesz, I., Lightowler, S., Leresche, N. and Crunelli, V. (1989b) On the properties and origin of the GABA$_B$ inhibitory postsynaptic potential recorded in morphologically identified projection cells of the cat dorsal lateral geniculate nucleus. *Neuroscience*, 33: 23–33.

Soltesz, I., Lightowler, S., Leresche, N. and Crunelli, V. (1989c) Optic tract stimulation evokes GABA$_A$ but not GABA$_B$ IPSPs in the rat ventral lateral geniculate nucleus. *Brain Res.*, 479: 49–55.

Soltesz, I., Roberts, J.D.B., Takagi, H., Richards, J.G., Mohler, H. and Somogyi, P. (1990) Cellular and subcellular localization of the benzodiazepine/GABA$_A$ receptor/Cl$^-$ channel complex using monoclonal antibodies in the dorsal lateral geniculate nucleus of the cat. *Eur. J. Neurosci.*, 2: 414–429.

Soltesz, I., Lightowler, S., Leresche, N., Jassik-Gerschenfeld, D., Pollard., C.E. and Crunelli, V. (1991) Two inward currents and the transformation of low frequency oscillations of rat and cat thalamocortical cells. *J. Physiol.*, 441: 175–197.

Spreafico, R., De Curtis, M., Frassoni, C. and Avanzini, G. (1988) Electrophysiological characteristics of morphologically identified reticular thalamic neurons from rat slices. *Neuroscience*, 27: 629–638.

Starke, K., Gothert, M. and Kilbinger, H. (1989) Modulation of neurotransmitter release by presynaptic autoreceptors. *Physiol. Rev.*, 69: 864–989.

Steriade, M., Deschenes, M., Domich, L. and Mulle, C. (1985) Abolition of spindle oscillations in thalamic neurons disconnected from the reticularis thalami. *J. Neurophysiol.*, 54: 1473–1497.

Steriade, M., Jones, E.G. and Llinas, R.R. (1990a) Thalamic oscillations and signaling. Wiley, London.

Steriade, M., Pare, D., Hu, B. and Deschenes, M. (1990b) The visual thalamocortical system and its modulation by the brainstem core. *Prog. Sens. Physiol.*, 10: 1–123.

Sterling, P. and Davis, T.L. (1980) Neurons in cat lateral geniculate nucleus that concentrate exogenous [$^3$H]-aminobutyric acid (GABA). *J. Comp. Neurol.*, 192:737–749.

Sumimoto, I., Nakamura, M. and Iwama, K. (1976) Location and function of the so-called interneurons of rat lateral geniculate boody. *Exp. Neurol.*, 51: 110–123

Sumimoto, I., Sugitani, M., Fukuda, Y. and Iwama, K. (1979) Properties of cells responding to visual stimuli in the rat ventral lateral geniculate nucleus. *Exp. Neurol.*, 66: 721–736.

Sumitomo, I., Takahashi, Y., Kayama, Y. and Ogawa, T. (1988) Burst discharges associated with phasic hyperpolarizing oscillations of rat ventrobasal relay neurons. *Brain Res.*, 447: 376–379.

Suzuki, S. and Rogawski, M.A. (1989) T-type calcium channels mediate the transition between tonic and phasic firing in thalamic neurons. *Proc. Natl. Acad. Sci. USA*, 86: 7228–7232.

Szentagothai, J. (1973) Neuronal and synaptic architecture of the lateral geniculate nucleus. In: R. Jung (Ed.), *Handbook of Sensory Physiology, Volume VII/3, Central Processing of Visual Information, Part B, Visual Centers in the Brain*. Springer-Verlag, Berlin, pp. 141–176.

Taylor, A.M. (1986) Experimental anatomical studies of the ventral lateral geniculate nucleus of the rat. PhD thesis, University of London.

Taylor, A.M. and Lieberman, A.R. (1987) Ultrastructural organisation of the projection from the superior colliculus to the ventral lateral geniculate nucleus of the rat. *J. Comp. Neurol.*, 256: 454–462.

Thomson, A.M. (1988) Inhibitory postsynaptic potentials evoked in thalamic neurons by stimulation of the reticularis nucleus evoke slow spikes in isolated rat brain slices-I. *Neuroscience*, 25: 491–502.

Thomson, A.M. (1990) IPSPs evoked by stimulation of the nucleus reticularis thalami can activate low threshold slow spikes in projection neurons. *Neurosci. Lett. Suppl.*, 38: S89.

Vidyasagar, T.R. (1984) Contribution of inhibitory mechanisms to the orientation sensitivity of cat dLGN neurons. *Exp. Brain Res.*, 55: 192–195.

Vitorica, J., Park, D., Chin, G. and de Blas, A.L. (1988) Monoclonal antibodies and conventional antisera to the GABA$_A$ receptor/benzodiazepine receptor/Cl$^-$ channel complex. *J. Neurosci.*, 8: 615–622.

Waldmeier, P.C. and Baumann, P.A. (1990) Presynaptic GABA receptors. In: Kalsner, S. and Westfall, T.C. (Eds.), *Presynaptic Receptors and the Question of Autoregulation of Transmitter Release. Ann. NY Acad. Sci.*, 604, 136–152.

Wilson, J.R., Friedlander, M.J. and Sherman, S.M. (1984) Fine structural morphology of identified X- and Y-cells in the cat's lateral geniculate nucleus. *Proc. R. Soc. London B*, 221: 411–436.

Yamamoto, C. (1974) Electrical activity recorded from thin sections of the lateral geniculate body, and the effects of 5-hydroxytryptamine. *Exp. Brain Res.*, 19: 271–281.

R.R. Mize, R.E. Marc and A.M. Sillito (Eds.)
Progress in Brain Research, Vol. 90

CHAPTER 9

# GABAergic circuits in the lateral geniculate nucleus of the cat

Daniel J. Uhlrich [1] and Josephine B. Cucchiaro [2]

[1] *Department of Anatomy, University of Wisconsin Medical School, Madison, WI 53706 and* [2] *Department of Neurobiology and Behavior, State University of New York at Stony Brook, Stony Brook, NY 11794, USA*

The primary visual afferent pathway from retina to cortex contains a station in the thalamus, the lateral geniculate nucleus (LGN). While the projection cells in the LGN receive their main visual drive from the retina, the overwhelming majority of the synaptic contacts onto these geniculate cells arises from extraretinal sources (Guillery, 1969; Wilson et al., 1984). These extraretinal inputs to the LGN control the visual information that is forwarded to the cortex, and thus must provide a neural basis for visual arousal and attention (Sherman and Koch, 1986; Steriade and Llinas, 1988).

The extraretinal input to LGN cells is extremely diverse, arising intrinsically from interneurons and extrinsically from widespread regions of the brain (e.g., thalamus, brainstem and cortex). These varied cell groups employ a variety of neurotransmitters, form distinctive neuroanatomical connections with LGN cells, and are likely to subserve different functions. A number of these extraretinal inputs to the LGN use the same neurotransmitter, gamma-aminobutyric acid (GABA). GABAergic terminals comprise about one-third of the synaptic terminals on LGN relay cells, and these are thought to underlie most of the inhibitory interactions in the LGN. GABA is known to dramatically affect the visual responsiveness and sensitivity of LGN cells, and it has also been implicated in binocular interactions, in

enhancing receptive field surrounds, and in subtle orientation tuning as described by other chapters in this volume (see Soltesz and Crunelli, Chapter 8, Norton and Godwin, Chapter 10, and Sillito, Chapter 17). The origin of and circuitry entered into by GABAergic terminals in the LGN, which provides the anatomical basis of these physiological processes, is the focus of this review.

## Organization of the cat's LGN

Although there are differences, the fundamental organization of the LGN is similar across species. The LGN of the cat is the focus of this review because its organization and its GABAergic circuitry have been most extensively studied. The LGN of the cat is a laminated and visuotopically organized nucleus that is located in the dorsal-lateral thalamus (Fig. 1). One half of each retina projects to the LGN in a retinotopic fashion. As a consequence, the LGN reflects a fairly precise map of the contralateral visual hemifield (Sanderson, 1971). For example, in the A laminae, visual field azimuths, from central to lateral visual fields, are mapped from medial to lateral in the LGN. This means that the vertical meridian and surrounding central visual field are found adjacent to the medial interlaminar nucleus (Fig. 1). Visual field elevations, uppermost to lowermost, are mapped from caudal to rostral. While the LGN is

172

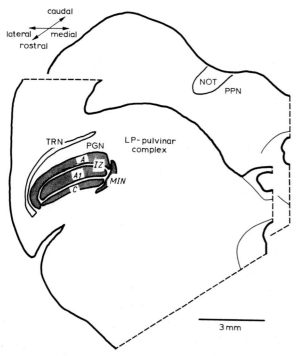

Fig. 1. The lateral geniculate nucleus (stippled) and the source of its known GABAergic innervation, in the coronal view. The front section through the thalamus is 1.5 mm rostral to the second section through the pretectum. IZ, interlaminar zone; MIN, medial interlaminar nucleus; NOT, nucleus of the optic tract; OPN, olivary pretectal nucleus; PGN, perigeniculate nucleus; PPN, posterior pretectal nucleus; TRN, thalamic reticular nucleus.

innervated by both retinas, the inputs remain segregated in different geniculate laminae. The two dorsal-most laminae, lamina A and A1, are innervated by the contralateral and ipsilateral eyes respectively, and they form a reasonably matched pair. Most of the studies related to GABAergic circuitry in the LGN have involved these laminae. Just ventral to the A layers are a group of C laminae, one magnocellular and four parvocellular. Other nuclei considered part of the geniculate complex include the medial interlaminar nucleus (which consists of three retinorecipient laminae and, despite its name, is often included as part of the LGN), the ventral lateral

geniculate nucleus and the perigeniculate nucleus. GABA clearly is used in these structures as well (e.g., Fitzpatrick et al., 1984; Montero and Zempel, 1985; Rinvik et al., 1987), but less is known about its organization there. Thus, this review is primarily limited to the discussion of GABAergic circuitry in the A laminae.

Cells in the cat's LGN have been divided into three distinct classes called X, Y and W cells. These cell types are distinguished on the basis of their visual receptive field properties, the conduction velocities of their retinal inputs, and their light and electron microscopic morphology (Friedlander et al., 1981; Sherman and Spear, 1982; Wilson et al., 1984). Each geniculate cell type is innervated by a retinal cell type of same name with similar receptive field properties. Thus the afferent visual pathway is composed of parallel X, Y and W "streams" that analyze and convey different aspects of the visual scene.

The parallel streams are channeled through different laminae of the LGN (Sherman and Spear, 1982). The A laminae contain X and Y cells. Y cells predominate in the magnocellular C lamina and the medial interlaminar nucleus, with small numbers of W and X cells. The parvocellular C laminae and ventral lateral geniculate nucleus contain W cells. Most LGN cells are relay cells, which project to cortex; however, about 25% of all the geniculate cells are putative interneurons that do not project out of the LGN. Many of these cells are GABAergic and are described below.

*Geniculate ultrastructural terminology*

Five major types of synaptic profiles have been described in the cat's LGN, and together, they comprise over 98% of the synaptic profiles that are seen in the A laminae (Guillery, 1969, 1971; Ide, 1982). Three types of profile form asymmetric synaptic contacts in the LGN. They are termed RLP (for *r*ound vesicles, *l*arge profile, and *p*ale mitochondria), RSD (for *r*ound vesicles, *s*mall profile, and *d*ark mitochondria), and RLD (*r*ound vesicles, *l*arge profile, and *d*ark mitochondria).

RLP terminals, which comprise about 10 to 20% of the terminals in the LGN, arise from the retina. They synapse onto the proximal dendritic shafts and somata of geniculate relay cells and also onto interneurons (see below). About half of the profiles in the LGN are RSD-like. Most of these probably originate from the visual cortex (Jones and Powell, 1969) but other sources are also known, including the parabrachial region of the brainstem, the dorsal raphe nucleus and intrinsic axon collaterals of some geniculate relay cells (Wilson et al., 1984; Weber and Kalil, 1987; DeLima and Singer, 1987; Cucchiaro et al., 1988). RLD terminals, which are rare in the LGN, may arise from axon collaterals of geniculate relay cells (Ide, 1982; Montero, 1989b).

About one-third of the synaptic profiles in the LGN form symmetrical synaptic contacts and are termed F profiles (for *f*lattened or pleomorphic vesicles). The F class of profile is fairly heterogeneous and often subdivided. Terminals of the F1 subtype have a dark cytoplasm, are densely packed with flattened vesicles, and have very thin postsynaptic densities. In contrast, F2 terminals have a pale cytoplasm, are more sparsely filled with pleomorphic vesicles, and have slightly thicker postsynaptic densities (Cucchiaro et al., 1988). F1 and F2 terminals are further distinguished by their connectivity and origin. F2 terminals are dendritic in origin (see below) and are postsynaptic to other synaptic terminals while F1 terminals arise from axons and are never postsynaptic. Finally, F2 terminals are usually involved in complex synaptic arrangements called synaptic *triads*. In a triad, one terminal (usually an RLP terminal) is presynaptic to an F2 terminal. Both the RLP and F2 terminals are presynaptic to a third profile in the triad, usually a dendritic appendage of a relay cell (e.g., Fig. 3a). Often several triads are associated with an RLP terminal, and this arrangement is called a *glomerulus* (e.g., Fig. 9e). Most F profiles in the LGN are immunoreactive for GABA (Montero and Singer, 1985; Montero, 1986), and they must be mediating some of the dramatic GABAergic effects that have been reported in the responses of geniculate cells.

## Interneurons

An obvious source of GABAergic innervation in the LGN is intrinsic. Approximately 25% of the cells in the LGN are immunoreactive for GABA. These cells have smaller somata than those of GABA-negative cells and are found in similar proportions in all laminae of the LGN. GABAergic cells do not appear to project to the visual cortex (Fitzpatrick et al., 1984; Montero and Zempel, 1985; Montero, 1989a) and thus are taken to be interneurons.

*Light microscopy*

Figure 2 shows *camera lucida* reconstructions of 2 interneurons. These cells have a characteristic somatodendritic morphology. They have small somata and thin, sinuous dendrites with many appendages. These dendrites often emit extremely fine, complexly-branched "axoniform" processes. Figure 2A illustrates the most common dendritic arbor morphology. It has a vertical columnar shape that spans the entire depth of lamina A, but only about 150 μm along the mediolateral and rostrocaudal axes. A small number of interneurons are radially symmetrical (Fig. 2B). They encompass the full depth of the lamina and have a 700 μm radius in the orthogonal orientation as well. EM analysis indicates that both cells in Fig. 2 have a myelinated axon, which appears to arborize within the dendritic arbor of the cell. However, at the light microscopic level, the axons cannot be unambiguously distinguished from the axon-like dendritic processes. The morphology of interneurons matches the description of geniculate type 3 cells by Guillery (1966, 1971), and it is clearly distinct from that of geniculate relay neurons, which have larger somata and stout, less elaborate dendrites. Montero (1986) has reported that, in the A laminae, only type 3 cells express GABA immunoreactivity, although it is not clear if all type 3 cells are GABAergic.

A

B

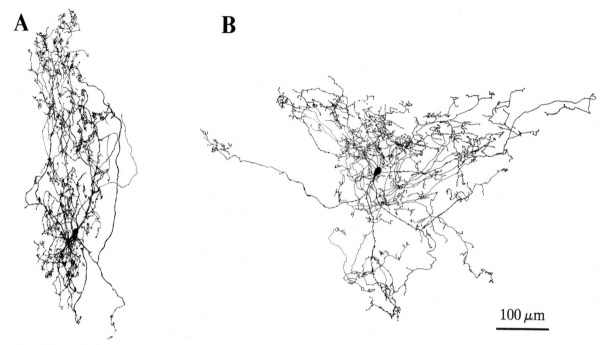

100 μm

Fig. 2. *Camera lucida* reconstructions of two geniculate interneurons. Both of these cells have class 3 morphology as described by Guillery (1971) and were physiologically classified as X cells. A. The most common form of interneuron. This cell has a narrow, columnar-shaped dendritic arbor. B. Interneuron with a radial dendritic arbor. The scale bar in B also applies to A.

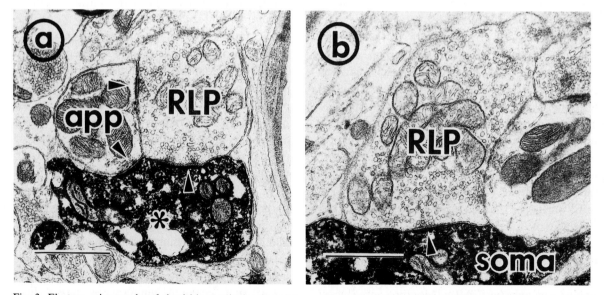

Fig. 3. Electron micrographs of dendritic terminals of an interneuron that was intracellularly filled with HRP. a. A labeled dendritic F2 terminal (asterisk) forms a synapse onto an appendage (app) of a geniculate relay cell. A retinal terminal (RLP) synapses onto both the relay cell appendage and the F2 terminal, forming a synaptic triad. b. The labeled soma of the geniculate interneuron receives a synapse from a retinal terminal (RLP). Scale bars are 1 μm. Adapted from Hamos et al. (1985).

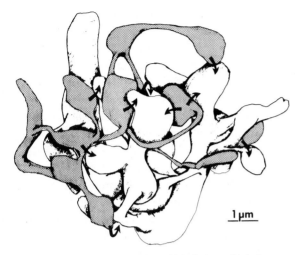

Fig. 4. Serial EM reconstruction of labeled terminals from an interneuron that was intracellularly filled with HRP (stippled) and the unlabeled dendrite (un-stippled) that was postsynaptic to these terminals. Arrows indicate the sites of synaptic contact made by the interneuron onto the relay cell. Redrawn from Hamos et al. (1985).

## Electron microscopy

Morphologically identified type 3 cells have been studied ultrastructurally after being labeled by the intracellular injection of HRP (Hamos et al., 1985) and Golgi-EM techniques (Montero, 1986). Although the labeling often obscures detail within the appendages, it is clear that the dendritic swellings are F2 profiles (Fig. 3a). They are sparsely filled with synaptic vesicles, which appear to be pleomorphic, they form symmetrical synapses, and they are both pre- and postsynaptic to other terminals. Further, they are often located in complex triadic synaptic arrangements (see above). Most of these triads involve RLP terminals and the dendritic appendages of relay cells (Wilson et al., 1984; Hamos et al., 1985). Thus, the F2 terminals of interneurons are ideally positioned to modulate retinogeniculate (primary visual) transmission.

Figure 4 further illustrates the relationship between the F2 appendages of an interneuron and the appendages of a relay cell. The labeled cluster of dendritic appendages received four RLP, one RSD and two F1 contacts. In turn, the interneuron cluster made nine F2 contacts with the dendritic appendages of a single relay cell. The labeled interneuron contacted no other targets in this part of the neuropil. However, the relay cell also received 23 unlabeled F2 and 17 unlabeled F1 synaptic contacts. Thus, while individual interneurons may selectively target postsynaptic cells, several interneurons and/or other inhibitory processes may converge onto single relay cells.

As mentioned above, geniculate interneurons also have axons (Hamos et al., 1985; Montero, 1987), and these axons tend to arborize within the dendritic arbor of the cells. The axonal terminals are F profiles that are slightly different from F1 or F2 terminals. Unlike F2 terminals, they are not postsynaptic to other terminals, but, unlike F1 terminals, they are not densely packed with synaptic vesicles. The axons of interneurons tend to terminate in two forms. Terminals on the axons are mostly *en passant*, although clawlike clusters of boutons are not uncommon (Famiglietti and Peters, 1972). These two forms have different postsynaptic targets. The *en passant* terminals contact small to medium sized dendritic shafts in extra-glomerular zones, while the clustered boutons contact putative relay cell appendages in glomeruli (Montero, 1987).

## Cable properties

Interneurons appear to have two output appendages, dendrites and axons, that enter into distinct geniculate circuitry. The reason for this design is not clear, but it suggests that these cells can perform two distinct functions. Bloomfield and Sherman (1989) addressed this issue by modeling the electrical current flow in the dendrites of geniculate interneurons and relay cells using linear steady-state cable theory (Rall, 1977). In brief, the model predicts the flow of electrical current down a dendrite, thereby estimating the electrical impact of synapses anywhere on the dendritic arbor. In such a passive model (i.e., assuming no active conductances), two primary morphological features of interneurons determine that they will conduct current less efficiently than relay cells. First, dendrites of interneurons are thinner and longer, and second, they do not follow the "3/2 branching rule," which states that the diameters of the daughter dendrites raised to the 3/2 power and summed equals the diameter of the parent dendrite raised to the 3/2 power. Such 3/2 power branching matches the impedance on both sides of the branch point and permits efficient current flow across it (Rall, 1977). Relay cell dendrites follow the 3/2 power rule, but the dendrites of interneurons do not; their daughter dendrites are too thin.

In Fig. 5, single dendritic branches from a geniculate X relay cell and an interneuron are schematized in a Sholl diagram. These data were derived from typical reconstructions of intracellularly filled neurons of these two types. The relay cell dendrite has a relatively unelaborate arbor,

while the interneuron displays many more orders of branching. Because the interneuron's dendritic branches are inefficient for current flow, synaptic currents should be severely attenuated as they travel down the thin dendrites with numerous branches. This suggestion is supported by computation of the cable theory model, whose results are shown in Fig. 5. When a voltage of 1.00 $V_{max}$ is applied to the distal part of a relay cell dendrite, a significant proportion of the voltage is conveyed to the soma and other parts of the dendritic arbor. Thus, relay cells are electrically compact. The soma can be influenced by synaptic input on all parts of the dendritic arbor, and axonal output of relay cells reflects the integration of these inputs. In comparison, the dendritic arbor of the interneuron is a poor conductor of current flow. The same voltage applied at the dendritic terminals is rapidly attenuated and little

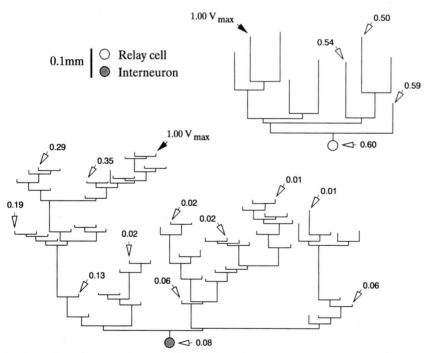

Fig. 5. Sholl diagrams illustrating cable modeling of current flow within the dendritic arbors of a geniculate relay cell and interneuron. Each diagram represents the branching pattern of a single dendrite branch. The locations of the somata are indicated by the circles. The lengths of all dendritic segments are drawn to the same anatomical scale, but dendritic thickness is not represented. In these examples, a voltage of 1.00 $V_{max}$ is applied at the tip of the dendrite indicated by the solid arrow. Voltage attenuation as a fraction of $V_{max}$ is indicated for the soma and selected parts of the dendritic arbor (open arrows). Redrawn from Bloomfield and Sherman (1989).

current is seen at the soma or other branches of the dendrite. This suggests that only those synapses on the soma (Fig. 3b) or in the proximal portions of the interneuron's dendritic arbor may significantly affect its soma and produce axonal output. By contrast, most parts of the dendritic arbors of interneurons, such as the synaptic triad shown in Fig. 3a, may be electrically isolated from the soma, thus serving autonomously with their own inputs and outputs. Therefore, interneurons may do double duty. The axon and dendrites of an interneuron can be considered separate processing systems with different synaptic inputs and producing different effects on postsynaptic cells. This implies that we cannot presume the effects of an input to an isolated dendritic arbor by recording from the cell body. Thus, if a neurotransmitter (e.g., acetylcholine) or a brainstem projection (e.g., one from the parabrachial region) is reported to inhibit interneurons, we cannot be sure the same is true at the glomerulus (cf, Pare et al., 1990; Steriade et al., 1990).

*Functional considerations*

Interneurons provide a substrate for feed-forward inhibition in the LGN. They receive direct retinal input and make axonal or dendritic synapses onto relay cells. Because most of this is accomplished within synaptic triads, conduction distances are minimized. Interneurons are thus ideally situated to control the transmission of primary visual information.

Interneurons are clearly involved in the X cell pathway. Thus far, all physiologically identified type 3 cells have X cell response properties (Sherman and Friedlander, 1988). Also, synaptic glomeruli and triadic input are the predominant feature of retinal input to X relay cells (Wilson et al., 1984; Hamos et al., 1987), and this is the form of retinal input onto cells that are postsynaptic to the studied interneurons. In contrast, retinal input to geniculate Y cells is mostly non-triadic and onto proximal dendritic shafts (Wilson et al., 1984).

The existence of Y interneurons has been proposed from electrophysiological recording experiments (Dubin and Cleland, 1977). Physiologically classified Y cells were identified as interneurons by failure to antidromically activate them from the cortex, but this classification relies on negative evidence. Other work has reported failure to antidromically activate geniculate cells that were subsequently labeled and had projection axons (Friedlander et al., 1981). Thus, the existence of Y interneurons has not been directly proven.

There is evidence that interneurons are involved in the Y cell pathway in the A laminae. Y cells receive some triadic input, albeit less than 10% (Wilson et al., 1984). It remains possible that there are only a few Y interneurons, and one has not yet been recovered using the intracellular HRP technique. Alternatively, the limited triadic input onto geniculate Y relay cells could be from the electrically isolated dendrites of the "X interneurons" described above, and the retinal Y input at the F2 terminal would not be seen at the soma (action potential) from which the recording was made. In addition, two putative local circuit profiles have been indirectly associated with the Y pathway. One is the relatively smooth dendritic shafts of unidentified cells that have been observed postsynaptic to retinogeniculate Y axons (Hamos, 1990). The shafts of these dendrites (not appendages) contain clusters of pleomorphic synaptic vesicles and are themselves presynaptic to large dendrites that have a Y-like morphology. These classic presynaptic dendrites are rare in the LGN, and their contribution may be correspondingly limited. In a study in the tree shrew LGN, these dendrites were termed "F3" and were shown to be GABA immunoreactive (Holdefer et al., 1988; see also Mize, Chapter 11). A second unidentified putative interneuron may be represented by the profiles that are postsynaptic to pretectal axons (see below). These *en passant* dendritic swellings are filled with vesicles but rarely form synaptic contacts. When they do form synapses, they are onto dendrites of geniculate cells with a Y-like ultrastructural morphology.

Thus, while the cell types that produce these two types of interneuron-like profiles have not been identified, they are potential candidates for GABAergic interneurons in the Y cell pathway.

*Interlaminar interneurons*

A second intrinsic source of GABAergic innervation in the LGN is from cells in the interlaminar zones between the geniculate laminae (Montero, 1989a). Like laminar interneurons, interlaminar cells are immunoreactive for GABA, and they do not appear to project to the cortex. However, in other ways, interlaminar cells are very different from laminar interneurons. In contrast to laminar interneurons, interlaminar cells are fewer in number, their mean soma size is larger, and they do not appear to receive direct retinal input. Their primary innervation appears to be thalamic, making them candidates for feedback rather than feedforward inhibition in the LGN. The physiological response properties of interlaminar cells are not known.

Montero (1989a) reported that interlaminar cells receive synaptic inputs from RLD, RSD, F, and some unclassified synaptic terminals, but not from retinal terminals. Interlaminar cells have axons, which may be their sole output because presynaptic dendrites have not been reported. The parent axons of some of these cells enter the A laminae, but their terminal targets are not known. Thus, the connectivity of interlaminar cells is incompletely understood. Further, because Montero was unable to examine the interlaminar dendrites to their distal ends, the entire synaptic relations of these cells is unknown. The complete picture might be very different. The distal dendritic segments could enter into the A laminae and receive retinal input or form presynaptic specializations, much like laminar interneurons. At present, however, the connections of interlaminar cells are quite different from those of laminar interneurons.

## Perigeniculate nucleus

The perigeniculate nucleus (PGN), which lies just dorsal to geniculate lamina A (Fig. 1), appears to be a major extrinsic source of GABAergic innervation to the LGN because most PGN cells are immunoreactive for GABA and project back to the LGN (Fitzpatrick et al., 1984; Rinvik et al., 1987; Montero, 1989a). PGN cells are visually responsive and display properties that are distinct from those of LGN relay cells and interneurons. That is, their receptive fields are relatively large or ill-defined and often binocular, and they appear to be di-synaptically activated by optic chiasm stimulation (i.e., di-synaptically innervated by the retina). This visual input, while often binocular, is usually dominated by one eye. PGN cells are innervated by the LGN and thus provide a recurrent GABAergic innervation to the LGN. The PGN is also innervated by the visual cortex and several ascending brainstem pathways and may thus serve as an intermediary to the LGN for other regions of the brain.

*Light microscopy*

Perigeniculate cells are among the largest cells in the thalamus in terms of soma size as well as dendritic spread, which may extend over 1 mm in the horizontal plane (Fig. 6). Thus, they may incorporate input from across a wide retinotopic extent of the LGN. Most PGN dendrites, particularly the distal portions, are beaded, and they often arborize into small elaborations (e.g., Fig. 6B) that may be the source of presynaptic dendrites that have been reported in the PGN (Ide, 1982). While perigeniculate dendritic arbors are mostly oriented horizontally, the dendrites of some PGN cells descend into geniculate lamina A (Szentágothai, 1972; Ide, 1982; Uhlrich et al., 1991). Neither the frequency nor the synaptic connections of these dendrites is known.

The dominant mode of interaction from the PGN to the LGN is axonal. The axons of individ-

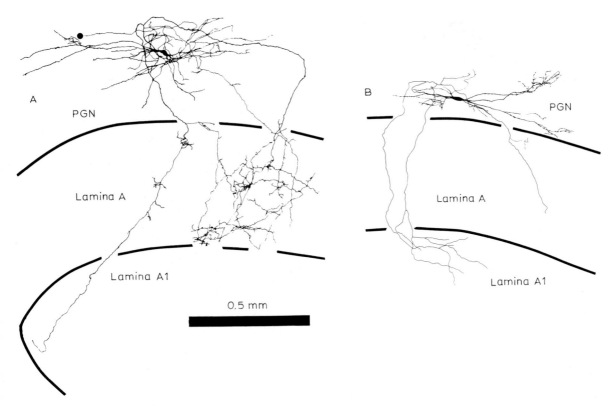

Fig. 6. *Camera lucida* reconstructions of two PGN cells intracellularly injected with HRP. A. Cell whose visual input was dominated by the contralateral eye. Medial is to the left. The filled circle in the PGN indicates a thin axon branch that extends medially and caudally away from the cell towards an unknown destination. Otherwise, the cell and axon are completely shown. B. Cell whose visual input was dominated by the ipsilateral eye. Medial is to the right. Although the dendritic arbor appears to be completely labeled, the axon is not. However, a preference for lamina A1 and a mediolateral organization are clear. Redrawn from Uhlrich et al. (1991).

ual PGN cells display many common features (Fig. 6A and B; Uhlrich et al., 1991). They originate from large dendrites and branch several times within the dendritic arbor of the cell. Some branches terminate locally, but most descend into the LGN to innervate a retinotopically restricted portion of the A laminae. This preference for the A laminae is evident at the single cell level (Fig. 6) and in material in which the projection is labeled *en masse* with *Phaseolus vulgaris* leuco-agglutinin (PHAL; Fig. 7). In the LGN, almost all of the terminal boutons of PGN axons are *en passant*, which gives the axons a beaded appearance (Fig. 8). Finally, within the LGN, the PGN axon arbors display medial and lateral components (Fig. 6). A relatively narrow medial compo-

nent innervates laminae A and A1, while a more robust lateral component is restricted to one of the A laminae, depending on the ocular dominance of the PGN cell. If the visual driving of the PGN cell is dominated by the contralateral eye, lamina A is targeted (Fig. 6A); lamina A1 is targeted if the ipsilateral eye dominates (Fig. 6B).

*Electron microscopy*

At the EM level, the swellings of beaded PGN axons form symmetrical synaptic contacts with geniculate dendrites (Fig. 9; Cucchiaro et al., 1991b). The labeled PGN profiles are never post-synaptic to other terminals and, in general, form only a single synaptic contact, although some form two synaptic outputs from a single terminal.

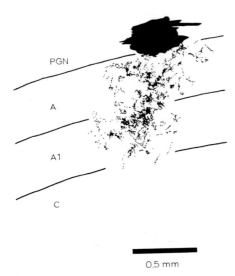

0.5 mm

Fig. 7. *Camera lucida* reconstructions of a PHAL injection in the PGN (solid filled area) and the location of axon terminal boutons in the LGN (dots). Redrawn from Uhlrich et al. (1991).

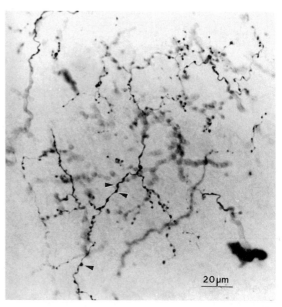

20 μm

Fig. 8. Photomicrograph of axon terminals in the LGN following an injection of PHAL in the PGN. Average size of PGN boutons (e.g., arrowheads) is $1.0 \pm 0.3$ μm in diameter. Adapted from Cucchiaro and Uhlrich (1990).

The terminals are densely filled with vesicles, although the dark label usually obscures vesicle shape and other internal details. These characteristics of PGN terminals are similar to F1 profiles, which confirms suggestions made from studies in the rat (Montero and Scott, 1981) that the PGN is a source of F1 terminals in the LGN.

Almost all ( > 90%) of the labeled PGN terminals synapse onto small caliber dendrites that also receive dense input from RSD profiles (Figs. 9C, D, and 10A, B). While the PGN input may be working in concert with the RSD (presumed cortical) input, the identity of all of the postsynaptic targets is unclear. The small caliber postsynaptic profiles that are contacted by PGN and RSD terminals may be the distal dendrites of geniculate relay cells (Wilson et al., 1984). In this case,

the PGN would be directly inhibiting relay cells. Because the distal portions of X and Y relay cells are ultrastructurally similar, the functional class of the postsynaptic cells is unclear. It is also possible that the small caliber postsynaptic dendrites are the dendritic shafts of interneurons (Weber et al., 1989). In this case, relay cells would be dis-inhibited via inhibition of interneurons. Both possibilities are conceivable, and this question needs to be addressed further to understand the influence of the PGN on geniculate transmission.

A minority of the perigeniculate synapses lie near retinal inputs onto large caliber dendrites

Fig. 9. Electron micrographs of PGN terminals labeled by intracellular injection of HRP. A and B. Labeled PGN terminals that synapse (arrowheads) onto geniculate cell appendages (a) and dendrites (d). These postsynaptic processes also receive synapses from retinal terminals (RLP), which leads us to classify these regions as retinal recipient zones. C and D. Two labeled PGN terminals that synapse onto geniculate dendrites that also receive input from RSD terminals (asterisks). Because the RSD profiles are presumably from the cortex, we classified these regions as corticorecipient zones. Scale bar in C applies to A–D. E. A synaptic glomerulus in which a central retinal terminal synapses onto several F2 terminals as well as onto dendritic appendages of a putative relay cell, forming synaptic triads. A labeled PGN terminal contacts the peripheral part of the glomerulus by synapsing onto an appendage of the relay cell. From Cucchiaro and Uhlrich (1990).

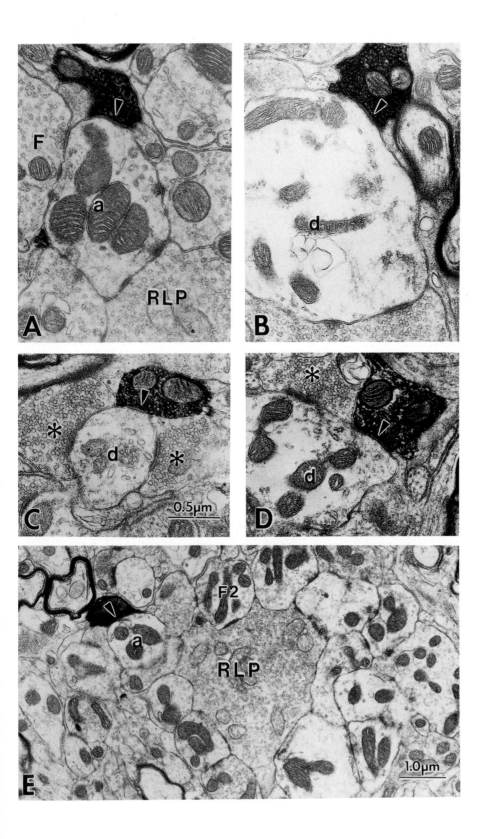

182

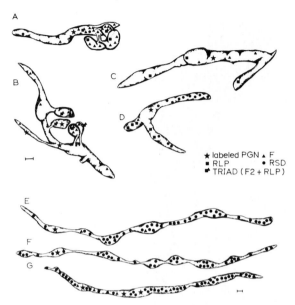

Fig. 10. Serial EM reconstructions of unlabeled geniculate dendrites that are postsynaptic to HRP-labeled PGN terminals (stars). A–D. Retinorecipient dendrites. The retinal input to the dendrites in A and B is through synaptic triads, a pattern most commonly associated with the retinogeniculate X pathway. The retinal input to the dendrites in C and D is not triadic, which is more common in the retinogeniculate Y pathway. E–G. Dendrites classified as corticorecipient because they are richly innervated by RSD terminals. Scale bars are 1 $\mu$m; the one in B applies to A–D, and the one in G applies to E–G. Adapted from Cucchiaro et al. (1991b).

and dendritic appendages (Figs. 9A, B, E and 10C, D). Based on analysis of our intracellularly filled HRP material (the cell in Fig. 6A), all perigeniculate synapses onto retinorecipient dendrites arise from the medial branch of the axon. This suggests that the medial and lateral axonal components enter into fundamentally different circuits. Further, all the retinal input to the geniculate dendrites is triadic, which suggests that the PGN cell in Fig. 6A participates in the X cell pathway. In the PHAL material, we have also seen labeled PGN contacts onto large dendrites that received non-triadic retinal input, which are presumably from Y cells. Thus, PGN terminals appear to contact both X and Y relay cells, but individual perigeniculate cells may be devoted to

one or the other pathway. Whether one of these pathways is favored is not known at this time.

*Functional considerations*

The perigeniculate nucleus is innervated by the LGN, and it reciprocates by providing recurrent inhibition to the A laminae of the LGN. Because most perigeniculate cells have extensive dendritic fields and large, binocular receptive fields, this recurrent inhibition was expected to be retinotopically diffuse and unrelated to ocular dominance. However, this no longer appears true. First, even though PGN cells are activated binocularly, one eye usually dominates, and this dominance is reflected in the target of the lateral component of the axon. Thus, although PGN cells are certainly involved with binocular inhibition, much of the recurrent inhibition remains in the same eye. Second, the medial/lateral pattern of perigeniculate axonal arborization is a completely unexpected feature of these cells. Because the LGN is so finely organized retinotopically, there must be a spatial correlate to this projection pattern. However, this has not yet been described, either in the visual responses of PGN cells or in the spatial pattern of visual inhibition that impinges on geniculate cells. Finally, the axon arbors of perigeniculate cells are surprisingly restricted. The medial or lateral components of the axons are often as narrow as the terminal arbors of retinogeniculate X axons (i.e., the most restricted retinal arbors). Thus the PGN projection may allow for the convergence of information from a large portion of the visual field onto a relatively restricted portion of the LGN. Alternatively, the PGN may serve a much more retinotopically restricted function than was previously thought. Why is this retinotopic precision not seen in the visual responses of PGN cells? It is possible that the appropriate visual stimuli have not been used to study PGN cells. Alternatively, PGN cells could be very susceptible to, and become unresponsive under, experimental conditions that use anesthesia or paralysis. Their receptive fields could be more restricted in an alert, behaving animal.

## Thalamic reticular nucleus (TRN)

The visual thalamic reticular nucleus (TRN) lies dorsal to the PGN, about 1 to 2 mm above the LGN (Fig. 1). Its cells are embedded in the optic radiations and are innervated by both the visual thalamus and the cortex (Jones, 1975). They are also GABAergic (Rinvik et al., 1987), including those that are retrogradely labeled from the LGN (Cucchiaro et al., 1990). In these ways, the TRN is very similar to the PGN, and the two nuclei are often grouped together functionally. However,

there are important differences between the two nuclei. As shown below, the axonal targets of the TRN are different from those of the PGN. Also, despite receiving visual input via the axon collaterals of geniculate relay cells, cells in the TRN have little or no visual response (Ahlsen et al., 1982), at least under acute experimental conditions. The anesthetized state of the preparation may affect TRN cells to a greater degree than PGN cells.

*Light microscopy*

Figure 11 illustrates TRN axon terminals in the LGN. TRN terminals are similar in morphology to PGN terminals; they are comparable in

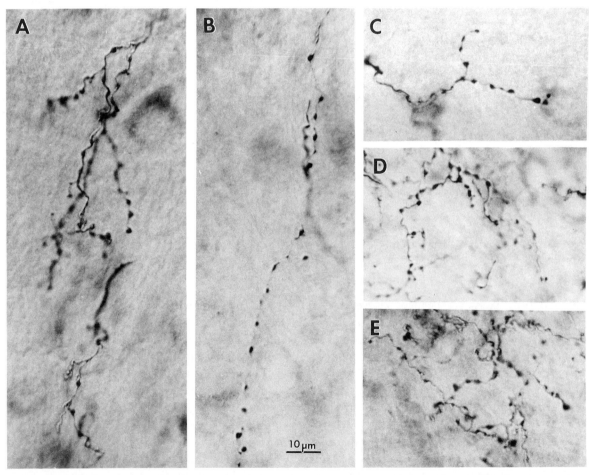

Fig. 11. Photomicrographs of axon terminals throughout the LGN following an injection of PHAL in the NRT. Average bouton size is $1.1 \pm 0.3$ $\mu$m. Scale bar in B also applies to A–E.

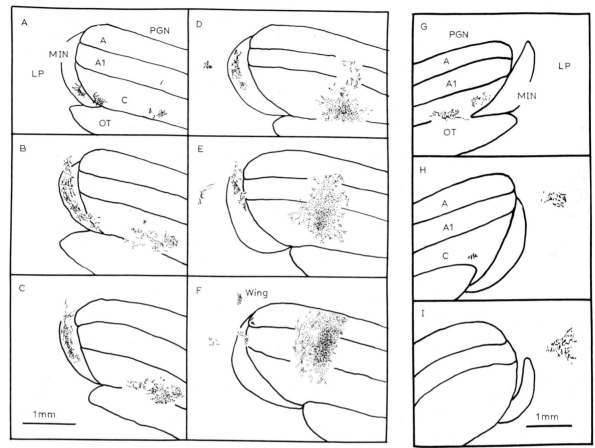

Fig. 12. *Camera lucida* drawings showing the distribution of terminals in the LGN (dots) labeled from injections of PHAL into the NRT. A–D. Results from a single injection into the NRT that spread ventrally to involve the PGN as well. A is the most caudal level and is about 2 mm behind the injection site. F is the most rostral. Scale bar in C applies to A–F. G–I. Results from a second injection of PHAL that was entirely restricted to the NRT, at its lateral boundary. G is the most caudal level of the projection (about 2 mm behind the injection) and I is the most rostral. Note that the number of thalamic targets is more restricted in the second experiment. Scale bar in I applies to G–I. MIN, medial interlaminar nucleus; LP, lateral posterior nucleus; PGN, perigeniculate nucleus; OT, optic tract; Wing, geniculate wing, a retinorecipient portion of the pulvinar.

size and their axons are beaded. However, the projection targets of the TRN differ from those of the PGN. Figure 12 shows the results of two experiments in which PHAL was injected into the TRN. In both cases, terminal label was found in the lateral posterior nucleus and the ventralmost geniculate C laminae (Fig. 12A–I). This labeling is not seen following injections limited to the PGN. In one case (Fig. 12A–F), beaded axons were found throughout all the C laminae, the medial interlaminar nucleus, the geniculate wing, the lateral posterior complex and also in the

geniculate A laminae. In this experiment, the injection site included a portion of the PGN. Thus, it is unclear what proportion of the projection to the A laminae is accounted for by the PGN and what portion by the TRN. In the second case (Fig. 12G–I), no beaded axons were evident in the geniculate A laminae, the medial interlaminar nucleus, the dorsal C laminae, or the geniculate wing. The pattern of labeling shown in Fig.12G–I resulted from a very small PHAL injection limited to the lateral aspect of TRN. Although these data are preliminary, it is clear that the PGN and TRN differ in their projection targets. The main question which we cannot answer at this time is whether TRN provides an innervation to the A laminae, in which case one might expect a different set of synaptic targets from those selected by the PGN (Cucchiaro et al., 1991b). However, based on the two injection cases we have to date, the TRN clearly provides innervation to some laminae and visual relay structures not innervated by the PGN, suggesting that the TRN may be providing complementary thalamic innervation (Cucchiaro et al., 1990).

*Electron microscopy*

The ultrastructure of TRN terminals in the LGN of the cat has not been studied. In the rat, EM autoradiography has shown that TRN terminals have an F1 morphology (Ohara et al., 1980; Montero and Scott, 1981). Like PGN terminals in the cat, most TRN terminals in rats contact small caliber dendrites. However, in the rat, many contacts onto F2 terminals and somata were also found. We did not observe these contacts from PGN cells in cat, although many unlabeled F1 terminals do form such contacts. These unlabeled F1 terminals presumably arise from a source other than the PGN, and one such possibility is the TRN.

*Functional considerations*

Very little is known about the projections and functional properties of visual TRN cells. These cells are often assigned roles similar to those of PGN cells because both cell groups lie dorsal to and provide recurrent inhibition to the LGN. However, there are important differences in their responsiveness. PGN cells are visually responsive, and they may serve to shape visual responses in the geniculate A laminae. In contrast, TRN cells do not have obvious visual responses. They may serve a more global, nonvisual role. One possible function is to control visual sensory transmission during sleep and arousal (Sherman and Koch, 1986; Steriade and Llinás, 1988; McCormick, 1989). Cells in the TRN have been implicated in

the genesis of rhythmic oscillations in the thalamus that are correlated with highly synchronized EEG spindles during sleep (Steriade and Llinás, 1988). This oscillatory behavior appears to entrain, *en masse*, geniculate relay cells through the resulting hyperpolarization, which de-inactivates a voltage-dependent $Ca^{2+}$ conductance. The relay cells then respond in a bursty fashion and do not faithfully reflect their retinal input. In contrast, during arousal, the TRN does not display this oscillatory behavior. Relay cells are released from the bursty firing mode, and their responses more faithfully relay their retinal input. Thus, the TRN may play a role in controlling the response state (i.e., faithful relay mode vs. burst mode) of geniculate cells. Whether the PGN and TRN serve such distinct functions remains to be determined. It is also possible that both nuclei perform both functions. Thus, PGN cells, which also display oscillatory behavior (Hue et al., 1990) may also assist in the control of response state of geniculate cells in the A laminae. In an unanesthetized, alert animal, the TRN may be more visually responsive and serve to shape the visual responses of geniculate cells.

**Pretectum**

Geniculate interneurons and cells in the PGN and TRN, because of their proximity, are expected sources of GABAergic innervation in the LGN. Recently, a more distant source of GABAergic terminals in the LGN has been demonstrated: one arising from the pretectum (Bickford et al., 1990; Cucchiaro et al., 1991a). In the cat, the pretectum consists of six nuclei, three of which receive direct retinal input and project to the LGN: these are the nucleus of the optic tract (NOT), the posterior pretectal nucleus, and the olivary pretectal nucleus (Fig. 1; Berman, 1977; Koontz et al., 1985; Kubota et al., 1987, 1988; Tamamaki et al., 1990; Cucchiaro et al., 1991a). The heaviest projection to the LGN arises from the nucleus of the optic tract (Fig. 13A and B; Itoh, 1977; Weber and Harting, 1980; Cuc-

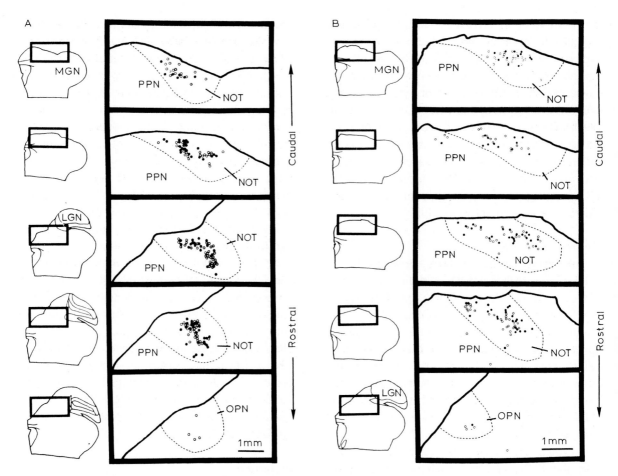

Fig. 13. Distribution of pretectal cells that were retrogradely labeled from a WGA–HRP injection in the LGN. A and B. The results from two separate experiments. The column on the left is a low-power series of drawings in the coronal plane through the pretectum. The rectangular enclosed region is shown at higher power in the drawings to the right. The location of pretectal cells that are double labeled both retrogradely and immunohistochemically for GABA is indicated by the filled circles. Cells labeled only retrogradely are indicated by open circles. MGN, medial geniculate nucleus; NOT, nucleus of the optic tract; PPN, posterior pretectal nucleus; OPN, olivary pretectal nucleus. Modified from Cucchiaro et al. (1991a).

chiaro et al., 1991a), where cells respond strongly to visual stimuli and are involved with eye movements (Hoffman, 1981).

*Light microscopy*

Numerous anterograde tracing studies have demonstrated that the pretectum innervates all laminae of the LGN and the PGN (Graybiel and Berson, 1980; Cucchiaro et al., 1989). Figure 14 shows labeled terminals following a PHAL injection in the NOT. This morphology is similar to that of all NOT axons that terminate in the LGN.

The boutons are mostly *en passant* and relatively larger in diameter than the axon terminals from the PGN or TRN.

The pretectal nuclei contain a large number of cells that are immunoreactive for GABA. Cucchiaro et al. (1991a) have reported roughly 40% of the pretectal cells that are retrogradely labeled from the LGN are immunoreactive for GABA (Fig. 13). These projection cells are among the largest GABAergic cells in the pretectum. This is a relatively rare type of projection, because most known GABAergic projections are local, rather than distant. However, the pretectum may be an exception. Appell and Behan (1990) have recently reported that the pretectum also has an extrinsic GABAergic projection to the superior colliculus.

Because the light and electron microscopic morphology of all pretectal axons are similar, it is conceivable that all pretectal cells that project to the LGN are GABAergic and some were simply not labeled for technical reasons. On the other hand, others have failed to find any GABAergic cells that project from the pretectum (Horn and Hoffmann, 1987), including the projection to the LGN (Nabors and Mize, 1991). These opposite results underscore the technical concerns that accompany immunohistochemical work (e.g., antibody sensitivity, antibody penetration, interaction of the retrograde HRP reaction with GABA immunoreactivity).

*Electron microscopy*

At the EM level, pretectal synaptic profiles terminating in the LGN (Fig. 15) are morphologically similar to GABAergic F1 profiles. Many cytoplasmic elements are obscured by the label, but the pretectal profiles form symmetrical synapses, contain dark mitochondria, are never postsynaptic to other synaptic profiles, and are densely filled with synaptic vesicles. In the LGN, these pretectal terminals selectively synapse onto dendritic profiles that in some ways resemble F2 profiles. These postsynaptic profiles have a pale cytoplasm, occasionally contain ribosomes, are sparsely filled with pleomorphic vesicles, and are connected to each other by extremely fine processes that, in unlabeled material, are difficult to reconstruct (Fig. 16). All of the postsynaptic "F2-like" profiles receive synaptic input in addition to that from the NOT, but only a single synaptic output has been seen. Thus, these "F2-like" profiles have features of interneurons, but are unlike the F2 terminals from the labeled X cell interneurons described above where a single F2

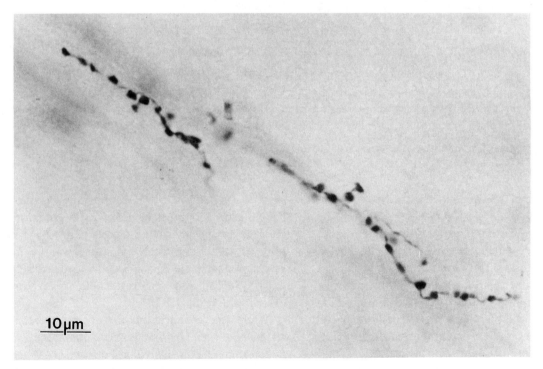

10 µm

Fig. 14. Photomicrographs of labeled pretectal terminals in the LGN following a PHAL injection into the nucleus of the optic tract. The average diameter of these terminals is 1.8 ±0.6 µm.

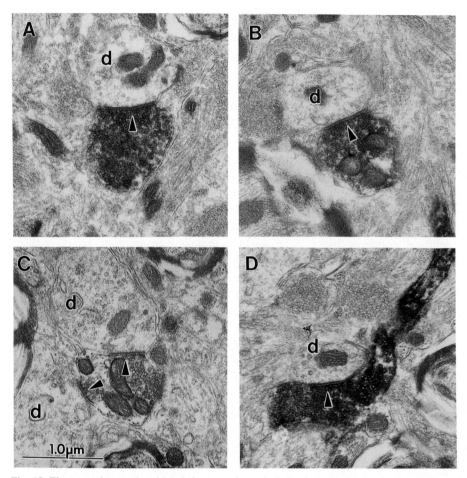

Fig. 15. Electron micrographs of labeled pretectal terminals in the geniculate A laminae labeled by a PHAL injection into the nucleus of the optic tract. The pretectal profiles have features of F1 terminals and make symmetrical synaptic contacts (arrows) onto dendrites (d) in the geniculate neuropil. Note the pleomorphic vesicles in the postsynaptic dendrites. Scale bar in C applies to A–D.

terminal both receives and makes synaptic contacts.

Figure 16 further illustrates the interconnections of a pretectal axon in the LGN. The labeled pretectal axon contacts several F2-like profiles of a putative interneuron dendritic arbor, and one of these profiles is presynaptic to a stout dendritic shaft of a putative relay cell. The relay cell receives non-triadic retinal input and is probably a Y cell (Wilson et al., 1984; Hamos, 1991). Thus, this pretectal axon appears to be affecting, via an interneuron, the Y cell pathway. Although the

source of the F2-like profiles is unknown, these data illustrate indirect evidence of interneurons involved in the geniculate Y cell pathway. It is possible that other pretectal axons will be involved in geniculate X cell circuitry, because retinal X cells also innervate the pretectum (Tamamaki et al., 1991).

While the chemical nature of the pretectal axons and their F2-like postsynaptic targets is undetermined, it is likely that both are GABAergic. Thus, the GABAergic projection from the pretectum may be inhibiting GABAergic in-

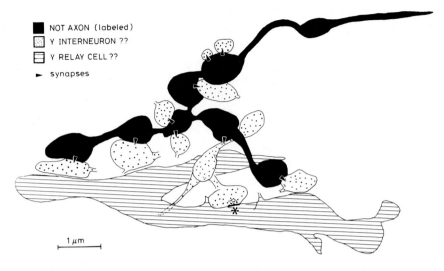

NOT AXON (labeled)
Y INTERNEURON ??
Y RELAY CELL ??
synapses

1 μm

Fig. 16. Serial EM reconstruction of a labeled pretectal axon and its postsynaptic geniculate targets. All of the swellings on the NOT axon formed synaptic contacts onto vesicle-filled dendritic profiles. Most of the postsynaptic profiles do not form synapses. In one case (asterisk), one of the profiles on the postsynaptic dendrite formed a synapse onto a large geniculate dendrite that also received non-triadic retinal inputs.

terneurons in the LGN, thereby dis-inhibiting geniculate relay cells. Because the pretectum also projects to the GABAergic cells in the PGN, two different dis-inhibitory circuits could exist.

*Functional considerations*

Cells in the pretectum respond well to visual stimuli. Many of them also project to eye movement centers in the pons and midbrain. Cells in the NOT, which provide the heaviest projection to the LGN, have been implicated in the generation of retinal slip signals and the slow phase of optokinetic nystagmus. They respond best to visual stimuli that are moving slowly toward the center of the visual field (Hoffmann and Schopmann, 1975, 1981; Ballas and Hoffmann, 1985). Thus, the pretectum may coordinate vision with eye movements. Through its descending projections, the pretectum may serve to elicit eye movements to maintain fixation on a target and, via disinhibition in the LGN, facilitate transmission of the visual information about the target.

## Conclusions

We have described four sources of GABAergic innervation to the LGN and the synaptic circuitry into which they enter, yet two observations suggest that this list is incomplete. First, the fact that the pretectum provides GABAergic innervation to the LGN suggests that other intermediate- or long-distance GABAergic projections to the LGN may exist. Second, the sources of many GABAergic terminals in the LGN have not been identified. Many are likely to be from intrinsic interneurons, such as the sources of F2 terminals and other presynaptic dendritic profiles that contact geniculate Y cells. However, the origin of other terminals is less clear. For example, many F1 terminals contact somata and proximal dendrites of relay cells and the F2 terminals of interneurons. Work done in rat (Ohara, 1980; Montero and Scott, 1981) suggests that the likely source of these F1 terminals is the PGN. However, in cat, PGN synaptic contacts have not been observed on these postsynaptic targets. The projection from the pretectum may account for some of the F1 contacts that have been described on some "F2-like" terminals, but it does not account for any of the many F1 contacts that are made onto F2 terminals of X interneurons. An obvious candidate is the projection from the TRN, which surely will give rise to F1 terminals and may account for all of the F1 terminals whose source is currently unknown. Another candidate is the axons of interlaminar cells. Although the locations of their terminal fields are unknown, the A laminae are a very likely target. However, unless the terminal fields of these axons are immense, they probably cannot account for all of the F1 terminals because there are only a few interlaminar cells.

Physiological evidence suggests that GABA plays a major role in modulating the transmission of visual information through the visual thalamus. Anatomical study reveals that the GABAergic circuitry in the LGN is complicated with a large cast of intrinsic and extrinsic players. The cast may be functionally expanded because some of these players assume more than one role. For example, interneurons have both dendritic and axonal outputs and perigeniculate cells have medial and lateral components, each of which enters into a different circuitry in the LGN. An additional tier of complexity is attained because some GABAergic terminals are presynaptic to other GABAergic terminals. The plot becomes even further complicated when different GABA receptors are considered. For example, $GABA_A$ and $GABA_B$ receptors have been demonstrated in the cat's LGN. These two receptors produce dramatically different postsynaptic effects (see Soltesz and Crunelli, Chapter 8). Obviously, to understand fully the role of GABA in the LGN, we must determine which single or combination of GABA receptors is involved in each GABAergic projection. Finally, almost all of the extrinsic projections to the LGN act, at least in part, through GABAergic circuitry. For example, axons from the cortex and brainstem synapse directly onto relay cells and interneurons. Thus, the GABAergic neurons serve as "invertors" for other projections. When it is passed through a GABAergic interneuron, an inhibitory projection becomes dis-inhibitory and an excitatory projection becomes inhibitory. The many levels of complexity in these GABAergic circuits suggest that the role of GABA in the LGN is an intricate one. Clearly, determining the function of these varied GABAergic circuits will go a long way towards understanding the role of the LGN in vision.

## References

Ahlsén, G., Lindström, S. and Lo, F.-S. (1982) Functional distinction of perigeniculate and thalamic reticular neurons in the cat. *Exp. Brain Res.*, 46: 118–126.

Ahlsén, G., Lindström, S. and Sybirska, E. (1978) Subcortical axon collaterals of principal cells in the lateral geniculate body of the cat. *Brain Res.*, 156: 106–109.

Appell, P.P. and Behan, M. (1990) Sources of subcortical GABAergic projections to the superior colliculus in the cat. *J. Comp. Neurol.*, 302: 143–158.

Ballas, I. and Hoffmann, K.-P. (1985) A correlation between receptive field properties and morphological structures in the pretectum of the cat. *J. Comp. Neurol.*, 238: 417–428.

Bickford, M.E., Cucchiaro, J.B. and Sherman, S.M. (1990) A GABAergic pretectal projection to the lateral geniculate nucleus in the cat. *Soc. Neurosci. Abstr.*, 16: 160.

Bloomfield, S.A. and Sherman, S.M. (1989) Dendritic current flow in relay cells and interneurons of the cat's lateral geniculate nucleus. *Proc. Natl. Acad. Sci USA*, 86: 3911–3914.

Cucchiaro, J.B. and Uhlrich, D.J. (1990) *Phaseolus vulgaris* leucoagglutinin (PHA-L): A neuroanatomical tracer for electron microscopic analysis of synaptic circuitry in the cat's dorsal lateral geniculate nucleus. *J. Electron Micros. Tech.*, 15: 352–368.

Cucchiaro, J.B., Uhlrich, D.J. and Sherman, S.M. (1989) Synapses from the pretectum in the geniculate A-laminae of the cat. *Soc. Neurosci. Abstr.*, 15: 1392.

Cucchiaro, J.B., Bickford, M.E. and Sherman, S.M. (1990a) A GABAergic projection from the pretectum to the dorsal lateral geniculate nucleus in the cat. *Neuroscience*, 41: 213–226.

Cucchiaro, J.B., Uhlrich, D.J. and Sherman, S.M. (1990b) A projection from the thalamic reticular nucleus to the dorsal lateral geniculate nucleus in the cat: A comparison with the perigeniculate projection. *Soc. Neurosci. Abstr.*, 16: 159.

Cucchiaro, J.B., Uhlrich, D.J. and Sherman, S.M. (1991) An electron-microscopic analysis of synaptic input from the perigeniculate nucleus to the A-laminae of the lateral geniculate nucleus in cats. *J. Comp. Neurol.*, 310: 316–336.

DeLima, A.D. and Singer, W. (1987) The serotoninergic fibers in the dorsal lateral geniculate nucleus of the cat. Distribution and synaptic connections demonstrated with immunocytochemistry. *J. Comp. Neurol.*, 258: 339–351.

Dubin, M.W. and Cleland, B.G. (1977) Organization of visual inputs to interneurons of the lateral geniculate nucleus of the cat. *J. Neurophysiol.*, 40: 410–427.

Famiglietti, E.V. and Peters, A. (1972) The synaptic glomerulus and the intrinsic neuron in the dorsal lateral geniculate nucleus of the cat. *J. Comp. Neurol.*, 144: 285–334.

Fitzpatrick, D, Penny, G.R., and Schmechel, D.E. (1984) Glutamic acid decarboxylase-immunoreactive neurons and terminals in the lateral geniculate nucleus of the cat. *J. Neurosci.*, 4: 1809–1829.

Friedlander, M.J., Lin, C.-S., Stanford, L.R. and Sherman, S.M. (1981) Morphology of functionally identified neurons in the lateral geniculate nucleus of the cat. *J. Neurophysiol.*, 46: 80–129.

Graybiel, A.M. and Berson, D.M. (1980) Autoradiographic evidence for a projection from the pretectal nucleus of the optic tract to the dorsal lateral geniculate complex in the cat. *Brain Res*, 195: 1–12.

Guillery, R.W. (1966) A study of Golgi preparations from the dorsal lateral geniculate nucleus of the adult cat. *J. Comp. Neurol.*, 128: 21–50.

Guillery, R.W. (1969) The organization of synaptic interconnections in the laminae of the dorsal lateral geniculate nucleus of the cat. *Z. Zellforsch.*, 96: 1–38.

Guillery, R.W. (1971) Patterns of synaptic interconnections in the dorsal lateral geniculate nucleus of cat and monkey. *Vision Res.*, 11: 211–227.

Hamos, J.E. (1990) Synaptic circuitry identified by intracellular labeling with horseradish peroxidase. *J. Electron Micros. Tech.*, 15: 369–376.

Hamos, J.E., Van Horn, S.C., Raczkowski, D. and Sherman, S.M. (1987) Synaptic circuits involving an individual retinogeniculate axon in the cat. *J. Comp. Neurol.*, 259: 165–192.

Hamos, J.E., Van Horn, S.C., Raczkowski, D., Uhlrich, D.J. and Sherman, S.M. (1985) Synaptic connectivity of a local circuit neurone in lateral geniculate nucleus of the cat. *Nature*, 317: 618–621.

Hoffman, K.-P. and Schopmann, A. (1975) Retinal input to direction selective cells in the nucleus tractus opticus of the cat. *Brain Res.*, 99: 359–366.

Hoffman, K.-P. and Schopmann, A. (1981) A quantitative analysis of the direction-selective response of neurons in the cat's nucleus of the optic tract. *Exp. Brain Res.*, 42: 146–157.

Holdefer, R.N., Norton, T.T. and Mize, R.R. (1988) Laminar organization and ultrastructure of GABA-immunoreactive neurons and processes in the dorsal lateral geniculate nucleus of the tree shrew (*Tupaia belangeri*). *Visual Neurosci.*, 1: 189–204.

Horn, A.K.E. and Hoffmann, K.-P. (1987) Combined GABA-immunocytochemistry and TMB-HRP histochemistry of pretectal nuclei projecting to the inferior olive in rats, cats and monkeys. *Brain Res.*, 409: 133–138.

Hu, B., Steriade, M. and Deschênes, M. (1989) The effects of brainstem peribrachial stimulation on perigeniculate neurons: The blockage of spindle waves. *Neuroscience*, 31: 1–12.

Ide, L.S. (1982) The fine structure of the perigeniculate nucleus in the cat. *J. Comp. Neurol.*, 210: 317–334.

Jones, E.G. (1975) Some aspects of the organization of the thalamic reticular complex. *J. Comp. Neurol.*, 162: 285–308.

Jones, E.G. and Powell, T.P.S. (1969) An electron microscopic study of the mode of termination of cortico-thalamic fibres within the sensory relay nuclei of the thalamus. *Proc. R. Soc. (London)*, 172: 173–185.

McCormick, D.A. (1989) Cholinergic and noradrenergic modulation of thalamocortical processing. *Trends Neurosci.*, 12: 215–221.

Montero, V.M. (1986) Localization of τ-aminobutyric acid (GABA) in type 3 cells and demonstration of their source to F2 terminals in the cat lateral geniculate nucleus: A Golgi-electron microscopic GABA-immunocytochemical study. *J. Comp. Neurol.*, 254: 228–245.

Montero, V.M. (1987) Ultrastructural identification of synaptic terminals from the axon of type 3 interneurons in the cat lateral geniculate nucleus. *J. Comp. Neurol.*, 264: 268–283.

Montero, V.M. (1989a) The GABA-immunoreactive neurons in the interlaminar regions of the cat lateral geniculate nucleus: light and electron microscopic observations. *Exp. Brain Res.*, 75: 497–512.

Montero, V.M. (1989b) Ultrastructural identification of synaptic terminals from cortical axons and from collateral axons of geniculocortical relay cells in the perigeniculate nucleus of the cat. *Exp. Brain Res.*, 75: 65–72.

Montero, V.M. and Scott, G.L. (1981) Synaptic terminals in dorsal lateral geniculate nucleus from neurons of the thalamic reticular nucleus. A light and electron microscope autoradiographic study. *Neuroscience*, 6: 2561–2577.

Montero, V.M. and Singer, W. (1985) Ultrastructural identification of somata and neural processes immunoreactive to antibodies against glutamic acid decarboxylase (GAD) in the dorsal lateral geniculate nucleus of the cat. *Exp. Brain Res.*, 59: 151–165.

Nabors and Mize, R.R. (1991) A unique neuronal organization in the cat pretectum revealed by antibodies to the calcium-binding protein calbindin-D 28K. *J. Neurosci.*, 11: 2460–2476.

Ohara, P.T., Sefton, A.J. and Lieberman, A.R. (1980) Mode of termination of afferents from the thalamic reticular nucleus in the dorsal lateral geniculate nucleus of the rat. *Brain Res.*, 197: 503–506.

Pape, H.C. and Eysel, U.T. (1986) Binocular interactions in the lateral geniculate nucleus of the cat: GABAergic inhibition reduced the dominant afferent activity. *Exp. Brain Res.*, 61: 265–271.

Paré, D., Curro Dossi, R. and Steriade, M. (1990) Genesis of inhibitory postsynaptic potentials (IPSPs) by interneurons in the feline anterior thalamic (AT) nuclei. *Soc. Neurosci. Abstr.*, 16: 467.

Rall, W. (1977) Core conductor theory and cable properties of neurons. In: E.R. Kandel (Ed.), *The Nervous System, Vol I: Cellular Biology of Neurons, Part 1*, Bethesda: American Physiological Society, 39–97.

Rinvik, E., Otterson, O.P. and Storm-Mathisen, J. (1987) Gamma-aminobutyrate-like immunoreactivity in the thalamus of the cat. *Neuroscience*, 21: 781–805.

Sanderson, K.J. (1971) The projection of the visual field to the lateral geniculate and medial interlaminar nuclei in the cat. *J. Comp. Neurol.*, 143: 101–118.

Sherman, S.M. and Koch, C. (1986) The control of retinogeniculate transmission in the mammalian lateral geniculate nucleus. *Exp. Brain Res.*, 63: 1–20.

Sherman, S.M. and Friedlander, M.J. (1988) Identification of X versus Y properties for interneurons in the A-laminae of the cat's lateral geniculate nucleus. *Exp. Brain Res.*, 73: 384–392.

Sherman, S.M. and Spear, P.D. (1982) Organization of the visual pathways in normal and visually deprived cats. *Physiol. Rev.*, 62: 738–855.

Sillito, A.M. and Kemp, J.A. (1983) The influence of GABAergic inhibitory processes on the receptive field structure of X and Y cells in cat dorsal lateral geniculate nucleus (dLGN). *Brain Res.*, 277: 63–78.

Steriade, M., Curro Dossi, R. and Paré, D. (1990) Cortically- and subcortically-evoked IPSPs in anterior thalamic (AT) cells are affected differentially by stimulation of a brainstem cholinergic nucleus. *Soc. Neurosci. Abstr.*, 16: 467.

Steriade, M. and Llinás, R.R. (1988) The functional states of the thalamus and the associated neuronal interplay. *Physiol Rev.*, 68: 649–742.

Tamamaki, N., Uhlrich, D.J. and Sherman, S.M. (1990) Morphology of physiologically identified retinal axons in the cat's thalamus and midbrain as revealed by intra-axonal injection of biocytin. *Soc. Neurosci. Abstr.*, 16: 711.

Uhlrich, D.J., Cucchiaro, J.B., Humphrey, A.L. and Sherman, S.M. (1991) Morphology and axonal projection patterns of individual neurons in the cat's perigeniculate nucleus. *J. Neurophysiol.*, 65: 1528–1541.

Weber, A.J. and Kalil, R.E. (1987) Development of corticogeniculate synapses in the cat. *J. Comp. Neurol.*, 264: 171–192.

Weber, A.J., Kalil, R.E. and Behan, M. (1989) Synaptic connections between corticogeniculate axons and interneurons in the dorsal lateral geniculate nucleus of the cat. *J. Comp. Neurol.*, 289: 156–164.

Weber, J.T. and Harting, J.K. (1980) The efferent projections of the pretectal complex: An autoradiograph and horseradish peroxidase analysis. *Brain Res.*, 194: 1–28.

Wilson, J.R., Friedlander, M.J. and Sherman, S.M. (1984) Fine structural morphology of identified X-and Y-cells in the cat's lateral geniculate nucleus. *Proc. R. Soc. (London)*, 221: 411–436.

R.R. Mize, R.E. Marc and A.M. Sillito (Eds.)
Progress in Brain Research, Vol. 90

CHAPTER 10

# Inhibitory GABAergic control of visual signals at the lateral geniculate nucleus

Thomas T. Norton [1] and Dwayne W. Godwin [2]

[1] Department of Physiological Optics and [1,2] Department of Psychology, The University of Alabama at Birmingham, Birmingham, AL 35294, USA

## Introduction

We all are subjectively aware that our ability to detect events occurring around us is influenced by whether we are asleep or awake and, if we are awake, by whether we are inattentive or, in contrast, focussing intently on something of interest. Numerous studies have documented that attentive phenomena exist in the visual system and that the thresholds for detecting visual stimuli differ with attention (see Posner and Petersen (1990) for review). For example, subjects cued to expect a stimulus to appear at a particular location in the visual field have an increased sensitivity for detecting targets that appear there (Downing, 1988).

Changes in the detectability of, and sensitivity to, visual stimuli require a neural substrate. As a synaptic relay on the path from the retina to the striate cortex, the lateral geniculate nucleus (LGN) may constitute the first central brain structure involved in the mechanisms that underlie visual attention. There appears to be little alteration at the LGN in the carefully constructed antagonistic center/surround organization of retinal ganglion cells (Bullier and Norton, 1979b) that are critical in setting up the receptive-field organization of primary visual cortical neurons (Palmer et al., 1991). However, alterations in the visual signal do occur at the LGN. In this chapter we will examine how the GABAergic circuits in the LGN control the flow of afferent information from the retina to the striate cortex. These circuits are in an excellent position to control retinogeniculate transfer which, in turn, controls both the detectability of visual signals and the contrast sensitivity of LGN relay neurons (a relay neuron is one that receives retinal input and sends its axon to primary visual cortex). Similar GABAergic mechanisms may exist at the thalamic level in other sensory modalities (Gottschaldt et al., 1983) and, within the visual system, throughout the cortical streams to which the LGN projects. Thus, GABAergic inhibition may play a general role in controlling afferent information flow.

There are at least two reasons for the nervous system to reduce sensory information flow at the LGN: one is to reduce unwanted or unnecessary information in a global manner (Sherman and Koch, 1986; Casagrande and Norton, 1991). This might be of assistance in falling asleep or in concentrating on a particular sensory modality such as occurs when one is reading instead of listening. A second reason for reducing information flow is to allow focal enhancement within a sensory modality, as when listening through one ear and ignoring information arriving through the other ear (Broadbent, 1958) or when attending to a region within the visual field (Posner, 1980).

One way to accomplish a focal enhancement is by reducing the transmission of information in all regions except the one of interest.

Any reduction in transmission should not be complete because the nervous system does not always know what will be of interest. Rather than excluding all afferent information, it must remain capable of detecting the presence of novel, unexpected events such as the calling of one's name or a tap on the shoulder. As will be noted later in this chapter, an initial portion of the visual response often passes through the LGN even when most of the message is blocked by GABAergic circuitry. This may provide a mechanism that can alert neurons within central structures to the presence of stimuli that may be of interest or importance so that the afferent flow through the LGN can be globally or focally increased.

**Circuitry**

As discussed in the preceding chapters of this volume, complex excitatory and inhibitory retinal circuitry produces the center-surround receptive-

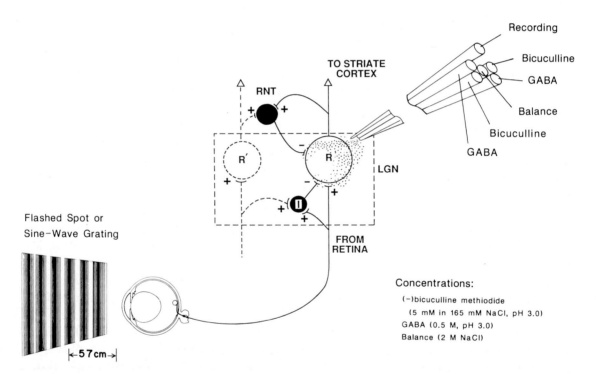

Fig. 1. Model and methods. *Model*. The simplified schematic diagram of the LGN shows the general projection scheme of retinal afferents, LGN relay cells (R), the feedforward pathway through interneurons (I) and the feedback pathway through the reticular nucleus of the thalamus (RNT). GABAergic inhibitory neurons are indicated in black. The circuits drawn with dashed lines indicate possible connections onto the feedforward inhibitory pathway from adjacent retinal afferents and onto the feedback inhibitory pathway from adjacent LGN relay cells (R'). Omitted are brainstem afferents to the LGN that are in a position to control in a global manner the activity of the GABAergic neurons. In addition, there is a retinotopically organized descending pathway from striate cortex (reviewed by Sillito, Chapter 17) that is in a position to focally control the activity of the GABAergic neurons and LGN relay cells. *Methods*. In the experiments that studied the effects of transmitter agonists and antagonists on LGN cells, a recording micropipette or tungsten-in-glass microelectrode was arranged so that it extended 5–15 $\mu$m beyond a multibarreled micropipette through which GABA, bicuculline and control solutions could be iontophoretically administered. Drug concentrations are given in the figure. Visual stimuli were presented to animals (cats or tree shrews) that were anesthetized with a nitrous oxide (70%)/oxygen (30%) mixture supplemented by halothane to maintain an anesthetized EEG, blood pressure and heart rate (see Bullier and Norton, 1979a; Humphrey and Norton, 1980; Norton et al., 1988; and Holdefer et al., 1989 for methodological details).

field organization of retinal cells and determines whether the presentation of a visual stimulus will cause the ganglion cells to increase the rate at which they produce action potentials. These action potentials constitute the visual input to the neurons in the LGN, which of course, have no information about whether the afferent action potentials were generated as a result of stimulation of the retinal cell's center or surround, or both. The center and the surround are thus determined principally, if not exclusively, by the retinal circuitry and not by the circuitry within the LGN. As shown in Fig. 1, retinal afferents project to the LGN and form excitatory synaptic contacts on the LGN relay cells which, in turn, project to the visual cortex. LGN relay cells generally receive input from only a few (1–5) retinal afferents (Cleland et al., 1971; Cleland and Lee, 1985; Mastronarde, 1987). As might be expected from this arrangement, the receptive-field organization of the LGN relay neuron is inherited from its retinal input. The sign (on- or off-center) and the type (W, X or Y) of the afferents define the sign and type of the recipient LGN cell such that, for example, an on-center LGN X cell receives its input from on-center retinal X cells (Cleland et al., 1971; Mastronarde, 1987). For simplicity, the model in Fig. 1 shows the LGN cell with input from only one retinal ganglion cell, although we and others (Cleland and Lee, 1985; Mastronarde, 1987; Tootle et al., 1989) have found examples of LGN cells with more than one retinal input. Examples shown in this chapter have been selected from LGN relay cells that appeared to have a single retinal excitatory input in order to simplify our analysis.

The feedforward and feedback circuits involving GABAergic neurons at the level of the LGN have been reviewed elsewhere in this volume (Soltesz and Crunelli, Chapter 8; Uhlrich and Cucchiaro, Chapter 9; Sillito, Chapter 17). As summarized in Fig. 1, there is a feedforward pathway through LGN interneurons and a feedback pathway through the reticular nucleus of the thalamus (RNT) (Lindström, 1982; Ahlsén et al.,

1985) which in cats, also appears to include the perigeniculate nucleus (PGN) (Cucchiaro et al., 1990). The feedforward pathway and, especially, the feedback pathway may receive excitatory inputs from other retinal afferents or LGN relay cells (Fig. 1).

The feedforward and feedback pathways are organized in a similar manner across species including nocturnal carnivore (cat) (Sterling and Davis, 1980; Fitzpatrick et al., 1984), primates (monkey and bush baby) (Fitzpatrick et al., 1982; Hendrickson et al., 1983) and in tree shrew (Holdefer et al., 1988), a diurnal mammal closely related to primates. Despite the dramatically different niches that these animals occupy and the specialized adaptations for nocturnal vision found in cat and bush baby, the basic LGN circuitry described in Fig. 1 seems to exist in each. Examples from both cat and tree shrew will be presented in this chapter to provide a broader view of LGN function. Looking across species is important because conclusions drawn from data in only one species might be limited to features that are specific to that species as the result of evolutionary specialization, rather than reflecting general organizational features of the LGN (Casagrande and Norton, 1991).

Although the feedforward and feedback pathways are similarly organized across a wide range of mammals, important species distinctions have been demonstrated between anatomical and physiological classes of cells. For instance, there are differences between the GABAergic connections onto W, X and Y cells in cat and onto magnocellular and parvocellular neurons in monkey (Wilson et al., 1984; Raczkowski et al., 1988; Fitzpatrick et al., 1982, 1984; Hendrickson et al., 1983). These differences undoubtedly play a role in controlling the responses of the cells, but the different roles have not been obvious in our studies. Partly, this may be due to the relatively small number of cells examined thus far in cat, preventing us from making meaningful distinctions between the effects on W, X and Y cell classes. Our discussion will focus on principles of GABAergic control in the LGN that appear to exist in most mammalian species and classes of cells.

*Functional implications*

At the physiological level, as expected from the circuits shown in Fig. 1, action potentials arriving from the retina will have two effects at the LGN: excitation and inhibition. Activity in the direct retinogeniculate excitatory synapse depolarizes the LGN relay cell toward threshold and may result in an action potential that proceeds to the cortex. In addition, the retinally-generated action potentials will activate the GABAergic feedforward inhibitory pathway through the interneuron. The GABAergic interneuron, after a synaptic delay, will have an inhibitory effect on the relay cell. A preceding chapter (Soltesz and Crunelli, Chapter 8) discusses the effects of GABA at both the $GABA_A$ receptors, which affect a chloride conductance and the $GABA_B$ receptors which affect a potassium conductance. Both types appear to be present on the relay cells (Soltesz et al., 1989) and presumably both are affected when GABA is released from the interneuron, producing inhibitory post-synaptic potentials that are several milliseconds in duration. Activation of these receptors thus reduces the likelihood that a subsequent retinal action potential arriving at the LGN cell during the IPSP will succeed in producing an action potential by the LGN cell.

An important implication of this feedforward GABAergic circuit is that the inhibition should be activity-dependent. For instance, when retinal cells are presented with a steady background luminance level, typical maintained discharge rates are about 20–40 spikes/s. At this rate, the average interspike interval would be 25–50 ms, long enough for the IPSP generated through the interneuron to dissipate before the next action potential arrives from the retina. However, when the retinal cell responds to a visual stimulus, the firing rate increases (instantaneous rates of 300–500 spikes/s can occur), decreasing the interspike interval to the point that subsequent retinal

action potentials will attempt to excite the LGN cell while the feedforward inhibition is strong. In addition, each new retinal action potential will produce further inhibition. Thus, the amount of inhibition should increase in proportion to the rate of arrival of action potentials from the retina.

In a similar manner, the feedback pathway through the reticular nucleus of the thalamus will also be activity dependent; however, here the amount of inhibition will depend upon the activity of LGN relay cells rather than retinal afferents. It should be noted that the feedback pathway (as well as the feedforward pathway) need not involve only one LGN relay cell. Even small visual stimuli must excite, in parallel, several adjacent retinal ganglion cells that can excite adjacent LGN relay cells (Fig. 1). These connections may contribute to the generation of a "pool" of inhibition (Bullier and Norton, 1979b) that could reduce the ability of excitatory retinal inputs to drive LGN relay cells, especially when large visual stimuli are used. Thus, while the feedback inhibitory pathway should also be activity dependent, its effect need not be solely dependent on the activity of the single LGN relay cell from which one is recording with a microelectrode.

*The transfer ratio*

A key decision made at the LGN is whether action potentials received from the retina will generate action potentials in the LGN cells and thus be transmitted, or relayed, to the striate cortex. The fraction of retinal afferent action potentials that generate output action potentials from the LGN relay cells is the transfer ratio:

transfer ratio

$$= \frac{\text{LGN output action potentials}}{\text{retinal input action potentials}}$$

At one extreme, if every retinal action potential generated an LGN action potential (transfer ratio = 1.0), the LGN would functionally disappear and retinal information could pass unchanged to activate cells in the striate cortex. At the other extreme, if none of the retinal action potentials were transferred on to the cortex (transfer ratio = 0), the retinal signal would end at the LGN and there would be no visual excitation of the cortical neurons. Examples in this chapter will show that both of these extremes are possible and that GABAergic inhibition can control the transfer ratio, with intermediate conditions between these end points generally occurring. In addition, we will show that, occasionally, high frequency bursts of action potentials can serve to increase the transfer ratio to above 1.0, providing possible amplification of retinally-generated signals (Lu et al., 1990).

*S-Potentials as a measure of retinogeniculate transfer*

In order to assess the transfer ratio in the LGN, it is necessary to have a measure of retinal input to compare with the output of the LGN as measured by relay cell action potentials. Such a measure is provided by the S (or slow) potential. As shown in Fig. 2, S-potentials are small, positive-going deflections recorded extracellularly by either tungsten electrodes or by micropipettes. Numerous studies have led to the conclusion that S-potentials are extracellularly recorded EPSPs from the LGN cell and that they faithfully represent the activity of the retinal input (Bishop et al., 1962; Kaplan and Shapley, 1984; Wang et al., 1985; Kaplan et al., 1987; Mastronarde, 1987). Not all S-potentials produce LGN action potentials (Fig. 2). In addition, sometimes action potentials can be seen arising from an S-potential that appears to have triggered it. Quite often, however no S-potential is seen when the LGN action potential occurs. Evidence presented later in this chapter (Figs. 3, 8, 9) suggests that most, if not all, of the LGN action potentials in our examples (except those in bursts, described later) were triggered by an S-potential that is masked by the action potential. Thus, even though the S-potential appears to be a postsynaptic event, it can serve as a monitor of the retinal input to the LGN cell that does not produce an output. The

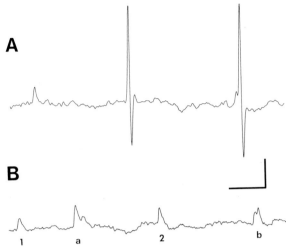

Fig. 2. A. LGN S-potentials and action potentials from a cat on-center X relay cell. On the left is an S-potential that does not produce an action potential. On the right, an action potential arises from an S-potential. In the middle, no S-potential is visible, but one probably occurred and is masked by the action potential. The transfer ratio in this example is 0.67 (2 LGN action potentials produced by 3 S-potentials). B. Two distinct S-potentials, labeled 1 and 2, recorded from another on-center LGN X relay cell, indicating the presence of input from at least two retinal afferents. The presence of two different inputs could be demonstrated by two criteria: the S-potentials were of two distinct waveforms and they could occur at extremely short intervals (i.e., <1 ms) from one another so that they could not have arisen from a single afferent (Coenen and Vendrik, 1972; Tootle et al., 1989). This second criterion also allows recognition of multiple retinal inputs in instances where the S-potentials from both sources are similar in shape and size. In this example, the S-potentials overlap temporally (marked a and b). On the left (a), it appears that S-potential 2 occurred slightly before S-potential 1 so that the two potentials overlapped. On the right (b), the reverse pattern occurred. The data presented in this chapter do not include cells in which there were S-potentials from more than one input. Initial examination of the data from multiple-input cells, however, suggests that conclusions derived from single-input cells extrapolates to cells with input from more than one retinal afferent. Vertical scale, 1 mV; horizontal scale, 5 ms in A, 6.4 ms in B.

LGN action potentials, of course, serve as a measure of retinal inputs that successfully produce an output from the LGN. Even if there are small errors in the use of S-potentials to calculate the transfer ratio, the measure is still of use as an index of changes in the amount of retinogeniculate transfer.

198

## Variations in the transfer ratio

### Response variability

When one records from cells in the lateral geniculate nucleus in anesthetized animals, it quickly becomes evident that repeated presentations of the same visual stimulus do not elicit identical responses to each stimulus repetition. Figure 3A shows a peristimulus time histogram of the response of an on-center X cell recorded in the LGN of an anesthetized cat. The stimulus produced a small average response from the cell over and above the maintained discharge that occurred during presentation of a homogeneously illuminated background. Figure 3B shows the responses of the cell to each of the 20 stimulus repetitions. Clearly, the response of the cell was quite variable, ranging from no response in the row marked 1 to a strong response in the row marked 3.

This cell was one in which the electrode recorded an S-potential as well as the LGN action potential, allowing us to examine the transfer ratio. Figure 3C shows the S-potentials and ac-

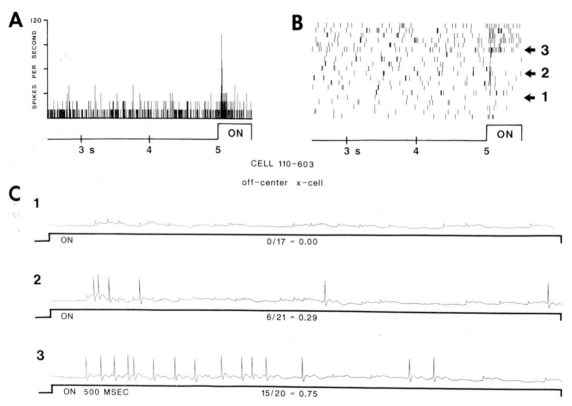

Fig. 3. A. Peristimulus time histogram (3 ms bin width, 20 stimulus repetitions) showing the response of a cat LGN relay cell to a flashed grating stimulus (contrast, 0.65). The spatial frequency of the grating (0.37 c/deg) was near the spatial frequency to which the cell was most responsive and was positioned to produce a maximum response. The grating was presented for 500 ms following a 5.5 s period of homogeneous 21 cd/m² background luminance. B. Raster display showing the variability of the responses of the LGN cell on the 20 stimulus presentations that produced the histogram in A. Each vertical mark indicates an action potential from the LGN cell. C. S-potentials and action potentials recorded on the three rows (1, 2, 3) indicated by the arrows in B. The responses that occurred only during the period the stimulus was on are shown. In the fraction below each trace, the numerator is the number of action potentials (LGN output) and the denominator is the sum of the action potentials and S-potentials (retinal input). Determination of S-potentials was performed at an expanded time scale that made S-potentials clearly distinguishable from changes in baseline voltage.

tion potentials on the three rows that were marked in Fig. 3B. In row 1, the LGN cell did not respond. The presence of retinal input is shown by the 17 S-potentials that occurred during the 500 ms period that the stimulus was presented. This clearly demonstrates that the absence of response by the LGN cell was not due to an absence of retinal driving. However, the afferent activity did not succeed in producing LGN responses; the transfer ratio was 0. Conversely, in row 3 where the LGN cell responded strongly, most retinal afferent spikes produced an LGN action potential, so that the transfer ratio was high (0.75). In row 2, there was an intermediate response and an intermediate transfer ratio.

It is important to note that although fewer S-potentials are visible in row 2 than in row 1 and that even fewer are visible in row 3, the total number of events (S-potentials and LGN spikes) remains statistically the same in this and in other LGN cells with S-potentials that we have examined under these conditions. The trade-off between visible S-potentials and LGN spikes and statistical invariance in the total number of events is convincing evidence that the LGN spikes in this record are triggered by S-potentials whose presence is masked by the LGN action potentials (see also Fig. 5). Except in the case of clear bursts of LGN action potentials (discussed later in this chapter) it appears that most, if not all, of the LGN spikes can be accounted for by retinal afferent spikes that can be visualized as S-potentials in records where the transfer ratio is zero.

We have observed in many cells that the number of LGN output spikes that occurred in response to repeated presentations of a stimulus is strongly related to the transfer ratio, suggesting that changes in transfer ratio account for most of the response variability. It is important to note that there may be additional "silent" retinal inputs that do not produce an S-potential but that may influence the LGN cell. However, as will be seen in subsequent figures, if such inputs occur, their ability to activate the LGN cells appears to be influenced by GABAergic circuitry in the same manner as are the inputs that do produce S-potentials.

*Variations in sleep and wakefulness*

The examples shown in Fig. 3 were recorded in an anesthetized animal, in which unknown factors produced the response variability of the LGN cells. Recordings in animals that were alternately awake or asleep (Coenen and Vendrik, 1972; Livingstone and Hubel, 1981) suggest that the transfer through the LGN and, hence, LGN cell responsiveness, may be controlled such that there is generally greater transfer and greater LGN cell responsiveness in waking states. During sleep the transfer ratio and, thus, LGN cell responsiveness, are lower.

Figure 4A illustrates the responses of an LGN cell studied by Livingstone and Hubel (1981) in a cat that alternated between a waking and a sleeping state. On the left is a histogram of the responses of the cell to a visual stimulus while the cat was awake, as indicated by the desynchronized EEG. In the middle panel, the response of the cell to the visual stimulus was reduced when the animal went briefly to sleep. On the right, the response increased when the animal reawoke. Importantly, the maintained activity when the stimulus was not present (the right half of each histogram) did not change dramatically in the three histograms (it may have increased slightly in the sleeping state), indicating that the visually-driven responses were more affected by the state of the animal than was the maintained activity.

Figure 4B, from a study by Coenen and Vendrik (1972), shows the changes in the transfer ratio in an animal that was awakened. During the period while the EEG record indicated that the animal was asleep, the transfer ratio in the two examples was about 0.5 (the number of output LGN spikes was about half of the retinal afferent input). When the animal was awakened, the transfer ratio rose toward 1.0.

Taken together, the studies of Coenen and Vendrik (1972) and of Livingstone and Hubel (1981) along with the data from the previous

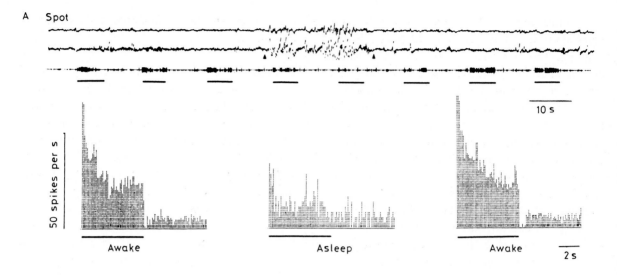

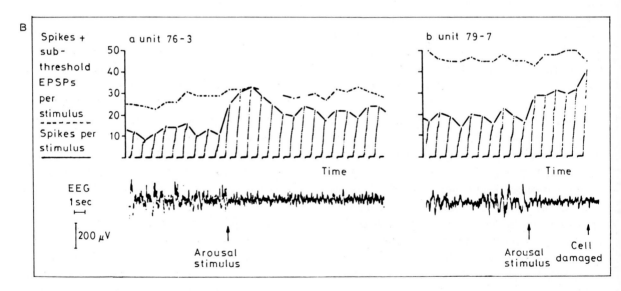

Fig. 4. A. Example of variations of the response of an LGN cell related to waking and sleeping. The upper two traces indicate the EEG recorded from the anterior and posterior cortex of a drowsy cat and show the animal moving from a desynchronized EEG to one indicating slow-wave sleep and back to the desynchronized pattern (arrows mark the approximate transitions). Below are pulses indicating the responses of an on-center LGN cell to a 0.25 ° light spot centered in the receptive field. The stimulus presentation times are indicated by the horizontal lines. Histograms taken before (left, 13 stimulus repetitions) during (center, 2 stimulus repetitions) and after (right, 16 repetitions) the animal went briefly to sleep demonstrate the reduced responsiveness of the LGN cell during the sleeping state (from Livingstone and Hubel, 1981). B. Two examples of increases in the transfer ratio of cat LGN cells related to arousal from sleep. In both graphs, the retinal input (the sum of "subthreshold EPSPs" (i.e., S-potentials) and LGN spikes) to the presentation of a visual stimulus is indicated by the dotted line at the top. The number of LGN action potentials is indicated by the solid line. Every vertical line indicates the response to a periodically presented stimulus. The EEG (displayed below each graph) changed from slow-wave sleep to a desynchronized pattern after an arousal stimulus and was accompanied by an increase in the transfer ratio (from Coenen and Vendrik, 1972).

section and from other investigators (Cleland and Lee, 1985; Kaplan et al., 1987), suggest that there is generally low transfer in anesthetized or sleeping animals, which produces a reduced responsiveness of the LGN cells in comparison with their retinal input (Bullier and Norton, 1979a,b). In the waking state, the transfer ratio increases, increasing the response of the LGN cells so that it more closely mimics the retinal afferent activity.

## GABAergic control of the transfer ratio

The previous sections of this chapter have noted the presence of GABAergic feedforward and feedback pathways and have described how changes in the transfer ratio control the responsiveness of LGN cells. In this section, we present evidence that the GABAergic circuitry can control the transfer ratio. The data have been obtained in anesthetized cats (Godwin and Norton, 1990; Norton and Godwin, 1990). As shown in Fig. 1, relay cells were studied in the LGN with tungsten-in-glass microelectrodes that recorded S-potentials and LGN action potentials. An oscilloscope monitor was placed so that the receptive field of each cell was centered on the screen (mean luminance 20–24 cd/m$^2$). Light or dark spots, or gratings of appropriate spatial frequency, contrast and phase were used to excite

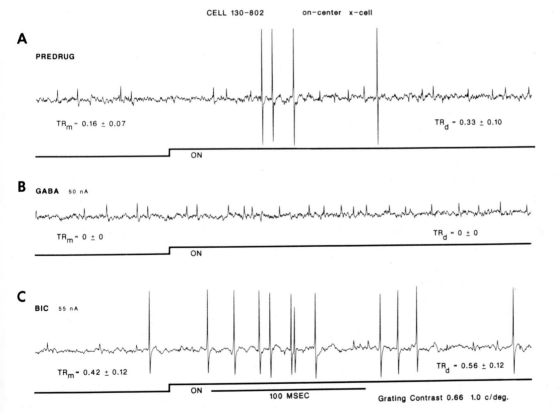

Fig. 5. The effects of GABA and bicuculline (BIC) on retinogeniculate transfer in a cat LGN cell are shown in representative recordings of S-potentials and action potentials. Stimulus duration was 500 ms, of which the first 235 ms are shown. The (mean ± standard deviation) transfer ratio during the 500 ms period of visual driving (TR$_d$) for 10 stimulus repetitions is displayed on the right. The transfer ratio during the immediately preceding maintained discharge period (TR$_m$) of homogeneous background luminance is indicated on the left. Iontophoretic currents were as indicated.

the cells. Following a predrug control record, GABA was iontophoretically applied through a multibarreled micropipette that was attached to the recording electrode. The stimulus remained the same during our iontophoretic manipulations, so that the retinal input, which, of course, exhibited some variability, remained relatively constant. Records taken when GABA was iontophoresed were designed to examine whether reductions in responsiveness and the transfer ratio were caused by the GABA. Then, following the protocols of Sillito and Kemp (1983) an appropriate ejection current for the $GABA_A$ antagonist bicuculline was individually determined for each cell such that it reversed the inhibition of a maximally effective GABA ejection current and records were taken using bicuculline alone. Finally, in cells that we were able to study for a long enough time (the effects of bicuculline dissipate slowly) post-drug control records were taken.

Figure 5 illustrates the effect of GABA and bicuculline on the transfer ratio of an on-center X cell recorded in cat LGN. In the predrug control record (Fig. 5A), S-potentials and action potentials are clearly visible. During the maintained discharge period, the transfer ratio ($TR_m$) across 10 trials was (mean $\pm$ standard deviation) $0.16 \pm 0.07$. Transfer was slightly higher ($0.33 \pm 0.10$) during the 500 ms period of visual driving ($TR_d$), which began after a latency of about 34 ms after stimulus onset. Figure 5B shows that GABA reduced the transfer to 0 both during the maintained discharge period and stimulus onset period. As in Fig. 3, the continued presence of retinal input is quite clearly demonstrated by the presence of the S-potentials. Across the 10 stimulus presentation trials, the number of S-potentials under GABA did not differ significantly ($t$-test, $P > 0.05$) from the number of events (S-potentials and action potentials) in the predrug condition, confirming that all of the LGN spikes could have been triggered by S-potentials. Figure 5C shows that bicuculline reversed the effects of GABA, increasing the transfer ratio. In this cell, the transfer ratio under bicuculline was significantly

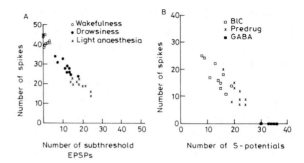

Fig. 6. A. Effects of arousal on the reciprocal relationship between the number of LGN spikes and "subthreshold EPSPs" (S-potentials) in cat LGN. During wakefulness the number of S-potentials was near zero and the number of LGN spikes was high, indicating a high transfer ratio. When the animal was drowsy or lightly anesthetized, the transfer ratio decreased as indicated by the reduced number of LGN spikes and the increased number of visible S-potentials (from Coenen and Vendrik, 1972). B. Effects of GABA and bicuculline on the relationship between LGN spikes and S-potentials in a cat on-center X relay cell measured during a 500 ms stimulus presentation period on 10 trials. In comparison to the anesthetized predrug control, GABA reduced the transfer to 0, so that S-potentials, but no LGN spikes were observed (some data points are obscured in the figure because they had the same values as others). Bicuculline increased the transfer ratio above the control level, yielding a greater number of action potentials and fewer S-potentials.

increased above that obtained during the pre-drug condition ($t$-test, $P < 0.0001$).

The data in Fig. 6 suggest that the decrease in the transfer ratio produced by GABA and the increase produced by bicuculline mimic the alterations in transfer ratio that occur with changes in arousal state (Coenen and Vendrik, 1972). Figure 6A illustrates the changes in the relative number of S-potentials and LGN action potentials in an LGN cell recorded from a cat that was alternately drowsy, aroused, and lightly anesthetized. During the period when a desynchronized EEG was recorded, indicating arousal, repeated presentation of a visual stimulus produced LGN action potentials almost exclusively (transfer ratio nearly 1.0). When the animal was drowsy or anesthetized, fewer LGN action potentials and more S-potentials occurred, indicating a lower transfer ratio. In Fig. 6B, an LGN cell in an anesthetized cat responded to a visual stimulus during the

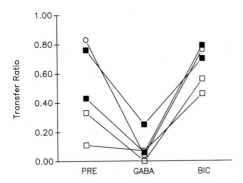

Fig. 7. Decrease in transfer ratio produced by administration of GABA and increase in transfer ratio produced by bicuculline (BIC) on 5 LGN cells in cat. GABA reduced the transfer ratio during the response to a visual stimulus. Bicuculline reversed the effects of GABA.

predrug control period with a mixture of S-potentials and action potentials similar to that seen under anesthesia in Fig. 6A. Application of GABA eliminated all action potentials, leaving only S-potentials (transfer ratio = 0). The effect of bicuculline was similar to that of arousal.

Figure 7 summarizes the effects of GABA and bicuculline on the transfer ratio in 5 cat LGN cells. Both during the period of maintained discharge (not shown) and during visual driving, GABA reduced the transfer ratio and bicuculline reversed the effect of GABA showing the specificity of its effect. It is also clear that the transfer ratio in the predrug control condition varied across cells. Cells with low initial transfer ratios were less affected by GABA (the transfer ratio could not be reduced below 0) and were more affected by bicuculline than were the cells that had a higher transfer ratio in the predrug condition.

We also found that, in the predrug condition, the transfer ratio during the maintained discharge period and during the period of visual driving were not particularly different. This is of interest because, as mentioned earlier, the amount of inhibition in the GABAergic feedforward and feedback pathways should be activity-dependent and, hence, should be greater during visual driving when the firing rate of the retinal

afferent is elevated. It would follow that the transfer ratio would be lower during visual driving than when the animal is presented with a homogeneous background luminance. That the transfer ratio is *not* uniformly lower during visual driving suggests that other influences may act to counteract any increased inhibition that occurs during the period of the visual response. Indeed, as may be seen in Fig. 3B and in row 2 of Fig. 3C, it is often the case that, if an LGN cell is unresponsive, either because of variations in transfer ratio in the predrug control record or when transfer is reduced by GABA, the occasional action potential that is generated nearly always occurs within the first 100 ms after stimulus onset and frequently occurs near the time of the peak response of the retinal afferent. The LGN spikes that occur under low transfer ratio conditions may be the result of temporal summation of the EPSPs generated by the retinal afferent, possibly coupled with a delay in the development of the feedforward and feedback inhibitory influences. It thus appears that the GABAergic inhibitory mechanisms at the LGN do not necessarily eliminate sensory afferent signals. Rather, the signals are attenuated but may still serve to convey information that a stimulus has occurred which, as noted earlier, is desirable in a mechanism underlying attention.

### GABAergic control of signal detectability

It was noted earlier (Fig. 4A) that when a cat shifted from a waking to a sleeping state, the response of the LGN neuron to a visual stimulus was reduced greatly, while there appeared to be only a slight change in the maintained discharge. The effect of such an alteration would be a reduction in the detectability of the visual stimulus, or the signal-to-noise ratio, because the visual response (the "signal") is reduced relative to the background activity (the "noise"). Indeed, Wilson et al. (1988) found that signal detectability was reduced in a sample of LGN X and Y cells in anesthetized cats in comparison with a sample of retinal X and Y cells. In tree shrew LGN cells we examined signal detectability using both ROC curves and another measure of detectability, a difference measure, $d$, (Fitzhugh, 1957) which is simply the difference in the average number of action potentials produced by the LGN cell during the maintained and during the visually-driven period. A large $d$ indicates a highly detectable signal that may have a stronger influence on cortical cells than would a small $d$. In tree shrews, S-potentials were not recorded, only the LGN action potentials. As may be seen in Fig. 8, bicuculline produced a very similar effect on LGN

relay cells in tree shrew as did awakening of the cat in Fig. 4A. The cell (Fig. 8A) gave a moderate response to the low contrast flashed stimulus during the predrug control period. During iontophoresis of bicuculline at 35 nA, there was an increase in the visual response that exceeded the increase in the maintained discharge. A higher iontophoresis rate (50 nA) greatly increased the visual response, with little effect on the maintained activity. The area under the ROC curves (on the right of Fig. 8A) also is a measure of signal detectability (Swets et al., 1964; Holdefer et al., 1989). Clearly, this measure of signal de-

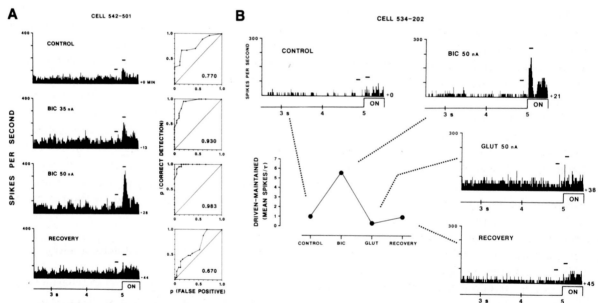

Fig. 8. Effect of microiontophoresis of bicuculline on maintained and visually-driven activity of LGN relay cells in tree shrew LGN. A. At the top is the control response of an on-center relay cell (center diameter 0.65°) to a flashed grating stimulus (0.5 c/degree at a contrast of 0.15). The grating was on for 0.5 s with a 5.5 s period of background luminance. To the right is a receiver operating characteristic (ROC) curve examining the detectability of the visually-driven activity (probability ($P$) of a correct detection, or signal) in comparison with the maintained activity ($P$ of a "false positive", or noise). The horizontal dark bars above the histograms denote the 100 ms time periods, tau ($\tau$) during which the maintained and driven activity were sampled. The area under the ROC curve (0.77 in the control record) is an index of the detectability of the visual stimulus against the background activity of the LGN cell. Microiontophoresis of bicuculline (BIC) at 35 and at 50 nA increased the visually-driven activity more than it increased the maintained discharge, thus increasing the area under the ROC curve to 0.93 and 0.983. The recovery record taken 44 min after the predrug control and 16 min after BIC offset shows a return to lower driven and maintained activity and a reduction in signal detectability to 0.67. B. In some cells there was no overlap in the number of spikes counted during $\tau$ for the maintained activity and the $\tau$ for the visually-driven activity. In these instances, the mean maintained discharge was simply subtracted from the mean visually-driven response. In comparison with the predrug control record, BIC increased the difference between the visually-driven and the maintained activity. Iontophoresis of glutamate generally raised both the maintained and driven activity, but did not change the difference between them, demonstrating the specificity of the BIC effect (from Holdefer et al., 1989).

tectability was also increased by the bicuculline and recovered to approximately the control level after discontinuation of the bicuculline administration. In another cell (Fig. 8B) the $d$ showed an increase in signal detectability under conditions of bicuculline iontophoresis.

In cat, we have found a similar increase in $d$ during bicuculline microiontophoresis (Fig. 9A). The $d$ value during bicuculline was significantly greater than the $d$ obtained during GABA administration, indicating that removal of $GABA_A$ inhibitory control increased the signal detectability (Godwin and Norton, 1990).

In the LGN cells in tree shrew, where only the LGN action potentials were recorded, it seemed likely that the increases in signal detectability were due to increases in the transfer ratio, but it was not possible to show this to be the case. The cat LGN cells shown in Fig. 9A, however, were the same ones shown in Fig. 7 in which the changes in the transfer ratio were observed. In each of these cells, it could be seen that the increase in the difference measure was indeed due to an increase in the transfer ratio produced by bicuculline iontophoresis, allowing the LGN cell to respond more like its retinal drive.

It was mentioned in the previous section that the transfer ratios we have observed during the maintained discharge period and during visual driving were quite similar and that the transfer ratios during both periods were decreased by GABA and increased by bicuculline. One then might ask why the difference between maintained and driven activity (signal detectability) increases under bicuculline. The answer lies in the amount of retinal afferent activity during the two periods. For example, the retinal afferents arriving at one on-center X relay cell, under conditions of maintained activity, responded at a relatively low rate (41 spikes/s). During visual driving the value increased to 64 spikes/s. When the transfer ratio was lowered by GABA, the output of the LGN cells fell to 0 spikes/s during the maintained activity and during visual driving, producing a difference measure of 0. When bicuculline raised

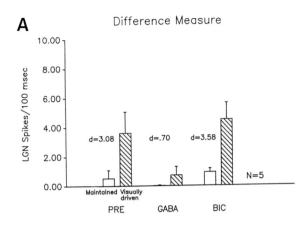

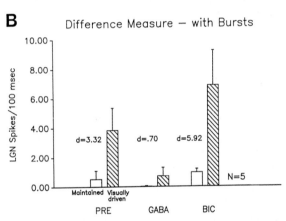

Fig. 9. Effect of microiontophoresis of GABA and bicuculline (BIC) on maintained and visually-driven activity of relay cells ($n = 5$) in cat LGN. For each cell, the number of LGN spikes were counted during a 100 ms period of maintained discharge and another 100 ms period that included the peak response of the cell to a flashed visual stimulus (10 stimulus repetitions). As in Fig. 8B, the difference between these two measures, $d$, is an indication of the strength or detectability of the LGN cell's response to the visual stimulus. As described in the text, the LGN cells occasionally produced high-frequency bursts (see Fig. 10). In A, only the first spike in any burst was included in the calculations of the maintained and visually-driven activity because it appeared that only the first spike could have been produced by a retinal input. In B, all spikes in the bursts were included in the calculations. Inclusion of bursts had only a small effect on the predrug control record, and no effect on the GABA record, since there were no bursts during that period. $d$ in B was significantly increased during bicuculline administration in comparison to the value without bursts in A.

the transfer ratio toward the full potential value of 1.0, the difference in the output of the LGN cell in the maintained and the visually-driven period increased because there were many more retinal afferent spikes during the period of visual driving than during the maintained discharge period. In this simple manner, controlling the transfer ratio can control the detectability of the visual signal at the LGN and, since a high rate of firing should have a stronger effect at the next synapse (Moore et al., 1966), control of the transfer ratio influences the impact of the visual signal on the striate cortex.

### Signal amplification

Earlier in this chapter it was noted that there was an exception to the general rule that all LGN spikes were produced by retinal afferents. This exception is illustrated in Fig. 10A in which a clear burst of LGN action potentials is seen. The interspike interval within the burst (2.0 ms in this example) was far shorter than the interspike intervals between any of the S-potentials seen in that cell, even during GABA administrations when the S-potentials were not obscured by the presence of action potentials and the minimum retinal interspike interval could be accurately measured. In this instance, as in other bursts, the number of output spikes from the LGN cell must have exceeded the number of input action potentials during this time interval, producing a transfer ratio greater than 1.0.

Bursts of spikes in the LGN are a well-known phenomenon that is characteristic of anesthetized or sleeping animals (Steriade et al., 1990) and are produced by de-inactivation of calcium spikes after a period of hyperpolarization of the cell membrane (Jahnsen and Llinas, 1984; Steriade and Llinás, 1988; McCormick and Feeser, 1990). Although cells respond less faithfully to visual stimuli when they are in the "burst mode" (McCormick and Feeser, 1990), Lu et al. (1990) recently suggested that bursts might actually serve, in some instances, to amplify visual signals. Data we have obtained in cat LGN cells offer some support for this suggestion. Figure 10B shows that bursts are clustered in the period 50–100 ms after cells begin to respond to a visual stimulus. Thus, many

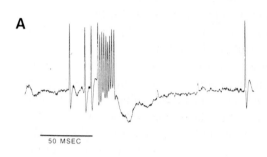

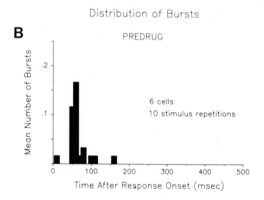

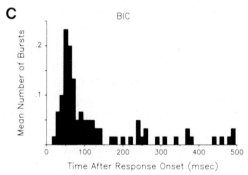

Fig. 10. A. Example of three LGN action potentials followed by a high-frequency burst in an on-center Y cell in cat from which S-potentials also were recorded. B. The distribution of the onset time of high-frequency bursts of LGN action potentials (defined as two or more spikes with interspike intervals of 4 ms or less (Lu et al., 1989)) in six cat LGN cells in the predrug control condition. For each cell, the onset time of each high-frequency burst was measured on each of 10 stimulus repetitions. To reduce scatter due to different response latencies between the cells, the burst onset was measured for each cell from the time at which that cell began to respond to the stimulus. C. Bicuculline administration increased the number of bursts while preserving their temporal distribution.

of the bursts could indeed serve to amplify the response to the visual signal. During bicuculline iontophoresis, there was a significant increase in the number of bursts (Fig. 10C) in comparison to the predrug condition ($t$-test, $P < 0.05$) and the bursts retained a similar time distribution to the predrug control pattern. Figure 9B shows that including the bursts in the calculations significantly increased the $d$ during bicuculline suggesting that removal of $GABA_A$ inhibition not only increases the transfer ratio, but also may increase the occurrence of LGN cell spike bursts, amplifying the visual signal at the LGN.

An important caveat to the suggestion that bursts may amplify the visual signal at the LGN is that these results were obtained in anesthetized animals and during bicuculline administration. It is not known whether high-frequency bursts occur frequently in the LGN of alert behaving animals and, thus, whether they could be part of a normal mechanism for enhancing visual signals. Whether or not bursts eventually prove to be important in the transmission of visual information, the results from both tree shrew and cat clearly demonstrate that GABAergic circuitry can control signal detectability at the LGN. GABA decreases detectability and bicuculline increases it. In cat we have shown directly that this is accomplished by control of the transfer ratio.

## GABAergic control of receptive-field sensitivity

An important aspect of visual function is the sensitivity of cells to visual stimuli. An increase in sensitivity (i.e., a decrease in threshold) of a cell increases the ability of the neuron to detect stimuli that might be of behavioral significance. An interesting result that has emerged from our studies of the GABAergic inhibitory circuitry in the LGN is the realization that, by controlling the transfer ratio, this circuitry controls the sensitivity of the LGN cells. Before presenting these results, it may be useful to review the difference of Gaussians model of the retinal receptive field and

its implications for the contrast sensitivity of cells responding to visual stimuli consisting of drifting sine-wave gratings.

### Difference of Gaussians model of retinal ganglion cell receptive-fields

Most of the retinal ganglion cells that project to the LGN are organized with an excitatory on- or off-center and an antagonistic surround. As is illustrated in Fig. 11A, it was recognized some years ago that the receptive fields of ganglion cells can be modeled as a difference of two Gaussian distributions (Rodieck and Stone, 1965; Enroth-Cugell and Robson, 1966). Although more complex models have been devised that deal more fully with misalignment of the center within the surround, center-surround phase differences and, in cat Y-cells, non-linear subunits (Hockstein and Shapley, 1976a,b; Dawis et al., 1984; Enroth-Cugell and Freeman, 1987; Soodak et al., 1987; see Kaplan, 1991, for review), the difference of Gaussians (DOG) model is a reasonable first approximation both in the retina and in the LGN, especially in primates and other animals, such as tree shrew, in which there are few spatially non-linear cells (Kaplan and Shapley, 1982; Troy, 1983; Sherman et al., 1984; Blakemore and Vital-Durand, 1986; Holdefer and Norton, 1986; Norton et al., 1988).

One virtue of the DOG model is its simplicity. The retinal receptive-field center is modeled by two parameters, the radius, $R_c$, and the sensitivity, $K_c$. Similarly, two parameters (radius, $R_s$ and sensitivity, $K_s$) define the surround. The center and surround are assumed to be opposed to each other so that stimulation of the surround, along with the center, produces a smaller response than would stimulation of the center alone. The result of this subtraction is a difference of Gaussians profile (Fig. 11B) which models the sensitivity of the cell to visual stimuli. Thus, if this were an on-center cell, it would have the lowest threshold to a spot of light presented precisely in the center of the field. The same size spot of light presented elsewhere within the center region in Fig. 11B

208

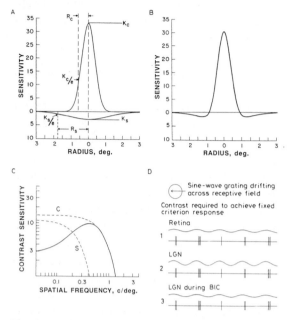

Fig. 11. A. Gaussian functions representing the center and surround mechanisms of a receptive field (Rodieck and Stone, 1965). The symbols represent the receptive-field center radius ($R_c$) and sensitivity ($K_c$) and the surround radius ($R_s$) and sensitivity ($K_s$). B. The center and surround mechanisms interact subtractively in the retina to produce the receptive-field sensitivity profile. For an on-center cell, light increments presented to the center and light decrements presented to the surround will produce an increase in the firing rate of the cell. C. Profiles from A transformed into the spatial frequency domain (Enroth-Cugell and Robson, 1966). The contrast sensitivity function, modeled by the difference of Gaussians function (solid line), represents the subtraction of the surround mechanism (S) from the center mechanism (C), indicated by the dotted lines. D. Modeled effects of the transfer ratio on contrast sensitivity. Panel 1 shows a criterion "threshold" visual response of a hypothetical retinal cell to a sine-wave grating drifted across the receptive field (indicated by the arrow and circle at the top). The contrast of the grating needed to produce this response is indicated by the amplitude of the sine wave. Panel 2 shows the criterion response of a hypothetical LGN cell that received input from the retinal cell. When the transfer ratio is low, as in anesthetized or sleeping animals, a higher contrast is needed for the LGN cell to produce the same criterion response as the retinal cell, as indicated by the higher amplitude of the sine wave (i.e., the contrast sensitivity of the LGN cell is less than that of its retinal input). In panel 3, when the transfer ratio is increased to 1.0 by the administration of bicuculline, the contrast required for the LGN cell to produce the criterion response is reduced to the same level as that of the retinal input in panel 1 (i.e., the contrast sensitivity of the LGN cell increases to equal that of its retinal input) (A, C and D from Norton et al., 1989).

would produce a response at light on, but only if a more intense spot were used (Rodieck and Stone, 1965). If the spot were presented in the surround, the cell would respond when the light was removed (or if a dark spot were presented) but again, the threshold would be relatively high because the surround sensitivity is low compared with that of the center.

An important contribution of the DOG model is that it also predicts the contrast sensitivities that would be expected of the retinal ganglion cell in response to a sine-wave grating (Enroth-Cugell and Robson, 1966). Transformed into the spatial frequency domain, the receptive-field center provides the sensitivity profile demarcated by the dashed line "C" in Fig. 11C. The surround profile is represented by the dashed line labeled "S". The predicted contrast sensitivity function for the cell, which is the center profile minus the surround profile, is indicated by the solid line.

Two important conclusions about retinal ganglion cells can be derived from Fig. 11C. First, the sensitivity of cells to high spatial frequencies is mediated by the receptive-field center. This is because the smaller radius of the center allows it to respond to finer gratings. The surround, with a larger radius, is insensitive to high spatial frequencies. The second point, and one that will be of particular interest later in this discussion, is that the lower sensitivity exhibited by many cells at low spatial frequencies (the "low spatial frequency roll-off") is produced by an interaction of the subtractive surround with the excitatory center. If the center sensitivity of the cell were greater (i.e., if the center sensitivity increased), the low spatial frequency roll-off would be reduced because the same surround would be subtracted from a more sensitive center. This would make the cell more sensitive to low spatial frequency stimuli. The same effect would also occur if the surround sensitivity were reduced. However, because the surround is insensitive to high spatial frequencies, changing the surround sensitivity should only affect the cell's sensitivity to lower spatial frequencies. In contrast, a change in center sensitivity should affect the cell's sensitivity at all spatial frequencies.

*Retinogeniculate transfer of contrast sensitivity*

In the retina, the interaction of the receptive-field center and surround determines the strength of the response to a visual stimulus. Thus, the surround has already been subtracted from the center before the action potentials are generated. As discussed earlier in this chapter, this retinal output spike train constitutes the input to the LGN relay cells.

In considering the expected effect of the transfer ratio on the contrast sensitivity of LGN cells, it is useful to consider the model shown in Fig. 11D. If, when determining a contrast sensitivity function, one begins with a drifting sine-wave grating of a particular spatial frequency and 0 contrast, the stimulus will not produce a response from the retinal afferent cell. If one increases the contrast of the stimulus (defined as $(L_{max} - L_{min})/(L_{max} + L_{min})$), eventually a contrast will be found that produces a threshold response. Panel 1 of Fig. 11D schematically indicates a threshold response from a retinal cell and the contrast of the grating required to produce the response. In practice, a variety of criteria have been used as a measure of threshold response (Enroth-Cugell and Robson, 1966; Kaplan and Shapley, 1982; Norton et al., 1988; Troy and Enroth-Cugell, 1989). Whatever criterion one selects, if the transfer ratio of the retinal afferent onto the LGN relay cell is 1.0, the LGN cell will respond identically to the retinal cell (assuming there are no visually-driven bursts) and the threshold contrast for the LGN cell will be the same as for the retinal drive. At the opposite extreme, if the transfer ratio is 0, the LGN cell will not respond at all, no matter how high the contrast of the grating stimulus. In such a situation, the threshold contrast for the LGN cell would be infinite and the contrast sensitivity would be 0. In the more usual situation, if the transfer ratio is not 0 but is less than 1.0, the stimulus contrast that evokes a threshold re-

sponse from the retinal cell will be below threshold for the LGN cell. In order to produce a response from the LGN cell that matches the threshold defined for the retinal cell, it will be necessary to use a higher contrast stimulus, as is indicated in panel 2 of Fig. 11D. It is evident that the lower the transfer ratio, the higher will be the contrast necessary to elicit a threshold response from the LGN cell.

As was demonstrated in the data presented earlier in this chapter (Figs. 2, 3, 5 and 6), transfer ratios in anesthetized cats have generally been between the extremes of 0 and 1. Since contrast sensitivity is the inverse of the threshold contrast, the LGN cell should have a reduced contrast sensitivity at each spatial frequency in comparison to its retinal input. If, as indicated in panel 3 of Fig. 11D, bicuculline blockade of the $GABA_A$ receptors is used to increase the transfer ratio, as it has been shown to do in previous sections of this chapter, it would be expected that the threshold contrast should be decreased. This, of course, would then increase the contrast sensitivity of the LGN cell.

Figure 12 presents examples of LGN relay cells recorded in tree shrew in which contrast sensitivity was determined for several spatial frequencies in the predrug control condition and again during iontophoretic application of bicuculline (Norton et al., 1989). With the exception of the cell shown in panel 4 (which also showed the lowest sensitivity to GABA), the sensitivity of the cells increased under bicuculline at most spatial frequencies. It is important to note that, as in the cell in panel 6, changes could occur in the sensitivity at high spatial frequencies, which, as noted earlier, must be detected by the receptive-field center. In addition, the cell in panel 5 had no low spatial frequency rolloff, suggesting that there may not have been a suppressive effect of the surround in that cell. The increased sensitivity at low spatial frequencies on that cell, therefore, most likely were due to an increase in receptive-field center sensitivity.

Averaging the center and surround values obtained from the difference of Gaussians fits to the data under both conditions across cells (Fig. 13A), there was a large, significant increase in the receptive-field center sensitivity ($K_c$) during bicuculline. The small decrease in surround sensitivity was not significant with this sample of 10 cells that was examined in tree shrew. Figure 13B shows the average center-surround profile for the 10 cells in the predrug and bicuculline conditions. The peak sensitivity nearly doubled under bicuculline.

As shown in Fig. 13C, the average contrast sensitivity function of the 10 cells was elevated under bicuculline at all spatial frequencies. Thus,

in tree shrew, bicuculline increased the contrast sensitivity of LGN cells to drifting sine-wave gratings. Based on the difference of Gaussians modeling, this increase appeared to be due to an increase in the sensitivity of the receptive-field center.

Studies of the effects of bicuculline on the responses of cat LGN cells (Berardi and Morrone, 1984) have found a similar result: the responsiveness of LGN cells to stimuli of a fixed contrast was increased. However, this increase was attributed to a decrease in "surround inhibition" at the LGN. As noted earlier in this section, an elevation of responsiveness or contrast

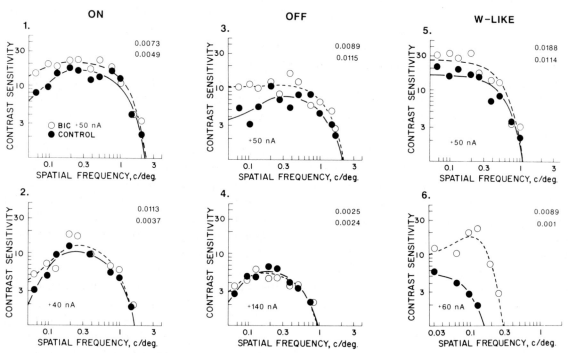

Fig. 12. Contrast sensitivity functions of 6 LGN relay cells in tree shrew taken before (predrug control, solid circles) and during (open circles) microiontophoretic administration of bicuculline. Ejection currents are as indicated in each panel. The solid (predrug) and dashed lines (bicuculline) are difference of Gaussians (DOG) curves that were fit to the data points by an interactive least-squares procedure as in previous experiments in cat retina and primate LGN (Linsenmeier et al., 1982; Norton et al., 1988). The error (mean error per data point) between the data points and the best-fitting DOG function (Linsenmeier et al., 1982; Irvin et al., 1986; Norton et al., 1988) is indicated at the top right of each panel for control (bottom) and bicuculline (top) conditions. An error of 0.01 indicates that each data point was, on average, 0.1 log units from the plotted curve. The low error for each cell indicates that a good fit of the curves to the data points was achieved both in the predrug control condition and during bicuculline. This means that the four receptive-field parameters: center radius ($R_c$) and sensitivity ($K_c$) and surround radius ($R_s$) and sensitivity ($K_s$) that produce the curves were accurately specified by the difference of Gaussians fits to the data under both conditions (from Norton et al., 1989).

sensitivity at low spatial frequencies might be due to a decrease in surround sensitivity. However, it could also be due to an increase in center sensitivity. To illustrate that an elevation in sensitivity to low spatial frequencies could have been achieved in the tree shrew cells simply by changing the center sensitivity, the dark solid line in Fig. 13C shows the effect of increasing just $K_c$, leaving all other parameters at the predrug levels. This change in only the center sensitivity matches the increase in the low spatial frequency roll-off.

In conclusion, microiontophoresis of bicuculline, which we have found increases the transfer ratio in the LGN in cats, increases the receptive-field center sensitivity of LGN cells in tree shrew in keeping with the predictions of the model shown in Fig. 11C. Thus, GABAergic circuitry at the LGN can control a parameter of fundamental importance to vision: the sensitivity of cells to stimuli.

*Effects of brainstem stimulation*

The possibility was raised earlier that the GABAergic inhibitory circuitry may, in turn, be regulated by brainstem or other afferent connec-

tions to the LGN such as the cholinergic connections from the parabrachial region (PBR) that were described in more detail earlier in this volume (Uhlrich and Cucchiaro, Chapter 9). Acetylcholine has been shown in in vitro slice preparations to directly excite the LGN relay cells and to inhibit interneurons and cells in the perigeniculate nucleus (McCormick and Prince, 1986, 1988; McCormick and Pape, 1988). Thus, activation of a major source of cholinergic input to the LGN from the PBR should reduce the GABAergic influences and increase the transfer ratio. This, in turn should increase the contrast sensitivity of the LGN cells. Recent experiments in anesthetized cats by Uhlrich et al. (1989) support this suggestion. For example, the cat LGN cell shown in Fig. 14A increased its responsiveness to a drifting sine-wave grating during electrical stimulation of the PBR. As also shown in Fig. 14B, the responses of the cell to a drifting grating of fixed contrast were increased during the PBR stimulation at all of the spatial frequencies examined. DOG curves were fit to the response data under the nonstimulated control condition and during brainstem stimulation. Comparison of the four

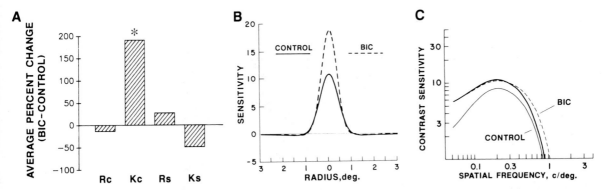

Fig. 13. Data from 10 tree shrew LGN relay cells before and during bicuculline administration. A. Average percent change of the center ($R_c$, $K_c$) and surround ($R_s$, $K_s$) parameters derived from the difference of Gaussians curves fit to the contrast sensitivity. Only the center sensitivity ($K_c$) was significantly changed during bicuculline ($t$-test, $P < 0.05$). B. Average receptive-field profiles (surround subtracted from center as in Fig. 11B) before (solid line) and during (dotted line) bicuculline. The primary change is that the center sensitivity was increased. C. Average contrast sensitivity functions showing the elevation in sensitivity during bicuculline (dashed line) in comparison to the predrug control level (solid line). The bold solid line models the effect on the predrug contrast sensitivity function of increasing only the receptive-field center sensitivity. At peak and at low spatial frequencies a change in this one parameter (leaving surround sensitivity constant) produced a change in the function that resembled the increase seen under bicuculline (from Norton et al., 1989).

receptive-field parameters under the two conditions (Fig. 14C) found that the receptive-field center sensitivity increased and that there was little change in the other parameters. Increased center sensitivity has been a consistent finding in other cells examined by Uhlrich et al. (1989). The effect of brainstem stimulation on surround sensitivity has been variable, increasing in some cells, decreasing in others and remaining approximately the same in still others.

The data both in tree shrew and in cat thus support the conclusion that GABAergic inhibitory circuitry controls the sensitivity of LGN cells to visual stimuli. As summarized in Fig. 15, the sensitivity profile of the ganglion cell is set by the retinal circuitry. If each retinal action potential were transferred through the LGN, the sensitivity profile would also be unchanged in the LGN. The GABAergic inhibitory pathways at the level of the LGN, by controlling the transfer ratio, modulate the sensitivity of the LGN cells, reducing it to 0 if the inhibition is sufficient to reduce the transfer ratio to 0. Brainstem inputs to the LGN, such as the cholinergic input, are in a position to act globally across the entire LGN, controlling the transfer ratio (and hence the sensitivity) throughout the visual field. Thus, in a sleeping or anesthetized animal, in which transfer might be expected to be low (Figs. 4B and 6), the sensitivity would be reduced at the LGN. Trans-

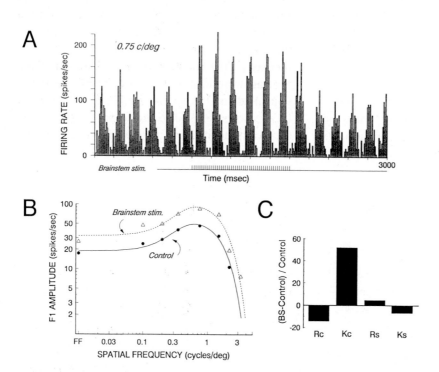

Fig. 14. Data from Uhlrich et al. (1989) showing the effect of stimulating the brainstem parabrachial region on the responses of an LGN X cell in cat. A. Responses to a drifting sine-wave grating (0.75 c/degree) before, during and after electrical stimulation (50 Hz) indicated by the vertical time marks. B. Responses to several spatial frequencies before (control, filled circles) and during brainstem electrical stimulation (open triangles). The amplitude of the response at the fundamental drift frequency (6 Hz) was determined for each spatial frequency and for full-field sinusoidal modulation of the oscilloscope screen (FF). At 3 c/degree the control response was within the noise and was not plotted. During brainstem stimulation, the responses during the first 200 ms after stimulation onset were not averaged to avoid initial transient responses. The data were fitted with a difference of Gaussians function (solid and dashed lines) as in Fig. 12. C. Changes during brainstem stimulation of the 4 receptive-field parameters that underlie the contrast sensitivity functions were examined. In this example, center sensitivity ($K_c$) was increased while other parameters showed little alteration. Figure kindly provided by Dr. D. Uhlrich.

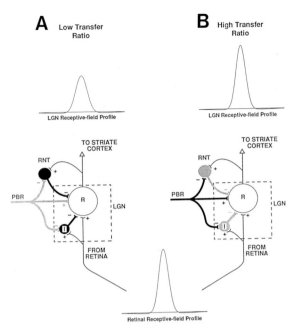

**A** Low Transfer Ratio

LGN Receptive-field Profile

TO STRIATE CORTEX

RNT

PBR

R

LGN

FROM RETINA

**B** High Transfer Ratio

LGN Receptive-field Profile

TO STRIATE CORTEX

RNT

PBR

R

LGN

FROM RETINA

Retinal Receptive-field Profile

Fig. 15. Schematic representation of the control of GABAergic inhibition at the LGN by brainstem cholinergic afferents from the parabrachial region (PBR) and their effect on the receptive-field sensitivity of LGN cells. A. When the brainstem afferents are less active, the GABAergic feedforward and feedback pathways act to reduce the transfer ratio at the LGN, reducing the sensitivity of the receptive-field profile of the LGN cell. B. When the brainstem inputs are active, as may occur during arousal, the GABAergic inhibitory pathways are inhibited and the relay neurons are facilitated (McCormick and Prince, 1986, 1988; McCormick and Pape, 1988), increasing the transfer ratio and, hence, the sensitivity profile of the LGN cell.

fer has not been measured in alert, behaving animals. Extrapolating from the data of Coenen and Vendrik (1972) transfer might be expected to be lower during inattentive states and higher when the animal is attending to visual stimuli.

As has been suggested by several authors (Tsumoto et al., 1978; Marrocco and McClurkin, 1985; Koch, 1987; Sillito and Murphy, 1988) the retinotopically organized corticogeniculate feedback pathway is in a position to control transfer focally within limited regions of the LGN. A focal elevation of transfer in a small LGN region against a background level of low transfer in the rest of the nucleus would increase the detectability of the visual signal that is passed on to the

striate cortex (Tsumoto et al., 1978; Koch, 1987). However, the effects of the corticogeniculate efferents on LGN cells are complex as is discussed in more detail in Chapter 17 of this volume (Sillito).

### Does the "inhibitory surround" get stronger at the LGN?

Previous studies of the LGN that have considered the responses of LGN and retinal cells have concluded that the receptive-field surround is strengthened at the LGN. Indeed, this is the one change that is generally attributed to the LGN in introductory textbooks. The data that lead to this conclusion are very clear. Hubel and Wiesel (1961) found that a small spot centered in the receptive field of an LGN cell produced a criterion response at a particular intensity. A stimulus of increased diameter that covered the center and the surround was then presented and the intensity of the larger spot was adjusted so that a retinal afferent (monitored by an opponent S-potential) produced a response comparable to the one induced by about the same as the small spot. Under these conditions, the LGN cell produced very few action potentials. The point was that the same, larger, spot that would drive the retinal afferent would not drive the LGN cell. This has been interpreted as a stronger effect of the surround upon the center, similar to the antagonistic effect of the retinal surround upon the center mechanism at the level of the bipolar or ganglion cell.

In considering the mechanisms that produced this change, it is important to remember that the antagonistic interaction between the retinal "center" and "surround" has already occurred in the retina before the action potentials are generated by the ganglion cell. Thus, the train of action potentials sent to the LGN already encodes a "center-minus-surround" message in which the number of action potentials emitted by the ganglion cell in response to a stimulus of a certain size and intensity is determined by its location in the receptive field (Fig. 11B). When these action potentials arrive at the LGN, what appears to change, depending on stimulus diameter, is the transfer ratio. With a small spot, the transfer ratio in the example shown by Hubel and Wiesel was about 0.3, and with the large spot, the transfer ratio was 0. The question then arises, what produces a lower transfer ratio when a larger stimulus is used? Although a complex pattern of "crossed inhibition" (Singer and Creutzfeldt, 1970) between on-center and off-center cells cannot be ruled out in cat, where on- and off-center cells are intermixed within LGN laminae, such a circuit seems most unlikely in tree shrew (Conway and Schiller, 1983; Holdefer and Norton, 1986) and other species (Zahs and Stryker, 1988) in which on- and off-center cells are segregated into separate laminae.

A simpler hypothesis is that the larger retinal spot used by Hubel and Wiesel (1961) excited additional retinal ganglion cells (dotted afferent connections in Fig. 1) that were not driven by the smaller spot. These additional ganglion cells could excite the feedforward and the feedback GABAergic pathways at the LGN, thereby reducing the transfer ratio of the cell that was being studied. The extent of the lateral connections of the feedforward inhibitory pathway is not known. However, in the feedback GABAergic pathway, it is known that the perigeniculate nucleus cells have large receptive fields that may integrate the output of many LGN cells and mediate a "long-range lateral inhibition" that has been measured by Eysel and Pape (1987). The activity of the additional retinal cells activated by the larger spot could readily excite additional LGN relay cells (R′ in Fig. 1) that would raise the activity in the feedback pathway, reducing the transfer ratio. Such an effect would not have been produced in the experiments we have reported in this chapter because the visual stimuli used to examine each cell always remained the same size.

Evidence that GABAergic inhibition produced Hubel and Wiesel's result has been provided by the data of Sillito and Kemp (1983). After repli-
cating the reduction in LGN cell response using a large diameter spot, they demonstrated that microiontophoretic administration of bicuculline increased the responses of LGN cells, to the same stimulus, in comparison with the predrug control condition. Based on the data shown in this chapter, this most likely was due to an elevation in the transfer ratio produced by the bicuculline. Thus, GABAergic regulation of the transfer ratio at the LGN appears to be the mechanism responsible for Hubel and Wiesel's effect.

Not only does control of the transfer ratio explain this classic result, it also explains why reduction of GABAergic influences with bicuculline iontophoresis "strengthens" the surround at least in one situation. When we and others (Sillito and Kemp, 1983; Eysel and Pape, 1987) have used an annulus to excite the LGN cell through its receptive-field surround, the response of LGN cells to this stimulus is increased by bicuculline. Once again, this occurs because the transfer ratio is increased. It matters not at all whether the retinal action potentials arriving at the LGN cell are produced by stimulating the retinal cell's center or its surround.

From the viewpoint of the cortical cells that receive the output of the LGN, it may not matter whether the reduced response received when a larger stimulus is used is due to a stronger retinal-type surround or to increased inhibition at the LGN which reduces the transfer; in either event, the cortical cell receives a weaker input, making the visual system less responsive to diffuse illumination. However, from the viewpoint of understanding the neural mechanisms that produce this reduction, it is indeed useful to know that this reduction is produced in the LGN by GABAergic circuitry controlling the transfer ratio.

In conclusion, the lateral geniculate nucleus appears to be organized to "set the stage" for the cortex in many ways, including retinotopic organization, laminar segregation and the relative representation of the parallel afferent pathways (Casagrande and Norton, 1991). As reviewed in this chapter, another important function that occurs at the LGN is control of the flow of visual information to the cortex. Recognition that the GABAergic inhibitory pathways can control the transfer ratio at the LGN provides a relatively simple explanation of a number of diverse changes that occur in the LGN and other thalamic relay structures (Gottschaldt et al., 1983). Control of the transfer ratio not only explains how changes in signal detectability and contrast sensitivity may occur, it also helps to explain the creation of a "strengthened inhibitory surround" at the LGN. Moreover, because the GABAergic circuitry at the LGN may itself be globally (Fig. 15) or focally controlled, it can serve as an early stage in the neural mechanisms that underlie attention.

## Note added in proof

We have now shown, and it has also been found by Hartveit and Heggelund (1991), that electrical stimulation of the parabrachial region of the brainstem increases the transfer ratio of LGN cells.

Hartveit, E. and Heggelund, P. (1991) The effect of brainstem peribrachial stimulation on the contrast-response properties of cells in the cat lateral geniculate nucleus. *Soc. Neurosci. Abstr.*, 17: 710.

## Acknowledgements

Much of the work reported in this chapter was supported by grants from the National Institutes of Health: R01 EY02909, T32 EY07033, F32 MH09693, BRSG RR05932, P30 EY03039 (CORE). We thank Mr. John T. Siegwart, Jr., for excellent technical assistance and Ms. Caroline W. Dunn for assistance in preparation of the manuscript. Mr. Ken Norris provided illustrations for some of the figures.

## References

Ahlsén, G., Lindström, S. and Lo, F.-S. (1985) Interaction between inhibitory pathways to principal cells in the lateral geniculate nucleus of the cat. *Exp. Brain Res.*, 58: 134–143.

Berardi, N. and Morrone, M.C. (1984) The role of gamma-aminobutyric acid mediated inhibition in the response properties of cat lateral geniculate nucleus neurones. *J. Physiol. (London)*, 357: 505–523.

Bishop, P.O., Burke, W. and Davis, R. (1962) The interpretation of the extracellular response of single lateral geniculate cells. *J. Physiol. (London)*, 162: 451–472.

Blakemore, C. and Vital-Durand, F. (1986) Organization and post-natal development of the monkey's lateral geniculate nucleus. *J. Physiol. (London)*, 380: 453–491.

Broadbent, D.E. (1958) *Perception and Communication*, Oxford: Pergamon Press, Inc.

Bullier, J. and Norton, T.T. (1979a) X and Y relay cells in the cat lateral geniculate nucleus: Quantitative analysis of receptive-field properties and classification. *J. Neurophysiol.*, 42: 244–273.

Bullier, J. and Norton, T.T. (1979b) Comparison of the receptive-field properties of X and Y ganglion cells with X and Y lateral geniculate cells in the cat. *J. Neurophysiol.*, 42: 274–291.

Casagrande, V.A. and Norton, T.T. (1991) The lateral geniculate nucleus: A review of its physiology and function. In: A.G. Leventhal (Ed.), *The Neural Basis of Visual Function, Vol. 4, Vision and Visual Dysfunction*, London: Macmillan, pp. 41–84.

Cleland, B.G. and Lee, B.B. (1985) A comparison of visual responses of cat lateral geniculate nucleus neurones with those of ganglion cells afferent to them. *J. Physiol. (London)*, 369: 249–268.

Cleland, B.G., Dubin, M.W. and Levick, W.R. (1971) Sustained and transient neurones in the cat's retina and lateral geniculate nucleus. *J. Physiol. (London)*, 217: 473–496.

Coenen, A.M.L. and Vendrik, A.J.H. (1972) Determination of the transfer ratio of cat's geniculate neurons through quasi-intracellular recordings and the relation with the level of alertness. *Exp. Brain Res.*, 14: 227–242.

Conway, J.L. and Schiller, P.H. (1983) Laminar organization of tree shrew lateral geniculate nucleus. *J. Neurophysiol.*, 50: 1330–1342.

Cucchiaro, J.B., Uhlrich, D.J. and Sherman, S.M. (1990) A projection from the thalamic reticular nucleus to the dorsal lateral geniculate nucleus in the cat: a comparison with the perigeniculate projection. *Soc. Neurosci. Abstr.*, 16: 159.

Dawis, S., Shapley, R., Kaplan, E. and Tranchina, D. (1984) The receptive field organization of X-cells in the cat: spatiotemporal coupling and asymmetry. *Vis. Res.*, 24: 549–564.

Downing, C.J. (1988) Expectancy and visual-spatial attention:

effects on perceptual quality. *J. Exp. Psychol. Hum. Percept. Perf.*, 14: 188–197.

Enroth-Cugell, C. and Robson, J.G. (1966) The contrast sensitivity of retinal ganglion cells of the cat. *J. Physiol. (London)*, 187: 517–552.

Enroth-Cugell, C. and Freeman, A.W. (1987) The receptive field spatial structure of cat retinal Y cells. *J. Physiol. (London)*, 384: 49–79.

Eysel, U.T. and Pape, H.-C. (1987) Lateral excitation in the cat lateral geniculate nucleus. *Exp. Brain Res.*, 67: 291–298.

Fitzhugh, R. (1957) The statistical detection of threshold signals in the retina. *J. Gen. Physiol.*, 40: 925–948.

Fitzpatrick, D., Penny, G.R. and Schmechel, D. (1984) Glutamic acid decarboxylase-immunoreactive neurons and terminals in the lateral geniculate nucleus of the cat. *J. Neurosci.*, 4: 1809–1829.

Fitzpatrick, D., Penny, G.R., Schmechel, D. and Diamond, I.T. (1982) GAD immunoreactive neurons in the lateral geniculate nucleus of the cat and *Galago*. *Soc. Neurosci. Abstr.*, 8: 261.

Godwin, D.W. and Norton, T.T. (1990) GABAergic modulation of the transfer ratio in cat lateral geniculate nucleus (LGN). *Soc. Neurosci. Abstr.*, 16: 160.

Gottschaldt, K.M., Vahle-Hinz, C. and Hicks, T.P. (1983) Electrophysiological and micropharmacological studies on mechanisms of input-output transformation in single neurones of the somatosensory thalamus. In G. Macchi, A. Rustioni and R. Spreafico (Eds.), *Somatosensory Integration in the Thalamus*, Amsterdam: Elsevier.

Hendrickson, A.E., Ogren, M.P., Vaughn, J.E., Barber, R.P. and Wu, J.Y. (1983) Light and electron microscopic immunocytochemical localization of glutamic acid decarboxylase in monkey geniculate complex: Evidence for GABAergic neurons and synapses. *J. Neurosci.*, 3: 1245–1262.

Hochstein, S. and Shapley, R.M. (1976a) Quantitative analysis of retinal ganglion cell classifications. *J. Physiol. (London)*, 262: 237–264.

Hochstein, S. and Shapley, R.M. (1976b) Linear and non-linear spatial subunits in Y cat retinal ganglion cells. *J. Physiol. (London)*, 262: 265–284.

Holdefer, R.N. and Norton, T.T. (1986) Laminar organization of receptive-field properties in the lateral geniculate nucleus of the tree shrew (*Tupaia belangeri*). *Soc. Neurosci. Abstr.*, 12: 8.

Holdefer, R.N., Norton, T.T. and Mize, R.R. (1988) Laminar organization and ultrastructure of GABA-immunoreactive neurons and processes in the dorsal lateral geniculate nucleus of the tree shrew (*Tupaia belangeri*). *Vis. Neurosci.*, 1: 189–204.

Holdefer, R.N., Norton, T.T. and Godwin, D.W. (1989) Effects of bicuculline on signal detectability in lateral geniculate nucleus relay cells. *Brain Res.*, 488: 341–347.

Hubel, D.H. and Wiesel, T.N. (1961) Integrative action in the cat's lateral geniculate body. *J. Physiol. (London)*, 155: 385–398.

Humphrey, A.L. and Norton, T.T. (1980) Topographic organization of the orientation column system in the striate

cortex of the tree shrew (*Tupaia glis*). I. Microelectrode recording. *J. Comp. Neurol.*, 192: 531–547.

Irvin, G.E., Norton, T.T. and Casagrande, V.A. (1986) Receptive-field properties derived from spatial contrast sensitivity measurements of primate LGN cells. *Invest. Ophthalmol. Vis. Sci. (Suppl.)* 27: 16.

Kaplan, E. (1991) The receptive field structure of retinal ganglion cells in cat and monkey. In A.G. Leventhal (ed.) *The Neural Basis of Visual Function, Vol. 4, Vision and Visual Dysfunction*, London: Macmillan, London, pp. 10–40.

Kaplan, E. and Shapley, R.M. (1982) X- and Y-cells in the lateral geniculate nucleus of macaque monkeys. *J. Physiol. (London)*, 330: 125–143.

Kaplan, E. and Shapley, R. (1984) The origin of the S (slow) potential in the mammalian lateral geniculate nucleus. *Exp. Brain Res.*, 55: 111–116.

Kaplan, E., Purpura, K. and Shapley, R.M. (1987) Contrast affects the transmission of visual information through the mammalian lateral geniculate nucleus. *J. Physiol. (London)*, 391: 267–288.

Koch, C. (1987) The action of the corticofugal pathway on sensory thalamic nuclei: A hypothesis. *J. Neurosci.*, 23: 399–406.

Lindström, S. (1982) Synaptic organization of inhibitory pathways to principal cells in the lateral geniculate nucleus of the cat. *Brain Res.*, 234: 447–453.

Linsenmeier, R.A., Frishman, L.J., Jakiela, H.G. and Enroth-Cugell, C. (1982) Receptive field properties of X and Y cells in the cat retina derived from contrast sensitivity measurements. *Vis. Res.*, 22: 1173–1183.

Livingstone, M.S. and Hubel, D.H. (1981) Effects of sleep and arousal on the processing of visual information in the cat. *Nature*, 291: 554–561.

Lu, S.-M., Lo, F.S. and Sherman, S.M. (1989) Burst discharges of neurons of the lateral geniculate nucleus in cats. *Soc. Neurosci. Abstr.*, 15: 1393.

Lu, S.-M., Guido, W. and Sherman, S.M. (1990) Low threshold calcium spikes in LGN cells during responses to visual stimuli. *Soc. Neurosci. Abstr.*, 16: 159.

Marrocco, R.T. and McClurkin, J.W. (1985) Evidence for spatial structure in the cortical input to monkey lateral geniculate nucleus. *Exp. Brain Res.*, 59: 50–56.

Mastronarde, D.N. (1987) Two classes of single-input X-cells in cat lateral geniculate nucleus. II. Retinal inputs and the generation of receptive-field properties. *J. Neurophysiol.*, 57: 381–413.

McCormick, D.A. and Feeser, H.R. (1990) Functional implications of burst firing and single spike activity in lateral geniculate relay neurons. *Neuroscience*, 39: 103–113.

McCormick, D.A. and Pape, H.C. (1988) Acetylcholine inhibits identified interneurons in the cat lateral geniculate nucleus. *Nature*, 334: 246–248.

McCormick, D.A. and Prince, D.A. (1986) Acetylcholine induces burst firing in thalamic reticular neurons by activating a potassium conductance. *Nature*, 319: 402–405.

McCormick, D.A. and Prince, D.A. (1988) Noradrenergic

modulation of firing pattern in guinea pig and cat thalamic neurons, in vitro. *J. Neurophysiol.*, 59: 978–996.

Moore, G.P., Perkel, D.H. and Segundo, J.P. (1966) Statistical analysis and functional interpretation of neuronal spike data. *Ann. Rev. Physiol.*, 28: 493–522.

Norton, T.T. and Godwin, D.W. (1990) Inhibitory control of visual signals at the lateral geniculate nucleus (LGN) by GABAergic circuitry. *Invest. Ophthalmol. Vis. Sci.* (*Suppl.*) 31: 174.

Norton, T.T., Casagrande, V.A., Irvin, G.E., Sesma, M.A. and Petry, H.M. (1988) Contrast sensitivity functions of W-, X- and Y-like relay cells in lateral geniculate nucleus of bush baby (*Galago crassicaudatus*). *J. Neurophysiol.*, 59: 1639–1656.

Norton, T.T., Holdefer, R.N. and Godwin, D.W. (1989) Effects of bicuculline on receptive-field center sensitivity of relay cells in the lateral geniculate nucleus. *Brain Res.*, 488: 352–358.

Palmer, L.A., Jones, J.P. and Stepnowski, R.A. (1991) Striate receptive fields as linear filters: characterization in two dimensions of space. In A.G. Leventhal (Ed.), *The Neural Basis of Visual Function, Vol. 4, Vision and Visual Dysfunction*, London: MacMillan, pp 246–265.

Posner, M.I. (1980) Orienting of attention. *Quart. J. Exp. Psychol.*, 32: 3–25.

Posner, M.I. and Petersen, S.E. (1990) The attention system of the human brain. *Ann. Rev. Neurosci.*, 13: 25–42.

Raczkowski, D., Hamos, J.E. and Sherman, S.M. (1988) Synaptic circuitry of physiologically identified W-cells in the cat's dorsal lateral geniculate nucleus. *J. Neurosci.*, 8: 31–48.

Rodieck, R.W. and Stone, J. (1965) Analysis of receptive fields of cat retinal ganglion cells. *J. Neurophysiol.*, 28: 833–849.

Sherman, S.M. and Koch, C. (1986) The control of retinogeniculate transmission in the mammalian lateral geniculate nucleus. *Exp. Brain Res.*, 63: 1–20.

Sherman, S.M., Schumer, R.A. and Movshon, J.A. (1984) Functional cell classes in the macaque's LGN. *Soc. Neurosci. Abstr.*, 10: 296.

Sillito, A.M. and Kemp, J.A. (1983) The influence of GABAergic inhibitory processes on the receptive field structure of X and Y cells in cat dorsal lateral geniculate nucleus (dLGN). *Brain Res.*, 277: 63–77.

Sillito, A.M. and Murphy, P.C. (1988) The modulation of the retinal relay to the cortex in the dorsal lateral geniculate nucleus. *Eye (Suppl.)*, 2: s221–s232.

Singer, W. and Creutzfeldt, O. (1970) Reciprocal lateral inhibition of On- and Off-center neurones in the lateral geniculate nucleus of the cat. *Exp. Brain Res.*, 10: 311–330.

Soltesz, I., Lightowler, S., Leresche, N. and Crunelli, V. (1989) On the properties and origin of the GABA$_B$ inhibitory postsynaptic potential recorded in morphologically identified projection cells of the cat dorsal lateral geniculate nucleus. *Neuroscience*, 33: 23–33.

Soodak, R.E., Shapley, R.M. and Kaplan, E. (1987) Linear mechanisms of orientation tuning in the retina and lateral geniculate nucleus of the cat. *J. Neurophysiol.*, 58: 267–275.

Steriade, M., Jones, E.G. and Llinas, R.R. (1990) *Thalamic Oscillations and Signalling.* New York: Wiley.

Sterling, P. and Davis, T.L. (1980) Neurons in cat lateral geniculate nucleus that concentrate exogenous [$^3$H]-γ-aminobutyric acid (GABA). *J. Comp. Neurol.*, 192: 737–749.

Swets, J.A., Tanner, W.P. and Birdsall, T.G. (1964) Decision processes in perception. In J.A. Swets (Ed.) *Signal Detection and Recognition by Human Observers*, New York: Wiley.

Tootle, J.S. Coleman, L.A. and Friedlander, M.J. (1989) Convergence and input-output relations in the cat dorsal lateral geniculate nucleus assessed by S potential recordings. *Soc. Neurosci. Abstr.*, 15: 174.

Troy, J.B. (1983) Spatial contrast sensitivities of X and Y type neurons in the cat's dorsal lateral geniculate nucleus. *J. Physiol.* (*London*), 344: 399–417.

Troy, J.B. and Enroth-Cugell, C. (1989) Dependence of center radius on temporal frequency for the receptive-fields of X retinal ganglion cells in cat. *J. Gen. Physiol.*, 94: 987–995.

Tsumoto, T., Creutzfeldt, O.D. and Legendy, C.R. (1978) Functional organization of the corticofugal system from visual cortex to lateral geniculate nucleus in the cat. *Exp. Brain Res.*, 32: 345–364.

Uhlrich, D.J., Tamamaki, N., Murphy, P.C. and Sherman, S.M. (1989) Brainstem modulation of geniculate cells in cats. *Soc. Neurosci. Abstr.*, 15: 175.

Wang, C., Cleland, B.G. and Burke, W. (1985) Synaptic delay in the lateral geniculate nucleus of the cat. *Brain Res.*, 343: 236–245.

Wilson, J.R., Bullier, J. and Norton, T.T. (1988) Signal-to-noise comparisons for X and Y cells in the retina and lateral geniculate nucleus of the cat. *Exp. Brain Res.*, 20: 399–405.

Wilson, J.R., Friedlander, M.J. and Sherman, S.M. (1984) Fine structural morphology of identified X- and Y-cells in the cat's lateral geniculate nucleus. *Proc. R. Soc. Lond.*, 221: 411–436.

Zahs, K.-R. and Stryker, M.P. (1988) Segregation of On and Off afferents to ferret visual cortex. *J. Neurophysiol.*, 59: 1410–1429.

R.R. Mize, R.E. Marc and A.M. Sillito (Eds.)
Progress in Brain Research, Vol. 90
© 1992 Elsevier Science Publishers B.V. All rights reserved

CHAPTER 11

# The organization of GABAergic neurons
# in the mammalian superior colliculus

R. Ranney Mize *

*Department of Anatomy and Neurobiology and the Center for Neuroscience, College of Medicine, The University of Tennessee,
Memphis, TN 38163, USA*

## Introduction

The superior colliculus (SC) plays an essential role in visuomotor behavior. The SC is involved in detecting moving objects in the visual field, in directing attention to and orienting towards those objects, and in generating voluntary and involuntary eye movements, particularly saccades (Schiller, 1972; Wurtz and Albano, 1980; Sparks and Mays, 1981; Chalupa, 1984; Hall and May, 1984). The inhibitory neurotransmitter gamma-aminobutyric acid (GABA) contributes to the control of these visuomotor behaviors. This function is well-understood in some of these behaviors, particularly the gating of saccadic eye movements (Wurtz and Hikosaka, 1986). The mechanism of GABA in other visuomotor behaviors is poorly understood even though we have a solid understanding of the anatomical organization and physiological actions of GABA in SC.

The superior colliculus has one of the highest concentrations of GABA found in the central nervous system. High levels of GABA are present as measured by biochemical analysis (Okada, 1974, 1976; Chapter 12; Lund Karlsen and Fonnum, 1978; Fonnum et al., 1979; Kvale et al., 1983; Fosse et al., 1989) and by immunocyto-

chemistry (Mugnaini and Oertel, 1985). Superior colliculus neurons contain both GABA and its synthetic enzyme, glutamic acid decarboxylase (GAD) (Okada, 1974; Houser et al., 1983; Mugnaini and Oertel, 1985; Mize, 1988). There is also a high affinity uptake system for GABA in SC (Mize et al., 1981). GABA can be released in SC tissue slices by potassium-dependent stimulation (Sandberg et al., 1982; Sandberg and Corazzi, 1983) and iontophoretic application of GABA can reduce stimulus evoked and spontaneous activity in some SC neurons (Kawai and Yamamoto, 1967; Straschill and Perwein, 1971; Okada and Saito, 1979; Kayama et al., 1980). GABA or GABA ligands also bind with specificity to both $GABA_A$ and $GABA_B$ receptors (Young and Kuhar, 1979; Bowery et al., 1984; 1987). GABA thus fulfills many of the criteria as an inhibitory neurotransmitter in the mammalian superior colliculus.

Much is also known about the anatomical organization of GABA neurons in the mammalian superior colliculus. The purpose of this chapter is to review this organization. I have attempted to answer the following questions regarding the organization of GABA in SC. First, is there a laminar pattern to the distribution of GABA containing neurons in SC and does this pattern differ in different mammalian species? Second, are there many separate classes of GABA neuron as is the case in visual cortex, or are there only

---

\* Current address: Department of Anatomy, Louisiana State University Medical Centre, New Orleans, LA 70112, USA.

one or two cell types as is thought to be the case in the lateral geniculate nucleus? Third, how are GABA neurons organized synaptically and how might these GABAergic synaptic circuits relate to the functions of these neurons? Fourth, how are GABA receptors distributed in SC and how are they related to GABA containing neurons? Fifth, do GABA containing neurons in the SC co-localize other neuroactive substances, which might distinguish these cell types or help explain their function? Finally, is GABA content in SC cells modified by manipulations of the environment such as monocular deprivation?

## General organization of the mammalian superior colliculus

The mammalian superior colliculus is a highly laminated structure, consisting of the zonal, superficial gray, optic, intermediate gray and white, and deep gray and white layers (Kanaseki and Sprague, 1974; Huerta and Harting, 1984). These layers can be divided into two functionally distinct units: a superficial subdivision and a deep subdivision (Harting et al., 1973; Edwards, 1980). The superficial subdivision is involved in the detection of purely visual stimuli and lesions of it produce deficits in some forms of visual discrimination (Casagrande et al., 1972). The superficial layers of SC receive significant inputs from both the retina and visual cortex, as well as several subcortical nuclei. These layers contain neurons which project to several targets in the diencephalon, including the dorsal and ventral lateral geniculate nuclei, the lateral posterior nucleus, and the pretectum (see Huerta and Harting, 1984, for review). Superficial neurons are movement sensitive and/or directionally selective and probably designed to detect or track moving objects in the visual field (Sterling and Wickelgren, 1969; Stein and Arigbede, 1972; Rosenquist and Palmer, 1971; Mize and Murphy, 1976).

The deep subdivision of the superior colliculus is multimodal and is involved in motor related behaviors. Lesions involving the deep layers produce profound deficits in visual orienting (Casagrande et al., 1972). The deep layers receive major inputs from extrastriate cortical areas, the substantia nigra, and a variety of other brainstem and oculomotor related regions of the brain. These layers in turn project principally to descending targets, including major pathways through the contralateral predorsal bundle to the medulla and spinal cord and through the ipsilateral tecto-ponto-bulbar pathway to the midbrain and pons (see Huerta and Harting, 1984, for review; Moschovakis and Karabelas, 1985; Redgrave et al., 1986). Many neurons in the deep layers respond to somatic and auditory as well as visual stimuli (Stein et al., 1975, 1976). Many cells also respond in relation to saccadic eye movements (Wurtz and Albano, 1980; Sparks and Mays, 1981). GABA has been shown to gate the response of these neurons (Hikosaka and Wurtz, 1985a,b).

The projection neurons of both the superficial and deep subdivisions are at least partially segregated by layer. Ascending projection neurons are located principally in the superficial layers while the descending projection neurons are found principally in the deep layers (Huerta and Harting, 1984). Even within a layer, projection neurons to particular targets vary in distribution. Thus, for example, neurons projecting to the dorsal and ventral lateral geniculate nuclei are most densely distributed within the upper superficial gray layer while those projecting to the lateral posterior nucleus complex are most densely concentrated within the deep superficial gray layer (Kawamura et al., 1980; Caldwell and Mize, 1981; Harrell et al., 1982; Abramson and Chalupa, 1988).

## Distribution of GABA neurons in the superior colliculus

Despite the impressive segregation of projection neurons, there is no apparent laminar segregation of GABA neurons in the superior colliculus of any mammal so far studied. GABA or GAD immunoreactive neurons are found throughout the superior colliculus of the rat, mouse, cat, rabbit, opossum, tree shrew and Rhesus and Cynomolgous monkey (Houser et al., 1983; Ottersen and Storm-Mathisen 1984; Penny et al., 1984; Mize and Norton, 1985; Mugnaini and Oertel, 1985; Horn and Hoffmann, 1987; Mize, 1988; Pinard et al., 1990a; Warton et al., 1990; Mize et al., 1991a). The density of these GABA neurons does vary in different layers, but this variability appears to be closely related to the density of the total population of neurons in a given layer.

Figure 1 shows the distribution of GABA neurons in the superior colliculus of the Rhesus monkey. Although GABA immunoreactive neurons are most densely concentrated within the zonal and upper superficial gray layer (SGL), labeled neurons can also be seen throughout the optic, intermediate and deep layers of SC (Fig. 1). Quantitative plots of this distribution in monkey show that about one-third (32.5%) of the labeled neurons fall within the zonal and superficial gray layers, about 16% within the optic layer, 13% in the intermediate gray layer and 38% in the deep gray and white layers (Mize et al., 1991a). The densest concentration of GABA-labeled neurons is also found in the superficial layers of the cat and tree shrew, although the precise distribution differs somewhat for each species (Mize and Norton, 1985; Mize, 1988). Regardless of these fine variations, a principal feature of organization in the SC of mammals is that GABAergic neurons are distributed throughout all layers of the structure.

The reason(s) for the differences in labeled neuron density in different laminae is uncertain. One possibility is that the density of GABA neurons reflects the density of the total neuron population in these layers. Figure 2 shows the density of GABA neurons at different depths within the SC of cat compared to the density of unlabeled neurons at those same depths. This figure illustrates two points. First, GABA-labeled neurons represent between 40–55% of all neurons within the zonal, superficial gray, optic and intermediate

gray layers. Second, GABA neurons are a fairly constant ratio of the total cell population within these four layers. This ratio does not hold for the deepest layers where the percentage of GABA neurons is lower. These data suggest that there is a constant relationship between GABA cells and unlabeled cells within the dorsal four layers of SC, a phenomenon also reported for the four parvicellular layers of the tree shrew lateral geniculate nucleus (Holdefer et al., 1988).

The different densities of GABA neurons in different layers is also reflected in biochemical assays which show that concentrations of GABA are highest within the zonal and SGL, are reduced by about one-third in the optic and intermediate gray, and are lowest in the deepest layers of SC in the cat, guinea pig and rabbit (Okada, 1974, 1976; Chapter 12; Arakawa and Okada, 1988; Kanno and Okada, 1988). The density of $GABA_A$ and $GABA_B$ receptors is also reported to be highest within the SGL and to decrease in the deepest layers (see below, GABA receptor distribution). There thus appears to be a close relationship between the intrinsic GABA neuron density and the concentration of GABA receptor sites in the superior colliculus of all mammals studied to date.

**Morphology of GABAergic neurons in SC**

Virtually all GABA neurons in the superior colliculus are small to medium sized cells (Fig. 1), as shown by GAD and GABA immunocytochemistry or by uptake of exogenous GABA (Mize et al., 1981, 1982; Houser et al., 1983; Mugnaini and Oertel, 1985; Mize, 1988; Mize et al., 1991a). A comparison of cell size in the cat, tree shrew and Rhesus monkey reveals that the vast majority of neurons range from 9–15 $\mu$m in diameter in each species (Mize and Norton, 1985; Mize, 1988; Mize et al., 1991a). Very few larger neurons are found, and these are widely scattered within the deep layers. Despite the relatively uniform size of these neurons, they clearly differ in morphology. At the light microscope level, horizontal, pyriform and

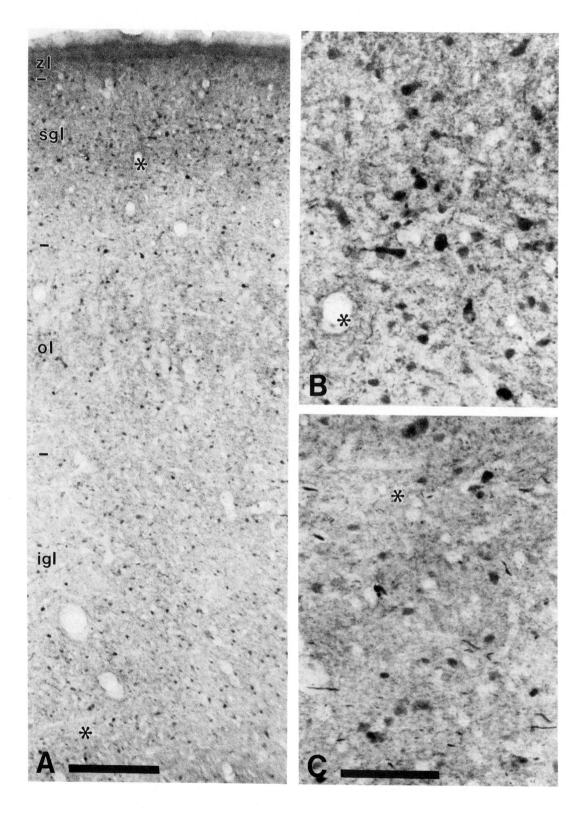

small stellate-like neurons have been identified in cat and monkey using GABA antibody immunocytochemistry (Mize, 1988; Mize et al., 1991a). Horizontal neurons have horizontally elongated fusiform cell bodies with stout dendrites coursing horizontally near the surface of the colliculus (Fig. 3A). These neurons are found mostly in the upper SGL, very rarely beneath that subdivision. Their number varies in different species. GABA immunoreactive horizontal neurons are fairly common in cat, less frequent in tree shrew, and relatively rare in the Rhesus monkey (Mize and Norton, 1985; Mize, 1988; Mize et al., 1991a).

GABA immunoreactive pyriform neurons have pear-shaped cell bodies often with a single thick, prominent dendrite directed superficially towards the surface of the colliculus (Fig. 3B,C). This type of cell is very common within the upper SGL in monkey, cat and tree shrew. The pyriform cell has also been described in Golgi studies in cat (Sterling, 1971; Langer, 1976), rat (Langer and Lund 1974) and monkey (Laemle, 1981).

Many GABA-labeled neurons found beneath the upper SGL are small round or stellate-shaped neurons whose morphologies are ill-defined in immunoreactive material (Fig. 3D,E). These cells are not distinctive in the light microscope because their dendrites are poorly filled with reaction product. However, electron microscope reconstructions of GABA-labeled neurons suggest these cells are a distinct cell type.

At least three separate GABA containing cell types can be recognized in electron microscope reconstructions (Mize et al., 1982). These neurons, identified by accumulation of exogenously applied GABA, were reconstructed from serial thin sections (Fig. 4). Neurons of similar morphologies have been shown to accumulate [³H]muscimol (Mize and White, 1989) and to be

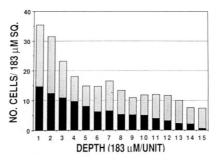

Fig. 2. Histogram illustrating the density and ratio of GABA-labeled and unlabeled neurons at different depths within the SC of the cat. GABA-labeled neurons range from 9 to 54% of the total population of neurons. The ratio of labeled to unlabeled cells is relatively constant within the zl, sgl, ol and igl (upper 10 depth units). From Mize, 1988.

labeled by antibodies to GABA (Mize, 1988), although they were not serially reconstructed in the latter studies.

The three GABA-labeled cell types were originally called horizontal, granule A and granule C cells (Mize et al., 1982). The horizontal cells had oblong fusiform somata and thick horizontally distributed dendrites (Fig. 4A). In extensive reconstructions they were found to have punctate accumulations of synaptic vesicles and to form dendro-dendritic synapses. Horizontal neurons received few synaptic inputs, over half of which came from Areas 17–18 of visual cortex. These cells are therefore distinguished by their soma and dendritic morphology, by the type of presynaptic dendrite, and by the source and density of their synaptic input.

GABA accumulating granule A neurons are probably pyriform neurons. These neurons had small round or pyriform cell bodies and thin dendrites with no consistent orientation (Fig. 4B). In one case, an initial segment was identified, suggesting that these neurons have axons and might give rise to some of the GABA containing

Fig. 1. Distribution of neurons labeled by gamma aminobutyric acid (GABA) antibodies in the superior colliculus (SC) of the Rhesus monkey. A. Neuron distribution at low magnification. B,C. Higher magnification showing cell size and density in the zonal and superficial gray layers (B) and in the intermediate gray layer (C). Asterisks indicate regions in A that are enlarged in B,C. zl: zonal layer; sgl: superficial gray layer; ol: optic layer; igl: intermediate gray layer; and dgl: deep gray layer. Scale bar in A = 300 μm; B,C = 100 μm. Modified from Mize et al., 1991a.

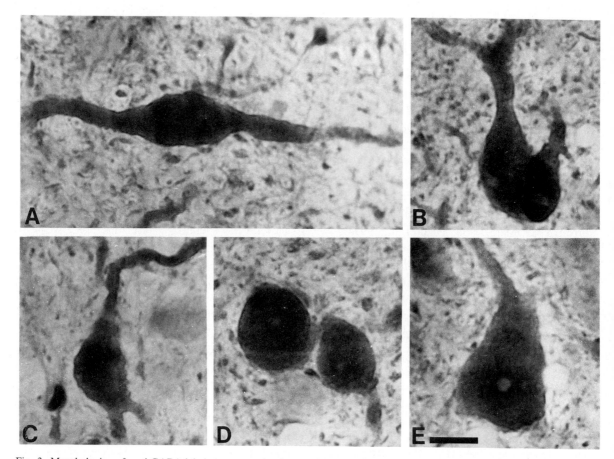

Fig. 3. Morphologies of anti-GABA-labeled neurons in the cat SC. A. Horizontal neuron with thick caliber dendrites. B,C. Pyriform neurons with pear-shaped cell bodies, ascending dendritic tree. D. Small round neurons with unclassified morphologies. E. Larger multipolar neuron with stellate-like cell body. Modified from Mize, 1988.

axon terminals within the SGL. Granule A neurons were shown to have a moderate synaptic input density, most of which came from unidentified sources and not from visual cortex. This cell type clearly differed from the horizontal cell in soma shape, dendritic morphology, the absence of proximal presynaptic dendrites, and a higher synaptic input density (Mize et al., 1982).

Granule C neurons are probably small stellate neurons (Mize et al., 1982). This cell type had a mean grain density lower than horizontal and granule A neurons but double that of any other reconstructed cell type (see Mize, 1988). Granule C neurons had somewhat larger somata and thicker dendrites than granule A cells. They had

a moderate synaptic input density, most of it from fibers other than those from visual cortex. The most distinctive feature of these neurons was the presence of somatic and dendritic spines which contained pleomorphic synaptic vesicles. Vesicle containing dendritic spines also were found to be labeled by GABA antibodies (Mize, 1988), confirming that this cell type is probably a third class of GABA neuron.

Several GABA-accumulating cell types have also been identified in the tectum of birds using autoradiographic uptake of tritiated GABA (Hunt and Kunzle, 1976). These cell types include: (1) horizontal cells with presynaptic dendrites located in sublayer IId; (2) a small stellate neuron

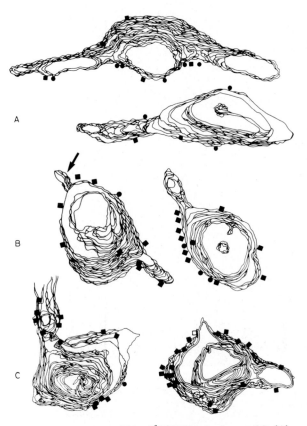

Fig. 4. Neurons accumulating [³H]GABA in the cat SC. (A) Horizontal neurons with fusiform cell bodies and thick horizontal dendrites. B. Granule A neurons with pyriform shaped cell bodies and obliquely oriented dendrites. Arrow indicates an initial axon segment. C. Granule C neurons with stellate-shaped cell bodies and somatic and dendritic spines. Symbols: circles, degenerating cortical terminals; squares, synapses of unknown origin. Modified from Mize et al., 1982.

nals, are labeled by GABA in both birds and mammals, suggesting that common cell types may exist in a variety of species.

## Ultrastructural organization of GABAergic neurons

At least three separate types of synaptic profile labeled by GABA can be identified in the superior colliculus. The first of these is one type of presynaptic dendrite (PSD) commonly found in relationship to retinal terminals. Retinal terminals in the SGL of the rat, cat, tree shrew and monkey are organized in a fashion similar to those seen in the W layers of the dorsal lateral geniculate nucleus and in the ventral LGN (Mize and Horner, 1984; Mize et al., 1986). They have characteristic pale mitochondria, round synaptic vesicles and a scalloped shape, and they form synaptic islands which are similar to the synaptic glomeruli found in the LGN (Lund, 1969, 1972; Sterling, 1971; Behan, 1981; Mize, 1983a,b; Mize and Norton, 1985; Carter et al., 1989). Retinal terminals in SC contact both conventional dendrites and presynaptic dendrites (Fig. 5). The conventional dendrites are small, thin dendritic thorns, some of which arise from the distal dendrites of vertical fusiform neurons lying deeper within the SGL (Mize and Sterling, 1976).

The presynaptic dendrites (PSDs) within the synaptic islands usually contain loose accumulations of pleomorphic synaptic vesicles which are scattered throughout the cytoplasm of the dendrite (Fig. 5). The vesicles are small and round or ovoid in shape but are rarely dramatically flattened. By definition, PSDs receive synaptic input from retinal or other vesicle containing terminals (Fig. 5A,B). PSDs also sometimes make postsynaptic contacts with conventional dendrites in the same plane of section (Fig. 5A).

The PSDs in the retinal synaptic islands are commonly labeled by GAD or GABA antibodies (Fig. 5B) (Houser et al., 1983; Mize, 1988; Pinard et al., 1990a; Mize et al., 1991a) and have been

in sublayer IIc with a superficial dendritic tree and descending axon; (3) a bipolar neuron in sublayer IIi with an axon thought to project to the thalamus (Hunt and Kunzle, 1976). Presynaptic dendrites and axon terminals in the pigeon optic tectum were also found to accumulate [³H]GABA (Streit et al., 1978). Although some of the morphological details of these cell types differ from those found in cat, at least two of the synaptic profiles, presynaptic dendrites and axon termi-

226

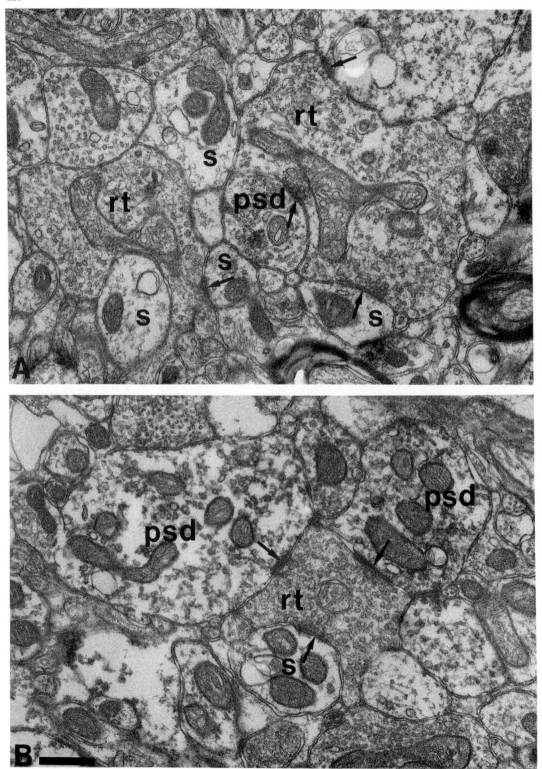

Fig. 5. Retinal terminals within the synaptic islands of the SGL of the Rhesus monkey SC. A. Two retinal terminals (rt) with pale mitochondria making synaptic contact with a presynaptic dendrite (psd) and a number of spine-like processes (s). Note that the psd contains pleomorphic synaptic vesicles. B. Retinal terminal (rt) making synaptic contact with two presynaptic dendrites (psd) labeled by anti-GABA and with an unlabeled spine (s). Scale bar = 0.5 $\mu$m. From Mize et al., 1991a.

shown to accumulate exogenous [$^3$H]GABA in autoradiography experiments (Mize et al., 1981, 1982). This type of PSD has been described in the SC of a variety of species (rat: Lund, 1969; hamster: Carter et al., 1989; cat: Sterling, 1971; mouse: Valderde, 1973; chimpanzee: Tigges and Tigges, 1975; monkey: Lund, 1972). These PSDs are quite similar to the F2 presynaptic dendrites originally described by Guillery (1969) in the cat LGN (see Uhlrich and Cucchiaro, Chapter 9). We hypothesize but have not proven that these PSDs arise from the spines of GABA-labeled granule C neurons which have vesicle containing somatic and dendritic spines (Mize et al., 1982). Many PSDs have a varicose spine-like appearance and they can sometimes be seen to extend from a parent dendrite (Fig. 6A,B).

Another type of GABA-labeled PSD arises from horizontal cells. These PSDs are large calibre dendrites, often containing ribosomes, which have small, punctate accumulations of synaptic vesicles that are clustered near the synaptic density (Fig. 6C). In cat, these dendrites have been reconstructed back to their soma of origin in the upper SGL (Mize et al., 1982). Horizontal PSDs have also been identified in monkey (Mize et al., 1991a). These dendrites are similar to a class of presynaptic dendrite recently identified in the lateral geniculate nucleus in the cat (Hamos et al., 1985; Montero, 1989) and tree shrew (Holdefer et al., 1988).

A third type of GABA immunoreactive profile in the upper SGL, called an F profile, is thought to be an axon terminal (Fig. 7A–C). These terminals have bulbous shapes, contain mostly flattened vesicles, and form symmetric synaptic contacts with other profiles, either dendrites or somata. They usually can be distinguished from PSDs because of their shape, their smaller size, and the more flattened morphology of their synaptic vesicles. In addition, the vesicles are often more densely packed than those in PSDs. F terminals are always presynaptic, never postsynaptic (Fig. 7). We think they arise from a variety of sources, some extrinsic, others intrinsic (see

below). They are never found within the center of a retinal island, although they are sometimes found at the edges of these islands.

Some myelinated axons also exhibit GABA immunoreactivity. These axons are usually small calibre, thinly myelinated fibers, often with dense reaction product coating the microtubules. Dendrites without synaptic vesicles also are sometimes labeled by GABA antibodies (Fig. 6D). We do not know whether these profiles are PSDs cut transversely where no vesicles are present or are conventional dendrites from cell types which do not have presynaptic dendrites.

Presynaptic dendrites labeled by GABA antibodies also are found in the intermediate gray layer of the cat and monkey SC. The organization is not unlike the retinal synaptic islands in the SGL, except that the PSDs are contacted by non-retinal axon terminals. Putative axon terminals labeled by GABA are also found within the intermediate gray layer where they are more varied in morphology than in the SGL. Many GABA-labeled axon terminals in the intermediate gray layer are larger than those seen in the SGL, although they also contain dense accumulations of flattened synaptic vesicles and form symmetric synaptic contacts (Fig. 7E). These profiles are often seen in synaptic contact with cell bodies and proximal dendrites as well as on smaller, more distal dendrites (Fig. 7E). By contrast, axons in the SGL only contact dendrites, not somata. The possible sources of these putative labeled axon terminals are discussed in the following section.

GABA-labeled synaptic profiles are sometimes also found in contact with one another. In serial reconstructions of retinal synaptic islands in the Rhesus monkey SC we have shown that vesicle containing horizontal dendrites receive synaptic input from both axon terminals that contain flattened vesicles and also from other PSDs that contain pleomorphic synaptic vesicles (Fig. 8) (Mize et al., 1991a) This flattened vesicle upon flattened vesicle synaptic circuitry could be the structural basis of the GABAergic disinhibition

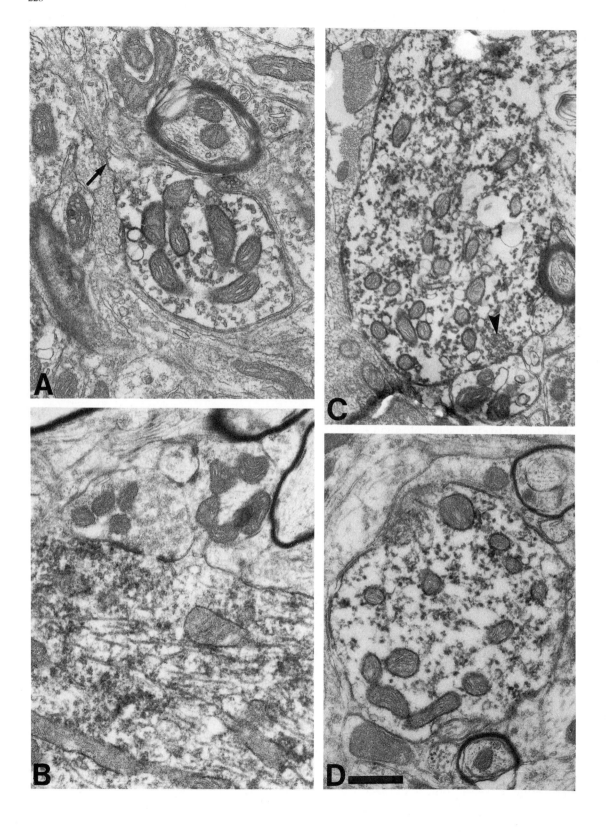

described by Okada (Chapter 12 and Arakawa and Okada, 1989).

## Extrinsic GABAergic projections to the superior colliculus

Superimposed upon the intrinsic GABA cell types are at least three well-defined GABAergic pathways to the superior colliculus. These are the pathways from the substantia nigra (Araki et al., 1984; Ficalora and Mize, 1989), the zona incerta (Araki et al., 1984; Ficalora and Mize, 1989) and the contralateral colliculus (Appell and Behan, 1990). Appel and Behan (1990) recently have shown that neurons in a variety of other diencephalic and brainstem structures that are labeled by GABA also send projections to the cat superior colliculus. These structures include the cuneiform nucleus, the subcuneiform area, the peri-parabigeminal area, the inferior colliculus, several nuclei of the lateral lemniscus, the perihypoglossal nucleus and several nuclei of the pretectal complex. However, the physiological action of these putative GABAergic projection neurons are unknown and the presence of light antibody labeling in some of these neurons suggests that they may not all use GABA as a neurotransmitter.

The SC pathway from the substantia nigra has long been thought to be inhibitory. Electrical or chemical stimulation of the SN inhibits neurons in the intermediate and deep gray layers of SC (Deniau et al., 1978; Chevalier et al., 1981a,b;). This inhibition can be reversibly blocked by biculline (Chevalier et al., 1981b; Hikosaka and Wurtz, 1983d). The same SC neurons can be inhibited by iontophoretic application of GABA into the deep layers of SC (Chevalier et al., 1981b). Recent evidence suggests that the SN pathway gates saccadic eye movements because SN cells tonically inhibit SC cells, an inhibition which is released just prior to saccades (Hikosaka and Wurtz, 1985a,b; reviewed further below and by Okada, Chapter 12). Biochemical studies also have shown that the SN pathway is GABAergic: electrolytic or kainic acid lesions of SN reduce biochemical levels of glutamic acid decarboxylase (GAD) in the deep layers of SC (Hattori et al., 1973; Vincent et al., 1978; DiChiara et al., 1979).

The inhibitory nature of the SN pathway is also supported by anatomical evidence. The hypertrophy of SN neurons that is induced by lesions of the frontal cortex and striatum leads to a concomitant increase in GABA-labeled fiber density in the rat SC (Pearson et al., 1987). Axon terminals in the deep layers of SC that are anterogradely labeled after injections into the SN of cats (Behan et al., 1987) and rats (Hattori et al., 1973; Vincent et al., 1978) have typical inhibitory morphologies, including pleomorphic vesicles and symmetric synaptic contacts. Immunocytochemical studies have shown that terminals with these characteristics are labeled by GAD or GABA in the deep layers of SC of cat (Mize, 1988) monkey (Mize et al., 1991a) and rat (Lu et al., 1985). These nigral synapses terminate primarily upon the distal dendrites of deep-layer efferent neurons (Lu et al., 1985; Behan et al., 1987), although some nigral terminals have also been shown to terminate directly upon the somata of tectospinal neurons.

Originally, the substantia nigra pathway was shown to project principally to the dorsal intermediate gray layer of the caudolateral SC where it formed distinctive patches of label (Graybiel, 1978; Illing and Graybiel, 1985). More recently, significant nigrotectal terminations have also been reported in other regions (Harting et al., 1988).

Fig. 6. Morphologies of presynaptic dendrites in the superior colliculus labeled by anti-GABA. A. Spine-like or varicose psd with pleomorphic synaptic vesicles found in the SGL of the Rhesus monkey SC. Arrow indicates thin stalk. B. Spine with pleomorphic synaptic vesicles attached to a GABA-labeled dendrite in the SGL of the cat SC. C. Non-varicose PSD with a small cluster of synaptic vesicles (arrowhead) from the SGL of the Rhesus monkey SC. D. Conventional dendrite with arrays of labeled microtubules in the cat SC. Scale bar = 0.5 $\mu$m. A,C taken from Mize et al., 1991a; B,D taken from Mize, 1988.

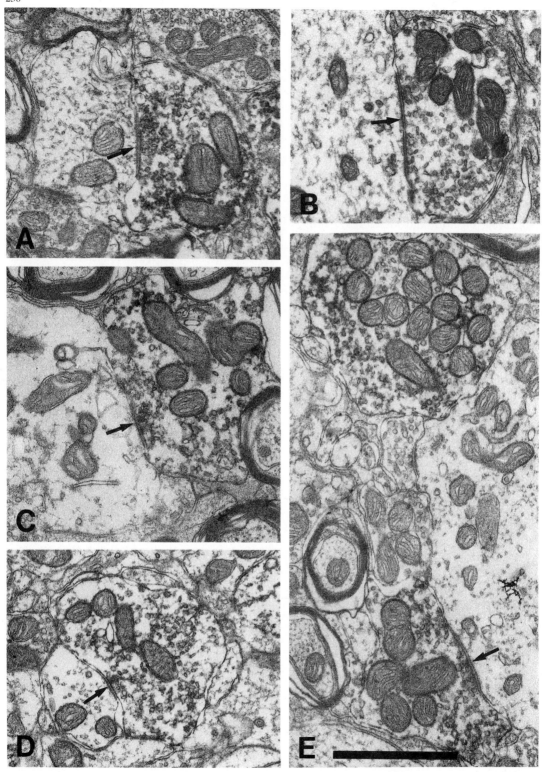

Fig. 7. Putative axon terminals labeled by anti-GABA in the Rhesus monkey SC. A–D show the relatively dense accumulation of flattened synaptic vesicles typical of axon terminal-like F profiles labeled by anti-GABA. E illustrates labeled F profiles found below the SGL of the Rhesus monkey SC. Scale bar = 1 $\mu$m. Modified from Mize et al., 1991a.

Harting et al. (1988), for example, have shown three separate tiers of input to the intermediate gray layer of the SC. These tiers probably arise from distinct regions or subdivisions of the substantia nigra complex.

Consistent with the evidence for multiple termination sites, the pathway from the substantia nigra has been shown to arise from both the pars reticulata and pars lateralis subdivisions in several species (May and Hall, 1986; Harting et al., 1988; Ficalora and Mize, 1989). Evidence that the cells in the pars lateralis and pars reticulata differ in size and morphology (Ficalora and Mize, 1989) further supports the notion that there are separate projections from the two subdivisions. Neurons in the pars lateralis are larger neurons with spindle shaped cell bodies and multipolar or bipolar dendrites while pars reticulata neurons are slightly smaller and have somewhat rounder cell bodies (Fig. 9). The significance of these differences in morphology is unknown.

Cells in both the pars reticulata and pars lateralis subdivisions are labeled by antibodies to GABA (Fig. 9) (Ficalora and Mize, 1989), GABA-T (Nagai et al., 1983) and GAD (Oertel et al., 1982). Earlier reports (Ottersen and Storm-Mathisen, 1984; Beckstead and Kersey, 1985) which failed to find significant labeling in SN to antibodies directed against GAD were apparently due to the low concentrations of the synthesizing enzyme in the somas of long projection neurons such as those in the substantia nigra.

The projection from the zona incerta (ZI) is a second major source of GABAergic input to the superior colliculus. This input arises primarily from neurons in the ventral ZI (Fig. 9) (Ficalora and Mize, 1989) which project both to the intermediate and deep gray layers (Ricardo, 1981; Rieck et al., 1986). Virtually all of these cells are labeled by GABA, GABA-T and GAD (Oertel et al., 1982; Araki et al., 1985; Ficalora and Mize, 1989). The function of this pathway is unknown, but its distribution appears to only partially overlap that of the substantia nigra. The morphology

of these neurons also differs from those in SN. Many neurons in ZI are smaller than those in SN and many GABA-labeled ZI neurons have a horizontal fusiform shape with dendrites extending mostly in a horizontal plane (Fig. 9).

The commissural projection from the opposite superior colliculus also apparently arises from neurons labeled by GABA antibodies (Appell and Behan, 1990). The cells of this pathway are located primarily within the intermediate gray layer of the rostral superior colliculus and terminate mainly within the intermediate gray layer in cat (Edwards, 1977; Edwards et al., 1979) and golden hamster (Fish et al., 1982)

These commissural cells were originally thought to mediate the Sprague effect. Behaviorally, cats receiving unilateral lesions of visual cortex show a profound neglect of the visual field contralateral to the lesion. This contralateral hemianopsia is ameliorated by lesioning the SC opposite the cortical lesion or by transecting the colliculus commissure (Sprague and Meikle, 1965; Sprague, 1966a,b). It was proposed that this recovery occurred because the commissural pathway was inhibiting the colliculus ipsilateral to the cortical lesion (Sprague, 1966b). However, recent evidence suggests that the effect is mediated by a pathway that originates in the substantia nigra. Neither transections of the rostral SC commissure, which cut all axons of tectotectal cells, nor ibotenic acid lesions of SC, which destroy tectotectal cells but spare fibers of passage, produce the expected recovery. Only transections of the caudal commissure ameliorate the effect (Wallace et al., 1989). Small ibotenic lesions of the lateral caudal portion of the pars reticulata appear to involve the critical site for the behavioral recovery, although the pathway mediating the effect is probably multisynaptic because SNR cells in this zone contribute few fibers to the caudal commissure (Wallace et al., 1990).

This behavioral phenomenon is consistent with the known tonic inhibition of tectal neurons produced by stimulation of the substantia nigra in monkey (Wurtz and Hikosaka, 1986) and cat

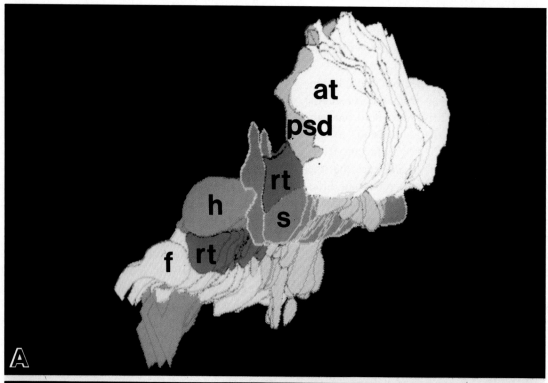

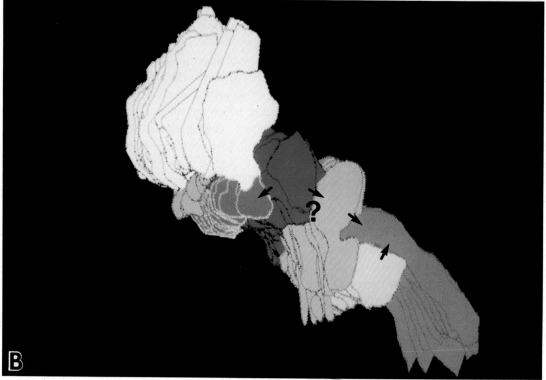

(Boussaoud and Joseph, 1985; Joseph and Boussaoud, 1985). The nigrotectal pathway plays an especially important role in the control of saccadic eye movements (see also Okada, Chapter 12). Cells in the substantia nigra pars reticulata of the monkey decrease their activity at the onset of a visual stimulus and increase their activity at the offset of that stimulus when fixated (Hikosaka and Wurtz, 1983a,b). The response of these cells is also decreased just prior to saccadic eye movements (Hikosaka and Wurtz, 1983a,b,c). These cells therefore appear to signal the initiation or termination of visually guided eye movements. Many of these cells can be antidromically activated from SC (Hikosaka and Wurtz, 1983c). In addition, a decrease in the discharge rate of SN cells is correlated with an increase in the discharge rate of SC cells which suggests that the two are linked synaptically (Hikosaka and Wurtz, 1983c).

Iontophoretic experiments show that this linkage is mediated by GABA. When injected into the substantia nigra pars reticulata, muscimol, a GABA agonist, facilitates saccades, while bicuculline, a GABA antagonist, inhibits saccades (Hikosaka and Wurtz, 1985b). In the SC the effect is reversed. Saccade related responses in SC cells as well as saccadic eye movements themselves are suppressed by muscimol and facilitated by bicuculline (Hikosaka and Wurtz, 1983d, 1985a). Based on this evidence, Hikosaka and Wurtz have proposed that the substantia nigra pars reticulata tonically inhibits saccade related cells in the superior colliculus via the neurotransmitter GABA. SC cells are released from this inhibition just prior to saccadic eye movements (Hikosaka and Wurtz, 1985b). More recent evidence from Hikosaka's laboratory (Hikosaka et al., 1989) has shown that the pathway controlling saccadic eye movements also involves the caudate nucleus.

## GABA receptor distribution in the superior colliculus

Two basic types of GABA receptor have been identified: $GABA_A$ and $GABA_B$ receptors. Several subtypes of each receptor are now recognized (see Brecha, Chapter 1, and Slaughter and Pan, Chapter 3, for details). These subtypes vary in their affinity to various agonists and antagonists, in their dissociation constants, in their membrane channel properties and in their distribution within the CNS. The specificity of various ligands to the GABA receptor subtypes is a rapidly evolving area of neuropharmacology (Bureau and Olsen, 1990; Mohler et al., 1990). In general, the high affinity $GABA_A$ receptor is thought to bind [$^3$H]muscimol, and to be bicuculline sensitive and baclofen insensitive. A low affinity $GABA_A$ receptor thought to be part of the benzodiazepine receptor, chloride channel complex may selectively bind [$^3$H]flunitrazepan. The $GABA_B$ receptor is activated by baclofen but is insensitive to bicuculline (Hill and Bowery, 1981). Other selective radiolabeled agonists and antagonists (phaclofen, saclofen) are also available to this receptor.

The binding of these agonists/antagonists in the superior colliculus has principally been studied in rat. Biochemically, [$^3$H]muscimol binds with high affinity in the rat superior colliculus with a $B_{max}$ about one-third that of visual cortex (Schliebs and Rothe, 1988). Receptor localization studies have shown that [$^3$H]muscimol binds with intermediate density to the superficial gray layer

---

Fig. 8. Computer reconstructions of a retinal synaptic island within the SGL of the Rhesus monkey SC. A. Profiles in the island include two retinal terminal boutons (rt, red), two spine-like conventional dendrites (s, blue), a PSD containing synaptic vesicles (psd, green), a horizonal PSD (h, purple), a putative axon terminal with flattened vesicles (f, yellow), and a large unidentified axon terminal (at, white). B. Reconstruction rotated approximately 90° from A. Arrows indicate synaptic contacts. The green varicose PSD and the yellow F profile both synapse on the purple horizontal PSD. These synaptic relationships represent a possible structural basis for GABA-mediated disinhibition.

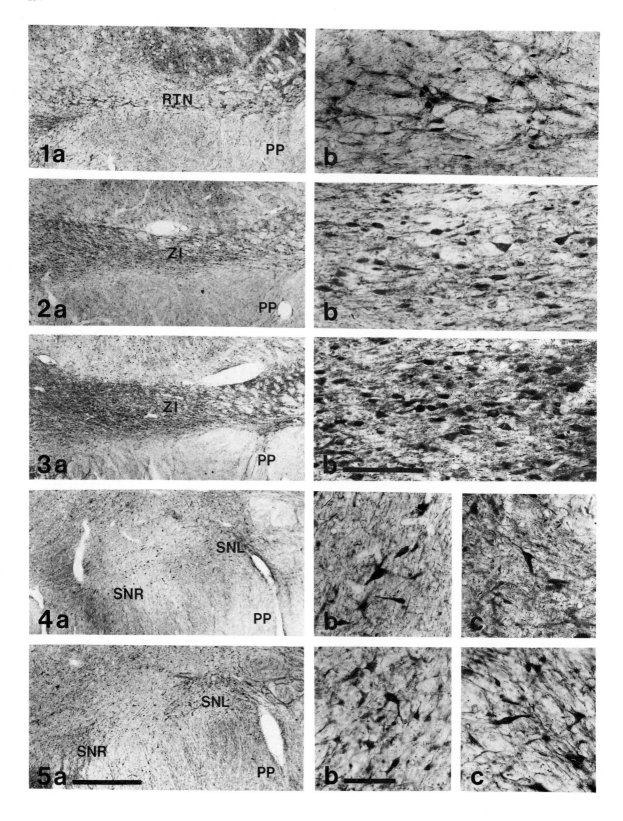

of the rat SC and with low density to the deep layers (Palacios et al., 1981). In cat, [³H]muscimol binds most intensely to the zonal and superficial gray layers, but lower levels of binding are also seen in the deeper layers (Skangiel-Kramska et al., 1986). In vivo injection of [³H]muscimol also results in dense neuropil labeling within the upper superficial gray with scattered grains found deeper (Mize and White, 1989). Cells throughout SC also accumulate muscimol in vivo, presumably due to a high affinity uptake of this agonist in GABAergic neurons (Mize and White, 1989).

GABA$_A$ sites identified by [³H]GABA binding after blocking GABA$_B$ sites with baclofen are most densely concentrated in the superficial layers, although they are also moderately distributed in the deep layers (Bowery et al., 1987). It also recently has been shown that the superficial layers of rat SC are labeled by an antibody to the $\beta_2$ and $\beta_3$ subunits of the putative GABA$_A$ benzodiazepine-receptor complex (Richards et al., 1987; Pinard et al., 1990b), a general pattern similar to that seen with [³H]muscimol. Ultrastructurally, the label is found within the cytoplasm and along the post-synaptic membranes of dendrites. Sometimes this label is opposite presynaptic terminals which contain pleomorphic vesicles, but this is not always the case (Pinard et. at, 1990b).

Benzodiazepine receptors also have been identified in SC using the ligand [³H]flunitrazepam, the antagonist [³H]clonazepam, the antagonist Ro-15-1788 and the specific partial reverse agonist Ro-15-4513 (see Richards et al., 1987, and Pinard et al., 1988). Specific binding of [³H]-flunitrazepam in rat SC, measured biochemically, is of high affinity and of similar density to that of visual cortex and about 3.5 times higher than in LGN (Rothe et al., 1985). In receptor autoradiograms, [³H]flunitrazepam is most densely bound to the superficial gray layer (Young and Kuhar, 1979; Young et al., 1981). The benzodiazepine agonist Ro-15-4513 also binds with high affinity to a single population of benzodiazepine receptors in rat SC ($B_{max}$ 650 fmol/mg dry weight.) Ultrastructurally, autoradiographic grains have been found primarily over varicose dendrites and at axo-dendritic appositions. Some labeling occurs at non-synaptic sites (Pinard et al., 1988).

GABA$_B$ receptors have been localized using either [³H]baclofen (Gehlert et al., 1985) or [³H]GABA after blocking GABA$_A$ receptors with isoguavacine (Bowery et al., 1984). The distribution of GABA$_B$ receptors is denser than that of GABA$_A$ receptors in rat SC (Bowery et al., 1984). GABA$_B$ receptor labeling also appears to be far more selective to the superficial layers, although light labeling is also seen deeper (Bowery et al., 1987; Gehlert et al., 1985). These results suggest differences in the distributions of the two basic GABA receptor types, although the detailed differences in distribution have not yet been worked out.

In our laboratory, (Mize and Butler, 1991) we have used an antibody selective to the $\beta_2$ and $\beta_3$ subunits of the GABA$_A$ receptor complex (De-Blas et al., 1988; Vitorica et al., 1988, 1990) to localize these receptor sites in the cat superior colliculus. Reaction product was found distributed through the zonal and superficial gray layers and throughout the deeper layers. Some neurons contained a halo of reaction product on their outer membrane surfaces. These cells included the very large predorsal bundle cells in the intermediate gray layer which are known to receive GABAergic terminal input (see above). At the ultrastructural level, label was found along the membrane surfaces of both cell bodies and dendrites. This label was most often found at

Fig. 9. GABA-antibody labeling in the thalamic reticular nucleus (RTN), the zona incerta (ZI) and the substantia nigra of the cat. (a) illustrates the distribution of GABA-labeled neurons at five rostro-cuadal levels through the thalamus and midbrain. (b,c) show the labeled cells at higher magnification. SNR, substantia nigra, pars reticulata; SNL, substantia nigra, pars lateralis; PP, pes penduculi. Scale bars: a = 500 μm; b,c = 100 μm.

236

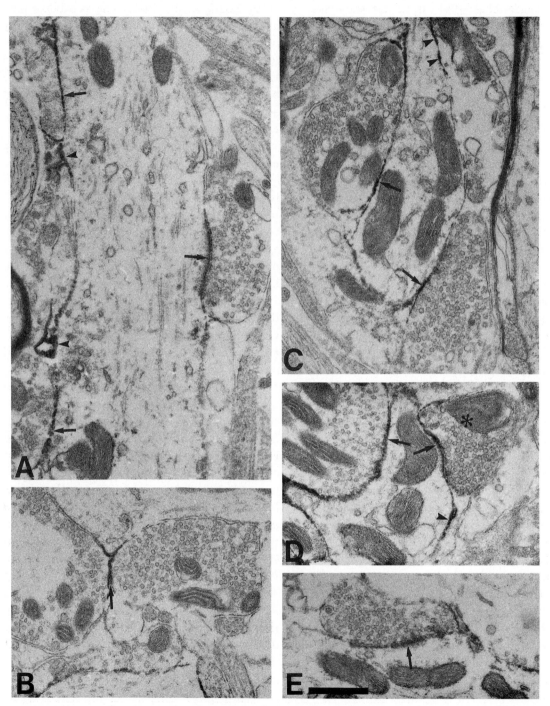

Fig. 10. Localization of the $\beta_2$ and $\beta_3$ subunits of the GABA$_A$ receptor in the cat SC. The label is distributed along membrane surfaces at sites of synaptic apposition. The presynaptic terminals at these sites contain pleomorphic or flattened vesicles (arrows, A,B,C,D,E) or round synaptic vesicles (asterisk, D). Label was also found at non-synaptic sites (arrowheads) and, rarely, coating the membranes of presynaptic profiles (arrow, B). Scale bar = 0.5 $\mu$m.

synaptic sites between axon terminals and dendrites (Fig. 10). Usually, the synaptic vesicles that were presynaptic to labeled membranes were pleomorphic and included small round, ovoid and flattened shapes (Fig. 10A–E). However, label could also be found adjacent to presynaptic terminals containing only round synaptic vesicles (Fig. 10D) and on membranes at non-synaptic sites (Fig. 10C,D). Rarely, membrane associated label was also found coating presynaptic vesicle-containing profiles (Fig. 10B). These results suggest that the $GABA_A$ receptor $\beta_2$ and $\beta_3$ subunits are often postsynaptic in location and associated with pleomorphic vesicle containing profiles which have been shown to be labeled by GABA antibodies (see above). However, it is clear that the $GABA_A$ receptor subunits can also be found at non-synaptic sites and can even be internalized in the cytoplasm of GABA receptive neurons (see Brecha, Chapter 1, for a further discussion).

## Colocalization of GABA with other chemical substances

Specific subclasses of GABA neuron have been distinguished by various molecular probes. In the visual cortex, for example, antibodies to cell surface molecules have been shown to label subpopulations of GABA neuron (Naegele and Barnstable, 1989; Barnstable et al., Chapter 23). GABA cell classes in visual cortex also have been distinguished by the peptides which they colocalize (Somogyi et al., 1984; Demeulemeester et al., 1988). Several calcium binding proteins have also been shown to distinguish different types of GABA neuron in visual cortex (Hendry and Carder, Chapter 22). The colocalization of GABA with peptides and calcium binding proteins is of particular interest because these other substances may reflect differences in the function of these GABA neurons.

Several peptides are present in neurons of the mammalian superior colliculus. The pentapeptides leucine and methionine enkephalin (ENK)

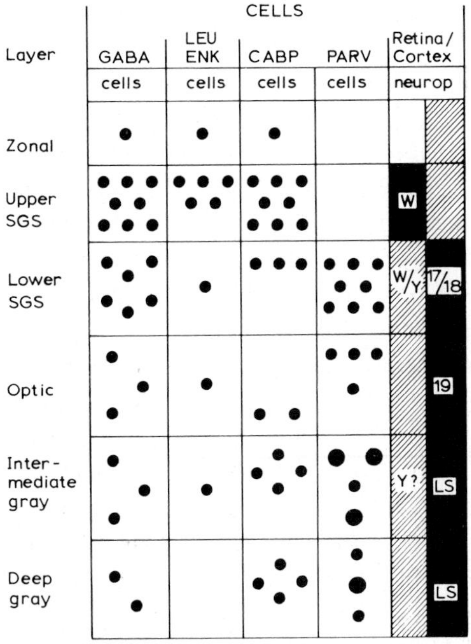

Fig. 11. Schematic diagram of the distribution of cells in the cat superior colliculus labeled by various antibodies. SC layers are shown to the left, the distribution of retinal and cortical terminals on the right. The density of labeled cells is indicated by the number of circles. GABA, gamma-aminobutyric acid; Leu Enk, leucine enkephalin; CABP, calbindin; PARV, parvalbumin. See text for details.

have been identified in the mammalian superior colliculus using biochemical, opiate receptor binding and immunocytochemistry techniques. Moderate levels of these peptides have been measured biochemically in rat (Palkovits and Brownstein, 1985). Binding to enkephalin-like receptors is especially dense within the superficial layers of this species (Pert et al., 1976; Atweh and Kuhar, 1977; Herkenham and Pert, 1980). Neurons labeled by antibodies to the enkephalins also are distributed most densely within the superficial layers of the rat SC (Watson et al., 1977; Khachaturian et al., 1983; Petrusz et al., 1985). In the cat, ENK immunoreactive cell bodies are confined largely to a thin band within the upper superficial gray layer (Graybiel et al., 1984; Mize, 1989; Berson et al., 1991). A dense band of immunoreactive fibers is also found in this same region of the cat SC (Fig. 11).

As this band overlaps the dense distribution of GABA immunoreactive neurons in the SGL, we determined whether the two substances are co-localized in the same neurons (Mize, 1989). ENK-labeled neurons in the cat SC were virtually all small neurons and had morphologies similar to GABA immunolabeled neurons, including horizontal and pyriform shapes. Electron microscope studies showed that the ENK antiserum labeled presynaptic dendrites whose ultrastructure was indistinguishable from that of GABA containing presynaptic dendrites. The distribution, size, morphology and ultrastructural features suggested to us that many if not all enkephalin immunoreactive neurons must therefore contain GABA (Mize, 1989). However, two-chromagen double labeling experiments revealed that only about one-fifth (18%) of ENK-labeled neurons were also labeled by GABA (Mize, 1989). These transmitter specific neurons therefore must be for the most part separate populations of neurons, although they are virtually indistinguishable in size and morphology. An alternative possibility is that the levels of the two substances vary and that only one substance is expressed in high concentration at any given time within a single cell.

The thin band of ENK immunoreactivity in fibers in the upper SGL also appears to arise from intrinsic sources. Some of these fibers probably also contain GABA. Some axon terminals with pleomorphic synaptic vesicles similar to F profiles are labeled by ENK antibodies (Mize, 1989). Ibotenic acid/$N$-methyl-D-aspartate chemical lesions practically eliminate ENK fiber labeling in the upper SGL, presumably by destroying the intrinsic ENK-labeled neurons in this region of SC (Berson et al., 1991).

ENK-labeled fibers that are found in patches within the dorsal intermediate gray layer probably also colocalize GABA (Graybiel et al., 1984; Mize, 1989; Berson et al., 1991). The origin of these fibers is unknown, but unlike the superficial fiber band, the IGL fibers survive excitotoxin lesions (Berson et al., 1991), suggesting they are of extrinsic origin. One likely source is the sub-stantia nigra pars reticulata. The ENK fibers match the periodicity and dorsoventral distribution of the SN pathway (Graybiel, 1978; Graybiel et al., 1984). Some cells in the SN pars reticulata of the cat are also ENK immunoreactive (Beckstead and Kersey, 1985). As the pathway from SN to SC is GABAergic (see above), it seems likely that this pathway colocalizes enkephalin.

Other peptides also co-occur with GABA in the CNS. For example, GAD has been shown to co-exist with somatostatin (SRIF), cholecystokinin (CCK) and corticotropin-releasing factor (CRF) in the cat visual cortex (Demeulemeester et al., 1988). Some of these peptides are also found in the superior colliculus. Somatostatin is found in some cells in the SC of both rat (Laemle and Feldman, 1985) and cat (Spangler and Morley, 1987). However, these cells are unlikely to be GABAergic. Somatostatin positive neurons in the cat SC are preferentially distributed within the deep SGL and within patches in the intermediate gray layer (Spangler and Morley, 1987). This distribution does not match that of GABA neurons in the cat SC. Their morphology also differs, as many somatostatin positive cells are reported to have a vertical fusiform morphology (Spangler and Morley, 1987). Substance P is also unlikely to co-occur with GABA in the cat SC because SP-labeled neurons are mostly medium to large cells, including the very large predorsal bundle neurons found in the intermediate gray layer (Mize, unpublished observations). Neurons of this size range are not labeled by GABA. In our laboratory, we have been unable to label any neurons in the cat SC using antibodies to vasoactive intestinal polypeptide (VIP), neuropeptide Y, or cholecystokinin (unpublished observations). In general, the co-existence of peptides and GABA seems far less prevalent in SC than in visual cortex

The calcium binding proteins parvalbumin and calbindin also commonly co-exist with GABA in many parts of the nervous system (Celio, 1986, 1990), including the visual cortex and lateral geniculate nucleus (Hendry and Carder, Chapter 22; Stichel et al., 1987, 1988; Demeulemeester et al., 1989; DeFelipe et al., 1989; Hendry et al., 1989). In cat visual cortex, separate classes of GABA neuron can be distinguished by their differential labeling by parvalbumin vs. calbindin (Hendry and Carder, Chapter 22). The laminar distribution of these cell types differs as well. The distribution of calbindin and parvalbumin in the superior colliculus also differs, but unlike visual cortex, co-localization with GABA occurs only in a small subpopulation of calbindin neurons and apparently not in any parvalbumin neurons.

Calbindin is distributed in three separate neuronal tiers within both the cat and monkey SC, one within the upper SGL, one that straddles the optic and intermediate gray layers, and one within the deep gray layer (Mize et al., 1991b; Luo and Mize, 1991) (Fig. 11). Although the cells vary in distribution, most are small neurons. By retrogradely filling neurons with HRP injected into both the ascending and descending projection targets of cat SC, we have shown that all but a few calbindin neurons are interneurons. The only projection neurons containing calbindin were a small group of cells that projected to the lateral geniculate nucleus. Many of these cells had morphologies roughly identical to those of GABA neurons, including distinctive horizontal, pyriform and stellate shapes (Mize et al., 1991b).

Despite the similarity in morphologies, double-labeling studies using two chromagens revealed very little co-localization of calbindin and GABA. Within the superficial dense band, only about 8% of calbindin neurons were also labeled by GABA (Mize et al., 1991b). This percentage must be treated as a rough estimate due to technical limitations of the double labeling procedure (suppression of one antibody by the other, incomplete penetration). However, GABA and calbindin neurons each represent about 40% of the total population of cells in the SGL which also suggests that they are separate cell populations. We believe the small interneurons in SC must represent a variety of chemically heterogeneous cell types, although there are only a few morphologically distinctive cell types.

In SC, parvalbumin labels a very different cell population (Mize et al., 1991c). Parvalbumin immunoreactive neurons are confined largely to the deep superficial gray and upper optic layers where they form a single dense band that fits between the two upper tiers of calbindin neurons (Fig. 11). The parvalbumin neurons also differ in that they are mostly larger neurons and many project to ascending and descending targets of SC (Mize et al., 1991c). This population differs from GABA immunoreactive neurons in distribution, cell size, morphology and cell type (projection vs. interneuron). These differences make it virtually impossible for parvalbumin and GABA to be colocalized in the cat SC. In summary, we find little evidence that the calcium binding proteins co-occur with GABA in the cat superior colliculus and neither calbindin nor parvalbumin distinguish separate classes of GABAergic neuron.

## Monocular deprivation and GABA content in the superior colliculus

There is increasing evidence that the content of GABA in individual neurons can be altered by visual deprivation in adult mammals. In monkey area 17, for example, short-term (2–11 weeks) enucleation, lid suture, or intravitreal injection of tetrodotoxin produce a significant reduction in the numbers of GABA or GAD immunoreactive neurons in the ocular dominance columns related to the deprived eye (Hendry and Jones, 1986; Hendry and Carder, Chapter 22). Reduction in GABA immunoreactive neurons also has been found in the affected laminae of the cat lateral geniculate nucleus (Luo et al., 1991). Calbindin and parvalbumin immunoreactivities are also affected by deprivation in the adult monkey visual cortex (Hendry and Carder, Chapter 22) and LGN (Luo et al., 1990; Tigges and Tigges, 1991).

Despite these dramatic effects in the geniculo-cortical system, monocular deprivation apparently has no effect in the adult monkey superior colliculus. To date, we have examined 10 monkeys, some with unilateral occlusion from birth, others with one eye removed 2 weeks to 6 years prior to sacrifice, and others with both long-term occlusion and short-term enucleation. Qualitatively, there were no obvious differences in GABA immunoreactivity in either cells or neuropil on the side opposite the removed and/or deprived eye. Neurons in the upper superficial gray were well-labeled by GABA on both sides, and there was no consistent reduction in the number of these neurons. In addition, no obvious reduction in calbindin labeling on the affected side was found.

To test this quantitatively, we measured the staining intensity of both the full field and individual cells within the upper superficial gray layer using an image analyzer (Luo and Mize, 1991). Field measures of optical density in the zonal and upper SGL revealed only very small differences between the contralateral and ipsilateral sides in GABA antibody labeling (Fig. 12). Measurements of the optical density and average diameter of individual labeled neurons also failed to show any large differences between the two SC (Fig. 12). There is thus no evidence that GABA content is consistently altered by short or long term deprivation in the adult monkey, a result strikingly different from that seen in the visual cortex and

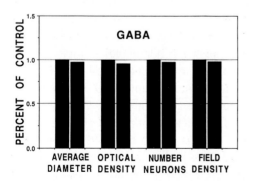

Fig. 12. Effects of monocular deprivation on anti-GABA immunoreactivity in the Rhesus monkey SC. Histogram illustrates the percent decrease in the average diameter, optical density, number of neurons and field density on the side ipsilateral to the occlusion/enucleation (bars on left) vs. the side contralateral to those procedures (bars on right). Data are summed from two animals that sustained combined long-term monocular occlusions and short-term enucleations of the same eye.

lateral geniculate nucleus. The significance of this difference is discussed below (Functional Considerations).

## Functional considerations

### Does GABA play a role in directional selectivity in SC?

In visual cortex, directional selectivity is generated at least in part by GABA mediated inhibition (see Sillito, Chapter 17, and Eysel, Chapter 19). Many cells in the superior colliculus of cat and some other species are directionally selective (Sterling and Wickelgren, 1969; Rosenquist and Palmer, 1971; Stein and Arigbede, 1972; Rhoades and Chalupa, 1978) and this mechanism could involve intrinsic GABAergic neurons. However, there are three reasons why GABA inhibition is probably not involved in directional selectivity in the mammalian superior colliculus. First, directional selectivity is primarily conveyed to the SC from extrinsic sources. In cat and hamster, this source is thought to be the visual cortex because corticotectal cells have directionally selective properties like those in SC (Palmer and Rosenquist, 1974) and lesions or inactivation of visual cortex reduce or eliminate directionally selective responses in SC (Wickelgren and Sterling, 1969; Rosenquist and Palmer, 1971; Mize and Murphy, 1976; Rhoades and Chalupa, 1978). In other species, such as rabbit, directional selectivity is probably generated in the retina itself.

Secondly, the same types of GABA synaptic circuits are found both in species that do and species that do not have directionally selective neurons in SC. In cat, over two thirds of neurons have directionally biased receptive fields (see references above). By contrast, very few directionally selective neurons are found in the superior colliculus of the Rhesus monkey (Cynader and Berman, 1972; Schiller et al., 1974; Updyke, 1974; Marrocco and Li, 1977). Nevertheless, GABA cells in both species have a similar distribution and morphology. The same GABA synaptic profiles are present in both monkey and cat (Mize,

1988; Mize et al., 1991a). Thus, intrinsic GABA circuitry in SC is unlikely to be involved in generating directionally selective receptive fields.

Third, some physiological studies have shown that the neurons in SC which display IPSPs are not directionally selective. In rabbit SC, Takahashi and Ogawa (1978) report that only narrow field vertical fusiform neurons have prolonged secondary IPSPs (however, cf. Grantyn et al., 1984). The receptive fields of narrow field vertical fusiform neurons respond vigorously to stationary lights but are rarely if ever directionally selective in either hamster (Mooney et al., 1985) or tree shrew (Irvin et al., 1983). In addition, some vertical fusiform cells within the upper SGL of rat SC are insensitive to iontophoretically applied GABA, although other narrow field vertical cells are responsive (Kayama et al., 1980). Stellate neurons, most of which are directionally selective in hamster (Mooney et al., 1985), do not generate IPSPs in rabbit (Takahashi and Ogawa, 1978) and may or may not be sensitive to iontophoretically applied GABA in rat (Kayama et al., 1980). Thus, neither the presence of IPSPs nor sensitivity to GABA is correlated with whether an SC neuron is or is not directionally selective. Although no study has carefully examined the effect of GABA or its analogues on directionally selective responses in the mammalian SC, there is little evidence to suggest that GABA is related to this receptive field property in the mammalian superior colliculus.

*What is the role of GABA in SC?*

What role or roles GABA does play in the superficial layers of the superior colliculus is unknown. The horizontal cell is well-suited by virtue of its dendritic spread to mediate lateral inhibition at some distance across the collicular surface. Consistent with this idea, Rizzolatti et al. (1974) have reported a form of remote inhibition in the cat superior colliculus in which stimuli can inhibit neurons whose receptive fields are several mm away from the location of the stimulus. As the horizontal cell dendrites are large, smooth profiles, one can assume that the action of these presynaptic dendrites may be like that of relay cell dendrites in the LGN where current spread passes down the dendrite without significant attenuation (Bloomfield and Sherman, 1989; Uhlrich and Cucchiaro, Chapter 9). In this case, synaptic input would probably influence the synaptic output sites at extended distances from the site of input. Horizontal cell dendrites probably are like the F3 dendritic profiles in LGN which have been hypothesized to mediate interocular inhibition across laminar borders (Ahlsen et al., 1985; Holdefer et al., 1988).

The GABA containing pyriform and stellate neurons in SC may have a very different action. According to Golgi studies, many small pyriform and stellate neurons in the SGL of cat have locally ramifying axons (Sterling, 1971; Langer, 1976). As the morphology of these neurons is similar to that of the GABAergic pyriform and stellate neurons, it is likely that these cells also have axons with short collaterals. These types of cell might mediate spatially localized forms of inhibition, such as the secondary response inhibition described by McIlwain and Fields (1971) in which there is a pronounced secondary response depression following initial excitation.

Vesicle-containing spines and/or varicose PSDs may act via a third mechanism. We believe, although we have not yet proven, that these profiles serve feed forward inhibition in SC analogous to the F2 profiles found in the lateral geniculate nucleus (Guillery, 1969; Famiglieti and Peters, 1971; Fitzpatrick et al., 1984; Montero, 1986; Uhlrich and Cucchiaro, Chapter 9). The PSDs found in the retinal synaptic islands of SC have many similarities to the F2 profiles in the retinal glomerulus of the LGN. Both are intermediate elements with a retinal terminal presynaptic and a conventional relay cell dendrite postsynaptic to the PSD. Both have sparse accumulations of pleomorphic vesicles spread throughout the profile. Both form symmetric synaptic contacts. Both participate in synaptic triads. The synaptic circuitry is thus identical. F2 profiles provide feed

242

forward inhibition to relay cells. Bloomfield and Sherman (1989) have modeled the cable properties of the dendrites giving rise to F2 profiles in LGN and have shown that they conduct current flow poorly and thus probably mediate localized inhibition. In the superior colliculus, it is not known how this synaptic circuitry influences the postsynaptic relay cells, but it is reasonable to hypothesize that the action would be like that found in the LGN.

*Why is GABA in SC unaffected by environmental alterations?*

As adult enucleation produces significant alterations in GABA content in both the LGN and visual cortex, it is surprising that there is no effect of enucleation or occlusion in the monkey superior colliculus. There are two likely reasons for this. First, the GABA system in SC is probably phylogenetically old because many of the same GABA containing cell types and synaptic components have been described in a variety of species, including pigeons (Hunt and Kunzle, 1976). Evolutionarily conserved systems are often less amenable to alteration by environmental manipulations. Secondly, the enucleation effects on GABA in LGN and visual cortex occur primarily in regions where input from the two eyes is strictly segregated. By contrast, the contralateral and ipsilateral retinal input to the monkey SC overlaps (Hubel et al., 1975) and probably terminates on the same cells. It seems likely in these cases that the activity of the remaining eye input would maintain the chemical environment of the postsynaptic cell in SC. This does not occur in the LGN or visual cortex, because these cells receive input primarily from one eye only.

**Summary**

GABA is an important inhibitory neurotransmitter in the mammalian superior colliculus. As in the lateral geniculate nucleus, GABA immunoreactive neurons in SC are almost all small and are distributed throughout the structure in all mammalian species studied to date. Unlike the LGN,

GABA-labeled neurons in SC have a variety of morphologies. These cells have been best characterized in cat, where horizontal and two granule cell morphologies have been identified. Horizontal cells give rise to one class of presynaptic dendrite while granule C cells give rise to another class of spine-like presynaptic dendrite. Granule A cells may be the origin of some GABAergic axon terminals. GABA containing synaptic profiles form serial synapses, providing a possible substrate for disinhibition.

The distribution of GABA$_A$ and GABA$_B$ receptor subtypes appears similar to that of GABA neurons, with the densest distribution found within the superficial gray layer. However, antibody immunocytochemistry of the $\beta_2$ and $\beta_3$ subunits of the GABA$_A$ receptor reveals that it is located at both synaptic and non-synaptic sites, and may be associated with membrane adjacent to terminals with either flattened or round vesicles.

A few GABA containing neurons in SC colocalize the pentapeptide leucine enkephalin or the calcium binding protein calbindin. However, none appear to co-localize parvalbumin, a situation different from GABA containing interneurons in the LGN and visual cortex. The diversity of GABA neurons in SC rivals that found in visual cortex, although unlike visual cortex, the pattern of co-occurrence does not distinguish GABA cell types in SC. The superior colliculus also differs from both LGN and visual cortex in that GABA and calbindin immunoreactivity is not altered by either long-term occlusion and/or short-term enucleation in adult Rhesus monkeys. No consistent differences have been found in the optical density of GABA labeling in either cells or neuropil.

To conclude, GABA neurons in the superior colliculus share some properties like those in LGN and others like those in visual cortex. In other properties, they differ from GABA neurons in both the LGN and visual cortex. The GABA systems in the superior colliculus are similar in all mammalian species studied, suggesting that they are phylogenetically conserved systems which are not amenable to plastic alterations, a situation different to that in the geniculostriate system.

## Acknowledgements

Foremost, I thank Dr. Robert Spencer who has collaborated on many of the projects reported in this review over the past fifteen years. I also thank Dr. Thomas Norton and Dr. Margarete Tigges for collaborating on the studies of GABA neurons in the tree shrew or Rhesus monkey superior colliculus. The Yerkes Regional Primate Center at Emory University provided the deprived monkey tissue. C.J. Jeon, Q. Luo, K. Troughton, G. Butler and O. Hamada collected much of the data related to this project. Drs. Piers Emson, Angel DeBlas and Robert Wenthold provided some of the antibodies used in these studies. The work reported in this chapter was supported by USPHS grant NIH EY-02973 from the National Eye Institute and the Neuroscience Center of Excellence of the State of Tennessee.

## References

Abramson, B.P. and Chalupa, L.M. (1988) Multiple pathways from the colliculus to the extrageniculate visual thalamus of the cat. *J. Comp. Neurol.*, 271: 397–418.

Ahlsen, G., Lindstrom, S. and Lo, F.S. (1985) Interaction between inhibitory pathways to principal cells in the lateral geniculate nucleus of the cat. *Exp. Brain Res.*, 58: 134–143.

Appell, P.P. and Behan, M. (1990) Sources of subcortical GABAergic projections to the superior colliculus in the cat. *J. Comp. Neurol.*, 302: 143–158.

Arakawa, T. and Okada, Y. (1988) Excitatory and inhibitory action of GABA on synaptic transmission in slices of guinea pig superior colliculus. *Eur. J. Pharmacol.*, 158: 217–224.

Araki, M., McGeer, P.L. and McGeer, E.G. (1984) Presumptive gamma-aminobutyric acid pathways from the midbrain to the superior colliculus studied by a combined horseradish peroxidase-gamma-aminobutyric acid transaminase pharmaco-histochemical method. *Neuroscience,* 13: 433–439.

Atweh, S.F. and Kuhar, M.J. (1977) Autoradiographic localization of opiate receptors in the rat brain. II. The brain stem. *Brain Res.*, 129: 1–12.

Beckstead, R.M. and Kersey, K.S. (1985) Immunohistochemical demonstration of differential substance P, met-enkephalin, and glutamic acid-decarboxylase-containing cell body and axon distributions in the corpus striatum of the cat. *J. Comp.Neurol.*, 232: 481–498.

Behan, M. (1981) Identification and distribution of retinocollicular terminals in the cat: An electron-microscopic autoradiographic analysis. *J. Comp. Neurol.*, 199: 1–16.

Behan, M., Lin, C.S. and Hall, W.C. (1987) The nigrotectal projection in the cat: An electron microscope autoradiographic study. *Neuroscience,* 22: 529–539.

Berson, D.M., Graybiel, A.M., Brown, W.D. and Thompson, L.A. (1991) Evidence for intrinsic expression of enkephalin-like immunoreactivity and opioid binding sites in cat superior colliculus. *Neuroscience,* in press.

Bloomfield, S.A. and Sherman, S.M. (1989) Dendritic current flow in relay cells and interneurons of the cat's lateral geniculate nucleus. *Proc. Natl. Acad. Sci. USA,* 86: 3911–3914.

Boussaoud, D. and Joseph, J.P. (1985) Role of the cat substantia nigra pars reticulata in eye and head movements. II. Effects of local pharmacological injections. *Exp. Brain Res.*, 57: 297–304.

Bowery, N.G., Price, G.W., Hill, D.R., Wilkin, G.P. and Turnbull, M.J. (1984) GABA receptor multiplicity. Visualization of different receptor types in the mammalian CNS. *Neuropharmacology,* 23: 219–231.

Bowery, N.G., Hudson, A.L. and Price, G.W. (1987) $GABA_A$ and $GABA_B$ receptor site distribution in the cat central nervous system. *Neuroscience,* 20: 365–383.

Bureau, M. and Olsen, R.W. (1990) Multiple distinct subunits of the gamma-amino butyric acid-A receptor protein show different ligand-binding affinities. *Mol. Pharmacol.*, 37: 497–502.

Caldwell, R.B. and Mize, R.R. (1981) Superior colliculus neurons which project to the cat lateral posterior nucleus have varying morphologies. *J. Comp. Neurol.*, 203: 53–66.

Carter, D.A., Bray, G.M. and Aguayo, A.J. (1989) Regenerated retinal ganglion cell axons can form well-differentiated synapses in the superior colliculus of adult hamsters. *J. Neurosci.*, 9: 4042–4050.

Casagrande, V.A., Harting, J.K., Hall, W.C. Diamond, I.T. and Martin, G.F. (1972) Superior colliculus of the tree shrew (*Tupaia glis*): Evidence for a structural and functional subdivision into superficial and deep layers, *Science,* 177: 444–447.

Celio, M.R. (1986) Parvalbumin in most gamma-aminobutyric acid-containing neurons of the rat cerebral cortex. *Science,* 231: 995–997.

Celio, M.R. (1990) Calbindin D-28K and parvalbumin in the rat nervous system. *Neuroscience,* 35: 375–475.

Chalupa, L.M. (1984) Visual physiology of the mammalian superior colliculus. In H. Vanegas (Ed.), *Comparative Neurology of the Optic Tectum,* New York: Plenum Press, pp. 775–818.

Chevalier, G., Deniau, J.M., Thierry, A.M. and Feger, J. (1981a) The nigrotectal pathway. An electrophysiological reinvestigation in the rat. *Brain Res.*, 213: 253–263.

Chevalier, G., Thierry, A.M., Shibazaki, T. and Feger, J. (1981b) Evidence for a GABAergic inhibitory nigrotectal pathway in the rat. *Neurosci. Lett.,* 21: 67–70.

Cynader, M. and Berman, N. (1972) Receptive-field organization of monkey superior colliculus. *J. Neurophysiol.,* 35: 187–201.

deBlas, A.L., Vitorica, J. and Friedrich, P. (1988) Localization of the $GABA_A$ receptor in the rat brain with a monoclonal antibody to the 57,000 Mr peptide of the $GABA_A$ receptor/ benzodiazepine receptor/ Cl-channel complex. *J. Neurosci.,* 8: 602–614.

Demeulemeester, H., Vandesande, F., Orban, G.A., Brandon, C. and Vanderhaeghen, J.J. (1988) Heterogeneity of GABAergic cells in the cat visual cortex. *J. Neurosci.,* 8: 988–1000.

Demeulemeester, H., Vandesande, F., Organ, G.A., Heizmann, C.W. and Pochet, R. (1989) Calbindin D-28K and parvalbumin immunoreactivity is confined to two separate neuronal subpopulations in the cat visual cortex, whereas partial coexistence is shown in the dorsal lateral geniculate nucleus. *Neurosci. Lett.,* 99: 6–11.

Deniau, J, M., Chevalier, G. and Feger, J. (1978) Electrophysiological study of the nigro-tectal pathway in the rat. *Neurosci. Lett.,* 10: 215–220.

DeFelipe, J., Hendry, S.H.C. and Jones, E.G. (1989) Synapses of double bouquet cells in monkey cerebral cortex visualized by calbindin immunoreactivity. *Brain Res.,* 503: 49–54.

Di Chiara, G., Porceddu, M.L., Morelli, M., Mulas, M.L. and Gessa, G.L. (1979) Evidence for a GABAergic projection from the substantia nigra to the ventromedial thalamus and to the superior colliculus of the rat. *Brain Res.,* 176: 273–284.

Edwards, S.B. (1977) The commissural projection of the superior colliculus in the cat. *J. Comp. Neurol.,* 173: 23–40.

Edwards, S.B. (1980) The deep cell layers of the superior colliculus: Their reticular characteristics and structural organization. In J.A. Hobson and M.A.B. Brazier (Eds.), *The Reticular Formation Revisited,* New York: Raven Press, pp. 193–209.

Edwards, S.B., Ginsburgh, C.L., Henkel, C.K. and Stein, B.E. (1979) Sources of subcortical projections to the superior colliculus in the cat. *J. Comp. Neurol.,* 184: 309–330.

Famiglietti, E.V. and Peters, A. (1972) The synaptic glomerulus and the intrinsic neuron in the dorsal lateral geniculate nucleus of the cat. *J. Comp. Neurol.,* 144: 285–334.

Ficalora, A.S. and Mize, R.R. (1989) The neurons of the substantia nigra and zona incerta which project to the cat superior colliculus are GABA immunoreactive: a double-label study using GABA immunocytochemistry and lectin retrograde transport. *Neuroscience,* 29: 567–581.

Fish, S.E., Goodman, D.K., Kuo, D.C., Plocer, J.D. and Rhoades, R.W. (1982) The intercollicular pathway in the golden hamster: An anatomical study, *J. Comp. Neurol.,* 204: 6–20.

Fitzpatrick, D., Penny, G.R., and Schmechel, D.E. (1984) Glutamic acid decarboxylase-immunoreactive neurons and terminals in the lateral geniculate nucleus of the cat. *Neuroscience,* 4: 1809–1829.

Fonnum, F., Lund Karlsen, R., Malthe-Sorenssen, D., Skrede, K. and Walaas, I. (1979) Localization of neurotransmitters, particularly glutamate, in hippocampus, septum, nucleus accumbens and superior colliculus. *Prog. Brain Res.,* 51: 167–191.

Fosse, V.M., Heggelund, P. and Fonnum, P. (1989) Postnatal development of glutamatergic, GABAergic, and cholinergic neurotransmitter phenotypes in the visual cortex, lateral geniculate nucleus, pulvinar, and superior colliculus in cats. *J. Neurosci.,* 9: 426–435.

Gehlert, D.R., Yamamura, H.I. and Wamsley, J.K. (1985) Gamma-aminobutyric acid B receptors in the rat brain: Quantitative autoradiographic localization using $^3$H-Baclofen. *Neurosci. Lett.,* 56: 183–188.

Grantyn, R., Ludwig, R. and Eberhardt, W. (1984) Neurons of the superficial tectal gray. An intracellular HRP-study on the kitten superior colliculus in vitro. *Exp. Brain Res.* 55: 172–176.

Graybiel, A.M. (1978) Organization of the nigrotectal connection: An experimental tracer study in the cat. *Brain Res.,* 143: 339–348.

Graybiel, A.M., Brecha, N. and Karten, H.J. (1984) Cluster-and-sheet pattern of enkephalin-like immunoreactivity in the superior colliculus of the cat. *Neuroscience,* 12: 191–214.

Guillery, R.W. (1969) The organization of synaptic interconnections in the laminae of the dorsal lateral geniculate nucleus of the cat. *Zschr. Zellforsch. Mikroskop. Anat.,* 96: 1–38.

Hall, W.C. and May, P.J. (1984) The anatomical basis for sensorimotor transformations in the superior colliculus. *Contrib. Sensory Physiol.,* 8: 1–40.

Hamos, J.E., Van Horn, S.C., Raczkowski, D., Uhlrich, D.J. and Sherman, S.M. (1985) Synaptic connectivity of a local circuit neuron in the lateral geniculate nucleus of the cat. *Nature,* 317: 618–621.

Harrell, J.V., Caldwell, R.B. and Mize, R.R. (1982) The superior colliculus neurons which project to the dorsal and ventral lateral geniculate nuclei in the cat. *Exp. Brain Res.,* 46: 234–242.

Harting, J.K., Hall, W.C., Diamond, I.T. and Martin, G.F. (1973) Anterograde degeneration study of the superior colliculus in *Tupaia glis:* Evidence for a subdivision between superficial and deep layers. *J. Comp. Neurol.,* 148: 361–386.

Harting, J.K., Huerta, M.F., Hashikawa, T., Weber, J.T. and Van Lieshout, D.P. (1988) Neuroanatomical studies of the nigrotectal projection in the cat. *J. Comp. Neurol.,* 278: 615–631.

Hattori T., McGeer P.L., Fibiger, H.C. and McGeer, E.G. (1973) On the source of GABA-containing terminals in the substantia nigra. Electron microscopic autoradiographic and biochemical studies. *Brain Res.,* 54: 103–114.

Hendry, S.H.C. and Jones, E.G. (1986) Reduction in number of GABA immunostained neurons in deprived-eye dominance columns of monkey area 17. *Nature,* 320: 750–53.

Hendry, S.H., Jones, E.G., Emson, P.C., Lawson, D.E., Heizmann, C.W. and Striet, P. (1989) Two classes of cortical

GABA neurons defined by differential calcium binding protein immunoreactivities. *Exp. Brain Res.*, 76: 467–472.

Herkenham, M. and Pert, C.B. (1980) In vitro autoradiography of opiate receptors in rat brain suggests loci of opiatergic pathways. *Proc. Natl. Acad. Sci. USA*, 77: 5523–5536.

Hikosaka, O. and Wurtz, R.H. (1983a) Visual and oculomotor functions of monkey substantia nigra pars reticulata. I. Relation of visual and auditory responses to saccades. *J. Neurophysiol.*, 49: 1230–1253.

Hikosaka, O. and Wurtz, R.H. (1983b) Visual and oculomotor functions of monkey substantia nigra pars reticulata. II. Visual responses related to fixation of gaze. *J. Neurophysiol.*, 49: 1254–1267.

Hikosaka, O. and Wurtz, R.H. (1983c) Visual and oculomotor functions of monkey substantia nigra pars reticulata. IV. Relation of substantia nigra to superior colliculus. *J. Neurophysiol.*, 49: 1285–1301.

Hikosaka, O. and Wurtz, R.H. (1983d) Effects on eye movements of a GABA agonist and antagonist injected into monkey superior colliculus. *Brain Res.*, 272: 368–372.

Hikosaka, O. and Wurtz, R.H. (1985a) Modification of saccadic eye movements by GABA-related substances. I. Effect of muscimol and bicuculline in monkey superior colliculus. *J. Neurophysiol.*, 53: 266–291.

Hikosaka, O. and Wurtz, R.H. (1985b) Modification of saccadic eye movements by GABA-related substances. II. Effects of muscimol in monkey substantia nigra pars reticulata. *J. Neurophysiol.*, 53: 292–308.

Hikosaka. O., Sakamoto, M. and Usui, S. (1989) Functional properties of monkey caudate neurons. I. Activities related to saccadic eye movements. *J. Neurophysiol.*, 61: 780–798.

Hill, D.R. and Bowery, N.G. (1981) $^3$H-baclofen and $^3$H-GABA bind to bicuculline-insensitive GABA$_B$ sites in rat brain. *Nature*, 290: 149–152.

Holdefer, R.N., Norton, T.N. and Mize, R.R. (1988) The organization of GABA immunoreactive cells and processes in the lateral geniculate nucleus of the tree shrew (*Tupaia Belangeri*). *Vis. Neurosci.*, 1: 189–204.

Horn, A.K.E. and Hoffmann, K.P. (1987) Combined GABA-immunocytochemistry and TMB-HRP histochemistry of pretectal nuclei projecting to the inferior olive in rats, cats and monkey. *Brain Res.*, 409: 133–138.

Houser, C.R., Lee, M. and Vaughn, J.E. (1983) Immunocytochemical localization of glutamic acid decarboxylase in normal and deafferented superior colliculus: Evidence for reorganization of gamma-aminobutyric acid synapses. *J. Neurosci.*, 3: 2030–2042.

Hubel, D.H., Levay, S. and Wiesel, T.N. (1975) Mode of termination of retinotectal fibers in macaque monkey: an autoradiographic study. *Brain Res.*, 96: 25–40.

Huerta, M.F. and Harting, J.K. (1984) The mammalian superior colliculus: Studies of its morphology and connections. In: H. Vanegas (Ed.), *Comparative Neurology of the Optic Tectum*, New York: Plenum Press, pp. 687–773.

Hunt, S.P. and Kunzle, H. (1976) Selective uptake and transport of label within three identified neuronal systems after injection of $^3$H-GABA into the pigeon optic tectum: An autoradiographic and Golgi study. *J. Comp. Neurol.*, 170: 173–190.

Illing, R.B. and Graybiel, A.M. (1985) Convergence of afferents from frontal cortex and substantia nigra onto acetylcholinesterase-rich patches of the cat's superior colliculus. *Neuroscience*, 14: 455–482.

Irving, G.E., Norton, T.T. and Kuyk, T.K. (1983) Morphology of physiologically identified neurons in the superior colliculus of the tree shrew. *Invest. Ophthalmol. Vis. Sci. (Suppl.)*, 24(3): 224.

Joseph, J.P. and Boussaoud, D. (1985) Role of the cat substantia nigra pars reticulata in the eye and head movements. I. Neural activity. *Exp. Brain Res.*, 57: 286–296.

Kanaseki, T. and Sprague, J.M. (1974) Anatomical organization of pretectal nuclei and tectal laminae in the cat. *J. Comp. Neurol.*, 158: 319–338.

Kanno, S. and Okada, Y. (1988) Laminar distribution of GABA (gamma-amino butyric acid) in the dorsal lateral geniculate nucleus, Area 17 and Area 18 of the visual cortex, and the superior colliculus of the cat. *Brain Res.*, 451: 172–178.

Kawai, N. and Yamamoto, C. (1967) Effects of gamma-aminobutyric acid on the potentials evoked in vitro in the superior colliculus. *Experientia (Basel)*, 23: 822–823.

Kawamura, S., Fukushima, N., Hattori, S. and Kudo, M. (1980) Laminar segregation of cells of origin of ascending projections from the superficial layers of the superior colliculus in the cat. *Brain Res.*, 184: 486–490.

Kayama, Y., Fukuda, Y. and Iwama, K. (1980) GABA sensitivity of neurons of the visual layer in the rat superior colliculus. *Brain Res.*, 192: 121–131.

Khachaturian, H., Lewis, M.E. and Watson, S.J. (1983) Enkephalin systems in diencephalon and brain stem of the rat. *J. Comp. Neurol.*, 220: 310–320.

Kvale, I., Fosse, V.M. and Fonnum, F. (1983) Development of neurotransmitter parameters in the lateral geniculate body, superior colliculus and visual cortex of the albino rat. *Brain Res.*, 283: 137–145.

Laemle, L.K. (1981) A Golgi study of cellular morphology in the superficial layers of superior colliculus in man, Saimiri, and Macaca. *J. Hirnforsch*, 22: 121–125.

Laemle, L.K. and Fieldman, S.C. (1985) Somatostatin (SRIF)-like immunoreactivity in subcortical and cortical visual centers of the rat. *J. Comp. Neurol.*, 233: 452–462.

Langer, T.P. (1976) Cellular and Fiber Patterns in the Superior Colliculus of the Cat. Ph.D. Dissertation, University of Washington, Seattle, WA.

Langer, T.P. and Lund, R.D. (1974) The upper layers of the superior colliculus of the rat: A Golgi study, *J. Comp. Neurol.*, 158: 405–432

Lu, S.M., Lin, C.S., Behan, M., Cant, N.B. and Hall, W.C. (1985) Glutamic acid decarboxylase immunoreactivity in the intermediate grey layer of the superior colliculus in the cat. *Neuroscience*, 16: 123–131.

Lund, R.D. Karlsen, R. and Fonnum, F. (1978) Evidence for glutamate as a neurotransmitter in the corticofugal fibers to the dorsal lateral geniculate body and the superior colliculus in rats. *Brain Res.*, 151: 457–467.

246

Lund, R.D. (1969) Synaptic patterns of the superficial layers of the superior colliculus of the rat. *J. Comp. Neurol.*, 135:179–208.

Lund, R.D. (1972) Synaptic patterns in the superficial layers of the superior colliculus of the monkey, Macaca mulatta. *Exp. Brain Res.*, 15: 194–211.

Luo, Q. and Mize, R.R. (1991) Calbindin and GABA immunoreactivities are not reduced by monocular deprivation in the superior colliculus of the Rhesus monkey. *Invest. Ophthalmol. Vis. Sci. (Suppl.)*, 32:1035.

Luo, Q., Mize, R.R. and Tigges, M. (1990) Anti-calbindin labeling in the lateral geniculate nucleus of the Rhesus monkey and its reduction by enucleation. *Neurosci. Abstr.*, 16:108.

Luo, X.G., Kong, X.Y. and Wong-Riley, M.T.T. (1991) Effect of monocular enucleation or impulse blockage on gamma-aminobutyric acid and cytochrome oxidase levels in neurons of the adult cat lateral geniculate nucleus. *Vis. Neurosci.*, 6: 55–68.

Marrocco, R.T. and Li, R.H. (1977) Monkey superior colliculus: properties of single cells and their afferent inputs. *J. Neurophysiol.*, 40: 844–860.

May, P.J. and Hall, W.C. (1986) The sources of the nigrotectal pathway. *Neuroscience*, 19: 159–180.

McIlwain, J.T. and Fields, H.L. (1971) Interactions of cortical and retinal projections on single neurons of the cat's superior colliculus. *J. Neurophysiol.*, 34: 763–772.

Mize, R.R. (1983a) Variations in the retinal synapses of the cat superior colliculus revealed using quantitative electron microscope autoradiography. *Brain Res.*, 269: 211–221.

Mize, R.R. (1983b) Patterns of convergence and divergence of retinal and cortical synaptic terminals in the cat superior colliculus. *Exp. Brain Res.*, 51: 88–96.

Mize, R.R. (1988) Immunocytochemical localization of gamma-aminobutyric acid (GABA) in the cat superior colliculus. *J. Comp. Neurol.*, 276: 169–187.

Mize, R.R. (1989) Enkephalin-like immunoreactivity in the cat superior colliculus: distribution, ultrastructure, and colocalization with GABA. *J. Comp. Neurol.*, 285: 133–55.

Mize, R.R. and Butler, G.D. (1991) GABA$_A$ subunit receptor distribution in the cat superior colliculus using antibody immunocytochemistry. *Neurosci. Abstr.*, 17: 112.

Mize, R.R. and Horner, L.H. (1984) Retinal synapses of the cat medial interlaminar nucleus and ventral lateral geniculate nucleus differ in size and synaptic organization. *J. Comp. Neurol.*, 224: 579–590.

Mize, R.R. and Murphy, E.H. (1976) Alterations in receptive field properties of superior colliculus cells produced by visual cortex ablation in infant and adult cats. *J. Comp. Neurol.*, 168: 393–424.

Mize, R.R. and Norton, T.T. (1985) GABA antiserum reactivity in the superior colliculus of the tree shrew (Tupaia Belangeri). *Invest. Ophthalmol. Vis. Sci. (Suppl.)*, 26: 163.

Mize, R.R. and Sterling, P. (1976) Synaptic development in the superficial gray layer of the cat superior colliculus analyzed by serial section cinematography. *Invest. Ophthalmol. Vis. Sci. (Suppl.)*, 15:47.

Mize, R.R. and White, D.A. (1989) [$^3$H]muscimol labels neurons in both the superficial and deep layers of cat superior colliculus. *Neurosci. Lett.*, 104: 31–37.

Mize, R.R., Spencer, R.F. and Horner, L.H. (1986) Quantitative comparison of retinal synapses in the dorsal and ventral (parvicellular C) laminae of the cat dorsal lateral geniculate nucleus. *J. Comp. Neurol.*, 248: 57–73.

Mize, R.R., Spencer, R.F. and Sterling, P. (1981) Neurons and glia in cat superior colliculus accumulate gamma-aminobutyric acid (GABA). *J. Comp. Neurol.*, 202: 385–396.

Mize, R.R., Spencer, R.F. and Sterling, P. (1982) Two types of GABA-accumulating neurons in the superficial gray layer of the cat superior colliculus. *J. Comp. Neurol.*, 206: 180–192.

Mize, R.R., Jeon, C.J., Hamada, O.L. and Spencer, R.F. (1991a) Organization of neurons labeled by antibodies to gamma-aminobutyric acid (GABA) in the superior colliculus of the Rhesus monkey. *Vis. Neurosci.*, 6: 75–92.

Mize, R.R., Jeon, C.J., Butler, G.D., Luo, Q. and Emson, P.C. (1991b) The calcium binding protein calbindin-D 28K reveals subpopulations of projection and interneurons in the cat superior colliculus. *J. Comp. Neurol.*, 307: 417–436.

Mize, R.R., Jeon, C.J., Luo, Q. and Nabors, B. (1991c) Parvalbumin antibodies label projection neurons in the cat superior colliculus. *Invest. Ophthalmol. Vis. Sci. (Suppl.)*, 32: 1036.

Mohler, H., Malherbe, P., Draguhn, A. and Richard, J.G. (1990) GABA$_A$ receptors: structural requirements and sites of gene expression in mammalian brain. *Neurochem. Res.*, 15: 199–207.

Montero, V.M. (1986) Localization of gamma aminobutyric acid (GABA) in type 3 cells and demonstration of their source of F2 terminals in the cat lateral geniculate nucleus: A golgi-electron microscopic GABA immunocytochemical study. *J. Comp. Neurol.*, 243: 117–138.

Montero, V.M. (1989) The GABA-immunoreactive neurons in the interlaminar regions of the cat lateral geniculate nucleus: light and electron microscopic observations. *Exp. Brain Res.*, 75: 497–512.

Mooney, R.D., Klein, B.G. and Rhoades, R.W. (1985) Correlations between the structural and functional characteristics of neurons in the superficial laminae and the hamster's superior colliculus. *J. Neurosci.* 5: 2989–3009.

Moschovakis, A.K. and Karabelas, A.B. (1985) Observation on the somatodendritic morphology and axonal trajectory of intracellularly HRP-labelled efferent neurons located in the deeper layers of the superior colliculus of the cat. *J. Comp. Neurol.*, 239: 276–308.

Mugnaini, E. and Oertel, W.H. (1985) An atlas of the distribution of GABAergic neurons and terminals in the rat CNS as revealed by GAD Immunohistochemistry. In: A. Bjorklund and T. Hokfelt (Eds.), *GABA and neuropeptides in the CNS, Handbook of Chemical Neuroanatomy, Vol. 4, Pt. 1*, Amsterdam: Elsevier, pp. 436–608.

Naegele, J.R. and Barnstable, C.J. (1989) Molecular determinants of GABAergic local-circuit neurons in the visual cortex. *TINS*, 12: 28–34.

Nagai, T., McGeer, P.L. and McGeer, E.G. (1983) Distribution of GABA-T-intensive neurons in the rat forebrain and midbrain. *J. Comp. Neurol.*, 218: 220–238.

Oertel, W.H., Tappaz, A., Berod, and Mugnaini, E. (1982) Two-color immuno-histochemistry for dopamine and GABA neurons in rat substantia nigra and zona incerta. *Brain Res. Bull.*, 9: 463–474.

Okada, Y. (1974) Distribution of gamma-aminobutyric acid (GABA) in the layers of superior colliculus of the rabbit. *Brain Res.*, 75: 362–365.

Okada, Y. (1976) Distribution of GABA and GAD activity in the layers of superior colliculus of the rabbit. In: E. Roberts, T.N. Chase and D.B. Tower (Eds.), *GABA in Nervous System Function.* New York: Raven Press, pp. 229–233.

Okada, Y. and Saito, M. (1979) Inhibitory action of adenosine, 5-HT (serotonin) and GABA (gamma-aminobutyric acid) on the postsynaptic potential (PSP) of slices from olfactory cortex and superior colliculus in correlation to the level of cyclic AMP. *Brain Res.*, 160: 368–371.

Ottersen, O.P. and Storm-Mathisen, J. (1984) Glutamate and GABA containing neurons in the mouse and rat brain, as demonstrated with a new immunocytochemical technique. *J. Comp. Neurol.*, 229: 374–392.

Palacios, J.M., Wamsley, J.K. and Kuhar, M.J. (1981) High affinity GABA receptors; autoradiographic localization. *Brain Res.*, 222: 285–307.

Palkovits, M. and Brownstein, J.J. (1985) Distribution of neuropeptides in the central nervous system using biochemical micromethods. In: A. Bjorklund and T. Hökfelt (Eds.), *Handbook of Chemical Neuroanatomy. GABA and Neuropeptides in the CNS, Vol. 4, Pt 1,* Amsterdam: Elsevier, pp. 436–595.

Palmer, L.P. and Rosenquist, A.C. (1974) Visual receptive fields of single striate cortical units projecting to the superior colliculus in the cat. *Brain Res.*, 67: 27–42.

Pearson, R.C.A., Neal, J.W. and Powell, T.P.S. (1987) Increase in immunohistochemical staining of GABAergic axons in the superior colliculus and thalamus of the rat following damage of the ipsilateral striatum and frontal cortex. *Brain Res.*, 412: 352–356.

Penny, G.R., Conley, M., Schmechel, D.E. and Diamond, I.T. (1984) The distribution of glutamic acid decarboxylase immunoreactivity in the diencephalon of the opossum and rabbit. *J. Comp. Neurol.*, 228: 38–56.

Pert, C.B., Kuhar, M.J., and Snyder, S.H. (1976) Opiate receptor: Autoradiographic localization in rat brain. *Proc. Natl. Acad. Sci. USA*, 73: 3729–3733.

Petrusz, P., Merchenthaler, I. and Maderdrut, J.L. (1985) Distribution of enkephalin-containing neurons in the central nervous system. In: A. Bjorklund and T. Hökfelt (eds): *Handbook of Chemical Neuroanatomy. GABA and Neuropeptides in the CNS. Vol.4, Pt 1,* Amsterdam: Elsevier, pp. 273–334.

Pinard, R., Segu, L., Cau, P. and Lanoir, J. (1988) Distribution of benzodiazepine receptors in the rat superior colliculus: A light and electron microscope quantitative autoradiographic study. *Brain Res.*, 474: 48–65.

Pinard, R., Benfares, J. and Lanoir, J. (1990a) Electron microscopic study of GABA-immunoreactive neuronal processes in the superficial gray layer of the rat superior colliculus: their relationships with degenerating retinal nerve endings. *J. Neurocytol.*, 20: 989–1003.

Pinard, R., Richards, J.G. and Lanoir, J. (1990b) Subcellular localization of GABA$_A$/benzodiazepine receptor-like immunoreactivity in the superficial gray layer of the rat superior colliculus. *Neurosci. Lett.*, 120: 212–216.

Redgrave, P., Odekunle, A. and Dean, P. (1986) Tectal cells of origin of predorsal bundle in the rat: location and segregation from ipsilateral descending pathway. *Exp.Brain Res.*, 63: 279–93.

Rhoades, R.W. and Chalupa, L.M. (1978) Functional and anatomical consequences of neonatal visual cortical damage in superior colliculus of the golden hamster. *J. Neurophysiol.*, 41: 1466–1494.

Ricardo, J.A. (1981) Efferent connections of the subthalamic region in the rat. II. The zona incerta. *Brain Res.*, 214: 43–60.

Richards, J.G., Schoch, P. Haring, P., Takacs, B. and Mohler, H. (1987) Resolving GABA$_A$/benzodiazepine receptors: cellular and subcellular localization in the CNS with monoclonal antibodies, *J. Neurosci.*, 7: 1866–1886.

Rieck R.W., Huerta M.F., Harting J.K. and Weber J.T. (1986) Hypothalamic and ventral thalamic projections to the superior colliculus in the cat. *J. Comp. Neurol.*, 243: 249–265.

Rizzolatti, G., Camarda, R., Grupp, L.A. and Pisa, M. (1974) Inhibitory effect of remote visual stimuli on visual responses of cat superior colliculus: Spatial and temporal factors. *J. Neurophysiol.*, 37: 1262–1275.

Rothe, T., Schliebs, R. and Bigl, V. (1985) Benzodiazepine receptors in the visual structures of monocularly deprived rats. Effects of light and dark adaptation. *Brain Res.*, 329: 143–150.

Rosenquist, A.C. and Palmer, L.A. (1971) Visual receptive field properties of cells of the superior colliculus after cortical lesions in the cat. *Exp. Neurol.*, 33: 629–652.

Sandberg, M., Jacobson, I. and Hamberger, A. (1982) Release of endogenous amino acids in vitro from the superior colliculus and the hippocampus. *Prog. Brain Res.*, 55: 157–166.

Sandberg, M. and Corazzi, L. (1983) Release of endogenous amino acids from superior colliculus of the rabbit: In vitro studies after retinal ablation *J. Neurochem.*, 40: 917–921.

Schiller, P.H. (1972) The role of the monkey superior colliculus in eye movement and vision. *Invest. Ophthalmol. Vis. Sci.*, 11: 451–460.

Schiller, P.H., Stryker, M., Cynader, M. and Berman, N. (1974) Response characteristics of single cells in the monkey superior colliculus following ablation or cooling of visual cortex. *J. Neurophysiol.*, 37: 181–194.

Schliebs, R. and Rothe, T. (1988) Development of GABA$_A$ receptors in the central visual structures of rat brain. Effects of visual pattern deprivation. *Gen. Physiol. Biophys.*, 7: 281–292.

Skangiel-Kramska, J., Cymerman, U. and Kossut, M. (1986) Autoradiographic localization of GABAergic and muscarinic cholinergic receptor sites in the visual system of the kitten. *Acta Neurobiol. Exp.*, 46: 119–130.

Somogyi, P., Hodson, A.J., Smith, A.D., Nunzi, M.G., Goiro,

A. and Wu, J.Y. (1984) Different populations of GABAergic neurons in the visual cortex and hippocampus of cat contain somatostatin or cholecystokinin-immunoreactive material. *J. Neurosci.*, 4: 2590–2603.

Spangler, K.M. and Morley, B.J. (1987) Somatostatin-like immunoreactivity in the midbrain of the cat. *J. Comp. Neurol.*, 260: 87–97.

Sparks, D.L. and Mays, L.E. (1981) The role of the monkey superior colliculus in the control of saccadic eye movements. In: A.F. Fuchs and W. Becker (Eds.), *Progress in Oculomotor Research:, Vol. 2,*, Amsterdam: Elsevier, pp. 137–144.

Sprague, J.M. (1966a) Visual, acoustic, and somesthetic deficits in the cat after cortical and midbrain lesions. In: D.P. Purpura and M.D. Yahr (Eds.), *The Thalamus*, New York, Columbia Univ. Press, pp. 391–417.

Sprague, J.M. (1966b) Interaction of cortex and superior colliculus in mediation of visually guided behavior in the cat. *Science,* 153: 1544–1547.

Sprague, J.M. and Meikle, T.H. Jr. (1965) The role of the superior colliculus in visually guided behavior. *Exp. Neurol.,* 11: 115–146.

Stein, B.E. and Arigbede, M.O. (1972) A parametric study of movement detection properties of neurons in the cat's superior colliculus. *Exp. Neurol.,* 36: 179–196.

Stein, B.E., Magalhaes-Castro, B. and Kruger, L. (1975) Superior colliculus: Visuotopic-somatopic overlap. *Science,* 189: 224–226.

Stein, B.E., Magalhaes-Castro, B. and Kruger, L. (1976) Relationship between visual and tactile representations in cat superior colliculus. *J. Neurophysiol.,* 34: 401–419.

Sterling, P. (1971) Receptive fields and synaptic organization of the superficial gray layer of the cat superior colliculus. *Vision Res. (Suppl.),* 3: 309–328.

Sterling, P. and Wickelgren, B.G. (1969) Visual receptive fields in the superior colliculus of the cat, *J. Neurophysiol.,* 32: 1.

Straschill, M. and Perwein, J. (1971) Effect of iontophoretically applied biogenic amines and of cholinomimetic substances upon the activity of neurons in the superior colliculus and mesenscephalic reticular formation of the cat. *Pflügers Arch.,* 324: 43–55.

Stichel, C.C., Singer, W., Heizmann, C. and Norman, A.W. (1986) Ontogeny of calcium-binding proteins, parvalbumin and calbindin-D28K, in the dorsal lateral geniculate nucleus (LGNd) of the cat. *Neurosci. Lett. Suppl.,* 26: S55.

Stichel, C.C., Singer W., Heizmann, C.W. and Norman, A.W. (1987) Immunohistochemical localization of calcium-binding proteins, parvalbumin and calbindin-D 28K, in the adult developing visual cortex of cats: a light and electron microscopic study. *J. Comp. Neurol.,* 262: 563–577.

Stichel, C.C., Singer, W. and Heizmann, C.W. (1988) Light and electron microscopic immunocytochemical localization of parvalbumin in the dorsal lateral geniculate nucleus of the cat: Evidence for coexistence with GABA. *J. Comp. Neurol.,* 268: 29–37.

Streit, P., Knecht, E., Reubi, J.C., Hunt, S.P. and Cuenod, M. (1978) GABA specific presynaptic dendrites in pigeon optic tectum: A high resolution autoradiographic study. *Brain Res.,* 149: 204–210.

Takahashi, Y. and Ogawa, T. (1978) Electrophysiological properties of morphologically identified neurons in the rabbit's superior colliculus. *Exp. Neurol.,* 60: 254–266.

Tigges, M. and Tigges, J. (1975) Presynaptic dendrite cells and two other classes of neurons in the superficial layers of the superior colliculus of the chimpanzee. *Cell Tissue Res.,* 162: 279–295.

Tigges, M. and Tigges, J. (1991) Parvalbumin immunoreactivity of the lateral geniculate nucleus in adult Rhesus monkeys after monocular eye enucleation. *Vis. Neurosci.,* 6: 375–382.

Updyke, B.V. (1974) Characteristic of unit responses in superior colliculus of the monkey. *J. Neurophysiol.,* 37: 896–909.

Valverde, F. (1973) The neuropil in superficial layers of the superior colliculus of the mouse. A correlated Golgi and electron microscopic study. *Z. Anat. Entwickl. Gesch.,* 142: 117–147.

Vincent, S.R., Hattori, T. and McGeer, E.G. (1978) The nigrotectal projection: A biochemical and ultrastructural characterization. *Brain Res.,* 151: 159–164.

Vitorica, J., Park, D., Chin, G. and de Blas, A.L. (1988) Monoclonal antibodies and conventional antisera to the GABA$_A$ receptor/benzodiazpeine receptor/Cl-channel complex. *J. Neurosci.,* 8: 615–622.

Vitorica, J., Park, D., Chin, G. and de Blas, A.L. (1990) Characterization with antibodies of the gamma-aminobutyric acid$_A$ / benzodiazepine receptor complex during development of the rat brain. *J. Neurochem.,* 54: 187–194.

Wallace, S.F., Rosenquist, A.C. and Sprague, J.M. (1989) Recovery from cortical blindness mediated by destruction of nontectotectal fibers in the commissure of the superior colliculus in the cat. *J. Comp. Neurol.,* 284: 429–450.

Wallace, S.F., Rosenquist, A.C. and Sprague J.M. (1990) Ibotenic acid lesions of the lateral substantia nigra restore visual orientation behavior in the hemianopic cat. *J. Comp. Neurol.,* 296: 222–252.

Warton, S.S., Perouansky, M. and Grantyn, R. (1990) Development of GABAergic synaptic connections in vivo and in cultures from the rat superior colliculus. *Dev. Brain Res.,* 52: 95–111.

Watson, S.J., Akil, H., Sullivan, S. and Barchas, J.D. (1977) Immunocytochemical localization of methionine enkephalin: Preliminary observations. *Life Sci.,* 21: 733–738.

Wickelgren, B.G. and Sterling, P. (1969) Influence of visual cortex on receptive fields in the superior colliculus of the cat. *J. Neurophysiol.,* 32: 16–23.

Wurtz, R.H. and Albano, J.E. (1980) Visual-motor function of the primate superior colliculus. *Annu. Rev. Neurosci.,* 3: 189–226.

Wurtz, R.H. and Hikosaka, O. (1986) Role of the basal ganglia in the initiation of saccadic eye movements. *Prog. Brain Res.,* 64: 175–190.

Young, W.S. III and Kuhar, M.J. (1979) Autoradiographic localization of benzodiazepine receptors in the brains of humans and animals. *Nature,* 280: 393–395.

Young, W.S. III, Niehoff, D., Kuhar, M.J. Beer. B. and Lippa, A.S. (1981) Multiple benzodiazepine receptor localization by light microscopic radiohistochemistry. *J. Pharm. Exp. Ther.,* 216: 425–430.

R.R. Mize, R.E. Marc and A.M. Sillito (Eds.)
Progress in Brain Research, Vol. 90

CHAPTER 12

# The distribution and function of gamma-aminobutyric acid (GABA) in the superior colliculus

Yasuhiro Okada

*Department of Physiology, School of Medicine, Kobe University, Kusunoki-cho, Chuo-ku, Kobe 650, Japan*

## Introduction

The superior colliculus (SC) plays an important role in the integration of visual, auditory and sensory-motor information, especially in relation to eye movements. GABA must be involved in the integrative action of the SC because the SC contains many GABAergic neurons and concentrations of GABA and GAD in the superficial grey layer (SGL) are the highest in the CNS. Here we report the fine distribution of GABA and GAD in the SC of different species and the dose-dependent excitatory and inhibitory biphasic action of GABA on neurotransmission in SGL of SC slices. GABA in the SC controls eye movements, especially saccades, and further regulates the activity of collicular neurons which suppresses the propagation of seizures. Long-term potentiation can be elicited in the SGL after tetanic stimulation applied to the optic nerve. It is argued that GABA may be involved in modulating the formation of LTP in SGL. This chapter reviews the evidence for these functional effects of GABA in the mammalian SC.

## Fine distribution of GABA and localization of GABA-sensitive neurons in the superior colliculus

Gamma-aminobutyric acid (GABA) is widely distributed in the nervous system of vertebrates and invertebrates. As regards the regional distribution of GABA in the central nervous system (CNS), the superior colliculus (SC) contains a high amount of GABA (Okada et al., 1971). Histologically, the superior colliculus is characterized by cells and fibers that are organized in a laminated pattern. Laminar analysis of the distribution of GABA as well as glutamate decarboxylase (GAD), a GABA synthesizing enzyme, was performed within the SC of the rabbit (Okada, 1974, 1976a), cat (Kanno and Okada, 1988) and guinea pig (Arakawa and Okada, 1988) using microassay methods (Okada et al., 1976). The regional distribution of GABA and GAD activity obtained for each layer of the superior colliculus is summarized in Table 1. The distribution pattern of GABA within the SC was similar in each species studied. The highest level of GABA was found in the superficial gray layer (SGL) averaging 37–40 mmol/kg dry weight. The GABA levels in the optic and intermediate gray layers were each only half that of the concentration in the SGL. GABA content in the intermediate white, deep gray and deep white layers was lower than the concentration in the optic layer, ranging from 10–22 mmol/kg dry weight. GABA concentration of the whole SC was 22.9 mmol/kg dry weight in the rabbit, 29.0 in the cat, and 18.0 in the guinea pig. These GABA values based upon dry weight are in good agreement with those by wet weight (Okada et al., 1971) if the dry weight of the tissue is assumed to be 20–25% of the wet weight.

250

## TABLE 1

GAD activity and GABA levels in the layers of the superior colliculus of rabbit (Okada, 1974), cat (Kanno and Okada, 1988) and guinea pig (Arakawa and Okada, 1989)

| | Rabbit | | Cat | Guinea pig |
| | GAD | GABA | GABA | GABA |
|---|---|---|---|---|
| SGL (U) | 239.4 | 43.6 ± 2.0 | (U) 40.3 | (U) 37.4 |
| (L) | | 34.8 ± 1.8 | (L) 36.8 | (L) 23.4 |
| OL | 108.8 | 22.3 ± 0.6 | 28.2 | 15.5 |
| IG | 95.5 | 22.1 ± 0.5 | 24.1 | 15.0 |
| IW | 85.3 | 17.7 ± 0.5 | 24.0 | 10.8 |
| DG | 82.4 | 19.1 ± 0.5 | 25.2 | 13.1 |
| DW | 72.1 | 17.1 ± 0.4 | 24.5 | 10.9 |

GABA, mmol/kg dry; GAD, ~ mmol produced GABA/kg dry/h; SGL, superficial gray layer ((U) upper half of SGL) ((L) lower half of SGL); OL, optic layer; IG, intermediate gray layer; IW, intermediate white layer; DG, deep gray layer; DW, deep white layer.

The SGL, which contained the highest level of GABA, was further dissected into 6 thin laminated layers (50–80 $\mu$m in width). Table 2 shows the GABA distribution within the SGL of the rabbit SC. The GABA concentration of the superficial half was in the range of 40–44 mmol/kg dry weight, while the GABA content in the deep layers was 26–35 mmol/kg. This was true for the cat and guinea pig as shown in Table 1. A dry weight level of GABA of 44 mmol/kg is the same as that in the substantia nigra (SN) and the medial forebrain bundle which have the highest

## TABLE 2

GABA concentrations within the superficial grey layer of the rabbit superior colliculus

| Dissected layer | mmol/kg (dry) ± S.E.M. |
|---|---|
| 1 | 44.3 ± 0.9 |
| 2 | 44.8 ± 1.0 |
| 3 | 40.7 ± 2.2 |
| 4 | 34.5 ± 1.6 |
| 5 | 33.3 ± 1.7 |
| 6 | 26.4 ± 1.3 |
| OL | 21.0 ± 1.5 |

The dissected SGL was further cut into 6 thin laminated pieces (50–80 $\mu$m width), and the GABA content in each tissue piece was determined.

amount of GABA in the mammalian brain (Okada et al., 1971; Okada, 1980). GAD activity parallels the GABA levels in each layer of the SC and is highest in the SGL, where the highest level of GABA was also found. The GAD activity of other layers ranged from 30 to 49% of that in the SGL. Thus the distribution of GAD activity in each layer agrees well with that of GABA.

The SC receives a substantial input from the visual cortex and retina as well as from other nuclei in the brain stem (Lund and Lund, 1971; Sprague, 1975; Wurtz and Albano, 1980). Fibers from the retina and visual cortex terminate in the SGL and optic layers in an orderly and precise fashion. Physiological studies have revealed that both retina and cortex exert an early facilitation and later inhibition on collicular neurons (McIlwain and Field, 1971). The SC on one side also exerts an inhibition on the contralateral tectum. To investigate whether the large amount of GABA in the SGL is contained in the afferent fibers terminating in the SC or originates intrinsically within interneurons, three major inputs to the SC of the rabbit were destroyed. In one group, the left visual cortex was ablated; in another group, the left optic nerve was transected just behind the eyeball; in a third group, the SC commissure was cut by knife. The GABA level and GAD activity in the SGL were determined in each animal at 12 days after these surgical operations. No decrease in GABA content in the SGL was found by comparison with that of unoperated controls as shown in Table 3. These results indicate that the GABA concentrated in the SGL is probably intrinsic to the layer and likely contained within interneurons in the SGL.

Numerous histological and immunohistochemical studies have indicated the existence of GABAergic interneurons in the SGL (Mize et al., 1981, 1982; Mize, 1988). Cajal (1955) designated the upper SGL the "zone of horizontal cells" and the lower SGL the "zone of vertical fusiform cells". Mize showed that 45% of the SGL neurons and 30% of the intermediate grey neurons in the cat SC are GABA-immunoreactive (Mize,

1988). Electron microscopic studies have also shown that there exist many nerve terminals with flattened vesicles in the SGL of the rat (Lund, 1969; Lund and Lund, 1971), suggesting that GABAergic neurons also are located within the SGL of this species. In this connection, it is to be noted that the secondary inhibition evoked from the optic tract and the visual cortex is mediated by a single mechanism intrinsic to the SGL, and that this mechanism is postsynaptic in nature (McIlwain and Fields, 1971).

In the intracellular recording studies of SGL neurons (Takahashi et al., 1977; Takahashi and Ogawa, 1978), units exhibiting distinct inhibitory postsynaptic potentials (IPSP) elicited by optic nerve stimulation were mainly found in the upper and middle part of the SGL. Iontophoretic application of GABA (Kayama et al., 1980) readily depressed the unitary discharges of Ia cells (vertical fusiform cells in the zone of horizontal cells, Lund, 1969) and IVb cells (stellate cells) whereas II (pyriform cells) and IIIa cells (narrow field vertical cells) were GABA-insensitive. Cultured SGL neurons also have been reported to be GABA sensitive (Warton et al., 1990). These biochemical, morphological, and electrophysiological studies thus suggest that there are GABA sensitive neurons in the SGL and that the inhibition is mediated by interneurons within the SGL, although some of the GABA contained in the intermediate gray layer also originates in the nerve terminals of the nigro-tectal pathway

(Vincent et al., 1978; Dichiara et al., 1979; Chevalier et al., 1981; Karabelas et al., 1985).

## Excitatory and inhibitory effects of GABA on synaptic transmission in superior colliculus slices

In in vivo studies, iontophoretic application of GABA and muscimol into the SC can depress the evoked discharge of SC neurons, an inhibition that is antagonized by bicuculline (Kayama et al., 1980, Hikosaka and Wurtz, 1985). However, in these studies, the concentration of GABA required to produce the effect was not determined. To investigate the dose-dependent action of GABA in SGL, we have used thin slices of the SC from the guinea pig and applied GABA and its agonists and antagonists to the perfusion medium in known concentrations (Arakawa and Okada, 1987, 1988).

To prepare SC slices, tissue blocks of the SC were dissected out from the brainstem and cut parasagittally into slices of between 400 and 500 $\mu$m thickness as shown schematically in Fig. 1. The postsynaptic potential was recorded from the SGL after stimulation of the optic layer (OL). The postsynaptic potentials have been recorded previously from the surface of SC slices in horizontal thin sections after stimulation of the optic nerve (Kawai and Yamamoto, 1969; Okada and Saito, 1979). However, in such experiments, only two slices could be prepared from each animal. In the slice preparation used here, cutting the SC

TABLE 3

GABA concentrations in the SGL after denervation of main input pathways to SC of the rabbit

| Treatment | No. of animals | GABA concentration (mmol/kg (dry)) | |
|---|---|---|---|
| | | right-SGL | left-SGL |
| No surgical operation (control) | 4 | 40.6 ± 1.5 (20) | 40.9 ± 1.3 (20) |
| Ablation of right visual cortex | 4 | 39.8 ± 1.1 (20) | 39.8 ± 1.3 (20) |
| Transection of left optic nerve | 3 | 38.2 ± 1.1 (18) | 39.4 ± 1.2 (20) |
| Sections of superior collicular commissure | 3 | 39.5 ± 1.0 (18) | 40.5 ± 0.9 (18) |

252

sagittally allowed us to produce 10 slices with a histologically homogeneous structure from one animal. Using this preparation, recording and stimulating sites within the laminated SC were easily visualized. The potentials elicited in the SGL after stimulation of the OL or optic nerve are composed of two responses, an early prepotential (Fig. 1C-f) and a late potential (Fig. 1C-s). The late component was reduced by high frequency stimulation and was completely blocked in $Ca^{2+}$-free medium, although the early potential was not affected. The potentials were also recorded from slices which contained only the SGL and the OL, and repetitive extracellular unitary discharges were often superimposed on the negative field potential. These results indicate that the late negative field potential with high amplitude represents the postsynaptic potential (PSP), probably a potential representing population spikes.

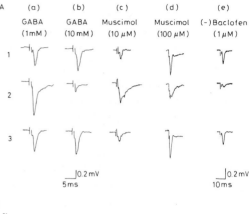

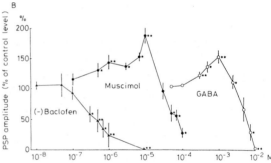

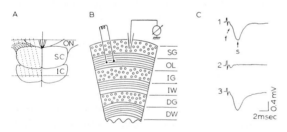

Fig. 1. A schematic drawing of a sagittal slice of the superior colliculus (SC) showing the placement of the stimulating and recording electrodes. A. A block of the brainstem containing the superior and inferior colliculus. The superior colliculus was cut sagittally into half at the centre. Five to 6 slices were obtained from each SC. It is important that the slices must be cut at a slightly oblique angle using the fibre input of the optic nerve as a guide. Cross-section slices of the SC do not result in good recording of the PSP.B. The arrangement of the recording and stimulating electrodes. C-1. Two kinds of negative potentials in the control response. Note the earlier deflection (f) in the declining phase of the large potential(s). C-2. 10 min after removal of $Ca^{2+}$ from the standard medium, the large potential(s) was abolished but not the earlier response (f). The early response (deflection) can now be clearly seen. C-3. The recovery of the later potential 10 min after reintroduction of $Ca^{2+}$ into the standard medium. In A and B. ON, optic nerve; SC, superior colliculus; IC, inferior colliculus; SG, superficial grey layer; OL, optic layer; IG, intermediate grey layer; IW, intermediate white layer; DG, deep grey layer; DW, deep white layer.

Fig. 2. Effects of GABA, muscimol, and ( − )-baclofen on the PSPs evoked in the SGL of SC slices after stimulation of OL.A. (1) Indicates the PSPs before the bath application of GABA (a, 1 mM; b, 10 mM), muscimol (c, 10 $\mu$M; 100 $\mu$M) or ( − )-baclofen (e, 1 $\mu$M), These conditions represent the control situation. (2) The PSPs recorded 10 min after the application of drugs. The PSPs were enhanced in both (a) and (c), while they were depressed in (b), (d) and (e). An early low presynaptic potential was not influenced in any of the cases. (3) Twenty minutes after removal of the drugs. Each PSP returned to the control level. A downward deflection indicates negativity. B. The dose-response curves of the effects of GABA (open circles), muscimol (filled circles), or ( − )-baclofen (filled triangles) on the amplitude of evoked PSPs. The changes in amplitude are expressed as changes compared to the original level taken as 100%. On the abscissa the concentrations of the drugs are expressed on a logarithmic scale. At the lower concentrations of GABA, up to 1 mM, the amplitude of the PSPs was augmented in a dose-dependent manner, while at concentrations greater than 1 mM the PSP amplitude was diminished in a dose-dependent manner. A similar tendency was observed with the application of muscimol. However only a decrease of the PSP was obtained with the application of ( − )-baclofen. Each plot indicates the mean value ± S.E.M. obtained from 5 slices. Asterisks indicate a significant difference from the control values (two-tailed $t$-test; * $P < 0.05$, ** $P < 0.01$).

Figure 2A shows the effect of GABA, muscimol, and ( − )-baclofen on the PSP amplitude evoked in the SGL. Bath application of GABA at a concentration of 1 mM enhanced the amplitude of the PSP. The amplitude returned to its initial level 20 min after the removal of GABA. Muscimol at 10 μM induced a similar increase in the PSP amplitude and again the PSP returned to its control level after muscimol was washed out. Figure 2B illustrates the dose-response curve of GABA, muscimol and ( − )-baclofen on the PSP evoked in SGL. When GABA was applied in the concentration range between 100 μM and 1 mM the amplitude of the evoked PSP increased in a dose-dependent fashion and a maximum increase in the amplitude of 54.2% was observed at 1 mM. A similar pattern was obtained with muscimol, a potent agonist for GABA$_A$ receptors, at concentrations between 0.1 and 10 μM. In this case, an 89.3% increase in the amplitude of the PSP was observed at a concentration of 10 μM. No enhancement of the amplitude of the PSP was observed when ( − )-baclofen, a potent agonist for GABA$_B$ receptors, was applied.

GABA at concentrations greater than 1 mM subsequently depressed the PSP in a dose-dependent manner and completely abolished it at 10 mM. Similarly, the PSP was depressed at concentrations of muscimol greater than 10 μM, and 0.1 μM ( − )-baclofen, and it almost disappeared at 100 μM muscimol and 1 μM ( − )-baclofen. Thus GABA and muscimol showed dose-dependent biphasic excitatory and inhibitory effects on neurotransmission whereas ( − )-baclofen had only an inhibitory effect.

Bicuculline is a specific antagonist for GABA$_A$ receptors. Bicuculline methiodide at concentrations greater than 10 μM elicited by itself a long-lasting negative wave following the wave of the PSP which was recorded in the standard medium. To test the effect of bicuculline methiodide on the response to GABA, we applied bicuculline methiodide at a concentration of 1 μM, which does not influence the PSP nor evoke the long-lasting negative wave. Figure 3 shows the

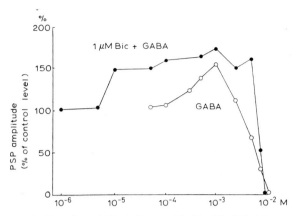

Fig. 3. The effect of bicuculline methiodide (filled circle) at a concentration of 1 μM on the dose-response curve of GABA. In the presence of bicuculline methiodide, the dose-response curve of GABA (open circle) at a concentration greater than 1 μM was shifted to the right, and the excitatory effect of GABA at lower concentrations was markedly enhanced. Bic, bicuculline methiodide.

dose-response curve of GABA in the presence of bicuculline methiodide at 1 μM. The dose-response curve for GABA inhibition was shifted slightly to the right, while the excitatory effect of GABA at lower concentrations was markedly enhanced.

It is interesting to note that both GABA and muscimol had a dual effect on neurotransmission in the SGL, i.e., excitation or inhibition depending upon their concentration. By contrast ( − )-baclofen had only an inhibitory effect. Bicuculline, a specific antagonist for GABA$_A$ receptors, shifted the inhibitory dose-response curve of GABA to the right at GABA concentrations over 1 mM (Fig. 3). These results indicate that GABA$_A$ and GABA$_B$ receptors are involved in the inhibitory action of GABA in the SGL.

GABA has been believed to function primarily as an inhibitory neurotransmitter in the CNS, although several reports have indicated the possibility of an excitatory action of GABA because GABA can cause cell depolarization in the hippocampus CA1 region of the guinea pig (Andersen et al., 1980), the guinea pig myenteric plexus ganglion (Charubini and North, 1984), the supraoptic nucleus (Ogata, 1987), the dorsal root ganglion of the rat (Deschenes et al., 1976) and the cat (Gallagher et al., 1978), and the superior cervical ganglia of the cat (De Groat, 1970) and rat (Bowery and Brown, 1974). In addition, there are reports indicating that GABA has an excitatory effect on neurotransmission in the isolated frog tectum (Nistri and Sivilotti, 1985; Sivilotti and Nistri, 1989; Mazda et al., 1990).

Concerning the mechanism of the excitatory effect of GABA in the SC slice reported here, at least three possibilities can be hypothesized. First, there could exist a network of GABAergic inhibitory interneurons which are depressed by GABA within the SGL. At lower concentrations of GABA, only those GABAergic inhibitory interneurons which possess classical GABA$_A$ receptors might be depressed. The postsynaptic neurons which give rise to the excitatory postsynaptic potential would then be free from tonic inhibition, and evoked PSPs could be facilitated by disinhibition. At higher concentrations of GABA, however, both the inhibitory interneurons and the postsynaptic neurons could be completely depressed. In fact, Lalley (1983, 1986) proposed this hypothesis for respiratory neurons of the pontine region concerned with inspiration and expiration during systemic infusion of ($-$)-baclofen. However, this hypothesis cannot explain the remarkable enhancement of the excitatory effect of the PSP at lower concentrations of GABA during the application of bicuculline methiodide at a concentration of 1 $\mu$M. Moreover, it is unlikely that the GABAergic interneurons are more sensitive to GABA than the postsynaptic cell for eliciting the PSP. In the second possibility, excitatory neurotransmitter release from the afferent optic nerve fibers might be modified presynaptically by GABAergic fibers terminating on the endings of the optic nerve fibers which would enhance the release of the excitatory transmitter used by the retinal afferents (probably glutamate). At lower concentrations of GABA, the presynaptic GABA receptors would be affected and release of the excitatory transmitter from the optic nerve terminal would be increas-

ed. At higher concentrations of GABA, the postsynaptic GABA receptor would be activated and the PSP would be depressed. Thus GABA could elicit a dual, excitatory and inhibitory action depending on its concentration. In the third possibility, there could exist two subtypes of GABA$_A$ receptors on postsynaptic sites responding to GABA and muscimol. One subtype could mediate excitation, responding to lower concentrations of GABA (high-affinity receptor for GABA), and the other could mediate inhibition, responding to greater doses of GABA (low-affinity receptor for GABA). At the lower concentrations of GABA, only high-affinity receptors would be activated and induce excitation. On the other hand, with the application of high amounts of GABA, low-affinity receptors would be activated, and the PSPs would be depressed as a result. Concerning the excitatory effect of GABA at the lower concentrations, bicuculline instead enhanced the amplitudes of PSPs (Fig. 3). In this case the existence of a new subtype of GABA$_A$ receptor could be suggested because this receptor (high-affinity) would be activated by muscimol but not blocked by bicuculline.

Concerning the dual effect of GABA, Andersen et al. (1980) and Thalmann et al. (1981) have reported a depolarizing and a hyperpolarizing effect of GABA in hippocampal CA1 neurons. Andersen et al. (1980) reported that iontophoretic application of GABA to the dendritic region depolarized the CA1 neuron, while application to the cell soma hyperpolarized the membrane potential, although it was not determined whether this depolarization actually induced excitation. This result could indicate the presence of two receptive regions on a single neuron for a single transmitter. Kandel and others (Wachtel and Kandel, 1967; Blankenship et al., 1971) reported that acetylcholine had a similar dual effect, excitation and inhibition on a single cell (L7) in the abdominal ganglion of Aplysia. These authors suggested that there are two different receptors for one transmitter, one related to excitation (easily desensitized) and another related to inhibition. Sivilotti and Nistri (1986) have also recently reported that glycine shows a biphasic excitatory and inhibitory effect on neurotransmission in the tectum of the frog. The mechanism of the dual effect of GABA in these experiments has not been fully determined. These novel excitatory and inhibitory effects of GABA in the SC may play important roles in regulating the integrative function of the SC.

## Functional aspects of GABA in the SC

*GABA-sensitive neurons in SC and modification of saccadic eye movements*

The superior colliculus is well known to be involved in eye movements, particularly saccadic eye movements (Wurtz and Albino, 1980). Cells in the intermediate layer are normally silent, but become active before saccades which are directed contralaterally. The information is sent to neurons in the brainstem reticular formation and is used for creating a motor signal for saccades. It has been shown that the saccade related cells within the SC are under tonic inhibition exerted by cells in the pars reticulata (SNr) of the substantia nigra. Before saccades to visual targets, SNr cells briefly reduce the inhibition, allowing a burst of spikes in SC cells that in turn lead to the initiation of a saccade.

Accumulating pharmacological studies support physiological evidence that the nigro-tectal pathway is GABAergic. The concentrations of GABA and GAD are high in the SC (this chapter) and GAD activity is significantly reduced after destruction of the SN (Vincent et al., 1978; Dichiara et al., 1979). Iontophoretic application of GABA readily suppresses the activity of SC cells. The synaptic inhibition induced by SN stimulation can be counteracted by the iontophoretic injection of bicuculline (Chevalier et al., 1981). On the basis of these results, Hikosaka and Wurtz (1985a) injected GABA agonists and antagonists into the monkey's SC to determine the role of GABA in saccade generation. GABA application disrupted saccadic eye movements. Muscimol delayed,

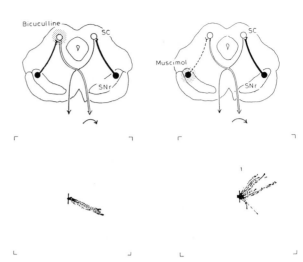

Fig. 4. Irrepressible saccade jerks induced by the blockade of the nigrocollicular tonic tonic inhibition. In (A) bicuculline was injected into the SC and in (B) muscimol into substantia nigra pars reticulata. The bottom figure below each scheme shows trajectories of saccade jerks during a fixation period after the drug injections. The monkey made irrepressible saccades toward the contralateral visual field. By injections, efferent neurons in the superior colliculus are released from the nigra-induced tonic inhibition, providing the brainstem saccade generator with continuous command signals as expressed by a thickened axon (arrow) of collicular cell in the scheme (data from Hikosaka and Wurtz, 1985a,b).

slowed, or shortened saccades made to visual or remembered targets. Injection of bicuculline facilitated the initiation of saccades (Fig. 4). Injection was followed almost immediately by stereotyped and apparently irrepressible saccades made toward the center of the movement field of SC neurons at the injection site. The eye position shifted toward the side contralateral to the injection, and saccades to the contralateral side increased in frequency. To investigate the involvement of other afferent GABAergic connections to SC or other GABA neurons within the SC, Hikosaka and Wurtz (1985b) modified the neural activity of SNr neurons which receive GABAergic input from the striatum (Okada, 1976b; DiChiara, 1980). Injections of muscimol into the SN showed the same general effect as bicuculline in the SC (Fig. 4). These results strongly suggest that the SN exerts a tonic inhibition on saccade-related neurons in SC and that the inhibition is mediated by GABA. These authors conclude that the basal ganglia contributes to the initiation of movements by a release of the target structure from tonic inhibition, and they suggest that this mechanism must be critical for generating movements that are based on stored or remembered signals that are not currently available to the animal.

*Involvement of SC in the propagation of seizures*

Because of the inhibitory action of GABA, the level of GABA helps control the neural activity in the brain. A decrease of GABA in the brain causes convulsions while the GABA agonists and drugs which increase GABA concentration have been used for clinical therapy as anticonvulsants.

Concerning transmission at the level of the colliculus, GABA may control the propagation of generalized seizures. Injection of GABA antagonists into the SC and the inferior colliculus resulted in the occurrence of running fits followed by tonic and clonic convulsions (Yamashita and Hirata, 1978; Millan et al., 1986). A decrease of GABA levels in the colliculus correlated well with the appearance of seizure afterdischarge in the slices of inferior colliculus (Yamauchi et al., 1989). Bilateral ablation of the SC abolished the anticonvulsant effects of the intranigral injection of muscimol (Galant and Gale, 1987) while the intracollicular application of bicuculline reduced seizure activity after maximal electroshock (Dean and Gale, 1989). A selective destruction of the SC facilitated the development of kindling and increased afterdischarges and motor seizures (N'gouemo and Rondouin, 1990).

Nitsch and Okada (1976) indicated the involvement of SN in the occurrence of generalized seizures, showing a correlation between the decrease of GABA concentration in discrete regions of brain and seizure discharges produced by application of methoxypyridoxine, a vitamin B6 antagonist. Gale and her colleagues found that the nigro-collicular GABAergic pathway is involved in the control of generalized convulsive seizure activity (Gale, 1985). Potentiation of GABAergic transmission within SN by bilateral

microinjections of muscimol or gamma-vinyl-GABA was found to suppress generalized convulsive seizures in the rat (Gale, 1985; Gonzalez and Hettinger, 1984; Iadarola and Gale, 1982). Bilateral injection of a GABA agonist in SN also suppressed generalized non-convulsive petit mal seizures (Depaulis et al., 1988; Depaulis et al., 1989). These reports indicate that the GABAergic nigrocollicular pathway may function as a gating mechanism for generalized seizures. The inhibition of SN efferents has an antiepileptic effect, presumably by disinhibiting the collicular cells which suppress the propagation of seizures. Which neurons in SC are responsible for anticonvulsant effects and which are the target cells of the nigrocollicular projection must be studied further.

*LTP formation in SGL and the role of GABA*

In, 1973, Bliss and Lomo (1973) discovered the phenomenon of long-term potentiation (LTP) in the hippocampus of the rabbit which was maintained for long periods after tetanic stimulation. LTP formation is interpreted to be a substantial increase in synaptic efficacy. The phenomenon has attracted great interest because of the possibility that LTP might underlie some aspect of memory storage. For this reason, research findings on the formation of LTP in the mammalian brain have mainly come from studies of the hippocampus (Teyler, 1987; Collingridge, 1987; Lynch et al., 1990).

On the other hand, it has been suggested that LTP might represent a general synaptic plasticity for modifying synapses throughout the brain. If this is so, it would be expected that LTP could be reliably recorded in many parts of the central and peripheral nervous system. Besides the hippocampus, the LTP phenomenon has been observed in several areas of cerebral cortex (Komatsu et al., 1983; Voronin, 1985, Kimura et al., 1989; Artola et al., 1990), the limbic forebrain (Racine et al., 1983), the medial geniculate body (Gerren and Weinberger, 1983), and the deep cerebellar nuclei (Racine et al., 1986). LTP also has been observed in non-mammalian neural tissue such as goldfish tectum (Lewis and Teyler, 1986). However, the properties and mechanism of LTP in tissues other than the hippocampus have not been studied extensively.

We have reported LTP formation in the SGL of the SC in in vitro (Okada, 1989; Okada and Miyamoto, 1989; Miyamoto et al., 1990) and in vivo (Shibata et al., 1990) preparations (Fig. 5 and Fig. 6) and shown that LTP formation can be modified by GABAergic interneurons within the SGL.

After electrical stimulation of the OL in SC slices, the PSP was recorded in the SGL of the SC as described previously (Fig. 1). Degeneration studies of retinotectal or corticotectal inputs to the SGL of the SC indicated that the PSP evoked in the SGL of SC slices was retinotectal in origin (Miyamoto et al., 1990). Neurotransmission in this pathway may be mediated by glutamate, be-

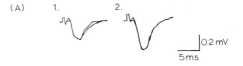

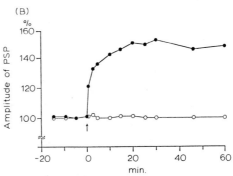

Fig. 6. An example showing the occurrence of LTP in the postsynaptic potential evoked in SGL of the rat in vivo after ablation of the ipsilatearl visual cortex. Before the experiment, the right visual cortical area was aspirated. The postsynaptic field potential was recorded at the surface of the right SC after stimulation of the optic nerve. Stimulus intensity was adjusted to obtain the negative wave at the surface whose amplitude was one-third of the maximum (evoked by the supramaximal stimulation). Twenty minutes after the tetanic stimulation (100 Hz for 10 sec), the amplitude of the negative wave increased to 150% of the original level. The line with closed circles in B shows a typical example of LTP formation. Tetanic stimulation was applied at the arrow. The line with the open circles represents the case in which no tetanic stimulation was applied. In the insert figures at the top, (AI) and (A2), the potentials just before and 20 min after tetanic stimulation are shown. The amplitude was measured from the peak of the negativity to the baseline. In the bottom figure, the amplitude just before the addition of tetanic stimulation was taken as 100%.

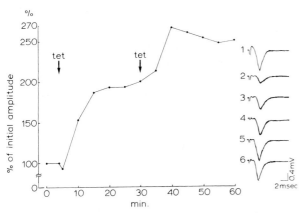

Fig. 5. The appearance of LTP in SGL of SC slice and the time course of a typical example of the LTP formation. Right panel shows the PSPs elicited in the SGL of the SC slice after the stimulation to OL. (1) indicates the PSP of maximum amplitude with one test stimulus. In (2) the stimulus intensity was adjusted to evoke PSP for the amplitude to be about 1/3 of the maximum amplitude. (3) and (4) show potentiated PSPs 5 and 15 min after the tetanic stimulation (50 Hz, 20 sec), respectively. Furthermore (5) and (6) show more potentiated PSPs 10 and 20 min after the second tetanic stimulation, respectively. Left panel indicates the time course of LTP formation of the slice shown in the right panel. In the figure the adjusted amplitude of PSP in (2) of right panel was taken as 100%. At tet↓, the tetanic stimulation was applied to OL.

cause the PSP amplitude was reduced or blocked by application of kynurenate or quinoxaline dione (DNQX) to the medium. Furthermore, the concentration of glutamate in the right SGL was significantly reduced by 32% after left optic tract denervation and by 30% after ablation of the right visual cortex, compared with that in the left SGL.

LTP in the SGL of SC slices was induced by tetanic stimulation to the OL. The optimal stimulation parameters for inducing LTP were 50 Hz frequency and 20 sec duration (Miyamoto and Okada, 1988). In the granular layer and CA1 region of hippocampus, activation of NMDA receptors has been reported to be essential for LTP (Collingridge and Bliss, 1987). However, this is not the case for LTP in the SC because NMDA receptor antagonists such as D-APV only mask the appearance of LTP during its application (Miyamoto et al., 1990). LTP formation in the hippocampus has been reported to be mediated by metabolic processes involving protein kinase C (PKC) (Lovinger et al., 1987; Malenka et al., 1987) and this is true for LTP in the SGL (Tomita et al., 1990).

In in vivo preparations in the rat, we could not induce LTP in the PSP by tetanic stimulation to the optic nerve of the intact animal. However, LTP was elicited by tetanic stimulation either when the ipsilateral visual cortex was removed (Fig. 6) or when picrotoxin, a GABA antagonist, was administered to the animal before tetanic stimulation (Shibata et al., 1990). In the SC slices, the application of GABA to the perfusion medium inhibited LTP formation and application of bicuculline facilitated the induction of LTP (Tomita and Okada, in preparation). These results indicate that GABAergic activity, whether it is extrinsic or intrinsic in the SC, can modulate the induction of LTP in the SGL.

Concerning the involvement of GABAergic neurons in modifying LTP formation, application of bicuculline and picrotoxin facilitate the induction of LTP in hippocampal slices (Wigstrom and Gustafasson, 1985). In study of LTP in slice preparations, bicuculline is usually applied to the medium (Kimura et al., 1989). In slices of visual cortex, application of low doses of bicuculline induces long-term depression by tetanic stimulation whereas bicuculline at high doses elicits LTP (Artola et al., 1990). The induction of LTP may thus be influenced by the excitability or the level of membrane potential of postsynaptic neurons which is modulated by GABAergic input.

The involvement of extrinsic GABAergic afferents to SC can not be completely excluded as sources of modulation of LTP formation in the SGL. However, the ablation of ipsilateral visual cortical areas or the application of picrotoxin in animals with an intact ipsilateral visual cortex both facilitate the formation of LTP in vivo preparations. The ipsilateral corticotectal pathway has been reported to exert an inhibitory action on the neural activity evoked by the retinotectal pathway (McIlwain and Fields, 1979). This inhibition is probably mediated by GABAergic interneurons located in the SGL because the corticotectal pathway is glutamatergic (Fosse and Fonnum, 1986; Sakurai et al., 1990) and many GABAergic interneurons located in the SGL receive corticotectal synapses (Mize, 1988). In the isolated slice preparation of the SC, LTP can be easily induced by tetanic stimulation and the formation of LTP is modified by GABA agonists and antagonists. These results strongly suggest that corticotectal afferents tonically inhibit the induction of LTP that is elicited by tetanic stimulation of the optic nerve, probably by activating GABAergic interneurons within SGL. This ability of neurons to induce LTP in the SC may depend upon the delicate balance between excitatory and inhibitory inputs through the retinotectal, corticotectal, or other extrinsic pathways. GABAergic systems thus may have an important role in maintaining a delicate balance of neural activity within SC. The true mechanism and function of LTP formation in the SC in connection with GABAergic inhibitory processes remains to be investigated in further studies.

## Summary

Laminer analysis of the distribution of GABA and GAD in the superior colliculus has shown that the distribution pattern of GABA within the SC is smilar in rabbit, cat, and guinea pig. The highest levels of GABA were found in the superficial gray layer (SGL), averaging 37–40 mmol/kg dry weight. The GABA concentrations in the deep layers were each only half that of the levels in the SGL. The concentrations of both GABA and GAD in the upper half of SGL are the same as those in the substantia nigra and medial forebrain bundle which have the highest amounts of GABA in the CNS. Denervation studies of the fibers projecting to SGL suggest that the GABA concentrated in the SGL is intrinsic to the layer. The results obtained from immunohistochemical and electron microscopic studies on the localization of GABA neurons corresponds well with the regional distribution pattern of GABA and GAD reported here. However, pharmacological and electrophysiological studies do not necessarily accord well with the GABA distribution studies because they indicate that there are many GABA sensitive neurons in both the SGL and DGL.

To investigate the role of GABA in the SGL, the effect of GABA and its agonists and antagonists on neurotransmission in SGL has been studied in SC slices in a perfusion system. Bath applied GABA (100 $\mu$M to 1 mM) enhanced the amplitude of postsynaptic field potentials (PSP) in SGL in a dose-dependent fashion and at concentrations above 1 mM it depressed the PSP in a dose-dependent fashion. A similar response pattern was obtained with muscimol (0.1–10 $\mu$M excitation; > 10 $\mu$M inhibition). However (−)-baclofen only inhibited the PSP. Bicuculline (1 $\mu$M) shifted the dose-response inhibitory curve of GABA to the right, while the excitatory effect was enhanced. These results indicate that GABA has an excitatory and inhibitory action on neurotransmission in the SGL.

The nigro-tectal GABAergic fibers terminate in the intermediate and deep layers of SC. Inhibition of GABAergic activity in the SC causes irrepressible saccades made toward the center of the movement field while GABA activation delays and slows saccadic eye movements. Thus, GABA in the SC plays an important role in the control of eye movements. The same GABAergic projection is also related to the propagation of generalized sezures. There exist collicular neurons which suppress the propagation of seizures. The activation of these neurons by disinhibition of the tonic action of the GABAergic nigro-tectal input to SC exerts antiepileptic effects. GABA in the SC thus appears to control the gating of

generalized seizures. Long-term potentiation (LTP), which has been extensively studied in the hippocampus, can also be evoked in the SGL of the superior colliculus after tetanic stimulation of the optic nerve. Application of GABA in the medium depresses the formation of LTP in the SGL of SC slices. In in vivo preparations, LTP in the SGL can be induced only when the ipsilateral visual cortex has been removed or when picrotoxin, a GABA antagonist, is administered to the animal before tetanic stimulation. GABA in the SC may be involved in the modification of LTP formation in SGL, probably through intrinsic GABA neurons.

In conclusion, GABA is found in high levels in the mammalian superior colliculus and plays an important role in integrating inputs from the cortex, retina, and brainstem. The neural circuits underlying this integration are as yet poorly understood.

## References

Andersen, P., Dingledine, R., Gjestad, L., Langmoen, I.A. and Mosfeldt Laursen, A. (1980) Two different responses of hippocampal pyramidal cells to application of gamma-aminobutyric acid. *J. Physiol.,* 305: 279–296.

Arakawa, T. and Okada, Y. (1987) Dual effect of γ-aminobutyric acid (GABA) on neurotransmission in the superior colliculus slices from the guinea pig. *Proc. Japan Acad.,* 63: Ser.B, 389–392.

Arakawa, T. and Okada, Y. (1988) Excitatory and inhibitory action of GABA on synaptic transmission in slices of guinea pig superior colliculus. *Eur. J. Pharmacol.,* 158: 217–224.

Artola, A., Brocher, S. and Singer, W. (1990) Different voltage-dependent thresholds for inducing long-term depression and long-term potentiation in slices of rat visual cortex. *Nature,* 347: 69–72.

Blankenship, J.E., Wachtel, H. and Kandel, E.R. (1971) Ionic mechanisms of excitatory, inhibitory, and dual synaptic actions mediated by an identified interneuron in abdominal ganglion of Aplysia. *J. Neurophysiol.,* 34: 76–92.

Bliss, T.V.P. and Lomo, T.J. (1973) Long-lasting potentiation of synaptic transmission in the dentate area of the anesthetized rabbit following stimulation of the perforant path. *J. Physiol.,* 232: 331–356.

Bowery, N.G. and Brown, D.A. (1974) Depolarizing actions of γ aminobutyric acid and related compounds on rat superior ganglia in vitro. *Br. J. Pharmacol.,* 50: 205–218.

260

Cajal, S. and Ramon, Y. (1955) *Histologie du System Nerveux de l'Homme et des Vertebres,* Vol.2, Consejo, Superior de Investigaciones Cientificas, Institute Ramon Cajal, Madrid.

Cherubini, E. and North, R.E. (1984) Actions of γ-aminobutyric acid on neurones of guinea-pig myenteric plexus. *Br. J. Pharmacol.,* 82: 93–100.

Chevalier, G., Thierry, A.M., Shibasaki, T. and Feger, J. (1981) Evidence for GABAergic inhibitory nigro-collicular pathway in the rat. *Neurosci. Lett.,* 21: 67–70.

Collingridge, G.L. and Bliss, T.V.P. (1987) NMDA receptors -their role in long-term potentiation. *Trends Neurosci.,* 10: 288–293.

Dean, P. and Gale, K. (1989) Anticonvulsant action of GABA receptor blockade in the nigro-collicular terget region. *Brain Res.,* 477: 391–395.

De Groat, W.C. (1970) The actions of γ aminobutyric acid and related amino acids on mammalian autonomic ganglia. *J. Pharmacol. Exp. Ther.,* 172: 384–396.

Depaulis, A., Vergnes, M., Marescaux, C., Lannes, B. and Warter, J.M. (1988) Evidence that activation of GABA receptors in the substantia nigra suppresses spontaneous spike-and-wave discharges in the rat. *Brain Res.,* 448: 20–29.

Depaulis, A., Snead, O.C., III. Marescaux, C. and Vergnes, M. (1989) Suppressive effects of intranigral injection of muscimol in three models of generalized non-convulsive epilepsy induced by chemical agents. *Brain Res.,* 498: 64–72.

Deschenes, M., Feltz, P. and Lamour, Y. (1976) A model for an estimate in vivo of the ionic basis of presynaptic inhibition: an intracellular analysis of the GABA-induced depolarization in rat dorsal root ganglia. *Brain Res.,* 118: 486–493.

DiChiara, G., Porceddu, M.L., Morelli, M.L., Mulas, M.L. and Gessa, G.L. (1979) Evidence for a GABAergic projection from the substantia nigra to the ventromedial thalamus and to the superior colliculus of the rat. *Brain Res.,* 176: 273–284.

DiChiara, G., Morelli, M., Porceddu, M.L. and Del Fiacco, M. (1980) Effect of discrete kainic acid induced lesions of corpus caudatus and globus pallidus on glutamic acid decarboxylase of rat substantia nigra. *Brain Res.,* 189: 193–208.

Fosse, V.M. and Fonnum, F. (1986) Effects of kainic acid and other excitotoxins in the rat superior colliculus: relations to glutamatergic afferents. *Brain Res.,* 383: 28–37.

Gale, K. (1985) Mechanisms of seizure control mediated by γ aminobutyric acid: role of the substantia nigra. *Fed. Proc.,* 44: 2414–2424.

Gallagher, J.P., Higashi, H. and Nishi, S. (1978) Characterization and ionic basis of GABA-induced depolarization recorded in vitro from cat primary afferent neurones. *J. Physiol.,* 275: 263–282.

Garant, D.S. and Gale, K. (1987) Substantia nigra-mediated anticonvulsant actions: role of nigral output pathways. *Exp. Neurol.,* 97: 143–159.

Gerren, R.A. and Weinberger, N.M. (1983) Long-term potentiation in themagnocellular medial geniculate nucleus of the anesthetized cat. *Brain Res.,* 265: 138–142.

Gonzalez, L.P. and Hettinger, M.K. (1984) Intranigral muscimol suppresses ethanol withdrawal seizures. *Brain Res.,* 298: 163–166.

Hikosaka, O. and Wurtz, R.H. (1985a) Modification of saccadic eye movements by GABA-related substances. I. Effect of muscimol and bicuculline in monkey superior colliculus. *J. Neurophysiol.,* 53: 266–291.

Hikosaka, O. and Wurtz, R.H. (1985b)) Modification of saccadic eye movements by GABA-related substances. II. Effects of muscimol in monkey substantia nigra pars reticulata. *J. Neurophysiol.,* 53: 292–308.

Iadarola, M.J. and Gale, K. (1982) Substantia nigra: site of anti-convulsant activity mediated by gamma-aminobutyric acid. *Science,* 218: 1237–1240.

Kanno, S. and Okada, Y. (1988) Laminar distribution of GABA (γ-aminobutyric acid) in the dorsal lateral geniculate nucleus, Area 17 and Area 18 of the visual cortex, and the superior colliculus of the cat. *Brain Res.,* 451: 172–178.

Karabelas, A.B. and Moschovakis, A.K. (1985) Nigral inhibitory termination on efferent neurons of the superior colliculus: An intracellular horseradish peroxidase study in the cat. *J. Comp. Neurol.,* 239: 309–329.

Kawai, N. and Yamamoto, C. (1969) Effect of 5-hydroxytryptamine, LSD and related compounds on electrical activities evoked in thin slices from the superior colliculus. *Int. J. Neuropharmacol.,* 8: 437–449.

Kayama, Y., Fukuda, Y. and Iwama, K. (1980) GABA sensitivity of neurons of the visual layer in the rat superior colliculus. *Brain Res.,* 192: 121–131.

Kimura, F., Nishigori, A., Shirokawa, T. and Tsumoto, T. (1989) Long-term potentiation and N-methyl-D-aspartate receptors in the visual cortex of young rats. *J. Physiol. (London),* 414: 125–144.

Komatsu, Y., Toyama, K., Maeda, J. and Sakaguchi, H. (1981) Long-term potentiation investigated in a slice preparation of striate cortex of young kittens. *Neurosci. Lett.,* 26: 269–274.

Lalley, P.M. (1983) Biphasic effect of baclofen, on phrenic motorneurons: possible involvement possible involvement of two types of aminobutyric acid (GABA) receptors. *J. Pharmacol. Exp. Ther.,* 226: 616–624.

Lalley, P.M. (1986) Effects of baclofen and γ aminobutyric acid on different types of medullary respiratory neurons. *Brain Res.,* 376: 392–395.

Lewis, D. and Teyler, T.J. (1986) Long-term potentiation in the goldfish optic tectum. *Brain Res.,* 375: 246–250.

Lovinger, D.M., Wong, K.L., Murakami, K. and Routtenberg, A. (1987) Protein kinase C inhibitors eliminate hippocampal long-term potentiation. *Brain Res.,* 436: 177–183.

Lund, R.D. (1969) Synaptic patterns of the superficial layers of the superior colliculus of the rat. *J. Comp. Neurol.,* 135: 179–208.

Lund, R.D. and Lund, J.S. (1971) Modifications of synaptic patterns in the superior colliculus of the rat during development and following deafferentation. *Vision Res., Suppl.,* 3: 281–298.

Lynch, G., Markus, K., Arai, A. and Larson, J. (1990) The Nature and causes of hippocampal long-term potentiation. In: J. Storm-Mathisen, J. Zimner and O.P. Ottersen (Eds.),

*Progress in Brain Research, Vol. 83*, Amsterdam: Elsevier, pp. 233–250.

Malenka, R.C., Ayoub, G.S. and Nicoll, R.A. (1987) Phorbol esters enhance transmitter release in rat hippocampal slices. *Brain Res.*, 403: 198–203.

Mazda, G.Y., Nistri, A. and Sivilotti, L. (1990) The effect of GABA on the frog optic tectum is sensitive to ammonium and to penicillin. *Eur. J. Pharmacol.*, 179: 111–118.

McIlwain, J.T. and Fields, H.L. (1971) Interactions of cortical and retinal projections on single neurons of the cat's superior colliculus. *J. Neurophysiol.*, 34: 763–772.

Millan, M.H., Meldrum, B.S. and Faingold, C.L. (1986) Induction of audiogenic seizure susceptibility by focal infusion of excitant amino acid or bicuculline into the inferior colliculus of normal rats. *Exp. Neurol.*, 91: 634–639.

Miyamoto, T. and Okada, Y. (1988) Effective stimulation parameters for the LTP formation in the superior colliculus slices from the guinea pig. *Proc. Japan Acad. Ser B*, 64: 256–259.

Miyamoto, T., Sakurai, T. and Okada, Y. (1990) Masking effect of NMDA receptor antagonists on the formation of long-term potentiation (LTP) in superior colliculus slices from the guinea pig. *Brain Res.*, 518: 166–172.

Mize, R.R., Spencer, R.F. and Sterling, P. (1981) Neurons and glia in cat superior colliculus accumulate [3H]-gamma-amminobutyric acid (GABA). *J. Comp. Neurol.*, 202: 385–396.

Mize, R.R., Spencer, R.F. and Sterling, P. (1982) Two types of GABA-accumulating neurons in the superficial gray layer of the cat superior colliculus. *J. Comp. Neurol.*, 206: 180–192.

Mize, R.R. (1988) Immunocytochemical localization of gamma-aminobutyric acid (GABA) in the cat superior colliculus. *J. Comp. Neurol.*, 276: 169–187.

N'gouemo, P. and Rondouin, G. (1990) Evidence that superior colliculi are involved in the control of amygdala kindled seizures. *Neurosci. Lett.*, 120: 38–41.

Nistri, A. and Sivilotti, L. (1985) An unusual effect of gamma-aminobutyric acid on synaptic transmission of frog tectal neurones in vitro. *Br. J. Pharmacol.*, 85: 917–921.

Nitsch, C. and Okada, Y. (1976) Differential decrease of GABA in the substantia nigra and other discrete regions of the rabbit brain during the preictal period of methoxypyridoxine-induced seizures. *Brain Res.*, 105: 173–178.

Ogata, N. (1987) γ-Aminobutyric acid (GABA) causes consistent depolarization of neurons in the guinea pig supraoptic nucleus due to an absence of GABAb recognition sites. *Brain Res.*, 403: 225–233.

Okada, Y., Nitsch-Hassler, C., Kim, J.S., Bak, I.J. and Hassler, R. (1971) Role of γ-aminobutyric acid (GABA) in the extrapyramidal motor system, I Regional distribution of GABA in rabbit, rat, guinea pig and baboon CNS. *Exp. Brain Res.*, 13: 514–518.

Okada, Y. (1974) Distribution of γ-aminobutyric acid (GABA) in the layers of superior colliculus of the rabbit. *Brain Res.*, 75: 362–365.

Okada, Y. (1976a) Distribution of GABA and GAD activity in the layers of superior colliculus of the rabbit. In: E. Roberts, T.N. Chase and D.B. Tower (Eds.), *GABA in Nervous System Function*, New York: Raven Press, pp. 229–233.

Okada, Y. (1976b) Role of GABA in the substantia nigra. In: E. Roberts, T.N. Chase and D.B. Tower (Eds.), *GABA in Nervous System Function,*, New York, Raven Press, pp. 235–243.

Okada, Y., Taniguchi, H. and Chimada, Ch. (1976) High concentration of GABA and high glutamate decarboxylase activity in rat pancreatic islets and human insulinoma. *Science,* 194: 620–622.

Okada, Y. and Saito M. (1979) Inhibitory action of adenosine, 5-HT (serotonin) and GABA (γ-aminobutyric acid) on the postsynaptic potential (PSP) of slices from olfactory cortex and superior colliculus in correlation to the level of cyclic AMP. *Brain Res.*, 160: 368–371.

Okada, Y. (1980) Regional distribution of GABA (γ-aminobutyric acid), GAD (glutamate decarboxylase), GABA-T (GABA-transaminase) and glutamate in the rat central nervous system. In: M. Ito, (Ed.), *Integrative Control Function of Brain III,* Tokyo: Kodansha, pp. 26–28.

Okada, Y. and Ozawa, S. (1982) The concentration of GABA required for its inhibitory action on the hippocampal pyramidal cell in vitro. In: Y. Okada and E. Roberts (Eds.), *Problems in GABA research from brain to bacteria*, Amsterdam: Excerpta Medica, pp. 87–95.

Okada, Y. and Miyamoto, T. (1989) Formation of long-term potentiation in superior colliculus slices from the guinea pig. *Neurosci. Lett.*, 96: 108–113.

Okada, Y. (1989) Long-term potentiation in the superior colliculus slices. In Rahmann (Ed.), Fortschritte der Zoologie /Progress in Zoology, Vol.37, *Fundamentals of Memory Formation: Neuronal Plasticity and Brain Function,* Stuttgart, New York: Gustav Fischer Verlag, pp. 190–196.

Racine, R.J., Milgram, N.W. and Hafner, S. (1983) Long-term potentiation phenomena in the rat limbic forebrain. *Brain Res.*, 260: 217–231.

Racine, R.J., Wilson, D.A., Gingell, R. and Sunderland, D. (1986) Long-term potentiation in the interpositus and vestibular nuclei in the rat. *Exp. Brain Res.*, 63: 158–162.

Sakurai, T., Miyamoto, T. and Okada, Y. (1990) Reduction of glutamate content in rat superior colliculus after retinotectal denervation. *Neurosci. Lett.*, 109: 299–303.

Shibata, Y., Tomita, H. and Okada, Y. (1990) The effects of ablation of the visual cortical area on the formation of LTP in the superior colliculus of the rat. *Brain Res.*, 537: 345–348.

Sivilotti, L. and Nistri, A. (1986) Biphasic effects of glycine on synaptic responses of the frog optic tectum in vitro. *Neurosci. Lett.*, 66: 25–30.

Sivilotti, L. and Nistri, A. (1989) Pharmacology of a novel effect of γ-aminobutyric acid on the frog optic tectum in vitro. *Eur. J. Pharmacol.*, 164: 205–212.

Sprague, J.M. (1975) Mammalian tectum: intrinsic organization, afferent inputs, and integrative mechanism. *Neurosci. Res. Prog. Bull.*, 13: 204–213.

Takahashi, Y., Ogawa, T., Takimori, T. and Kato, H. (1977)

Intracellular studies of rabbit's superior colliculus. *Brain Res.*, 123: 170–175.

Takahashi, Y. and Ogawa, T. (1978) Electrophysiological properties of morphologically identified neurons in the rabbit's superior colliculus. *Exp. Neurol.*, 60: 254–266.

Teyler, T.J. and Discenna, P. (1987) Long-term potentiation. *Annu. Rev. Neurosci.*, 10: 131–161.

Thalmann, R.H., Peck, E.J. and Ayala, G.F. (1981) Biphasic response of hippocampal pyramidal neurons to GABA. *Neurosci. Lett.*, 21: 319.

Tomita, H., Shibata, Y., Sakurai, T. and Okada, Y. (1990) Involvement of a protein kinase C-dependent process in long-term potentiation formation in guinea pig superior colliculus slices. *Brain Res.*, 536: 146–152.

Vincent, S.R., Hattori, T. and McGeer, E.G. (1978) The nigrotectal projection: a biochemical and ultrastructural characterization. *Brain Res.*, 151: 159–164.

Voronin, L.L. (1985) Synaptic plasticity at archicortical and neocortical levels. *Neurofiziologiya*, 16: 651–665.

Wachtel, H. and Kandel, E.R. (1967) A direct synaptic con-nection mediating both excitation and inhibition. *Science*, 158: 1206–1208.

Warton, S.S., Perouansky, M. and Grantyn, R. (1990) Development of GABAergic synaptic connections in vivo and in cultures from the rat superior colliculus. *Dev. Brain Res.*, 52: 95–111.

Wigstrom, H. and Gustafasson, B. (1985) Facilitation of hippocampal long-term potentiation by GABA antagonists. *Acta Physiol. Scand.*, 125: 159–172.

Wurtz, R.H. and Albano, J.E. (1980) Visual motor function of the primate superior colliculus. *Annu. Rev. Neurosci.*, 3: 189–226.

Yamashita, J. and Hirata, Y. (1978) Running fits induced by direct administration of semicarbazide into the SC of the mouse. *Neurosci. Lett.*, 8: 89–92.

Yamauchi R., Amatsu, M. and Okada, Y. (1989) Effect of GABA (γ-aminobutyric acid) on neurotransmission in inferior colliculus slices from the guinea pig. *Neurosci. Res.*, 6: 446–455.

R.R. Mize, R.E. Marc and A.M. Sillito (Eds.)
Progress in Brain Research, Vol. 90

CHAPTER 13

# Behavioural consequences of manipulating GABA neurotransmission in the superior colliculus

Paul Dean and Peter Redgrave

*Department of Psychology, University of Sheffield, P.O. Box 603, Sheffield, S10 2UR, England, UK*

The superior colliculus, situated on the roof of the midbrain, not only receives a massive visual input from the retina, but projects directly to premotor and motor areas of brainstem and spinal cord. Its non-mammalian homologue, the optic tectum, shares a similar organisation: there are striking resemblances between optic tectum and superior colliculus in animals as diverse as lizards and monkeys (Gaither and Stein, 1979). These observations suggest that the structure is concerned with basic, essential visuomotor competences. Traditionally its main role in mammals has been thought to be in orienting, that is identifying the spatial location of a novel stimulus and pointing the eyes, head or body towards it. However, recent behavioural and physiological data (for review see Dean et al., 1989) indicate that the superior colliculus, at least in rodents, is associated with initiating a wide range of appropriate behavioural and physiological reactions to stimuli suddenly appearing in the spatial map. For example, escape responses to the sight of a moving predator, critical to the survival of small animals such as rats, appear to require an intact superior colliculus.

An interesting feature of these 'appropriate' behavioural and physiological reactions is that they can be elicited not only by sensory stimuli, but also by appropriate manipulation of GABA-ergic neurotransmission within the superior colliculus. Why should this be? The present chapter attempts to answer that question by reviewing evidence concerning the behavioural consequences of manipulating GABA in the superior colliculus. It is divided into four main sections. The first describes the wide range of behavioural and physiological reactions that have been obtained by microinjecting drugs that affect GABA-ergic neurotransmission into the superior colliculus. The second reviews what is known of the collicular output mechanisms which mediate the reactions. The third considers to what extent the collicular behaviours produced pharmacologically are under control by GABAergic afferent projections in the normal animal. The final section discusses functional implications of the behavioural findings, in particular attempting to relate GABAergic disinhibitory control within the superior colliculus to the more general issues of forebrain control mechanisms and cerebral architecture.

This chapter concentrates on work carried out on rats, because not only have many of the relevant experiments been carried out in this species, but also the range of behavioural reactions obtained from collicular manipulation appears to be much greater in rodents than in cats or monkeys. Results obtained from manipulating collicular GABAergic transmission in species other than the rat are mentioned in the main body of the chapter where appropriate, and reviewed briefly at its end.

the nature of these physiological responses depended on the location of the injection site limits any contribution from non-specific effects of activating tectal tissue.

Finally, and possibly related to the EEG effects, interference with GABAergic neurotransmission in the superior colliculus can have effects on epileptic seizures. Bilateral injections of picrotoxin can produce mild clonic convulsions (Redgrave et al., 1981a), and bicuculline can potentiate seizures induced by the chemoconvulsant pentylenetetrazol (unpublished data). However, bilateral microinjections of bicuculline can also prevent tonic hindlimb extension in the MES (maximal electroshock) model of human grand mal seizures (Dean and Gale, 1989; Shehab et al., 1990).

### GABA related responses and collicular function

The above array of reactions produced by interfering with collicular GABAergic systems appears confusing when considered in the light of the classical view of the superior colliculus as a structure controlling orienting behaviour (Schneider, 1969; Schiller, 1972; Sprague et al., 1973). However, as mentioned above, more recent studies of the rodent superior colliculus indicate that it can mediate a wide range of species-specific responses appropriate to novel sensory events (Dean and Redgrave, 1984; Dean et al., 1989). In rodents, who have many predators, a high proportion of such responses are defensive. Thus, the mixture of behavioural effects obtained by reducing GABAergic transmission within the rat superior colliculus makes sense for a structure that can produce either approach or avoidance reactions to an unexpected stimulus (depending on the nature of the stimulus, the context and so forth).

Orienting and defensive movements, when elicited by natural stimuli, are accompanied by changes in heart rate, blood pressure and the cortical EEG. The similar autonomic changes produced by stimulation of the superior colliculus itself (including electrical stimulation and mi-

croinjection of excitatory amino acids, as well as of GABA-acting drugs) suggest that the superior colliculus can trigger a full integrated reaction to a novel stimulus, not just the movements alone (Dean et al., 1984, 1991; Redgrave and Dean, 1985; Keay et al., 1988, 1990a). The observations that (a) more than one pattern of autonomic response can be evoked from the superior colliculus and (b) different patterns of autonomic reaction accompany natural orienting and defensive movements, are consistent with this general view. However, the precise relationship between the behaviours and the autonomic reactions evoked from the superior colliculus remains to be determined (for further discussion see Keay et al., 1988).

It is not so easy to make functional sense of the pro- and anti-convulsant effects of manipulating GABAergic neurotransmission within the superior colliculus. Further studies are needed to clarify the relationship between these effects and the behavioural effects of individual microinjections.

## Distribution of responses within the superior colliculus: possible mediation by collicular efferents

A number of variables are likely to contribute to explaining why different microinjections of GABA-acting drugs produce different behavioural and physiological effects. Some of these variables, such as dose of drug, volume of injection or the particular pharmacological action a drug has on different classes of GABA-receptor, have been little investigated. The main variable of interest to date has been site of injection. Figure 1 illustrates how changing the injection site can have a major effect on the pattern of cardiovascular response obtained. Similar dramatic effects can be obtained for behaviour (e.g., Kilpatrick et al., 1982): for example, if a bilateral injection is by mistake made asymmetrically, it is possible to obtain a Jekyll and Hyde animal that approaches a stimulus on one side of its body, yet violently

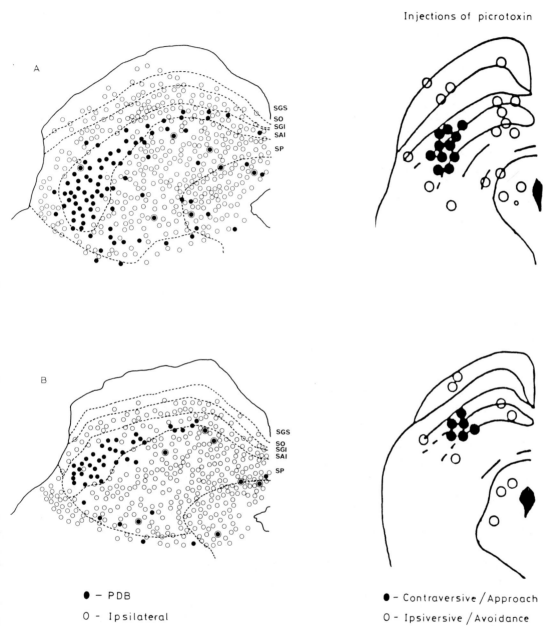

Injections of picrotoxin

A

SGS
SO
SGI
SAI

SP

B

SGS
SO
SGI
SAI

SP

● – PDB

O – Ipsilateral

● – Contraversive / Approach

O – Ipsiversive / Avoidance

Fig. 3. A comparison of anatomical data with results from behavioural experiments. A. Rostral colliculus (about 6.3 mm caudal to bregma). B. Caudal colliculus (about 7.3 mm caudal to bregma). *Labelled Cells.* Shows cell plots from a single animal used in a double label retrograde tracing study (Redgrave et al., 1986) in which different fluorescent tracers were injected simultaneously into the ipsilateral and contralateral descending pathways of the superior colliculus. Each black dot represents 5 cells labelled with True Blue after multiple injections into the contralateral predorsal bundle; these cells were concentrated in SAI (the intermediate white layer). Each unfilled circle represents 5 cells labelled with Diamidino Yellow after multiple injections into rostral parts of the ipsilateral descending pathway; these cells were concentrated in SO, SGI and SP layers of the superior colliculus (see legend to Fig. 1 for abbreviations). *Injections of Picrotoxin.* The distribution of sites giving contralateral/approach and ipsilateral/avoidance movements following microinjections of picrotoxin (40 ng in 200 nl) into rostral and caudal superior colliculus. Adapted from Redgrave et al. (1986); behavioural data from Kilpatrick et al. (1982).

retreats from the same stimulus presented on the opposite side.

The most plausible basis for these striking effects is the anatomical organisation of collicular output pathways. The superior colliculus projects to a wide variety of structures, located in the diencephalon, midbrain, pons, medulla and spinal cord (Huerta and Harting, 1984; Redgrave et al., 1987a). It is apparent that at least some of these projections arise from distinct populations of collicular output cells (Redgrave et al., 1986, 1987b, 1990a; Sahibzada et al., 1987) located in particular sub-regions of the superior colliculus. Thus, it has been suggested that the superior colliculus should be considered as an anatomical and functional 'mosaic', with interleaving groups or clusters of output cells (each of which may also have its own particular pattern of input connections) acting as functional sub-units (Huerta and Harting, 1984; Illing and Graybiel, 1985, 1986; Dean et al., 1989; Jeon and Mize, 1990).

Given this kind of organisation within the superior colliculus, it is to be expected that microinjections would vary in their effects, depending on which particular group of output cells they influenced. An early attempt to assess this idea compared the most complete map for unilateral injections of picrotoxin (66 pmol/200 nl: Kilpatrick et al., 1982) with the distributions of collicular cells that projected either ipsilaterally or contralaterally to the brainstem (Redgrave et al., 1986). As Fig. 3 indicates, there appears to be an approximate correspondence between (a) the location of sites giving responses resembling orientation or approach and the location of cells projecting contralaterally into the predorsal bundle and (b) sites giving defence-like movements and cells projecting ipsilaterally through the tecto-ponto-bulbar pathway (Redgrave et al., 1987a). This correspondence is consistent with evidence from other studies indicating that the crossed projection from the superior colliculus is concerned with approach movements whereas the ipsilateral descending projection mediates defensive responding (Dean et al., 1988, 1989).

However, the data illustrated in Fig. 3 represent only a crude first step towards understanding the effects of manipulating collicular GABAergic neurotransmission in terms of the organisation of collicular output pathways. On the one hand, each major descending projection is composed of a number of tracts ending in widely varying target structures. Among the targets of the ipsilateral projection, the cuneiform area and the dorsolateral pons receive from distinct sets of collicular cells (Redgrave et al., 1987b), and similarly within the crossed pathway there are independent projections to the caudal medulla/spinal cord and to the periabducens area (Keay et al., 1990b; Redgrave et al., 1990a). On the other hand, each major group of collicularly-mediated responses can be broken down into separate components, for example orienting movements of different parts of the body (whiskers, pinnae, eyes, head or the body itself), or different defence-like reactions such as freezing, directed avoidance, or undirected running. At this greater level of precision it is not well understood how anatomy and behaviour are related. For example, more recent work indicates that the crossed descending pathway mediates only some kinds of approach or orienting movements: other kinds depend on an as yet unidentified collicular efferent pathway (Dean et al., 1988).

Similarly, the collicular efferent pathways responsible for physiological reactions are not well understood; there are only weak direct links between the superior colliculus and the brainstem structures that control cardiovascular and respiratory systems in the ventrolateral medulla (Willet et al., 1983; Redgrave et al., 1987a), and these do not arise from the regions of the colliculus where cardiovascular changes can be most readily obtained by chemical stimulation (Keay et al., 1990a). The superior colliculus does project strongly to structures such as caudal central gray (Redgrave et al., 1988) and hypothalamus (Fallon and Moore, 1979) that both project directly to the ventrolateral medulla, and also have been associated with cardiovascular function (Hilton and

Smith, 1984; Li and Lovick, 1985). The hypothesis that these areas mediate the autonomic reactions produced by collicular stimulation awaits experimental test.

A second problem with interpreting the effects of altering collicular GABA-systems is the possibility that a given microinjection will interfere with more than one set of collicular output neurons. This possibility, long suggested by calculations concerning flow and diffusion from the injection site (e.g., Nicholson, 1985; Rice et al., 1985), has recently received more direct support from a method allowing visualisation of some of the cells activated by a particular treatment. Certain stimuli known to increase the activity of neurons also activate the nuclear proto-oncogene *c-fos* (see Dragunow and Faull, 1989 for review). One such example is presented in Fig. 4 which shows the location of cells expressing *c-fos* in the immediate vicinity of an injection of bicuculline methiodide into the lateral superior colliculus (Fig. 4B); *c-fos* surrounding a control injection of saline is included for comparison (Fig. 4A). In the colliculus injected with bicuculline, *c-fos* reaction product can be seen in areas known to contain cells of origin of both the ipsilateral and contralateral descending pathways (Redgrave et al., 1986). It is interesting, therefore, to note that the behavioural effects of this injection comprised a mixture of both ipsilaterally and contralaterally directed movements. In summary, it seems plausible that the behavioural effects of microinjections affecting GABA transmission will eventually be explicable in terms of the alterations that they produce in the properties of the relevant output neurons of the superior colliculus. However, considerable further work in understanding the properties of both the output pathways, and the local actions of the microinjections themselves, will be required before this goal can be achieved.

## GABAergic pathways afferent to the superior colliculus

The fact that behavioural responses can be obtained by interfering with GABAergic neuro-

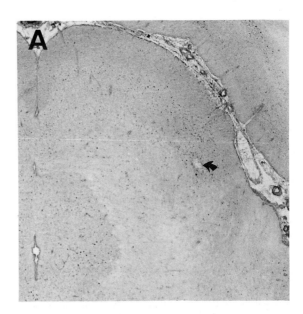

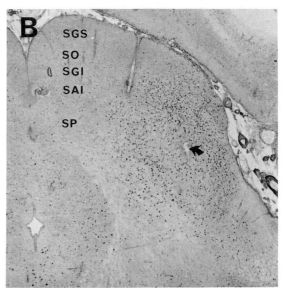

Fig. 4. Induction of *c-fos* protein in the immediate vicinity of microinjections into rat superior colliculus. A. *C-fos* surrounding an injection site (arrow) where 400 nl of saline vehicle was injected. B. Substantial induction of *c-fos* extending approximately 0.75 mm spherically from a site (arrow) where bicuculline methiodide (50 pmol in 400 nl) was injected. Labelled neurons can be seen in all layers of the superior colliculus. Calibration bar = 0.5 mm. For abbreviations see legend to Fig. 1.

transmission within the superior colliculus suggests that the neurons which mediate the responses are normally under tonic GABAergic

270

inhibitory control. Broadly speaking this could arise from either or both of (i) intrinsic GABAergic neurons (Mize et al., 1981, 1982; Mize, 1988) or (ii) extrinsic GABAergic afferents (Chevalier et al., 1981; Di Chiara et al., 1979; Vincent et al., 1978; Ficalora and Mize, 1989). There is now an accumulation of evidence identifying one such afferent pathway, namely the projection from substantia nigra pars reticulata to the superior colliculus: the nigrotectal pathway. Some of the evidence, and what it reveals about how the nigrotectal projection normally controls the superior colliculus, is reviewed in the main section below. A second brief section then considers the more recent and fragmentary evidence for an additional GABAergic projection to the superior colliculus, arising from cells in the substantia nigra pars lateralis and adjacent peripeduncular area.

*The nigrotectal projection: anatomy and physiology*

A number of lines of evidence indicate that the projection from the substantia nigra pars reticulata (SNR) to the superior colliculus is GABAergic. (i) Neurons in SNR that project to the superior colliculus stain for gamma-aminobutyric acid transaminase (rat: Araki et al., 1984), and are immunoreactive to a GABA antibody (cat: Ficalora and Mize, 1989). (ii) The morphology of nigrotectal terminals is consistent with their being GABAergic and inhibitory (rat: Vincent et al., 1978; cat: Behan et al., 1987). (iii) Destruction of the nigrotectal pathway depletes collicular GABAergic markers (Vincent et al., 1978; DiChiara et al., 1979). (iv) Nigral stimulation produces short latency inhibition in collicular cells (Deniau et al., 1978; Chevalier et al., 1981a,b); this inhibition is mimicked by GABA injected into the colliculus and reversibly blocked by bicuculline into the SC (Chevalier et al., 1981a).

Electrophysiological recordings from cells in SNR indicate that they normally fire continuously and vigorously (rat: Chevalier et al., 1985; cat: Joseph et al., 1985; monkey: Hikosaka and Wurtz, 1983a), thereby apparently subjecting the collicu-

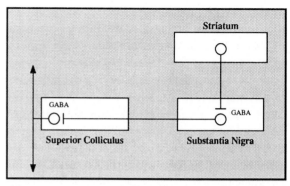

Fig. 5. Schematic diagram illustrating the double GABAergic link between the striatum and the superior colliculus via substantia nigra pars reticulata. A major component of the striatonigral pathway, and almost all nigrotectal neurons are GABAergic (see text). The majority of nigrotectal fibres arising from pars reticulata terminate in the intermediate layers of the superior colliculus, a region which contains cells of origin of both contralateral and ipsilateral descending pathways.

lar target cells of the nigrotectal pathway to a tonic inhibitory influence (Fig. 5). Thus, the firing rate for nigral cells is inversely related to that of collicular target cells (monkey: Hikosaka and Wurtz, 1983d), and if the nigral cells are themselves inhibited by intranigral microinjection of GABA, cells in the superior colliculus increase their firing rate (Chevalier et al., 1985). A plausible natural mechanism for inhibiting nigral cells is the action of the GABAergic striatonigral projection (Fig. 5), and indeed Chevalier et al. (1985) have shown that activating a small area of the caudate nucleus with glutamic acid can inhibit SNR cells and excite collicular cells. They and others have therefore proposed that disinhibition is a basic process whereby the striatum controls movement (Chevalier and Deniau, 1990; Hikosaka et al., 1989a,b,c; Hikosaka and Wurtz, 1989).

SNR cells project to a limited region of the rat superior colliculus, namely the intermediate layers (Fig. 6). One of these layers (the intermediate white layer) contains the bulk of the cells that project into the contralateral descending pathway (Fig. 3). Electron micrographic data indicate that nigrotectal terminals form synapses with contralaterally projecting tectospinal cells (Williams and Faull, 1988), and electrophysiological recordings show that antidromically identified tectospinal cells can be inhibited by nigral stimulation (Chevalier et al., 1984) and excited by nigral inhibition (Chevalier et al., 1985). One target of striatal disinhibitory control therefore appears to be cells of origin of the spinal component of the crossed descending pathway from the superior colliculus.

However, these are not the only target cells of the nigrotectal projection. First, the intermediate grey layer, to which the nigra also appears to project (Gerfen et al., 1982; Rhoades et al., 1982; Redgrave et al., 1990b), contains cells of origin of

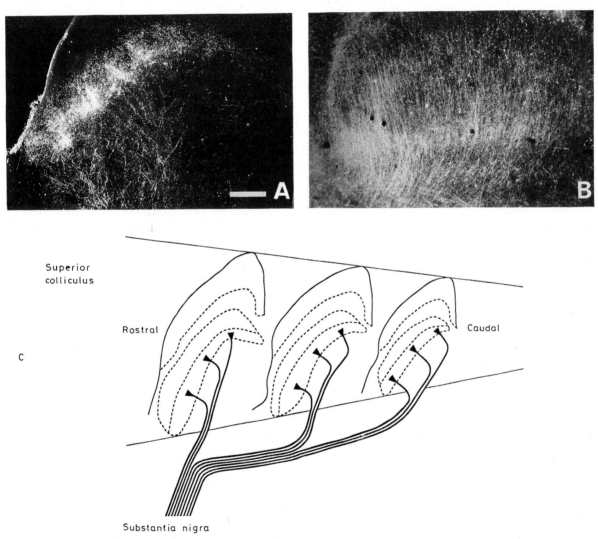

Fig. 6. Afferent nigrotectal fibres from ventral and medial SNR appear to form a spatial grid accessing the ventral surface of SAI (intermediate white layer). The photomicrographs in A and B illustrate the orthograde transport of WGA-HRP (20–50 nl of 1%) from injections into ventromedial pars reticulata. A. Coronal section showing afferent nigrotectal fibres entering caudal superior colliculus. B. Sagittal section (approximately 1.5 mm lateral to the midline; rostral, left; caudal, right) showing dorsally projecting nigrotectal fibres traversing the collicular deep layers and underlying midbrain reticular formation Bar: A, B = 0.55 mm. (This photograph was slightly underexposed to highlight the rising nigrotectal fibres.) C. A schematic 3-dimensional representation of the nigrotectal fibres arising from ventral and medial substantia nigra pars reticulata.

the ipsilateral descending pathway (Redgrave et al., 1986). Secondly, as described above, the contralateral cells in the intermediate white layer are not homogeneous: cells projecting to the spinal cord are found mainly in rostrolateral colliculus, whereas cells projecting to the periabducens area are found further medially and caudally (Redgrave et al., 1990a; Keay et al., 1990b). This distinction may be an important one for understanding the organisation of the nigrotectal projection, because recent anterograde and retrograde tracing data (Redgrave et al., 1990b) indicate that it consists of two separate channels: one with little if any topography from dorsolateral pars reticulata to the rostrolateral enlargement of the intermediate layers, and the other, which may be topographic, from ventral and medial pars reticulata to the medial and caudal intermediate layers. It appears, therefore, that the nigrotectal projection is structured to influence different classes of collicular output cell in different modes, although at present the functional significance of this arrangement remains to be elucidated (see below).

*The nigrotectal projection: behaviour*

As discussed above, the contralateral descending pathway from the superior colliculus appears to be involved in approach or orienting rather than defensive movements. Thus, unilateral microinjections of bicuculline or picrotoxin into the lateral intermediate and deep layers give contralaterally directed movements (e.g., circling), or a fixed contralateral head posture (Imperato and Di Chiara, 1981; Kilpatrick et al., 1982). Unilateral injections also give brief periods of gnawing (Kilpatrick et al., 1982), which become almost continuous when the injections are made bilaterally (Imperato and Di Chiara, 1981; cf. Redgrave et al., 1981b). It has been argued that in rodents gnawing is related to orienting, in the sense that pointing the muzzle towards a novel tactile stimulus allows it to be grasped in the mouth - the perioral reflex, a form of 'oral grasp' reflex as opposed to the more familiar visual grasp (Keay

et al., 1990b; Rhoades and DellaCroce, 1980; Stein, 1984; Wiener and Hartline, 1987).

Consistent with the anatomical and electrophysiological evidence that the nigrotectal pathway can exert disinhibitory control over the cells of origin of the crossed descending projection, behavioural evidence indicates that the SNR can influence the same responses that are mediated by the crossed projection, and that this influence is exercised by the nigrotectal projection. The behavioural evidence is as follows.

(i) Unilateral microinjections of muscimol into the SNR produce a range of contralaterally directed movements or postures including saccadic eye movements (Sakamoto and Hikosaka, 1989) head movements and rotational behaviour (Reavill et al., 1979; Kilpatrick and Starr, 1981; Olpe et al., 1977); bilateral microinjections produce continuous biting or gnawing (Scheel-Kruger et al., 1977; Olianas et al., 1978; Taha et al., 1982).

(ii) These behaviours are still obtained from SNR even if the thalamus and forebrain are missing (Welzl and Huston, 1981), suggesting that they can be mediated by descending nigral projections (for review see Scheel-Kruger, 1986).

(iii) Nigral-induced oral behaviour is abolished by lesions of the superior colliculus (Taha et al., 1982; Redgrave et al., 1984; Baumeister et al., 1987). Nigral circling or posturing is reduced (but not abolished) by collicular damage (Imperato et al., 1981; Kilpatrick et al., 1982; Leigh et al., 1983; Scheel-Krüger, 1986).

It therefore appears likely that some of the behaviours resulting from interfering with GABAergic neurotransmission in the superior colliculus arise because tonic inhibition from the GABAergic nigrotectal pathway is blocked. This is a particularly interesting conclusion insofar as the forebrain itself makes use of such a disinhibitory mechanism to produce movement (see below). Moreover, since the nigrotectal projection appears to contain anatomically segregated channels (see above) it is probable that the substantia nigra is able to exert differential control over several collicular output functions. In view of the well established roll of the paramedian reticular formation in the control of head and eye movements (see Grantyn, 1988 for review), our finding that ventral and medial nigral cells project to that part of the superior colliculus which contains cells projecting to the periabducens area (Redgrave et al., 1990a,b; Keay et al., 1990b) suggests that this basal ganglia output may exert control over movements of the head and eyes directed towards a novel stimulus. In contrast, the output from dorsolateral pars reticulata makes primary contact with that part of the superior colliculus receiving a major somatosensory input from the whiskers and mouth (Rhoades and DellaCroce, 1980; Wiener and Hartline, 1987): it is therefore possible that this nigrotectal channel is more concerned with 'oral' orienting (Keay et al, 1990b). However, the precise behavioural role of the nigrotectal channels in different forms of orienting and approach reactions awaits detailed experimental investigation.

*Projection from substantia nigra pars lateralis / peripeduncular area*

The projection from SNR to the superior colliculus seems to be involved primarily in approach and related responses; nigrotectal manipulations have not been reported to enhance defensive reactions (although muscimol applied to the nigra, for example, can enhance approach responses to the extent that normal defensive behaviour is severely curtailed). Is there perhaps some other GABAergic projection to the superior colliculus, which controls defensive responding in a manner analogous to that used by the nigrotectal pathway for orienting and approach?

Several lines of evidence, some preliminary, provide hints that there may be such a projection.

(i) Injections of retrograde tracers into some regions of the superior colliculus that mediate defence-like responding label cells in the substantia nigra pars lateralis (SNL) and adjoining peripeduncular area (PPA) (Arnault and Roger, 1987; Redgrave et al., 1990b). For example, bilateral injections of bicuculline (50 pmol) into the caudolateral deep layers produce a range of defensive reactions including cringing, vocalisation, wild biting attack and explosive running (Redgrave et al., 1989). Small injections of WGA-HRP into the same region of colliculus (Redgrave et al., 1990b) produce a pattern of retrograde labelling which is confined to SNL and adjoining PPA, with very few cells in SNR (Fig. 7). Unlike SNR, SNL and adjacent PPA in rat have major reciprocal connections with several structures associated with defensive behaviour including the amygdala, ventromedial hypothalamus, periaqueductal grey and cuneiform nucleus (Arnault and Roger, 1987; Gonzales and Chesselet, 1990; Bernard et al., 1989).

(ii) Cells in both rat and cat SNL that project to the superior colliculus either stain heavily for GABA transaminase (Nagai et al., 1983) or are immunoreactive to a GABA-antibody (Ficalora and Mize, 1989).

(iii) Preliminary electrophysiological data from our laboratory indicate the presence in SNL of spontaneously firing cells similar to those found in SNR. This observation suggests that if SNL/PPA cells are indeed GABAergic then target structures are likely to be tonically inhibited by SNL/PPA afferents.

(iv) Previously, we showed that certain treatments appear to increase the GABAergic-related inhibitory control over defensive behaviour initiated at the level of the superior colliculus; the threshold for eliciting defensive reactions with intracollicular injections of GABA antagonists was significantly raised after intranigral application of the catecholamine neurotoxin 6-hydroxydopamine (Redgrave and Dean, 1981b). In addition, some preliminary behavioural observations made in our laboratory indicate that injections of muscimol into caudolateral substantia nigra can elicit exaggerated withdrawal responses to tactile stimulation.

Although not compelling, these findings serve to encourage the search for pathways originating close to the ventrolateral junction between midbrain and diencephalon which in appropriate cir-

274

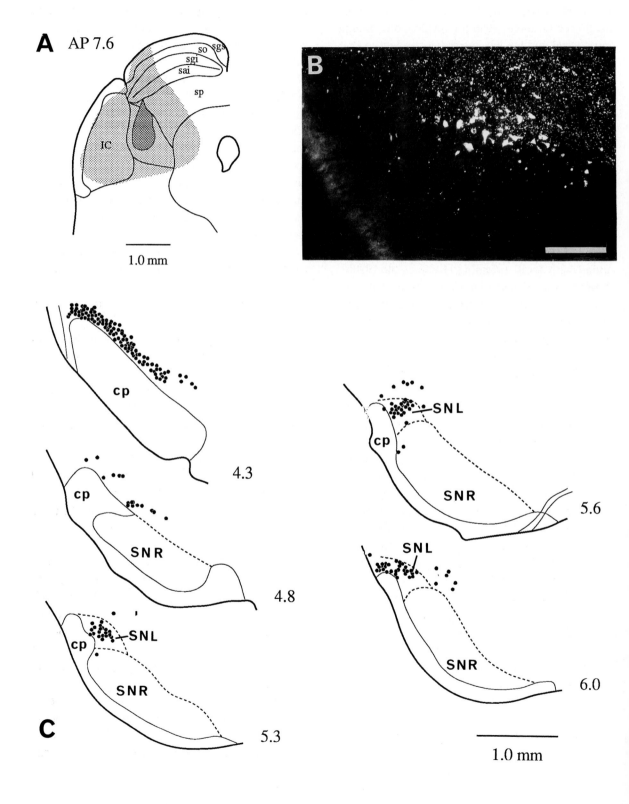

A  AP 7.6

so sgs
sgi
sai
sp

IC

1.0 mm

B

cp

4.3

cp

SNR

4.8

SNL

cp

SNR

5.3

SNL

cp

SNR

5.6

SNL

SNR

6.0

C

1.0 mm

cumstances can hold collicular defence mechanisms under inhibitory control. Whether a similar relationship holds for other species is unclear: projections from SNL to the SC have been demonstrated in other species (May and Hall, 1986; Harting et al., 1988; Ficalora and Mize, 1989), but it remains to be determined whether specific SNL terminal regions within the SC are particularly involved in defensive reactions.

## Functional implications

At first sight disinhibition seems an odd mechanism for producing movements. Why go to the trouble of having a tonically inhibitory pathway (from nigra to colliculus) that is itself under inhibitory control (from the striatum via the striato-nigral projection)? It would appear simpler to have excitatory projections throughout.

However, disinhibition as a control mechanism fits rather well with both well-established (Hughlings Jackson, 1932) and more recent views (Brooks, 1987) concerning the evolution of intelligence. The essential feature of these views is that evolution does not start from scratch, but builds on what it has got. For example, once the brain has evolved a mechanism for accurately directing movements of the head towards a suddenly appearing target, the next step is to add on 'higher' mechanisms which utilise the already established competence but do not replace it. These higher mechanisms would then be able to direct head movements towards some targets but not others, or towards targets that were not physically present. But to achieve such a redirection it is necessary that the higher mechanism be able to over-

ride the straightforward sensory trigger mechanisms utilised by the primitive competence. One over-ride mechanism is the maintenance of tonic inhibitory control, released only at the higher mechanism's command (cf. Chevalier et al., 1985; Goldberg and Segraves, 1990; Hikosaka and Wurtz, 1989).

The view that lower, evolutionarily more ancient centres are kept under inhibitory lock and key finds its expression in the idea that there are 'positive' clinical signs representing the 'release' from higher-order control (cf. Graybiel, 1990). Indeed, the appearance of circling, gnawing etc. after nigral inactivation (see above) seems to constitute a textbook example of such signs. However, the issue is of interest not only from a clinical perspective, but from a more general and abstract one to do with control in complex systems. Brooks has been concerned with the design of mobile robots that, unlike many existing models, have multiple functions and perhaps the ability to survive on their own in neutral or even hostile environments (Brooks, 1987, 1989). The design framework chosen is similar to the one outlined above: a module lower in the hierarchy retains its sensory and motor connections, but these can be modified by messages from higher modules. In particular, a higher module may supplement or replace the sensory inputs of a lower one with its own commands. The advantages and disadvantages of this approach are currently under very active scrutiny (e.g., Waldrop, 1990).

If disinhibitory control is indeed a mechanism of fundamental importance, for animal if not artificial intelligence, then it is necessary to understand in detail exactly how it works. Just what

Fig. 7. An example of the retrograde transport of WGA-HRP (10 nl of 1%) from an injection located in caudolateral deep layer/intercollicular region of the dorsal midbrain to the substantia nigra pars lateralis/peripeduncular area of the ventral midbrain. A. Schematic representation of the WGA-HRP injection site. B. A photomicrograph of retrogradely labelled cells in substantia nigra pars lateralis (approximate AP level, 5.3). Calibration bar = 0.2 mm. C. Quantitative plot of cells in the ventral midbrain following the injection of WGA-HRP illustrated in (A). Recent experiments in our laboratory (to be published) have shown that injections of bicuculline into this region of the dorsal midbrain induce a range of defensive responses including fast running, cringing, biting attack and vocalisation.

messages can be passed down to the superior colliculus from the forebrain? At present there appear to be two main possibilities.

(1) Altering the gain of sensory input. One of the effects of blocking GABAergic transmission within the superior colliculus is to exaggerate responses to sensory stimuli. A related phenomenon has been observed electrophysiologically in the superior colliculus as a consequence of nigral manipulation: Chevalier et al. (1985) found that after microinjection of GABA into SNR, tectospinal output neurons gave an increased response to stimulation of the snout. Related, but more striking effects, have been found in cat (Dunning et al., 1990), and recent recordings in our laboratory show that after local manipulation of GABA neurotransmission the sensory specificity of collicular cells can be altered. Thus, our initial results show that in the presence of nearby injections of bicuculline (25–50 pmol in 200–400 nl), extracellularly recorded intermediate layer cells which were previously exclusively sensitive to somatosensory input from the mouth and whiskers ($n = 8$ out of 8) became visually responsive (Westby, personal communication).

There are a number of possible mechanisms that could underlie these effects. Some nigral cells themselves respond to sensory stimuli, especially (in monkey) to visual stimuli (Hikosaka and Wurtz, 1983a,b,c,d). Secondly, nigral disinhibition could alter the responsivity of the target cells to sensory input from elsewhere, for example from the trigeminal nucleus (Killackey and Erzurumlu, 1981; Bruce et al., 1987; Rhoades et al., 1989a) or from the superficial visual layers of the colliculus (Rhoades et al., 1989b). Thirdly, direct projections from substantia nigra pars lateralis to the the superficial layers of the superior colliculus have been demonstrated in both cat (Harting et al., 1988) and rat (Redgrave et al., 1990b). The relative importance of these mechanisms remains to be established.

A related issue is whether the nigrotectal path-way is capable of biasing sensory input only in a global manner, or whether it can alter responsiveness selectively within a particular region of space. Anatomical investigations of the nigrotectal projection in rat (Redgrave et al., 1990b) (Fig. 6) favour the latter possibility, in that they suggest that part of it may be topographically organised. Electrophysiological evidence for (weak) topography has also been found for the primate nigrotectal pathway (Hikosaka and Wurtz, 1983a,d, 1989).

(2) Direct production of movement in the absence of a sensory trigger. Both microinjections of muscimol into SNR, and GABA blockers into the superior colliculus, produce movements that appear to occur without any immediately preceding sensory stimulus. Moreover, some cells in the primate substantia nigra respond before saccades to remembered targets, i.e., targets that are no longer physically present (Hikosaka and Wurtz, 1983c). Again Chevalier et al.'s (1985) electrophysiogical data provide a clue to the mechanism: nigral GABA can cause collicular output cells to become spontaneously active. The source of this activity is at present obscure; one possibility is the frontal cortex (e.g., Goldberg and Segraves, 1990), and another, suggested by preliminary behavioural observations from our laboratory, is the deep cerebellar nuclei that project to the same parts of the superior colliculus as the nigrotectal pathway (Faull and Carman, 1978; May and Hall, 1986). But whatever the source, the ability of the nigrotectal pathway to increase the firing of collicular output cells in the absence of specific sensory stimulation gives it the potential to produce movements directly.

In summary, the alterations in collicular GABAergic transmission that are produced crudely by microinjections in the laboratory, may be achieved more subtly by the brain itself to implement forebrain control of collicular competences. A major question is precisely how that control is exercised. Answering it may contribute to our understanding of a very general issue, namely the evolution of intelligence.

## Other species

The behavioural effects of manipulating GABA-ergic neurotransmission in the superior colliculus (or its homologue, the optic tectum), and their relation to the nigrotectal projection, are in some respects similar in a range of animals. In all cases orienting and related approach and prey catching responses are involved. Although these vary in form from animal to animal (e.g., prey-catching in frogs versus saccadic eye movements in primate), in each case they appear subject to forebrain disinhibitory control exercised via the nigrotectal projection or its analogue (Frog: Ewert, 1991; Cat: Boussaoud and Joseph, 1985, Cools, 1985; Monkey: Hikosaka and Wurtz, 1985a,b). In primates, one function of this projection seems to be the initiation of saccades to remembered targets (e.g., Hikosaka and Wurtz, 1983c, 1989). It may also be involved, together with frontal cortex and the caudate nucleus, in predictive saccades or saccades away from a target (Hikosaka et al., 1989; Goldberg and Segraves, 1990). These observations have been very important in suggesting how alterations in GABAergic neurotransmission within the superior colliculus may be used naturally to achieve sophisticated control of basic movement patterns (cf. previous section).

The main difference from the effects described here is that, so far, only in rodents has enhancement of *defence-like* responses been reported. For example, in monkey microinjection of either muscimol into the substantia nigra, or bicuculline into the superior colliculus, appears to affect only saccadic movements of the eyes (Hikosaka and Wurtz, 1985a,b). There may be several reasons for this difference, which have been discussed in detail elsewhere (Dean et al., 1989). First, it is possible that in animals like cats and monkeys the decision to investigate or escape is taken exclusively in the forebrain, so that the superior colliculus mediates orienting responses only. It is not clear, though, how well this explanation fits with evidence suggesting that basic architectural features such as the general organization of output pathways, discontinuous distribution of input terminals, and enzyme-related patches is shared by all mammals so far investigated including cat and monkey (Huerta and Harting, 1984; Stein, 1984; Illing and Graybiel, 1985, 1986; Dean et al., 1989). An alternative explanation of the stimulation data rests on the idea that the costs and benefits of decisions to look at or retreat from a novel event differ between species. A heavily predated species with poor central vision is likely to benefit from a bias towards defensive responding. In contrast, animals with relatively well-developed central vision and few predators (e.g., cats and monkeys) probably benefit from a tendency to look at a novel stimulus before deciding what to do. If these response biases were reflected in collicular organization, marked differences in the movements elicited by stimulation of the superior colliculus in different species would be predicted. However, in environments known to be dangerous, i.e. where sudden novel events normally elicit defensive responses, we would expect collicular stimulation also to produce avoidance movements in animals such as cats and monkeys. To date investigators using these animals have worked hard to avoid such conditions in their experiments.

### Acknowledgement

To Dr. S. Shehab for making available the micrographs presented in Fig. 4.

### References

Araki, M., McGeer, G.L. and McGeer, E.G. (1984) Presumptive $\gamma$-aminobutyric acid pathways from the midbrain to the superior colliculus studied by a combined horseradish peroxidase-$\gamma$-aminobutyric acid transaminase pharmacohistochemical method. *Neuroscience,* 13: 433–439.

Arnault, P. and Roger, M. (1987) The connections of the peripeduncular area studied by retrograde and anterograde transport in the rat. *J. Comp. Neurol.*, 258: 463–476.

Boussaoud, D. and Joseph, J.P. (1985) Role of the cat substantia nigra pars reticulata in eye and head movements. II. Effects of local pharmacological injections. *Exp. Brain Res.*, 57: 297–304.

Baumeister, A.A., Frye, G.D. and Moore, L.L. (1987) An investigation of the role played by the superior colliculus and ventromedial thalamus in self-injurious behaviour produced by intranigral microinjection of muscimol. *Pharmacol. Biochem. Behav.*, 26: 187–189.

Behan, M. (1987) The nigrotectal projection in the cat: an electron microscope autoradiographic study. *Neuroscience*, 21: 529–539.

Bernard, J.F., Peschanski, M. and Besson, J.M (1989) Afferents and efferents of the rat cuneiformis nucleus: an anatomical study with reference to pain transmission. *Brain Res.*, 490: 181–185.

Brooks, R.A. (1987) Autonomous mobile robots. In: Grimson, W.E.L. and Patil R.S. (Eds.), *AI in the, 1980's and beyond*, Cambridge, Massachusetts: MIT press, pp. 343–365,

Brooks, R.A. (1989) A robot that walks: Emergent behaviors from a carefully evolved network. *Neural Computation*, 1: 253–262.

Bruce, L.L, McHaffie, J.G. and Stein, B.E. (1987) The organization of trigeminotectal and trigeminothalamic neurons in rodents: A double-labeling study with fluorescent dyes. *J. Comp. Neurol.*, 262: 315–330.

Chevalier, G. and Deniau, J.M. (1990) Disinhibition as a basic process in the expression of striatal functions. *Trends Neurosci.*, 13: 277–280.

Chevalier, G., Deniau, J.M., Thierry, A.M. and Féger, J. (1981a) The nigro-tectal pathway. An electrophysiological reinvestigation in the rat. *Brain Res.*, 213: 253–263.

Chevalier, G., Thierry, A.M., Shibazaki, T. and Féger, J. (1981b) Evidence for a GABAergic inhibitory nigrotectal pathway in the rat. *Neurosci. Lett.*, 21: 67–70.

Chevalier, G., Vacher, S. and Deniau, J.M. (1984) Inhibitory nigral influence on tectospinal neurons, a possible implication of basal ganglia in orienting behavior. *Exp. Brain Res.*, 53: 320–326.

Chevalier, G., Vacher, S., Deniau, J.M. and Desban, M. (1985) Disinhibition as a basic process in the expression of striatal functions. I. The striato-nigral influence on tecto-spinal/tecto-diencephalic neurons. *Brain Res.*, 334: 215–226.

Cools, A.R. (1985) Brain and behavior: hierarchy of feedback systems and control of input. In: Bateson, P.P.G. and Klopfer, P.H. (Eds.), *Perspectives in Ethology, Vol. 6 Mechanisms*, New York: Plenum Press, pp. 109–168,

Dean, P. and Gale, K. (1989) Anticonvulsant action of GABA receptor blockade in the nigrotectal target region. *Brain Res.*, 477: 391–395.

Dean, P. and Redgrave, P. (1984) Superior colliculus and visual neglect in rat and hamster. III. Functional implications. *Brain Res. Rev.*, 8: 155–163.

Dean, P., Redgrave, P. and Lewis, G. (1982) Locomotor activity of rats in open field after microinjection of procaine into superior colliculus or underlying reticular formation. *Behav. Brain Res.*, 5: 175–187.

Dean, P., Redgrave, P. and Mitchell, I.J. (1988) Organisation of efferent projections from superior colliculus to brainstem in rat: evidence for functional output channels. In: Hicks, I.P. and Benedek, G. (Eds.), *Progress in Brain Research, Vol. 75*, Amsterdam: Elsevier, pp. 27–36.

Dean, P., Redgrave, P. and Molton, L. (1984) Visual desynchronization of cortical EEG impaired by lesions of superior colliculus in rats. *J. Neurophysiol.*, 52: 625–637.

Dean, P., Redgrave, P. and Westby, G.W.M. (1989) Event or emergency? Two response systems in the mammalian superior colliculus. *Trends Neurosci.*, 12: 137–147.

Dean, P., Simkins, M., Hetherington, L., Mitchell, I.J. and Redgrave, P. (1991) Tectal induction of cortical arousal: Evidence implicating multiple output pathways. *Brain Res. Bull.*, 26: 1–10.

Deniau, J.M., Hammond, C., Riszk, A. and Féger, J. (1978) Electrophysiological properties of identified output neurones of the rat substantia nigra (pars compacta and pars reticulata); Evidence for the existence of branched neurons. *Exp. Brain Res.*, 32: 409–422.

Di Chiara, G., Porceddu, M.L., Morelli, M., Mulas, M.L. and Gessa, G.L. (1979) Evidence for a GABAergic projection from the substantia nigra to the ventromedial thalamus and to the superior colliculus of the rat. *Brain Res.*, 176: 273–284.

Dragunow, M. and Faull, R. (1989) The use of *c-fos* as a metabolic marker in neuronal pathway tracing. *J. Neurosci. Methods*, 29: 261–266.

Dunning, D.D., Stein, B.E. and McHaffie, J.G. (1990) Effects of cortical and nigral deactivation of visual neurones in cat superior colliculus. *Neurosci. Abstr.*, 16: 47.11.

Ewert, J.-P. (1991) Modulation of visual stimulus responses in toads by loops involving the forebrain. In: Arbib, M.A. and Ewert, J.-P. (Eds.), *Visual Structures and Integrated Function, Research Notes in Neural Computing*, Berlin: Springer-Verlag, in press.

Faull, R.L.M. and Carman, J.B. (1978) The cerebellofugal projection in the brachium conjunctivum of the rat. I. The contralateral ascending pathway. *J. Comp. Neurol.*, 178: 495–518.

Ficalora, A.S. and Mize, R.R. (1989) The neurones of the substantia nigra and zona incerta which project to the cat superior colliculus are GABA immunoreactive: a double-label study using GABA immunocytochemistry and lectin retrograde transport. *Neuroscience*, 29: 567–581.

Gaither, N.S. and Stein, B.E. (1979) Reptiles and mammals use similar sensory organizations in the midbrain. *Science*, 205: 595–597.

Gerfen, C.R., Staines, W.A., Arbuthnott, G.W. and Fibiger, H.C. (1982) Crossed connections of the substantia nigra in the rat. *J. Comp. Neurol*, 207: 283–303.

Goldberg, M.E. and Segraves, M.A. (1990) The role of the frontal eye field and its corticotectal projection in the generation of eye movements. In: Cohen, B. and Bodis-Wollner, I. (Eds.), *Vision and the Brain. The Organisation of the Central Visual System*, New York: Raven Press, pp. 195–209.

Gonzales, C. and Chesselet, M-F. (1990) Amygdalonigral pathway: An anterograde study in the rat with *Phaseolus vulgaris* leucoagglutinin (PHA-L). *J. Comp. Neurol.*, 297: 182–200.

Graybiel, A.M. (1990) The basal ganglia and the initiation of movement. *Rev. Neurol. (Paris)*, 146: 570–574.

Hikosaka, O., Sakamoto, M. and Usui, S. (1989a) Functional

properties of monkey caudate neurons. I. Activities related to saccadic eye movements. *J. Neurophysiol.,* 61: 780–798.

Hikosaka, O., Sakamoto, M. and Usui, S. (1989b) Functional properties of monkey caudate neurons. II. Visual and auditory responses. *J. Neurophysiol.,* 61: 799–813.

Hikosaka, O., Sakamoto, M. and Usui, S. (1989c) Functional properties of monkey caudate neurons. III. Activities related to expectation of target and reward. *J. Neurophysiol.,* 61: 814–832.

Hikosaka, O. and Wurtz, R.H. (1983a) Visual and oculomotor functions of monkey substantia nigra pars reticulata. I. Relation of visual and auditory responses to saccades. *J. Neurophysiol.,* 49: 1230–1252.

Hikosaka, O. and Wurtz, R.H. (1983b) Visual and oculomotor functions of monkey substantia nigra pars reticulata. II. Visual responses related to fixation of gaze. *J. Neurophysiol.,* 49: 1254–1267.

Hikosaka, O. and Wurtz, R.H. (1983c) Visual and oculomotor functions of monkey substantia nigra pars reticulata. III. Memory-contingent visual and saccade responses. *J. Neurophysiol.,* 49: 1268–1284.

Hikosaka, O. and Wurtz, R.H. (1983d) Visual and oculomotor functions of monkey substantia nigra pars reticulata. IV. Relation of substantia nigra to superior colliculus. *J. Neurophysiol.,* 49: 1285–1301.

Hikosaka, O. and Wurtz, R.H. (1985a) Modification of saccadic eye movements by GABA-related substances. I. Effect of muscimol and bicuculline in monkey superior colliculus. *J. Neurophysiol.,* 53: 266–291.

Hikosaka, O. and Wurtz, R.H. (1985b) Modification of saccadic eye movements by GABA-related substances. II. Effects of muscimol in monkey substantia nigra pars reticulata. *J. Neurophysiol.,* 53: 292–308.

Hikosaka, O. and Wurtz, R.H. (1989) The basal ganglia. In: Wurtz, R.H. and Goldberg, M.E. (Eds.), *Neurobiology of saccadic eye movements. Reviews of oculomotor research Vol 3.,* Amsterdam: Elsevier, pp. 257–282,

Hilton, S.M. and Smith, P.R. (1984) Ventral medullary neurones excited from hypothalamic and midbrain defense areas. *J. Autonom. Nerv. Syst.,* 11: 35–42.

Huerta, M.F. and Harting, J.K. (1984) The mammalian superior colliculus: studies of its morphology and connections. In: Vanegas, H. (Ed.), *Comparative neurology of the optic tectum,* New York: Plenum Press, pp. 687–773.

Hughlings Jackson, J. (1932) Relations of different divisions of the central nervous system to one another and to parts of the body. In: Taylor, J. (Ed.), *Selected writings of John Hughlings Jackson,* London: Hodder and Stoughton, pp. 422–443.

Illing, R-B. and Graybiel, A.M. (1985) Convergence of afferents from frontal cortex and substantia nigra onto acetylcholinesterase-rich patches of the cat's superior colliculus. *Neuroscience,* 14: 455–482.

Illing, R-B. and Graybiel, A.M. (1986) Complementary and non-matching afferent compartments in the cat's superior colliculus: Innervation of the acetylcholinesterase-poor domain of the intermediate gray layer. *Neuroscience,* 18: 373–394.

Imperato, A. and Di Chiara, G. (1981) Behavioural effects of GABA-agonists and antagonists infused in the mesencephalic reticular formation - deep layers of superior colliculus. *Brain Res.,* 224: 185–194.

Imperato, A., Porceddu, M.L., Morelli, M., Faa, G. and Di Chiara, G. (1981) Role of dorsal mesencephalic reticular formation and deep layers of superior colliculus as out-put stations for turning behaviour elicited from the substantia nigra pars reticulata. *Brain Res.,* 216: 437–443.

Jeon, C.J. and Mize, R.R. (1990) Efferent cell clusters within the cholinergic patches in the intermediate gray layer of the cat superior colliculus. *Neurosci. Abstr.,* 16: 47.4.

Joseph, J.P., Boussaoud, D. and Biguer, B. (1985) Activity of neurons in the cat substantia nigra pars reticulata during drinking. *Exp. Brain Res.,* 60: 375–379.

Keay, K.A., Dean, P. and Redgrave, P. (1990a) N-methyl-D-aspartate (NMDA) evoked changes in blood pressure and heart rate from the rat superior colliculus. *Exp. Brain Res.,* 80: 148–156.

Keay, K.A., Redgrave, P. and Dean, P. (1988) Cardiovascular and respiratory changes elicited by stimulation of rat superior colliculus. *Brain Res. Bull.,* 20: 13–26.

Keay, K., Westby, G.W.M., Frankland, P., Dean, P. and Redgrave, P. (1990b) Organization of the crossed tecto-reticulo-spinal projection in rat. 2. Electrophysiological evidence for separate output channels to the periabducens area and caudal medulla. *Neuroscience,* 37: 585–601.

Killackey HP and Erzurumlu RS. (1981) Trigeminal projections to the superior colliculus of the rat. *J. Comp. Neurol.,* 201: 221–242.

Kilpatrick, I.C., Collingridge, G.L. and Starr, M.S. (1982) Evidence for the participation of nigrotectal γ-aminobutyrate-containing neurones in striatal and nigral-derived circling in the rat. *Neuroscience,* 7: 207–222.

Kilpatrick, I.C. and Starr, M.S. (1981) Involvement of dopamine in circling responses to muscimol depends on intranigral site of injection. *Eur. J. Pharmacol.,* 69: 407–419.

Leigh, P.N., Reavill, C., Jenner, P. and Marsden, C.D. (1983) Basal ganglia outflow pathways and circling behaviour in the rat. *J. Neural Trans.,* 58: 1–41.

Li, P. and Lovick, T.A. (1985) Excitatory projections from hypothalamic and midbrain defence region to nucleus paragigantocellularis in the rat. *Exp. Neurol.,* 89: 543–553.

May, P.J. and Hall, W.C. (1986) The cerebellotectal pathway in the grey squirrel. *Exp. Brain Res.,* 65: 200–212.

Mize, R.R. (1988) Immunocytochemical localization of gamma-aminobutyric acid (GABA) in the cat superior colliculus. *J. Comp. Neurol.,* 276: 169–187.

Mize, R.R., Spencer, R.F. and Sterling, P. (1981) Neurones and glia in cat superior colliculus accumulate [$^3$H]gamma-aminobutyric acid (GABA). *J. Comp. Neurol.,* 202: 385–396.

Mize, R.R., Spencer, R.F. and Sterling, P. (1982) Two types of GABA-accumulating neurones in the superficial gray layer of the cat superior colliculus. *J. Comp. Neurol.,* 206: 180–192.

Nagai, T., McGeer, P.L. and McGeer, E.G. (1983) Distribu-

280

tion of GABA-T intensive neurones in the rat forebrain and midbrain. *J. Comp. Neurol.*, 218: 220–238.

Nicholson, C. (1985) Diffusion from an injected volume of a substance in brain tissue with arbitrary fraction and tortuosity. *Brain Res.*, 333: 325–329.

Olianas, M.C., De Montis, G.M., Mulas, G. and Tagliamonte, A. (1978) The striatal dopaminergic function is mediated by the inhibition of a nigral, non-dopaminergic neuronal system via a striao-nigral GABAergic pathway. *Eur. J. Pharmacol.*, 49: 233–241.

Olpe, H-R., Schellenberg, H. and Koella, W.P. (1977) Rotational behaviour induced in rats by intranigral application of GABA-related drugs and GABA antagonists. *Eur. J. Pharmacol.*, 45: 291–294.

Paxinos, G. and Watson, C. (1982) *The rat brain in stereotaxic coordinates*, Sydney, Australia: Academic Press.

Reavill, C., Jenner, P., Leigh, N. and Marsden,C.D. (1979) Turning behaviour induced by injection of muscimol or picrotoxin into substantia nigra demonstrates dual GABA components. *Neurosci. Lett.*, 12: 323–328.

Redgrave, P. and Dean, P. (1981a) Collicular picrotoxin alleviates akinesia but not sensory neglect in rats with bilateral 6-hydroxydopamine lesions of ventral midbrain. *Psychopharmacology*, 75: 204–209.

Redgrave, P. and Dean, P. (1985) Tonic desynchronisation of cortical electroencephalogram by electrical and chemical stimulation of superior colliculus and surrounding structures in urethane-anaesthetised rats. *Neuroscience*, 16: 659–671.

Redgrave, P., Dean, P., Mitchell, I.J., Odekunle, A. and Clark, A. (1988) The projection from superior colliculus to cuneiform area in the rat. I. Anatomical studies. *Exp. Brain Res.*, 72: 611–625.

Redgrave, P., Dean P, Simkins, M. and Marrow, L. (1989) Systematic mapping of nigrotectal terminal zones with bicuculline for anticonvulsant effects in the electroshock model of generalised seizures. *Europ. J. Neurosci. Suppl.*, 2: 57.

Redgrave, P., Dean, P., Souki, W. and Lewis, G. (1981b) Gnawing and changes in reactivity produced by microinjections of picrotoxin into the superior colliculus of rats. *Psychopharmacology*, 75: 198–203.

Redgrave, P. Dean, P. and Taha, E.B. (1984) Feeding induced by injections of muscimol into the substantia nigra of rats: Unaffected by haloperidol but abolished by large lesions of the superior colliculus. *Neuroscience*, 13: 77–85.

Redgrave, P. Dean, P. and Westby, G.W.M. (1990a) Organization of the crossed tecto-reticulo-spinal projection in rat.1. Anatomical evidence for separate output channels to the periabducens area and caudal medulla. *Neuroscience*, 37: 571–584.

Redgrave, P., Marrow, L.P. and Dean, P. (1990b) Topographical organization of the nigrotectal projection in rat: Evidence for segregated channels. *Europ. J. Neurosci. Suppl.*, 3: 4253

Redgrave, P., Mitchell, I.J. and Dean, P. (1987a) Descending projections from the superior colliculus in rat: a study using orthograde transport of wheatgerm-agglutinin conjugated horseradish peroxidase. *Exp. Brain Res.*, 68: 147–167.

Redgrave, P., Mitchell, I.J. and Dean, P. (1987b) Further evidence for segregated output channels from superior colliculus in rat: ipsilateral tecto-pontine and tecto-cuneiform projections have different cells of origin. *Brain Res.*, 413: 170–174.

Redgrave, P., Odekunle, A. and Dean, P. (1986) Tectal cells of origin of predorsal bundle in rat: location and segregation from ipsilateral descending pathway. *Exp. Brain Res.*, 63: 279–293.

Rhoades, R.W. and DellaCroce, D.R. (1980) Cells of origin of the tectospinal tract in the golden hamster: An anatomical and electrophysiological investigation. *Exp Neurol.*, 67: 163–180.

Rhoades, R.W., Fish, S.E., Chiaia, N.L., Bennett-Clarke, C. and Mooney, R.D. (1989a) Organization of the projections from the trigeminal brainstem complex to the superior colliculus in the rat and hamster: Anterograde tracing with *Phaseolus vulgaris* leucoagglutinin and intra-axonal injection. *J. Comp. Neurol.*, 289: 641–656.

Rhoades, R.W., Kuo, D.C., Polcer, J.D., Fish, S.E. and Voneida, T.J. (1982) Indirect visual cortical input to the deep layers of the hamster's superior colliculus via the basal ganglia. *J. Comp. Neurol.*, 208: 239–254.

Rhoades, R.W., Mooney, R.D., Rohrer, W.H., Nikoletseas, M.M. and Fish, S.E. (1989b) Organization of the projection from the superficial to the deep layers of the hamster's superior colliculus as demonstrated by the anterograde transport of *Phaseolus vulgaris* leucoagglutinin. *J. Comp. Neurol.*, 283: 54–70.

Rice, M.E., Gerhardt, G.A., Hierl, P.M., Nagy, G and Adams, R.N. (1985) Diffusion coefficients of neurotransmitters and their metabolites in brain extracellular fluid space. *Neuroscience*, 15: 891–902.

Sahibzada, N., Yamasaki, D. and Rhoades, R.W. (1987) The spinal and commissural projections from the superior colliculus in rat and hamster arise from distinct neuronal populations. *Brain Res.*, 415: 242–256.

Sakamoto, M. and Hikosaka, O. (1989) Eye movements induced by microinjection of GABA agonist in the rat substantia nigra pars reticulata. *Neurosci. Res.*, 6: 216–233.

Scheel-Krüger, J. (1986) Dopamine-GABA interactions: evidence that GABA transmits, modulates and mediates dopaminergic functions in the basal ganglia and the limbic system. *Acta Neurol. Scand. Suppl.*, 107, 73: 54.

Scheel-Kruger, J., Arnt, J. and Magelund, G. (1977) Behavioural stimulation induced by muscimol and other GABA agonists injected into the substantia nigra. *Neurosci. Lett.*, 4: 351–356.

Schiller, P.H. (1972) The role of the monkey superior colliculus in eye movement and vision. *Invest. Opthalmol.*, 11: 451–460.

Schneider, G.E. (1969) Two visual systems. *Science*, 163: 895–902.

Shehab, S., Simkins, I., Dean, P. and Redgrave, P. (1990) Chemical stimulation of rat superior colliculus has anticonvulsant effects in the MES model of generalised seizures. *Eur. J. Neurosci. Suppl.*, 3: 2191

Sprague, J.M., Berlucchi, G. and Rizzolatti, G. (1973) The role of the superior colliculus and pretectum in vision and visually guided behavior. In: R. Jung (Ed.), *Handbook of Sensory Physiology, Vol. VIII / B*, Berlin: Springer, pp. 27–101.

Stein, B.E. (1984a) Multimodal representation in the superior colliculus and optic tectum. In: H. Vanegas (Ed.), *Comparative Neurology of the Optic Tectum*, New York: Plenum, pp. 819–841.

Stein, B.E. (1984b) Development of the superior colliculus. *Annu. Rev Neurosci.*, 7: 95–125.

Taha, E.B., Dean, P. and Redgrave, P. (1982) Oral behavior induced by intranigral muscimol is unaffected by haloperidol but abolished by large lesions of superior colliculus. *Psychopharmacology*, 77: 272–278.

Vincent, S.R., Hattori, T. and McGeer, E.G. (1978) The nigrotectal projection: a biochemical and ultrastructural characterization. *Brain Res.*, 151: 159–164.

Waldrop, M.M. (1990) Fast, cheap, and out of control. *Science*, 248: 959–961.

Wiener, S.I. and Hartline, P.H. (1987) Perioral somatosensory but not visual inputs to the flank of the mouse superior colliculus. *Neuroscience*, 21: 557–564.

Welzl, H. and Huston, J.P. (1981) Sensitization of the perioral biting reflex by intranigral GABA agonist after detelencephalization. *Neurosci. Lett.*, 21: 351–354.

Willette, R.N., Barcas, P.P., Krieger, A.J. and Sapru, H.N. (1983) Vasopressor and depressor area in the rat medulla. *Neuropharmacology*, 22: 1071–1079.

Williams, M.N. and Faull, R.L.M. (1988) The nigrotectal projection and tectospinal neurones in the rat. A light and electron microscopic study demonstrating a monosynaptic nigral input to identified tectospinal neurons. *Neuroscience*, 25: 533–562.

R.R. Mize, R.E. Marc and A.M. Sillito (Eds.)
Progress in Brain Research, Vol. 90

CHAPTER 14

# GABAergic neurons and circuits in the pretectal nuclei and the accessory optic system of mammals

J.J.L. van der Want, J.J. Nunes Cardozo and C. van der Togt

*Department of Morphology, The Netherlands Ophthalmic Research Institute, P.O. Box 12141, 1100 AC Amsterdam, The Netherlands*

## Introduction

During the last few decades there has emerged an increasing interest in the functional anatomy of the pretectum and the accessory optic system (AOS), in mammals and in non-mammalian species. In particular, the physiological studies of Maekawa and Simpson (1972, 1973), Simpson et al. (1979) and Hoffmann (1986) have given new spirit to a hitherto relatively unexplored area in the brain. Simultaneously, anatomical tracing studies by Giolli and co-workers have revealed details on the connectivity and the interrelationships of both systems (Blanks et al., 1982; Giolli et al., 1984, 1985, 1988, 1989). In addition, recent pharmacological and behavioral studies have emphasized the role of the pretectum and AOS in the processing of movements in the whole visual field (Grasse and Cynader, 1988, 1991; Ariel, 1989; Yücel et al., 1989; Schuerger et al., 1990). Components of the pretectal and the AOS nuclei convey retinal slip information that is integrated with vestibular input to stabilize a visual image on the retina during self generated motion of the body and motion of the visual surround (Graf et al., 1988, Leonard et al., 1988; Simpson et al., 1988b). Given that the physiological and structural relationships of the pretectal and AOS nuclei are known in some detail, it is possible to study the ultrastructural organization of their

neurons in relation to their physiology and thus describe the synaptic circuitry which underlies their function.

This chapter is concerned with the ultrastructural organization of the inhibitory components of this system mediated by gamma-aminobutyric acid (GABA). There is a growing body of evidence that the inhibitory neurotransmitter GABA is involved in transmission in many regions of the visual system. In the visual cortex it has been demonstrated that GABA plays a role in directional sensitivity (Sillito, 1977) and at the level of the retinal ganglion cells, properties such as speed and direction selectivity are generated in part by inhibitory, presumably GABAergic, mechanisms (Barlow and Levick, 1965; Caldwell et al., 1978; Grzywacz and Koch, 1987; Ariel, 1989). In the retina of the frog it has been suggested that GABA might be involved in reducing the slip velocity of images on the retina during the slow component of optokinetic nystagmus (OKN) (Bonaventure et al., 1983; Yücel et al., 1990). The observations in retina and cortex indicate the importance of GABAergic mechanisms in the regulation of speed and direction selectivity in these two structures. Whether the large numbers of GABAergic neurons and terminal profiles observed in the pretectum and the AOS also contribute to speed and directional selective properties, awaits further physiological investigation. In this chapter, we will describe the ultrastructural components of GABAergic neurons, with special attention paid to the following questions.

(1) Do GABAergic efferent systems exist that originate in the pretectum and AOS and reach the vestibular nuclei or other visually related nuclei that play a role in OKN? A number of different efferent pathways that originate from cell bodies located in the pretectum and the AOS are known to carry optokinetic information that converges upon secondary vestibular neurons. In particular, optokinetic information is mediated through the nucleus of the optic tract (NOT) and the dorsal terminal nucleus (DTN)* by the visual olivocerebellar pathway (Maekawa and Simpson, 1972, 1973). Barmack and Hess (1980a,b) have indicated that through the modulatory activity of the NOT and the DTN, eye-velocity signals are greatly reduced in the Inferior Olive (IO). The morphological substrate for this phenomenon could be formed by an inhibitory projection from the NOT/DTN to precerebellar brain stem nuclei. In this chapter a survey will be presented of the tracing studies that have been performed to demonstrate the possible involvement of GABAergic projection neurons in the NOT/DTN in this circuit.

(2) How are the afferent GABAergic projections and the local GABAergic terminals distributed and could that organization explain the significance of the GABAergic connections in speed and direction selectivity? Recent immunocytochemical studies have indicated significant GABAergic connections between several components of the subcortical primary visual centers. These include a GABAergic projection from the pretectum to the SC (Appell and Behan, 1990; Van der Want et al., 1991) and the LGN (Cuc-

chiaro et al., 1991) and an inhibitory projection from the AOS to the pretectum that accounts, at least in part for the GABAergic terminals in the NOT/DTN (Van der Togt et al., 1991). The ultrastructural characteristics and the distribution of these GABAergic terminals also will be presented in this chapter.

(3) How is the main sensory input from the retina related to the GABAergic circuit and does it use GABA itself? Electrophysiological studies have demonstrated high spontaneous activity in the NOT/DTN complex that can be modulated by retinal and other inputs to this region (Simpson et al., 1988b). This modulatory activity is highly specific. A close interaction between retinal terminals (R) and GABAergic terminals, is thought to be involved in the modulation of this spontaneous activity. This means that a spatial configuration is required that permits GABAergic and R synapses to interact directly and that the relative position of the synapses largely determines the strength and the intensity of the effect. This would be in accordance with the hypothesis presented by Somogyi (1990), formulated for the visual cortex, which postulates that neurons always contact both putative excitatory and inhibitory terminals, and that by differential placement of excitatory and inhibitory synapses a basic synaptic design is established which controls the flow of activity through various channels. In this chapter an analysis will be made of the complexity of the ultrastructural relations of the inhibitory GABAergic circuits that are formed by interneurons, GABAergic projection neurons and nonGABAergic neurons in the pretectum and the AOS.

### Anatomy and structural organization

The pretectal region of mammals includes a number of distinct nuclei located between the superior colliculus (SC) and the dorsal thalamus (Rose, 1935, 1942; Kühlenbeck and Miller, 1942; Rodieck, 1979). These nuclei include the anterior

---

* In physiological studies in rabbits on the functional properties of the NOT and DTN a distinction between these nuclei has never been indicated and as their boundaries can only arbitrarily be given, we consider the NOT/DTN as a single neuronal complex (Gregory, 1985).

pretectal nucleus (APN), the nucleus of the optic tract (NOT), the olivary pretectal nucleus (OPN), the posterior pretectal nucleus (PPN) and the suprageniculate pretectal nucleus (Scalia, 1972; Simpson et al., 1988a). Classically, the AOS comprises three nuclei: the dorsal terminal nucleus (DTN), the lateral terminal nucleus (LTN) and the medial terminal nucleus (MTN). Recently, a fourth nucleus has been described by Giolli et al. (1988), the interstitial nucleus of the superior fasciculus posterior fibers (inSFp). Except for the APN, all of these nuclei receive a retinal projection. In rat and rabbit the visual input originates predominantly (Giolli and Guthrie, 1969) or exclusively from the contralateral retina (Scalia, 1972; Klooster et al., 1983). The pretectal and AOS nuclei form extensive connections with other midbrain structures and preoculomotor centers and are therefore considered as highly important in the processing of visual input to these structures (Berman, 1977; Blanks et al., 1982; Holstege and Collewijn, 1982; Giolli et al., 1984, 1988; Korp et al., 1990). Figure 1 demonstrates transverse sections through the diencephalon of a pigmented rabbit showing the termination pattern of retinal fibers in the pretectal nuclei and the AOS nuclei. One interesting feature of this organization, first described by Scalia and Arango (1979) in rat, is that the retinal input to these nuclei appears to be organized in horizontally oriented parallel slabs that extend through the rostrocaudal dimensions of the pretectum. This appears to be a common feature in many species as it has also been shown that the retinal input forms parallel slabs in the cat (Koontz et al., 1985). These slabs correspond to specific calbindin labeled cell clusters in the cat (Nabors and Mize, 1991).

*Cellular distribution and morphology*

A number of cell types have been described in the pretectal nuclei at the light microscopic level (Kanaseki and Sprague, 1974; Berman, 1977; Scalia and Arango, 1979). These cells include large multipolar and medium to small multipolar

neurons with the larger neurons located more superficially (Gregory, 1985). In Golgi material, it has been shown that neurons in the NOT/DTN complex range in size from 10–25 $\mu$m in diameter. From their soma, three to seven dendrites emerge and traverse the neuropil to bifurcate extensively in adjacent pretectal nuclei thus forming a strongly interconnected system between different pretectal nuclei and the AOS system (Nunes Cardozo and Van der Want, 1987). Besides the dendritic arborizations, loosely arranged optic tract fibers pass perpendicularly through the NOT/DTN complex, resulting in a patchwork-like appearance of electron lucent areas intermingled with electron dense myelinated fibers (Fig. 2).

Neurons in the NOT/DTN complex in the cat are amongst the largest cells in the pretectal region and they are topographically distributed with respect to their efferent projection patterns: the large neurons project in a caudal direction and the smaller neurons project in a rostral direction (Weber and Harting, 1980). Separate groups of neurons are arranged according to their projection area, one to the lateral dorsal nucleus of the thalamus and another to the IO (Robertson, 1983). In the rat, Schiff and Schmidt (1990) have demonstrated that the efferents of the NOT are probably composed of at least three populations: an ipsilateral projection to the IO, a contralateral projection to the opposite NOT, and a bilateral projection to the LGN. It was further observed, in contrast to the cat, that these populations of projection neurons are homogeneously distributed throughout the nuclear complex.

Interspersed with these projection neurons are local circuit or interneurons. It is generally assumed that local circuit neurons have specific morphological (Lieberman, 1973; Hamori et al., 1983; Braak and Bachmann, 1985; Campbell and Lieberman, 1985) and immunocytochemical properties (Fitzpatrick et al., 1984; Montero and Singer, 1984; Ottersen and Storm-Mathisen, 1984; Giolli et al., 1985; Montero and Zempel, 1986; Horn and Hoffmann, 1987). Giolli et al. (1985)

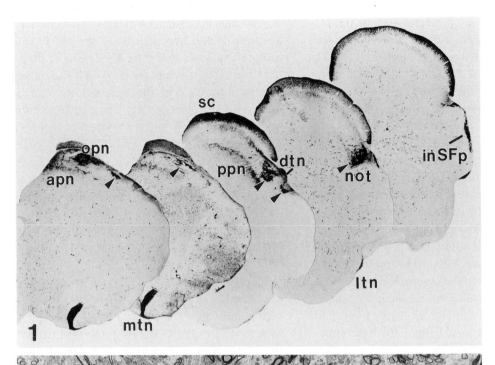

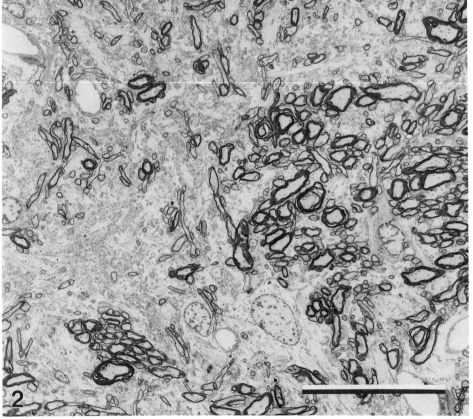

observed light microscopically high densities of GAD reactive neurons in the NOT/DTN of rat and gerbil, that could reach up to 27% of the total number of neurons. These GAD positive neurons are stastistically smaller than the mean size of a neuron from the total population, and they are more spherical, but otherwise indistinguishable from the total neuron population. According to Horn and Hoffmann (1987) GABAergic neurons in the NOT/DTN in cat, rat and monkey also are significantly smaller than retrogradely labeled cells from the IO that are nonGABAergic (Fig. 3a). Interneurons are generally considered as inhibitory and predominantly GABA positive. However, there is increasing evidence that GABAergic neurons can also be projection neurons (Fitzpatrick et al., 1984; Mugnaini and Oertel, 1985; Giolli et al., 1985; Appell and Behan, 1990; Cucchiaro et al., 1991; Van der Togt et al., 1991).

## GABAergic neurons and circuits

### Methodological considerations

GABA containing profiles have been identified using several techniques. In the earlier studies on the distribution of GABA in the central nervous system, tritiated GABA uptake was used to selectively label GABAergic neurons (Sotelo et al., 1972; Mize et al., 1982; Somogyi et al., 1983; Solnick et al., 1984). More recently, antibodies to glutamic acid decarboxylase (GAD), the synthesizing enzyme for GABA, have been used to identify GABAergic neurons, using immunocytochemical techniques (Oertel et al., 1982; Hendrickson et al., 1983; Houser et al., 1983). In GAD immunostaining, application of colchicine is often necessary to detect the enzyme in somata

(Tappaz et al., 1982). The application of colchicine enhances only the amount of GAD in cell bodies and does not increase the amount in terminals (Gabbott et al., 1986) and additionally deteriorates the ultrastructure considerably. The development of GABA antibodies conjugated to glutaraldehyde and the application of these antibodies in postembedded tissues, together with the use of immunogold to identify the immunoreactivity, permits sensitive detection in well preserved tissue in cell bodies, axons, dendrites and terminals (Van der Want and Nunes Cardozo, 1988).

## GABAergic and nonGABAergic cell bodies

A direct correlation between GABAergic and nonGABAergic neurons based on morphologically defined criteria, e.g., the size of the neuron, the shape of the nucleus or cytoplasmic stainability is often arbitrary and a classification based simply on ultrastructural criteria is not reliable (Van der Want and Nunes Cardozo, 1988). GABAergic neurons, although distributed throughout the whole NOT, tend to be more numerous in the caudal part than in the rostral part. The somata are small and spherical and the nuclei have smooth contours (Fig. 4a,b). However, there are also GABAergic neurons with medium sized somata and highly irregular shaped nuclei observed in the rabbit NOT/DTN complex (Fig. 4c,d). We have, therefore concluded that ultrastructural criteria cannot reliably distinguish GABAergic neurons in the absence of specific markers of this transmitter. However, the presence of two populations of GABAergic neurons, one with medium sized somata and one with small somata suggests the existence of two

Fig. 1. A series of transverse sections through the meso-diencephalon of a pigmented rabbit demonstrating the labeling pattern of retinal terminals after anterograde WGA-HRP transport from the retina, visualized with the tetramethylbenzidine method. Arrowheads indicate different parts of the NOT. See list for abbreviations.

Fig. 2. Low power electron micrograph of part of the NOT. The electron lucent neuropil is transsected by myelinated and unmyelinated axons. Bar = 5 $\mu$m.

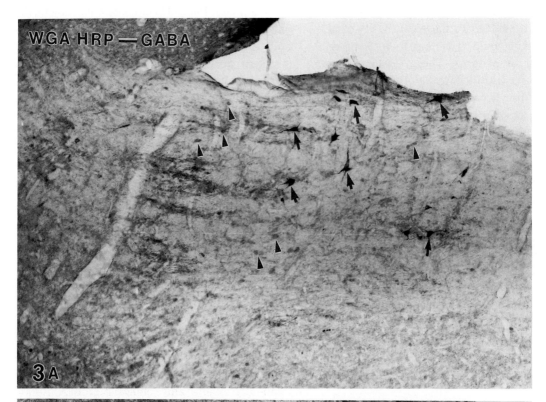

3A

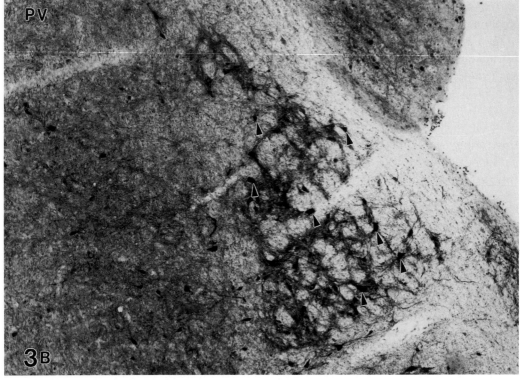

3B

separate GABAergic populations. The smaller cells could belong to the GABAergic interneurons and the larger ones to the GABAergic projection neurons (compare Fig. 6). In the rat and rabbit NOT/DTN complex, somata and neuropil show large variations in GABA immunoreactivity. Some neurons reveal a dense reaction product, others show much weaker staining. In the neuropil dendrites and terminal profiles also reveal intense reactivity, but areas with less reactivity were also noted. The different reactivities seem not related to gradients in the diffusion of the antibodies, but rather indicate true differences in GABA reactivity.

There have been several targets proposed for GABAergic projection neurons. The IO receives a strong input from the NOT/DTN and is one of the likely candidates to receive GABAergic input. To substantiate this, projection neurons in the NOT/DTN were selectively identified with retrograde tracers combined with GABA immunocytochemistry. In rabbit, rat, cat and monkey retrogradely transported WGA-HRP, injected into the IO, labeled cell bodies in the pretectum, but GABA reactivity could not be demonstrated in the labeled cell bodies (Horn and Hoffmann, 1987; Nunes Cardozo and Van der Want, 1990). The projection neurons to the dorsal cap of the inferior olive are found mainly in the rostral part of the NOT/DTN (Fig. 3a). The outlines of the somata and the primary dendrites of these projection neurons are rather smooth and densely studded with terminal profiles (Fig. 5). In recent tracing studies, in cat, GABA immunoreactive neurons were demonstrated to project from the APN, NOT and PPN to the SC (Appell and Behan, 1990). In an electron microscopical study we could demonstrate GABA reactivity in cell bodies that were retrogradely labeled after small iontophoretic injections of WGA-HRP in the superficial and deeper layers of the rat SC (Fig. 6). The identified GABAergic neurons are large to medium sized and show indented nuclei; these neurons are partly surrounded by glial envelopes, but on somatic surfaces that are free synaptic contacts with F terminals can be found. Until now we have not observed R terminals in contact with these somata (Van der Want et al., 1991).

Cucchiaro et al. (1991) observed that over 45% of the retrogradely labeled pretectal cells from the LGN were GABAergic and that those neurons were similar in size to the nonGABAergic neurons that were also labeled from the LGN. These results suggest the existence of two populations of GABA positive neurons in the cat's pretectum: projection neurons and interneurons. Those neurons are randomly distributed without evidence for clustering or segregation. These observations differ from that of Nabors and Mize (1991) who found, after HRP injection in the LGN, retrogradely labeled neurons in the cat pretectum that did not show GABA reactivity. Another important difference concerns the distibution of the projection neurons. In the latter study, HRP labeled neurons could be found arranged in clusters and these clusters correspond with calbindin reactivity. Further studies are necessary to resolve this conflicting data, but there are several factors that might explain the differences noted in these studies: (1) different sensitivity at the level of detection of the retrograde tracers in these studies will give rise to different numbers of retrogradely labeled neurons, (2) size of the injection and uptake of passing fibers, (3) different sensitivity and specificity of the antibodies used in double labeling experiments and (4) differences in defining the boundaries of the nuclei under investigation. Due to the location of

Fig. 3. a. Transverse section through the NOT/DTN immunostained for GABA and demonstrating retrogradely labeled WGA-HRP neurons that project to the inferior olive (arrows). GABAergic cell bodies (arrowheads) are relatively faintly stained, compared with the WGA-HRP labeled cell bodies. b. Transverse section at about the same level as in a, incubated for parvalbumin-immunoreactivity (PV) (arrowhead). PV reactivity is localized in the deeper parts of the NOT. Note that areas with retrogradely labeled and nonGABAergic projection neurons (in 3a) are observed in areas that are relatively free of PV reactivity.

290

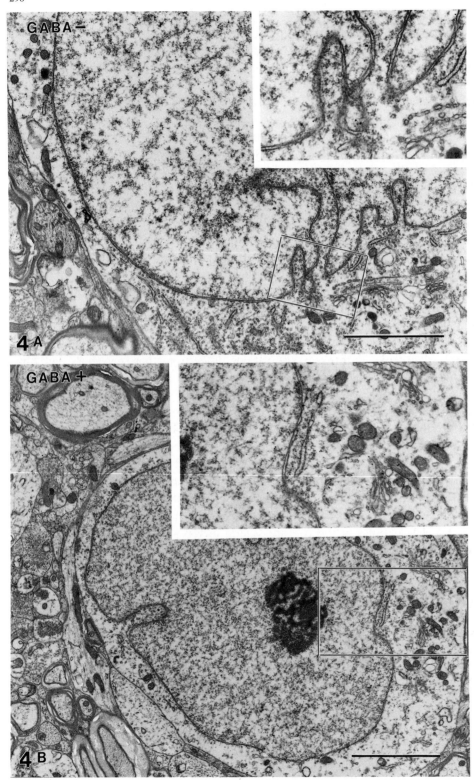

Fig. 4. For legend see p. 292.

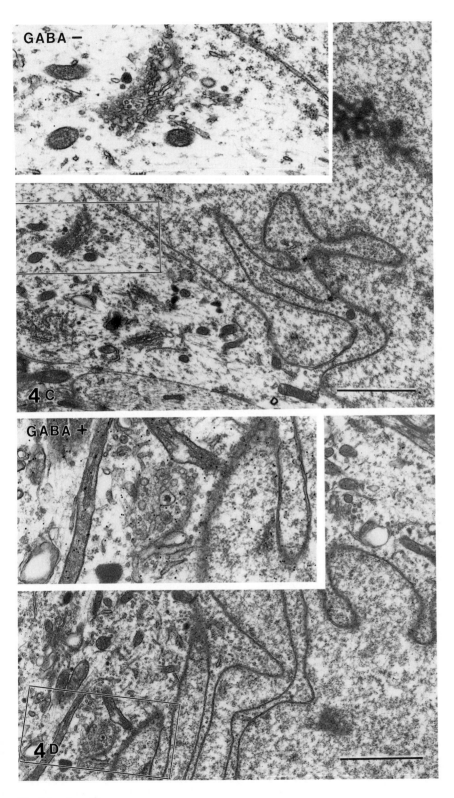

Fig. 4 (continued).

the pretectal nuclei within the myelinated fibers of the optic tract the penetration of antibodies and stains is rather limited and hence could easily cause conflicting results.

## Synaptology

### General description

The neuropil of the pretectal nuclei and the AOS is composed of axon terminals and dendritic profiles that are arranged either in glomerular-like configurations with a glial envelope or in free, loosely arranged terminal areas that are interspersed by dendrites and axons. The neuropil can be divided roughly into areas that receive retinal axon terminals (R) and areas that are devoid of R terminals. The retinal terminal organization described in the LGNd (Guillery, 1969; Hamori et al., 1974; Robson and Mason, 1979; Rapisardi and Miles, 1984) and the SC (Sterling, 1971; Vrensen and de Groot, 1977; Behan, 1981; Mize, 1983), resembles the glomeruli of R terminals in the NOT/DTN complex. A retinal glomerulus is formed by a centrally located R terminal that makes synaptic contacts on one or more profiles (Fig. 9). The R terminal and its postsynaptic elements usually are separated from the surrounding neuropil by a glial envelope. R terminals in the NOT/DTN are generally smaller than those in the LGN, they are easily identified on the basis of their electron lucent, "pale", mitochondria, spherical vesicles and asymmetric synapses (Figs. 7b, 9). R terminals synapse on nonGABAergic somata and dendrites and also on GABAergic terminals (F type,

see below), but they are never observed in synaptic contact with GABAergic somata (Fig. 7b). R terminals never show GABA immunoreactivity, but exhibit glutamate-like immunoreactivity (Nunes Cardozo et al., 1991).

### GABAergic terminals on identified cell bodies

Two different types of GABAergic terminals are found in the pretectum, the F and P type terminals. The F type contains clusters of flattened vesicles, but no ribosomes, and these are thought to be of axonal origin. There are two main varieties of F terminals that are classified according to the density of synaptic vesicles, the size of the terminal and the density of the cytoplasmic staining (Figs. 8a,b, 9). The larger F terminal has been observed throughout the neuropil and is often located at the periphery of complex arrangements of terminals and dendrites. These profiles contain loose accumulations of pleomorphic ovoid and flattened synaptic vesicles. A second, smaller type of F terminal is more often observed within such an arrangement. These terminals often contain more dense clusters of small ovoid or flattened vesicles. The F terminals are presynaptic to GABA immunonegative somata (Figs. 5, 7b) and dendrites and GABA positive dendrites. In an electron microscopic study in rabbits it was noted that the projection neurons to the IO, although not GABAergic themselves, receive a substantial GABAergic F type input on their somata (Nunes Cardozo and Van der Want, 1990), an observation that is in conflict with the light microscopic observations of Horn and Hoffmann (1987). In contrast with GABA immuno-

---

Fig. 4. a,b. Electron micrographs of two small neurons with spherical nuclei and electron lucent cytoplasm that is relatively free of organelles. These neurons resemble interneurons and have been incubated for GABA reactivity. The insets show higher magnifications, 4a does not contain 15 nm gold particles, localizing GABA reactivity. In b these particles can be seen. In c,d examples are given of large neurons with indented nuclei and extensive cytoplasm in which in c no GABA could be demonstrated, in d numerous particles indicate the presence of GABA. Bar = 1 μm.

---

Fig. 5. Composite electron micrograph of a soma of a retrogradely identified neuron in the NOT that projects to the dorsal cap of the inferior olive. The label in the cell body is composed of irregular gold precipitates, in the terminals GABA immunolabeling can be observed (visualised with 15 nm gold particles that are highly uniform in size). Labeled F-type terminals are indicated with +; some retinal (R) terminals contact the soma. Bar = 1 μm.

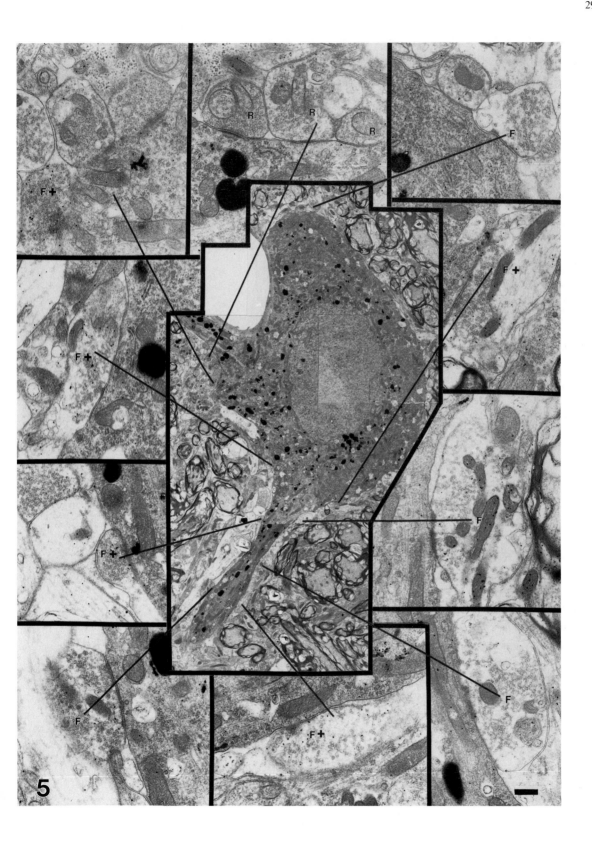

5

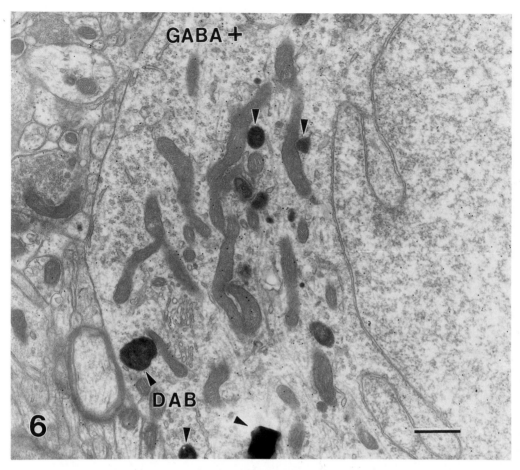

Fig. 6. Medium sized, WGA-HRP identified cell body (DAB arrowheads) in the rat NOT after retrogade labeling from the SC. The specimen has been incubated for GABA reactivity, that is visualized by 15 nm gold particles conjugated to the second antibody. In this part of the cell body no synaptic contacts are found. Bar = 1 μm.

positive cell bodies, which are almost devoid of terminals on their somata, GABA negative cell bodies receive a considerable number of GABA positive terminals on their cell bodies (Figs. 5, 7a, b). F terminals also can be postsynaptic to R terminals (Fig. 9).

The second type of GABA positive terminal exhibits pleomorphic vesicles (P terminal), contains ribosomes and is of dendritic origin (Figs. 8b, 9). The GABAergic dendrites have a wide distribution. There are two types of neurons from which they could originate: the GABAergic projection neuron or the GABAergic interneuron. From ultrathin sections this distinct origin could not be determined. Occasionally nonGABAergic

F and P terminals have also been found. Some differences in the terminal arrangement pattern of F type boutons in the NOT/DTN compared with the LGN, SC and OPN have been noted (Nunes Cardozo and Van der Want, 1987). In the OPN, triadic arrangements of F and P profiles and dendrites were frequently observed (Campbell and Lieberman, 1985). In the OPN triad, direct feedforward inhibition may be achieved through the F terminal that is in close vicinity to the R terminal. In the NOT/DTN, F terminals are only rarely found to participate in triadic arrangements.

The F terminals show structural features that resemble axon terminals (Montero and Singer,

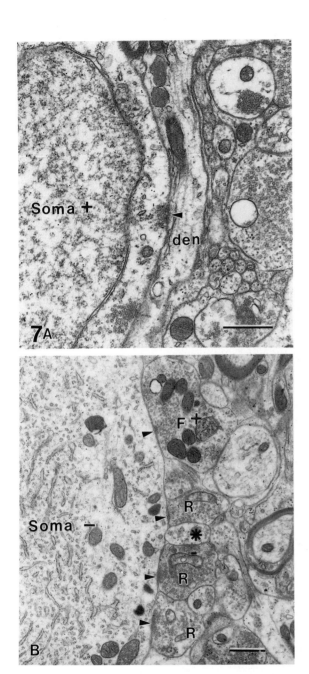

1985). The differences in characteristic fine structural details of the GABA immunopositive boutons suggest these GABAergic profiles may arise from multiple sources. Several projection areas could provide the NOT/DTN with these GABAergic terminals. Among these are the contralateral NOT, the ipsilateral MTN, the LGN, the SC and other pretectal and AOS nuclei. However, as yet there is only firm immunocytochemical support for the presence of GABA in terminals from the MTN to the NOT (Van der Togt et al., 1991). There is no evidence that the morphologically distinct F types that contain GABA (Fig. 8a,b, 9) correspond to different projection systems. It seems likely that the GABAergic F type terminals form part of the inhibitory system that connects visually related nuclei and that the P terminals belong to the local inhibitory systems.

## GABAergic circuit: projection from the MTN to the NOT/DTN complex

Immunocytochemical studies by Giolli et al. (1985, 1989) provide strong anatomical evidence for a GABAergic input to the NOT/DTN from the MTN. To investigate this GABAergic projection in more detail, a study, with anterograde labeling of the lectin *Phaseolus vulgaris* leucoagglutinin (PHA-L) and postembedding GABA immunocytochemistry of the same material, was performed. Many MTN terminals in the NOT/DTN were labeled by PHA-L (Fig. 10a,b). Preterminal fibers branch extensively and form small groups of varicosities near cell bodies and dendrites, covering most of the NOT/DTN. The PHA-L identified MTN terminals in the NOT/DTN contain GABA. Both labels can be clearly distinguished (Fig. 10b). The terminals belong to the F type and they form symmetrical synapses on nonGABAergic cell bodies and dendrites. MTN terminals are not contacted by R terminals. In fact, areas of the NOT/DTN that receive MTN terminals contain few R terminals and R terminals and MTN terminals were never seen in synaptic contact. This suggests that the terminal organization of the

Fig. 7. a,b. Electron micrographs of GABAergic (+) and nonGABAergic (−) somata, note that the GABAergic cell body receives few, if any terminals on its surface whereas the nonGABAergic neuron is studded with terminals that are either positive or negative for GABA. Asterisk indicates GABApositive dendrite and arrowheads indicate synapses. R indicates R terminals and * denotes a GABAergic P profile. The GABApositive soma is presynaptic to a dendrite (den). Bar = 1 μm.

296

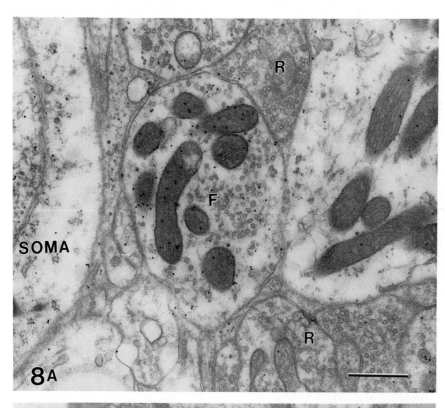

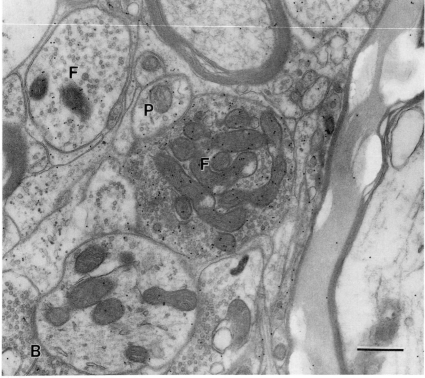

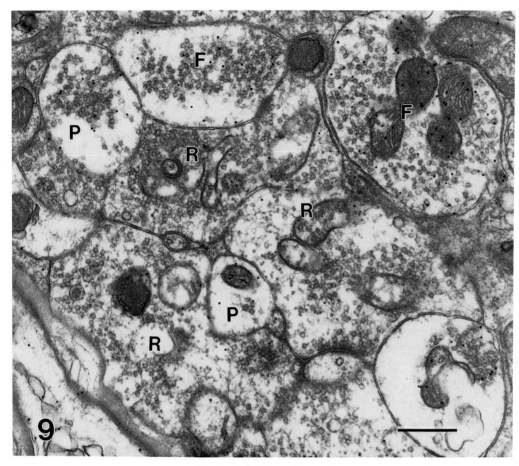

Fig. 9. Part of the NOT neuropil in the rabbit demonstrating the terminal organization of large retinal terminals (R) in close apposition with F and P terminals. Note that the R terminal does not contain GABA reactivity which is present in the F and P profiles. Bar = 1 μm.

GABAergic MTN input differs from local GABAergic terminals and that in this distinct terminal organization R terminals occupy a specific position. The segregation of GABAergic systems may provide the basis for the altered reactivity in OKN during MTN stimulation (Clement and Magnin, 1984). On the basis of electrophysio-logical evidence an inhibitory control by MTN neurons over the NOT has been suggested by Maekawa and Simpson (1972, 1973), Maekawa et al. (1984) and Clement and Magnin (1984). Our present data provide a structural basis for the existence of a strong and direct inhibitory input from the MTN on NOT/DTN neurons. The

Fig. 8. a,b. High magnification of different GABAergic F-type terminals (F) in the NOT neuropil of the rabbit, in 8a an F type with loosely arranged flattened vesicles can be seen and two retinal terminals (R) with clear and electron lucent mitochondria in comparison with the F terminal, in 8b an example is shown of an F terminal with dense accumulation of flattened vesicles. A dendritic P profile (P) is in synaptic contact with this F terminal. Bar = 1 μm.

298

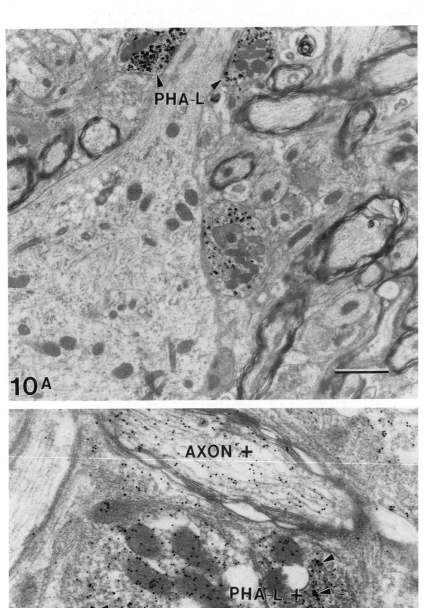

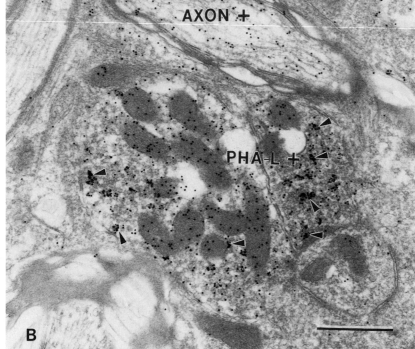

NOT/DTN neurons that are in receipt of these GABAergic F terminals are themselves nonGABAergic.

## Colocalization of the neuropeptide parvalbumin and GABA

Classically, the release of GABA has been thought to be mediated by a $Ca^{2+}$-dependent process (Llinas et al., 1976). However, recently, Pin and Bockaert (1989) suggested that depolarization induced GABA release mechanisms can occur in two ways: either via a tetanus toxin sensitive, voltage dependent $Ca^{2+}$ channel mechanism which is probably vesicular in nature, or through an inward $Na^+$-flux in the absence of $Ca^{2+}$ that is triggered by glutamate and which is tetanus toxin insensitive. This latter mechanism alters the equilibrium of the inward and outward transport of GABA and results in a reverse uptake system, that allows a nonvesicular and possibly extrasynaptic GABA release (Pin and Bockaert, 1989). These data suggest that one type of GABA neuron may contain large amounts of $Ca^{2+}$ and thus also require the presence of $Ca^{2+}$ binding proteins, such as parvalbumin (PV) and calbindin (CaBP) (Celio, 1986, 1990; Celio and Heizmann, 1981). PV and CaBP are closely associated with GABA containing interneuronal elements (Celio, 1986) and are found almost exclusively in a subpopulation of GABAergic neurons in some regions of the central nervous system (Stichel et al., 1988; Celio, 1990). PV and CaBP are considered to play a role in the modulatory activity of inhibitory neurons presumably through the control of $Ca^{2+}$ homeostasis in neurons with high firing rates (Kawaguchi et al., 1987). Specific PV immunoreactivity is present in somata and punctae in the NOT/DTN in rabbit (Fig. 3b). Its distribution closely resembles the distribution of GABA immunoreactivity (compare Fig. 3a). In the cat pretectum the calcium binding protein calbindin-D 28K preferentially labels clusters of neurons that correspond to the retinal termination fields (Nabors and Mize, 1991). Stichel et al. (1988) could demonstrate in the cat LGN coexistence of PV immunolabeling with GABA in F terminals at the ultrastructural level. These results strongly suggest that the abundance of calcium binding proteins in GABAergic systems, like in the NOT/DTN, is required to reduce $Ca^{2+}$ levels which in turn promotes GABA release. The absence of colocalization of CaBP and GABA immunoreactive neurons in the pretectum, as observed by Nabors and Mize (1991) seems in conflict with the observations by Stichel et al. (1988) in the LGN. Further studies are necessary to resolve these discrepancies.

## Functional implications

Physiological studies indicate that direction selectivity at the level of the retina does not differ from that observed at the pretectal and AOS-level (Ballas and Hoffmann, 1988), except that the receptive fields in the pretectum and AOS are much larger. Application of GABA in the cat NOT does not affect direction selectivity (K.-P. Hoffmann, personal communication). One can therefore tentatively conclude that GABA in the pretectum does not modify the transfer of speed and direction selective information from the retina to precerebellar brain stem nuclei. Mize (Chapter 11) also argues that GABAergic systems in the mammalian SC are unlikely to be involved in directional selectivity.

A specific class of neurons in the NOT/DTN complex has been described to respond vigorously to speed and directionally selective move-

Fig. 10. a,b. Electronmicrograph of PHA-L immunolabeled terminals in the NOT of the rat after an PHA-L injection in the MTN. Irregular gold deposits due to the gold substituted silver peroxidase application, identify PHA-L labeling (arrowheads). At higher magnification it can be noticed that the PHA-L terminal also contains strong GABA-labeling (15 nm gold particles). A GABApositive axon is indicated (axon + ). Bar = 1 $\mu$m.

ments of textured patterns in the full visual field (Sprague et al., 1973; Collewijn, 1975a,b; Hoffmann and Schoppmann, 1975, 1981; Cazin et al., 1980a,b; Precht and Strata, 1980; Grasse and Cynader, 1984; Kato et al., 1987). In the NOT/DTN complex, neurons have a preference for horizontal movements in the temporo-nasal direction and in the medial terminal nucleus (MTN) for movements in the vertical direction (for further details, see reviews of Simpson, 1984; Simpson et al., 1988a). An important difference, however, has been noted in the function of OKN between frontal eyed species and those with laterally placed eyes. According to Hoffmann (1989), in frontal eyed species (e.g., cat and monkey) a cortical loop that conveys indirect visual information to the NOT/DTN is essential for the generation of OKN and is even dominant over the direct retinal input in the NOT/DTN (Grasse and Cynader, 1991; Grasse et al., 1990). The excitatory cortical input will require a prominent position in the spatial configuration, as predicted in Somogyi's hypothesis (1990), formed by the excitatory R terminal and the inhibitory GABAergic input. This difference is also reflected in the connectivity in species that have laterally placed eyes (e.g., rat and rabbit) and where cortical ablation does not interfere with speed and direction selectivity of OKN (Ter Braak, 1936; Collewijn, 1975a). Unfortunately there are no fine structural studies on the organization of the cortical input available to compare the retinal and cortical inputs.

The pretectum and the AOS are undoubtedly involved in the generation of oculomotor reflexes since even partial lesioning of one of them results in a severe disturbance of OKN in rabbit (Collewijn, 1975a), cat (Hoffmann and Schoppmann, 1975) and monkey (Pasik and Pasik, 1973). A direct inhibitory connection between the MTN and the NOT/DTN has recently been demonstrated by Van der Togt et al. (1991). Such an inhibitory connection seems appropriate; slow movements in the horizontal plane that are modulated in the NOT will suppress activity in the

MTN. Vertical movements will activate MTN neurons which will in turn inhibit NOT/DTN activity. This latter effect has been demonstrated by Natal and Britto (1987) who lesioned the NOT in rat and found alterations in direction selectivity of MTN neurons. Inhibitory projections have also been demonstrated between other visually related nuclei, e.g., the pretectal nuclei and the SC (Appell and Behan, 1990; Van der Want et al., 1991) and from the pretectum to the LGN (Cucchiaro et al., 1991). It is likely that this intricate system that is formed by GABAergic projection neurons and their F terminals between the primary visual centres is involved in the fine tuning of oculomotor activity.

## Summary and conclusions

Two classes of GABAergic cell bodies have been described. They probably can be divided into GABAergic local interneurons and GABAergic projection neurons. GABAergic cell bodies receive few terminals which is in contrast to nonGABAergic somata, which receive many synaptic contacts. GABAergic dendrites that originate from GABAergic cell bodies, however, receive numerous terminals, both GABAergic and nonGABAergic. It can therefore be concluded that somatic inhibition is not present on GABAergic neurons, but does occur on nonGABAergic neurons. Furthermore, dendrites traverse large parts of the NOT/DTN forming a complex network that enables sampling and integration from a wide area. The projection to the IO is not GABAergic itself, but cells projecting to the IO receive a substantial GABAergic input, that probably originates in part from the MTN. Further investigation on the distribution of this input over a completely identified neuron would provide the quantitative data that are required to verify the above mentioned hypothesis. A GABAergic projection that originates in the pretectal nuclei is directed towards the superficial layers of the SC in the cat (Appell and Behan, 1990) and rat (Van der Want et al., 1991). A second

GABAergic projection derives from the pretectum and reaches the LGN (Cucchiaro et al., 1991). Whether this projection originates from the same GABAergic cell bodies that project to the SC and the LGN or is derived from different populations remains to be determined.

The ultrastructural studies of the NOT/DTN complex have shown that GABAergic terminals with different morphological characteristics are present and that the GABA positive F and P terminals are widely distributed over somata and the adjacent neuropil. The P terminals probably originate from dendrites of GABAergic interneurons while the F types originate from GABAergic projection and interneurons (Van der Want and Nunes Cardozo, 1988). One of these sources is located in the MTN. The GABAergic projection terminals from the MTN differ from the intrinsic GABAergic terminals with respect to their relation to R terminals. GABAergic MTN terminals were never observed to receive R terminal input. This is in contrast with other GABAergic terminals which frequently do receive direct contact from R terminals. Within glomeruli triadic arrangements, formed by a single retinal terminal, a dendritic profile and second axonal profile synapsing with the dendrite, were frequently encountered in the OPN (Campbell and Lieberman, 1985), but only occasionally in the NOT/DTN (Nunes Cardozo and Van der Want, 1987). The presence of excitatory R terminals, which are presynaptic to GABAergic terminals in the NOT/DTN neuropil, permits direct modulation of GABAergic synaptic activity by means of glutamate release. A similar neuromodulatory effect of glutamate on GABA release has also been demonstrated in cultures of prenatal rat SC (Perouansky and Grantyn, 1990).

## Abbreviations

| | |
|---|---|
| AOS, | accessory optic system |
| APN, | anterior pretectal nucleus |
| DTN, | dorsal terminal nucleus |
| GAD, | glutamic acid decarboxylase |
| HRP, | horseradish peroxidase |
| inSFp, | interstitial nucleus of the superior fasciculus posterior fibers |
| IO, | inferior olive |
| LGNd, | lateral geniculate nucleus dorsalis |
| LTN, | lateral terminal nucleus |
| MTN, | medial terminal nucleus |
| NOT, | nucleus of the optic tract |
| OPN, | olivary pretectal nucleus |
| OKN, | optokinetic nystagmus |
| PHA-L, | *Phaseolus vulgaris* leucoagglutinin |
| PPN, | posterior pretectal nucleus |
| R, | retinal terminal |
| SC, | superior colliculus |

## Acknowledgements

The authors thank Professor G. Vrensen, Department of Morphology, the Netherlands Ophthamic Research Institute and Professor R.A. Giolli, Department of Anatomy and Neurobiology, University of California, Irvine, California, USA, for helpful suggestions on the manuscript. Mr. N. Bakker is acknowledged for photographic assistance. The GABA antibody was kindly provided by Dr. R.M. Buijs, The Netherlands Institute for Brain Research, Amsterdam, The Netherlands and the Parvalbumin antibody by Professor Dr. M.R. Celio, Department of Histology, University of Fribourgh, Switzerland.

## References

Appell, P.P. and Behan, M. (1990) Sources of subcortical GABAergic projections to the superior colliculus in the cat. *J. Comp. Neurol.*, 302: 143–158.

Ariel, M. (1989) Analysis of vertebrate eye movement following intravitreal drug injections, Spontaneous nystagmus is modulated by the GABA-a receptor. *J. Physiol.*, 62: 469–480.

Ariel, M., Robinson, F.R. and Knapp, A.G. (1988) Analysis of vertebrate eye movements following intravitreal drug injections. II. Spontaneous nystagmus induced by picrotoxin is mediated subcortically. *J. Neurophysiol.*, 60: 1022–1035.

Ballas, I. and Hoffmann, K.-P. (1985) A correlation between receptive field properties and morphological structures in the pretectum of the cat. *J. Comp. Neurol.*, 238: 417–428.

Barlow, H.P. and Lewick, W.R. (1965) The mechanism of directionally selective units in rabbit's retina. *J. Physiol.*, 178: 477–504.

Barmack, N.H. and Hess, D.T. (1980a) Multiple-unit activity evoked in the dorsal cap of inferior olive of the rabbit by visual stimulation. *J. Neurophysiol.*, 43: 151–164.

Barmack, N.H. and Hess, D.T. (1980b) Eye movements evoked by micro stimulation of dorsal cap inferior olive in the rabbit. *J. Neurophysiol.*, 43: 165–181.

Berman, N. (1977) Connections of the pretectum in the cat. *J. Comp. Neurol.*, 174: 227–254.

Blanks, R.H.I., Giolli, R.A. and Pham, S.V. (1982) Projections of the medial terminal nucleus of the accessory optic system upon pretectal nuclei in the pigmented rat. *Exp. Brain Res.*, 48: 228–237.

Bonaventure, N., Wioland, N. and Bigenwald, J. (1983) Involvement of GABAergic mechanisms in the optokinetic nystagmus of the frog. *Exp. Brain Res.*, 50: 433–441.

Braak, H. and Bachmann, A. (1985) The percentage of projection neurons and interneurons in the human lateral geniculate nucleus. *Human Neurobiol.*, 4: 91–95.

Caldwell, J.H., Daw, N.W. and Wyatt, H.J. (1978) Effects of picrotoxin and strychnine on rabbit retinal ganglion cells: lateral interactions for cells with more complex receptive fields. *J. Physiol.*, 276: 277–298.

Campbell, G. and Lieberman, A.R. (1985) The olivary pretectal nucleus: Experimental anatomical studies in the rat. *Phil. Trans. R. Soc. London (Biol.)*, 310: 573–609.

Cazin, L., Prechtl, W. and Lannou, J. (1980a) Firing characteristics of neurons mediating optokinetic responses to rat's vestibular neurons. *Pflügers Arch. Physiol.*, 386: 221–230.

Cazin, L., Prechtl, W. and Lannou, J. (1980b) Pathways mediating optokinetic responses of vestibular neurons in the rat. *Pflügers Arch.*, 348: 19–29.

Celio, M.R. (1986) GABA neurons contain the calcium binding protein parvalbumin. *Science*, 232: 995–997.

Celio, M.R. (1990) Calbindin D-28k and Parvalbumin in the rat nervous system. *Neuroscience*, 35: 375–475.

Celio, M.R. and Heizmann, C.W. (1981) Calcium binding protein parvalbumin as a neuronal marker. *Nature (London)*, 293; 300–302.

Clement,G., and Magnin, M. (1984) Effects of accessory optic system lesions on vestibulo-ocular and optokinetic reflexes in the cat. *Exp. Brain Res.*, 55: 49–59.

Collewijn, H. (1975a) Direction-selective units in the rabbit's nucleus of the optic tract. *Brain Res.*, 100: 489–508.

Collewijn, H. (1975b) Oculomotor areas in the rabbits midbrain and pretectum. *J. Neurobiol.*, 6:3–22.

Cucchiaro, J.B., Bickford, M.E. and Sherman, S.M. (1991) A GABAergic projection from the pretectum to the dorsal lateral geniculate nucleus in the cat. *Neuroscience*, 41: 213–226.

Famiglietti, E.V. and Peters, A. (1972) The synaptic glomerulus and the intrinsic neuron in the dorsal geniculate nucleus of the cat. *J. Comp. Neurol.*, 144: 285–334.

Fitzpatrick, D., Penny, G.R. and Schmechel, D.E. (1984) GADimmunoreactive neurons and terminals in the lateral geniculate nucleus of the cat. *J. Neurosci.*, 4: 1809–1829.

Gabbott, P.L.A., Somogyi, J., Stewart, M.G. and Hamori, J. (1986) GABA-immunoreactive neurons in the rat cerebellum: a light and electron microscopic study. *J. Comp. Neurol.*, 251: 474–490.

Giolli, R.A. and Guthrie, M.D. (1969) The primary optic projections in the rabbit. An experimental degeneration study. *J. Comp. Neurol.*, 136: 99–126.

Giolli, R.A., Blanks, R.H.I., Torigoe, Y. (1984) Pretectal and brain stem projections of the medial terminal nucleus of the accessory optic system of the rabbit and rat as studied by anterograde and retrograde neuronal tracing methods. *J. Comp. Neurol.*, 27: 228–251.

Giolli, R.A., Clarke, R.J., Blanks, R.H.I., Torigoe, Y. and Fallon, J.H. (1989) Organization of the rat medial terminal accessory optic nucleus: Axon collateralization of neurons and its GABAergic neuron. *Anat. Rec.*, 223: 43A (Abstract).

Giolli, R.A., Peterson, G.M., Ribak, C.E., McDonald, H.M., Blanks, R.H.I. and Fallon, J.H. (1985) GABAergic neurons comprise a major cell type in rodent visual relay nuclei: an immunocytochemical study of pretectal and accessory optic nuclei. *Exp. Brain Res.* 61., 30: 9–31.

Giolli, R.A., Torigoe, Y., Blanks, R.H.I. and McDonald, H.M. (1988) Projections of the dorsal and lateral terminal accessory optic nuclei and of the interstitial nucleus of the superior fasciculus (posterior fibers) in the rabbit and rat. *J.Comp. Neurol.*, 277: 608–620.

Graf, W., Simpson, J.I. and Leonard, C.S. (1988) Spatial organization of visual messages of the rabbit's cerebellar flocculus. II. Complex and simple spike responses of Purkinje cells. *J. Neurophysiol.*, 60: 2091–2121.

Grasse, K.L. and Cynader, M.S. (1984) Electrophysiology of lateral and dorsal terminal nuclei of the cat accessory optic system. *J. Neurophysiol.*, 51: 276–293.

Grasse, K.L. and Cynader, M.S. (1988) The effect of visual cortex lesions on vertical optokinetic nystagmus in the cat. *Brain Res.*, 455: 385–389.

Grasse, K.L. and Cynader, M.S. (1991) The accessory optic system in frontal-eyed animals. In: A. Leventhal (Ed.), *Vision and Visual Dysfunction, Vol. IV, The Neuronal Basis of Visual Function*. New York: Macmillan, pp. 111–139.

Grasse, K.L., Ariel, M. and Smith, I.D. (1990) Direction-selective responses of units in the dorsal terminal nucleus of the cat following intravitreal injection of bicucculine. *Vis. Neurosci.*, 4: 605–617.

Gregory, K.M. (1985) The dendritic architecture of the visual pretectal nuclei of the rat: a study with the Golgi-Cox method. *J. Comp. Neurol.*, 234: 122–135.

Grzywacz, N.M. and Koch, C. (1987) Functional properties of models for direction selectivity in the retina. *Synapse*, 1: 417–434.

Guillery, R.W. (1969) The organization of synaptic interconnections in the laminae of the dorsal lateral geniculate nucleus of the cat. *Zeitschr. Zellforsch. Mikroskop. Anat.*, 96: 1–38.

Hamori, J., Pasik, T., Pasik, P. and Szentagothai, J. (1974) Triadic synaptic arrangements and their possible significance in the lateral geniculate nucleus of the monkey. *Brain Res.*, 80: 379–393.

Hamori, J., Pasik, P. and Pasik, T. (1983) Differential frequency of P-cells and I-cells in magnocellular and parvocellular laminae of monkey lateral geniculate nucleus: an ultrastructural study. *Exp. Brain Res.*, 52: 57–66.

Hendrickson, A.E., Ogren, M.P. Vaughn, J.E. Barber, R.P. and Wu, J.Y. (1983) Light and electron microscopic immunocytochemical localization of glutamic acid decarboxylase in monkey geniculate complex: evidence for GABAergic neurons and synapses. *J. Neurosci.*, 3: 1245–1262.

Hoffmann, K.-P. (1986) Visual inputs relevant for the optokinetic nystagmus in mammals. The oculomotor and skeletalmotor systems; differences and similarities. In: Freund, H.J., Büttner, U., Cohen, B. and Noth, J. (Eds.), *Progress in Brain Research, Vol. 64*, Amsterdam: Elsevier, pp. 75–84.

Hoffmann, K.-P. (1989) Functional organization of the optokinetic system of mammals. In: E. Rahmann (Ed.), Fortschr. Zool./ Progr. Zool. Band 37., pp.261–271. *Fundamentals of Memory Formation: Neuronal Plasticity and Brain Function.* Stuttgart, New York: G. Fisher Verlag.

Hoffmann, K.-P. and Schoppmann, A. (1975) Retinal input to direction selective cells in the nucleus tractus opticus of the cat. *Brain Res.*, 99: 146–159.

Hoffmann, K.-P. and Schoppmann, A. (1981) A quantitative analysis of the direction-specific response of neurons in the cat's nucleus of the optic tract. *Exp. Brain Res.*, 42: 146–159.

Holstege, G. and Collewijn, H. (1982) The efferent connections of the nucleus of the optic tract and superior colliculus in the rabbit. *J. Comp. Neurol.*, 209: 139–175.

Horn, A.K.E. and Hoffmann, K.-P. (1987) Combined GABA-immunocytochemistry and TMB-HRP histochemistry of pretectal nuclei projecting to the inferior olive in rats, cats and monkeys. *Brain Res.*, 409: 133–138.

Houser, C.R., Hendry, S.H.C., Jones, E.G. and Vaughn, J.E. (1983) Morphological diversity of immunocytochemically identified GABA neurons in the monkey sensory-motor cortex. *J. Neurocytol.*, 12: 617–638.

Kanaseki, T. and Sprague, J.M. (1974) Anatomical organization of pretectal nuclei and tectal laminae in the cat. *J. Comp. Neurol.*, 158: 339–362.

Kato, I., Harada, K., Hasegawa, T., Igarashi, T., Koike, Y. and Kawasaki, T. (1987) Role of the nucleus of the optic tract in monkeys in visually induced eye movements. In: M.D. Graham and J.L. Kemink, (Eds.), *The Vestibular System: Neurophysiologic and Clinical Research*, New York: Raven Press, pp. 623–632.

Kawachugi, Y., Katsumaru, H., Kosaka, T.,Heizmann, C.W. and Hama, K. (1987) Fast spiking cells in the in rat hippocampus (CA1 region) contain the calcium-binding protein parvalbumin. *Brain Res.*, 416: 369–374.

Kayama, Y., Fukuda, Y and Iwama, K. (1980) GABA sensitivity of neurons of the visual layer in the rat superior colliculus. *Brain Res.*, 192: 121–131.

Klooster, J., Van der Want, J.J.L. and Vrensen, G. (1983) Retinopretectal projections in albino and pigmented rabbits: An autoradiographic study. *Brain Res.*, 288: 1–12.

Korp, B.G., Blanks, R.H.I. and Torigoe, Y. (1989) Projections of the nucleus of the optic tract to the nucleus reticularis tegmenti pontis and prepositus hypoglossi nucleus in the pigmented rat as demonstrated by anterograde and retrograde transport methods. *Vis. Neurosci.*, 2: 275–286.

Koontz, M.A., Rodieck, R.W. and Farmer, S.G. (1985) The retinal projection to the cat pretectum. *J. Comp. Neurol.*, 236: 42–59.

Kühlenbeck, H. and Miller, R.N. (1942) The pretectal region of the rabbits brain. *J. Comp. Neurol.*, 76: 323–365.

Leonard, C.S., Simpson, J.I. and Graf, W. (1988) Spatial organization of visual messages of the rabbits cerebellar flocculus. I. Typology of inferior olive neurons of the dorsal cap of Kooy. *J. Neurophysiol.*, 60: 2073–2090.

Lieberman, A.R. (1973) Neurons with presynaptic perikarya and presynaptic dendrites in the rat lateral geniculate nucleus. *Brain Res.*, 59: 35–59.

Llinas, R., Steinberg, I.Z. and Walton, K. (1976) Presynaptic calcium currents and their relation to synaptic transmission: voltage clamp study in the squid giant synapse and theoretical model for the calcium gate. *Proc. Nat. Acad. Sci. USA*, 73: 2918–2922.

Maekawa, K. and Simpson, J.I. (1972) Climbing fiber activation of Purkinje cells in flocculus by impulses transferred through visual pathway. *Brain Res.*, 39: 245–251.

Maekawa, K. and Simpson, J.I. (1973) Climbing fiber responses evoked in vestibulocerebellum of rabbit from visual system. *J. Neurophysiol.*, 36: 649–666.

Maekawa, K., Takeda, T. and Kimura, M. (1984) Responses of the nucleus of the optic tract neurons projecting to the nucleus reticularis tegmenti pontis upon optokinetic stimulation in the rabbit. *Neurosci. Res.*, 2: 1–25.

Mize, R.R. (1983) Variations in the retinal synapses of the cat superior colliculus revealed using quantitative electron microscope autoradiography. *Brain Res.*, 269: 211–221.

Montero, V.M. and Singer, W. (1984) Ultrastructure and synaptic relations of neural elements containing glutamic acid decarboxylase (GAD) in the perigeniculate nucleus of the cat: A light and electron microscopic immunocytochemical study. *Exp. Brain Res.*, 59: 115–125.

Montero, V.M. and Singer, W. (1985) Ultrastructural identification of somata and neuronal processes immunoreactive to antibodies against glutamic acid decarboxylase (GAD) in the dorsal lateral geniculate nucleus of the cat. *Exp. Brain Res.*, 59: 151–165.

Montero, V.M. and Zempel, J. (1986) The proportion and size of GABA immunoreactive neurons in the magnocellular and parvocellular layers of the lateral geniculate nucleus of the rhesus monkey. *Exp. Brain Res.*, 62: 215–223.

Mugnaini, E. and Oertel, W.H. (1985) An atlas of the distribution of GABAergic neurons and terminals in the rat CNS as revealed by GAD immunohistochemistry. GABA and neuropeptides in the CNS. Part I. In: A. Björklund, and T. Hökfelt (Eds.), *Handbook of Chemical Neuroanatomy, Vol. 4*, Amsterdam: Elsevier, pp. 436–608.

Nabors, L.B. and Mize, R.R. (1991) A unique neuronal organization in the cat pretectum revealed by antibodies to the calcium-binding protein calbinding-D 28K. *J. Neurosci.*,

304

11: 2460–2476.

Natal, C.L. and Britto, L.R.G. (1987) The pretectal nucleus of the optic tract modulates the direction selectivity of accessory optic neurons in rats. *Brain Res.*, 419: 320–323.

Nunes Cardozo, J.J. and Van der Want, J.J.L. (1987) Synaptic organization of the nucleus of the optic tract in the rabbit: A combined Golgi-electron microscopic study. *J. Neurocytol.*, 16: 389–401.

Nunes Cardozo, B. and Van der Want, J. (1990) Ultrastructural organization of the retino-pretectal-olivary pathway in the rabbit: A combined WGA-HRP tracing and GABA immunocytochemical study. *J. Comp. Neurol.*, 291: 313–327.

Nunes Cardozo, B., Buijs, R. and Van der Want, J. (1991) Glutamate-like immunoreactivity in retinal terminals in the nucleus of the optic tract in rabbits. *J. Comp. Neurol.*, 309: 261–270.

Oertel, W.H., Mugnaini, E., Schmechel, D.E., Tappaz, M.L., and Kopin, I.J. (1982) The immunocytochemical demonstration of gamma-aminobutyric acidergic-neurons: methods and application. In: V. Chan-Palay and S.L. Palay (Eds.), *Cytochemical Methods in Neuroanatomy*, New York: Alan R. Liss, pp. 297–329.

Ottersen, O.P. and Storm-Mathisen, J. (1984) GABA-containing neurons in the thalamus and pretectum of the rodent. An immunocytochemical study. *Anat. Embryol.*, 170: 197–211.

Pasik, P. and Pasik, T. (1973) Extrageniculostriate vision in the monkey. V. Role of the accessory optic system. *J. Neurophysiol.*, 36: 450–457.

Perouansky, M. and Grantyn, R. (1990) is GABA release modulated by presynaptic excitatory amino acids receptors? *Neurosci. Lett.*, 113: 292–297.

Pin, J.-P. and Bockaert, J. (1989) Two distinct mechanisms, differentially affected by excitatory amino acids, trigger GABA release from fetal mouse striatal neurons in primary culture. *J. Neurosci.*, 9: 648–656.

Precht, W. and Strata, P. (1980) On the pathway mediating optokinetic responses in vestibular nuclear neurons. *Neuroscience*, 5: 777–787.

Rapisardi, S.C. and Miles, T.P. (1984) Synaptology of retinal terminals in the dorsal lateral geniculate nucleus of the cat. *J. Comp. Neurol.*, 223: 515–534.

Robertson, R.T. (1983) Efferents of the pretectal complex: separate populations of neurons project to lateral thalamus and to inferior olive. *Brain Res.*, 258: 91–95.

Robson, J.A. and Mason, C.A. (1979) The synaptic organization of terminals traced from individual labeled retinogeniculate axons in the cat. *Neuroscience*, 4: 99–111.

Rodieck, R.W. (1979) Visual pathways. *Ann. Rev. Neurosci.*, 2: 193–225.

Rose, J.E. (1942) The ontogenetic development of the rabbit's diencephalon. *J. Comp. Neurol.*, 77: 61–129.

Rose, M. (1935) Das zwischenhirn des Kaninchens. *Mem. Acad. Pol. Sci. Lett.*, 6: 1–108.

Scalia, F. (1972) The termination of retinal axons in the pretectal regions of mammals. *J. Comp. Neurol.*, 145: 223–258.

Scalia, F. and Arango, V. (1979) Topographic organization of the projections of the retina to the pretectal region in the rat. *J. Comp. Neurol.*, 186: 271–292.

Schiff, D. and Schmidt, M. (1990) Anatomical and histochemical characterization of nucleus of the optic tract (NOT) efferent populations in rat. *Eur. J. Neurosci. Suppl.*, 3: 243.

Schuerger, R.J., Rosenberg, A.F. and Ariel, M. (1990). Retinal direction sensitive input to the accessory optic system: an in vitro approach with behavioral relevance. *Brain Res.*, 522: 161–164.

Sillito, A.M. (1977) Inhibitory processes underlying the directional specificity of, simple, complex and hypercomplex cells in the cat s visual cortex. *J. Physiol. (London)*, 271: 699–720.

Simpson, J.I. (1984) The accessory optic system. *Ann. Rev. Neurosci.*, 7: 13–41.

Simpson, J.I., Giolli, R.A. and Blanks, R.H.I. (1988a) The pretectal nuclear complex and the accessory optic system. In: J.A. Büttner-Ennever (Ed.), *Neuroanatomy of the Oculomotor System, Reviews of Oculomotor Research, Vol. 2*, Amsterdam, New York, Oxford: Elsevier, pp. 335–364.

Simpson, J.I., Leonard, C.S. and Soodak, R.E. (1988b) The accessory optic system of rabbit. II. spatial organization of direction selectivity. *J. Neurophysiol.*, 60: 2055–2072.

Simpson, J.I., Soodak, R.E. and Hess, R. (1979) The accessory optic system and its relation to the vestibulocerebellum. In: R. Granit and O. Pompeiano (Eds.), *Reflex Control of Posture and Movement, Progress in Brain Research, Vol. 50*, Amsterdam: Elsevier, pp. 715–724.

Solnick, B., Davis, T.L and Sterling, P. (1984) Numbers of specific neurons in layer IVab of cat striate cortex. *Proc. Natl. Acad. Sci. USA*, 81: 3898–3900.

Somogyi, P. (1990) Synaptic organization of GABAergic neurons and GABAa receptors in the lateral geniculate nucleus and visual cortex. In: Lam, D.K.T., Gilbert, C.D. (Eds.), *Neural Mechanisms of Visual Perception, Proc. Ret. Res. Found. Symp., Vol. 2*, Houston: Portfolio Publ. Co., pp. 35–62.

Somogyi, P., Cowey, A., Kisvarday, Z.F., Freund, T.F. and Szentagothai, J. (1983) Retrograde transport of ($^3$H)GABA reveals specific interlaminar connections in the striate cortex of monkey. *Proc. Natl. Acad. Sci. USA*, 20: 2305–2309.

Sotelo, C., Privat, A. and Duran, M.J. (1972) Localization of ($^3$H)-GABA in tissue cultures of rat cerebellum using electron microscopy autoradiography. *Brain Res.*, 45: 302–308.

Sprague, J.M., Berlucchi, G. and Rizzolatti, G. (1973) The role of the superior colliculus and pretectum in vision and visually guided behavior. In: R. Jung (Ed.), *Visual Centers in the Brain, Handbook of Sensory Physiology VII/3B*, Heidelberg/New York: Springer Verlag, pp. 27–101.

Sterling, P. (1971) Receptive fields and synaptic organization of the superficial gray layer of the cat superior colliculus. *Vis. Res. (Suppl.)*, 3: 309–328.

Stichel, C.C., Singer, W. and Heizmann C.W. (1988) Light and electron microscopic immunocytochemical localization of parvalbumin in the dorsal lateral geniculate nucleus of the cat: evidence for coexistence with GABA. *J. Comp. Neurol.*, 268: 29–37.

Tappaz, M.L., Oertel, W.H., Wassef, M. and Mugnaini, E. (1982) Central GABAergic neuroendocrine regulations. Pharmacological and morphological evidence. *Prog. Brain Res.*, 55: 77–96.

Ter Braak, J.W.G. (1936) Untersuchungen über optokinetischen Nystagmus. *Arch. Neerl. Physiol.*, 21:309–376.

Van der Togt, C., Nunes Cardozo, B., Van der Want J.J.L. (1991) Medial terminal nucleus terminals in the Nucleus of the Optic Tract contain GABA. An electron microscopical study with immunocytochemical double labeling of GABA and PHA-L. *J. Comp. Neurol.*, 312: 231–241.

Van der Want, J.J.L. and Nunes Cardozo, J.J. (1988) GABA immuno-electron microscopic study of the nucleus of the optic tract in the rabbit. *J. Comp. Neurol.*, 272: 229–242.

Van der Want, J.J.L., Nunes Cardozo, J.J. and Van der Togt, C. (1991) The synaptic organization of the rat pretecto-collicular system. An ultrastructural demonstration of GABAergic and nonGABAergic projection neurons. *Soc. Neurosci. Abstr.*, 17.

Vrensen, G. and De Groot, D. (1977) Quantitative aspects of the synaptic organization of the superior colliculus in control and dark-reared rabbits. *Brain Res.*, 134: 417–428.

Weber, J.T. and Harting, J. (1980) The efferent projections of the pretectal complex: an autoradiographic and horse radish peroxidase analysis. *Brain Res.*, 194: 1–18.

Yücel, Y.H., Jardon, B. and Bonaventure, N. (1989) Involvement of ON and OFF retinal channels in the eye and head horizontal optokinetic nystagmus of the frog. *Vis. Neurosci.*, 2: 357–365.

Yücel, Y.H., Jardon, B., Kim, M.-S. and Bonaventure, N. (1990) Directional asymmetry of the horizontal monocular head and eye optokinetic nystagmus: Effects of picrotoxin. *Vis. Res.*, 30: 549–555.

R.R. Mize, R.E. Marc and A.M. Sillito (Eds.)
Progress in Brain Research, Vol. 90
© 1992 Elsevier Science Publishers B.V. All rights reserved

CHAPTER 15

# The pathways and functions of GABA in the oculomotor system

Robert F. Spencer [1], Shwu-Fen Wang [1] and Robert Baker [2]

[1] Department of Anatomy, Medical College of Virginia Richmond, VA 23298 and [2] Department of Physiology and Biophysics, New York University Medical Center, 550 First Avenue, New York, NY 10016, USA

## Introduction

Our present understanding of the mammalian oculomotor system has evolved from correlated morphological, physiological and behavioral studies of the neurons, nuclei and pathways that are related to five types of eye movement (vestibulo-ocular, saccadic, smooth pursuit, optokinetic and vergence). Conjugate eye movement involves co-ordinating the action of at least one pair of extraocular muscles in each eye. In horizontal eye movement, one muscle (for example, the medial rectus) must be excited and its antagonistic muscle (the lateral rectus) inhibited. In vertical eye movement this reciprocal relationship includes the superior and inferior recti. Actually, quite direct and simple circuits appear to mediate most eye movements. The final common premotor pathways originate from identifiable vestibular and reticular nuclei. Not unexpectedly, the pre-motor circuitry appears to involve the reciprocal excitatory regulation of at least *one pair* of ex-traocular motoneurons and the inhibition of the antagonistic pair of oculomotor neurons. Thus, one fundamental observation regarding premo-toneuronal organization is that each synaptic con-nection is well defined and it differs according to brain stem location and its putative role in hori-zontal and vertical eye movement. It is now well established that different types of neurotransmit-ters are involved and these can be related to a differential role in horizontal and vertical eye movement. Moreover it is the inhibitory synaptic connections that have been best documented and they clearly involve two neurotransmitters, GABA and glycine. Thus, it is the intent of this chapter to review the evidence underlying the anatomical and physiological organization of GABA inhibi-tion and then contrast that functional profile with glycine.

This chapter will review first the anatomical connections involved in vertical and horizontal vestibulo-ocular reflexes including vertical and horizontal gaze. Second, experimental evidence (heretofore unpublished) will be cited demon-strating GABA to be involved as the major neu-rotransmitter of inhibitory premotor neurons in the oculomotor system. Third, data will be com-pared between the monkey and the cat regarding the distribution and synaptic connections of GABA labeled neurons with a summary of their putative inhibitory role in eye movement.

## Organization of premotor neurons in the oculomotor system

### Vertical eye movements

Motoneurons in the extraocular motor nuclei are the final common pathway upon which affer-ents converge from brainstem premotor areas that are intimately related to the control of vertical and horizontal eye movements. Reciprocal excitatory and inhibitory synaptic connections of second-order vestibular neurons with motoneurons in the oculomotor and trochlear nuclei provide the physiological basis for the vertical vestibulo-ocular reflex (Highstein, 1973a; Highstein and Ito, 1971; Precht and Baker, 1972; Berthoz et al., 1973; Uchino et al., 1978; Iwamoto et al., 1990b). Most, if not all, of the inhibitory vestibular neurons that are related to the anterior and posterior vertical semicircular canals are located in the superior vestibular nucleus (Highstein and Ito, 1971; Yamamoto et al., 1978; Uchino et al., 1981, 1986; Baker et al., 1982; Graf et al., 1983; Mitsacos et al., 1983; Uchino and Suzuki, 1983; Hirai and Uchino, 1984; Graf and Ezure, 1986; McCrea et al., 1987a). The axons of these neurons ascend in the ipsilateral medial longitudinal fasciculus (MLF; McMasters et al., 1966; Gacek, 1971; Mitsacos et al., 1983; Carpenter and Cowie, 1985; McCrea et al., 1987a) and establish synaptic connections predominantly on the somata and proximal dendrites of motoneurons in the oculomotor and trochlear nuclei (Bak et al., 1976; Demêmes and Raymond, 1980; Spencer and Baker, 1983). Excitatory second-order vestibular neurons are located in the medial and ventral lateral vestibular nuclei (Highstein and Ito, 1971; Uchino et al., 1978, 1982; Baker et al., 1982; Carpenter and Cowie, 1985; Graf et al., 1983; Isu and Yokoto, 1983; Graf and Ezure, 1986; Highstein et al., 1987; McCrea et al., 1987a). Their axons ascend in the contralateral MLF (Iwamoto et al., 1990a) and terminate predominantly on the distal dendrites of oculomotor motoneurons (Demêmes and Raymond, 1980; Spencer and Baker, 1983). Some excitatory vestibular neurons that are related to the anterior vertical semicircular canal, however, are located in the superior vestibular nucleus, and their axons traverse the brachium conjunctivum and ascend in the ventral tegmentum (Yamamoto et al., 1978; Lang et al., 1979; Carpenter and Cowie, 1985; Hirai and Uchino, 1984) or in the ipsilateral MLF (Iwamoto et al., 1990a). The connections of excitatory and inhibitory sec-

ond-order vestibular neurons with motoneurons in the oculomotor and trochlear nuclei, to a certain extent, are specific to the semicircular canal from which they receive synaptic inputs. Excitatory second-order vestibular neurons that are related to the posterior vertical semicircular canal establish synaptic connections with superior oblique and inferior rectus motoneurons, while those that are related to the anterior vertical semicircular canal establish connections with inferior oblique and superior rectus motoneurons.

In addition to vestibulo-ocular reflex connections, vertical motoneurons in the oculomotor and trochlear nuclei also receive input from accessory oculomotor nuclei in the mesencephalic reticular formation that are related to the control of vertical saccadic eye movements (Büttner-Ennever et al., 1982; Fukushima, 1987). The interstitial nucleus of Cajal projects to the contralateral oculomotor nucleus via the posterior commissure and bilaterally to the trochlear nucleus (Carpenter et al., 1970; Graybiel and Hartwieg, 1974; Büttner-Ennever and Büttner, 1978; Steiger and Büttner-Ennever, 1979; Labandeira-Garcia et al., 1989). The rostral interstitial nucleus of the MLF projects ipsilaterally to the oculomotor nucleus (Büttner-Ennever and Büttner, 1978; Steiger and Büttner-Ennever, 1979; Nakao and Shiraishi, 1985; Labandeira-Garcia et al., 1989; Moschovakis et al., 1991a,b). Neurones in both locations discharge prior to vertical eye movements (Büttner et al., 1977; King and Fuchs, 1979; King et al., 1981; Vilis et al., 1989; Fukushima et al., 1990) and establish both excitatory and inhibitory synaptic connections with oculomotor and trochlear motoneurons (Schwindt et al., 1974; Nakao and Shiraishi, 1985).

*Horizontal eye movements*

The horizontal vestibulo-ocular reflex is mediated predominantly by reciprocal excitatory and inhibitory synaptic connections of second-order vestibular neurons with lateral rectus motoneurons and internuclear neurons in the abducens nucleus (Baker et al., 1969, 1980; Highstein,

1973b; Baker and Highstein, 1975; Uchino et al., 1982; Ishizuka et al., 1980; McCrea et al., 1980). Both the inhibitory and excitatory second-order vestibular neurons that project to the abducens nucleus are located in the medial and ventral lateral vestibular nuclei (Maciewicz et al., 1977; Ishizuka et al., 1980; McCrea et al., 1980; Uchino et al., 1981, 1982; Nakao et al., 1982; Carleton and Carpenter, 1983; Uchino and Suzuki, 1983; Langer et al., 1986; McCrea et al., 1987b; Belknap and McCrea, 1988; Ohgaki et al., 1988; Escudero and Delgado-García, 1988). A direct excitatory second-order vestibular input to medial rectus motoneurons originates from neurons in the ventral portion of the lateral vestibular nucleus whose axons course ipsilaterally via the ascending tract of Deiters (Baker and Highstein, 1978; Furuya and Markham, 1981; Reisine et al., 1981; Carleton and Carpenter, 1983; Carpenter and Carleton, 1983; Markham et al., 1986).

In addition to horizontal vestibulo-ocular reflex connections, abducens neurons also receive reciprocal excitatory and inhibitory synaptic inputs from neurons in the pontomedullary reticular formation that are related to horizontal gaze. Premotor excitatory burst neurons are located in the ipsilateral paramedian pontine reticular formation (nucleus reticularis pontis caudalis) ventral and rostral to the abducens nucleus (Büttner-Ennever and Henn, 1976; Highstein et al., 1976; Graybiel, 1977; Maciewicz et al., 1977; Grantyn et al., 1980a,b; Igusa et al., 1980; Curthoys et al., 1981; Kaneko et al., 1981; Langer et al., 1986; Strassman et al., 1986a; Escudero and Delgado-García, 1988). By contrast, inhibitory burst neurons are located in the contralateral dorsomedial pontomedullary reticular formation medial and caudal to the abducens nucleus (Hikosaka and Kawakami, 1977; Maciewicz et al., 1977; Hikosaka et al., 1978; Grantyn et al., 1980a,b; Hikosaka and Igusa, 1980; Yoshida et al., 1982; Langer et al., 1986; Strassman et al., 1986b; Escudero and Delgado-García, 1988; Scudder et al., 1988).

The prepositus hypoglossi nucleus potentially represents one site of interaction between the visual and vestibular systems. Neurons in the prepositus hypoglossi nucleus have visual receptive fields and exhibit eye movement-related activity (Baker and Berthoz, 1975; Baker et al., 1976; Gresty and Baker, 1976; Blanks et al., 1977; López-Barneo et al., 1982; Delgado-García et al., 1989). Lesions of the prepositus disrupt horizontal optokinetic, vestibulo-ocular, and saccadic integration processing (Cheron et al., 1986a,b; Cannon and Robinson, 1987). The prepositus hypoglossi nucleus has extensive interconnections with the vestibular nuclei and pontomedullary reticular formation (McCrea and Baker, 1985; Belknap and McCrea, 1988) and efferent connections with the extraocular motor nuclei (Graybiel and Hartwieg, 1974; Baker et al., 1977; Graybiel, 1977; Maciewicz et al., 1977; Steiger and Büttner-Ennever, 1979; Hikosaka and Igusa, 1980; López-Barneo et al., 1981; McCrea and Baker, 1985; Langer et al., 1986; Belknap and McCrea, 1988). Like the vestibular and reticular inputs to abducens neurons, those from the prepositus hypoglossi nucleus also have excitatory and inhibitory components (Escudero and Delgado-García, 1988).

## Early evidence for the role of GABA as an inhibitory neurotransmitter in the vestibulo-ocular system

Inhibition mediated by premotor afferent neurons is a fundamentally important aspect of the organization of the reciprocal excitatory and inhibitory synaptic inputs to extraocular motoneurons. This concept is underscored by the strategic proximal location of most inhibitory synaptic endings on the soma-dendritic surface of the motoneurons (Bak and Choi, 1974; Bak et al., 1976; Tredici et al., 1976; Spencer and Sterling, 1977; Destombes et al., 1979; Waxman and Pappas, 1979; Demêmes and Raymond, 1980; Destombes and Rouvière, 1981; Spencer and Baker, 1983). Electrophysiological, pharmacological and biochemical studies have established that GABA is the inhibitory neurotransmitter utilized by second-order vestibular neurons that establish synaptic connections with motoneurons in the oculomotor and trochlear nuclei. Systemic administration of picrotoxin, an antagonist of GABA, abolishes the depression of the antidromic field potential recorded extracellularly in the oculomotor nucleus following IIIrd nerve stimulation and eliminates the extracellular positive field potentials that represent the inhibitory postsynaptic currents resulting from ipsilateral VIIIth nerve stimulation (Ito et al., 1970). Iontophoresis of GABA in the vicinity of the oculomotor nucleus depresses the antidromic field potential elicited by IIIrd nerve stimulation and decreases or completely suppresses the spike generation of motoneurons in a manner similar to that produced by electrical stimulation of the ipsilateral VIIIth nerve (Obata and Highstein, 1970). The inhibitory responses elicited by VIIIth nerve stimulation and GABA iontophoresis furthermore are blocked by iontophoresis of picrotoxin in the vicinity of the motoneurons. Picrotoxin also blocks the slow muscle potential recorded from the extraocular muscles in a manner similar to removal of the second-order vestibular input to oculomotor motoneurons following lesions of the dorsolateral brainstem that effectively interrupt the inhibitory vestibular pathway (Ito et al., 1976). These electrophysiological and pharmacological findings are supported further by anatomical studies that have demonstrated synaptic endings in the oculomotor nucleus labelled autoradiographically by high affinity uptake of [$^3$H]GABA (Lanoir et al., 1982; Soghomonian et al., 1989) or immunohistochemically using an antibody to GABA (Soghomonian et al., 1989).

In the trochlear nucleus, systemic administration of picrotoxin significantly reduces or abolishes both the inhibitory synaptic current recorded extracellularly (Fig. 1A–D) and the IPSPs recorded intracellularly (Fig. 1E–H) from motoneurons following electrical stimulation of the ipsilateral VIIIth nerve (Precht et al, 1973). A similar depressant action on vestibular-evoked inhibition is obtained by systemically administered

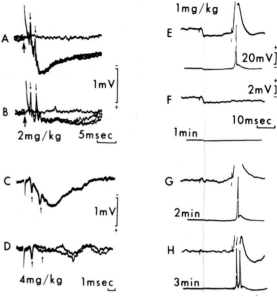

Fig. 1. Effect of picrotoxin on vestibular-evoked potentials recorded in cat trochlear motoneurons. A,B and C,D illustrate extracellular field potentials recorded in two different experiments in the trochlear nucleus following electrical stimulation of the ipsilateral VIIIth (Vi) nerve before (A and C) and after (B and D) intravenous administration of 2 mg/kg (B) and 4 mg/kg (D) of picrotoxin. E–H are intracellular records from a single trochlear motoneuron before (E) and 1 min (F), 2 min (G) and 3 min (H) after administration of 2 mg/kg picrotoxin. Note reduction of the IPSP following Vi stimulation (first stimulus; dotted line drawn at peak of IPSP), whereas no effect is observed on the EPSP and action potential generated by contralateral vestibular nerve stimulation. (Reproduced from Precht et al. (1973) with permission.)

bicuculline. Unilateral section of the MLF, which abolishes the vestibular-evoked inhibitory synaptic currents, reduces the concentration of GABA in the trochlear nucleus. Lesions of the superior vestibular nucleus also produce a marked decrease in GABA synthesis in the ipsilateral trochlear nucleus (Roffler-Tarlov and Tarlov, 1975).

GABA also was thought initially to be the inhibitory neurotransmitter mediating vestibular-evoked inhibition in the abducens nucleus. Both the antidromic field potentials and orthodromic synaptic currents recorded extracellularly following VIth and VIIIth nerve stimulation, respectively, were reduced when picrotoxin was administered systemically in the rabbit (Highstein, 1973b). A more recent comprehensive autoradiographic, immunohistochemical, and electrophysiological-pharmacological analysis in the cat, however, has revealed that, in contrast to the oculomotor and trochlear nuclei, inhibitory inputs to the abducens nucleus from second-order neurons in the vestibular nucleus, as well as from neurons in the dorsolateral medullary reticular formation and the prepositus hypoglossi nucleus, utilize glycine as a neurotransmitter (Spencer et al., 1989). These different populations of premotor neurons are labelled selectively by retrograde transport of [$^3$H]glycine injected into the abducens nucleus. Correlated with these findings, the abducens nucleus contains a high density of glycine-immunoreactive synaptic endings, and the vestibular inhibition of abducens motoneurons evoked by selective horizontal canal nerve electrical stimulation is abolished by strychnine, but is unaffected by picrotoxin or bicuculline administered systemically. Furthermore, glycine-immunoreactive neurons are located in the same areas as neurons labelled by retrograde transport of [$^3$H]glycine from the abducens nucleus. These findings are correlated with a distinctive pattern of immunoreactive staining in the MLF. GABA is associated predominantly with ascending axons that project to the oculomotor and trochlear nuclei. By contrast, glycine is localized predominantly in descending axons that project to the abducens nucleus and the spinal cord. These paradoxical differences in inhibitory neurotransmitters utilized by vertical and horizontal canal-related vestibular neurons may be correlated with the differential roles of GABA and glycine in vestibular commissural inhibition (Precht et al., 1973) and the differential association of GABA$_A$ and strychnine-sensitive glycine receptors with neurons in the vestibular nucleus (Smith et al., 1991).

Immunohistochemical studies of GABA localization also do not fully support the substantive physiological, biochemical and pharmacological data cited above regarding the role of GABA as the inhibitory neurotransmitter in vestibulo-ocular reflex connections. For example, few or no GABA-immunoreactive neurons have been found in the superior vestibular nucleus (Nomura et al., 1984; Kumoi et al., 1987; Walberg et al., 1990), despite evidence that both anterior and posterior vertical canal-related inhibitory second-order vestibular neurons reside in this region. By contrast, GABA-immunoreactive neurons have been observed predominantly in the medial and inferior vestibular nuclei. Neurons in the medial and inferior vestibular nuclei that project to the spinal cord also are immunoreactive toward glutamate decarboxylase (GAD), the synthesizing enzyme of GABA (Blessing et al., 1987). On the other hand, other evidence suggests that glycine is involved in these connections. First, the vestibular-evoked disynaptic IPSPs in neck motoneurons are effectively blocked by strychnine, a glycine antagonist (Felpel, 1972). Second, presumed glycinergic inhibitory vestibular neurons that project to the ipsilateral abducens nucleus have axonal branches that descend in the MLF toward the spinal cord (McCrea et al., 1980; Isu and Yokota, 1983). Third, spinal cord ventral horn motoneurons exhibit a high density of glycine receptors (Triller et al., 1985; Geyer et al., 1987). It is thus possible that neurons may colocalize GABA and glycine (Walberg et al., 1990) or that GABAergic synaptic endings are associated with glycine receptors (Triller et al., 1987).

At present, it is difficult to resolve these apparent disparate findings in regard to the locations of known populations of inhibitory vestibular neurons and the neurotransmitters with which they are associated. On the one hand, since vertical canal-related inhibitory second-order vestibular neurons are projection neurons, it is possible that, like cerebellar Purkinje cells, the concentration of GABA within the somata of the neurons is significantly less than that at their synaptic endings in the oculomotor and trochlear nuclei and cannot be detected immunohistochemically. Consequently, the above studies may not have identified the total population of GABAergic

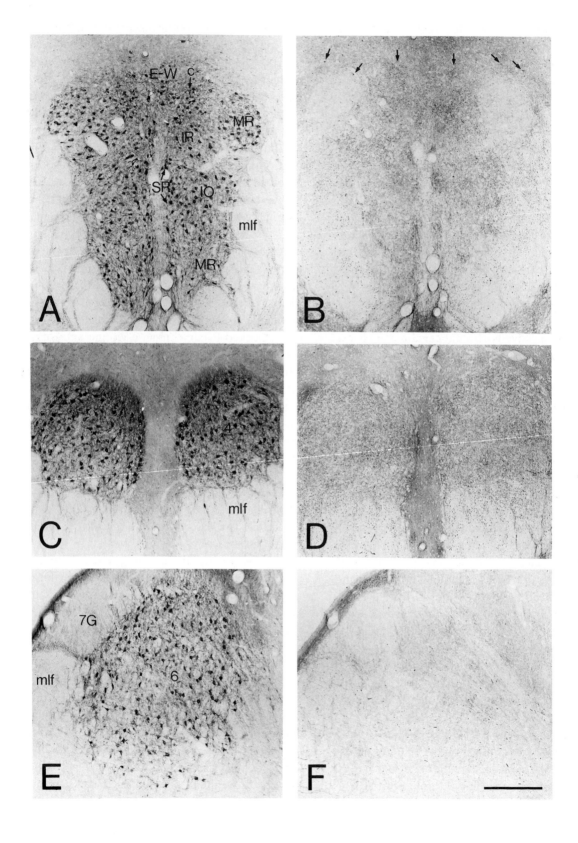

neurons in the vestibular nuclei, particularly within the superior vestibular nucleus. On the other hand, neurons in all of the vestibular nuclei may exhibit GABA or GAD immunoreactivity irrespective of whether they utilize GABA as a neurotransmitter. In this regard, the colocalization of GABA and glycine, as well as their colocalization with putative excitatory amino acid neurotransmitters, may indicate a metabolic pool of one that is unrelated to the neurotransmitter function of another. Despite the colocalization of GABA and glycine in single vestibular neurons, in most instances only one or the other appears to have a synaptic effect, as indicated by the specificity of pharmacological antagonism, and this effect presumably is dictated by the type and presence of the postsynaptic receptor with which the input is associated.

## Immunohistochemical localization of GABA and GAD in the extraocular motor nuclei

In continuation of our previous studies of glycine and to further resolve the issue of GABA as a neurotransmitter in the oculomotor system, we recently have localized GABA (Wenthold et al., 1986) and GAD (Oertel et al., 1981) in the extraocular motor nuclei of the Rhesus monkey and the cat using light and electron microscopic immunohistochemistry. The procedures used for these analyses are essentially similar to those previously described in detail (Spencer et al., 1989).

### Light microscopic observations of GABA and glycine in the rhesus monkey

The extraocular motor nuclei in the monkey are particularly illustrative of the patterned distribution of GABA in relation to different populations of motoneurons. In the oculomotor nucleus, the subgroups of motoneurons can be identified clearly by both retrograde labelling with horseradish peroxidase (HRP; Büttner-Ennever and Akert, 1981; Spencer and Porter, 1981; Porter et al., 1983) and immunohistochemical staining with choline acetyltransferase (ChAT), the synthesizing enzyme of the motoneuron neurotransmitter acetylcholine (Fig. 2A). GABA-immunoreactive terminals are found predominantly within the inferior rectus, superior rectus, inferior oblique, and dorsomedial (subgroup c) medial rectus subdivisions (Fig. 2B). Both the ventral (subgroup a) and dorsal (subgroup b) subdivisions of medial rectus motoneurons, however, apparently lack GABA-immunoreactive terminals. This negative finding is particularly significant, since both subgroups are the major target of the excitatory abducens internuclear projection that is responsible for conjugate horizontal eye movements (Carpenter and Batton, 1980; Carpenter and Carleton, 1983; McCrea et al., 1986; Belknap and McCrea, 1988). Furthermore, at least in the cat, medial rectus motoneurons lack IPSPs elicited by VIIIth nerve stimulation (Baker and Highstein, 1978). By contrast, the presence of GABA-immunoreactive terminals in the dorsomedial (subgroup c) medial rectus subdivision is consistent

Fig. 2. Light micrographs of the immunohistochemical localization of ChAT and GABA in Rhesus monkey extraocular motor nuclei. In A, the distribution of ChAT-immunoreactive neurons delineates the motoneuron subdivisions of the oculomotor nucleus (IR, inferior rectus; SR, superior rectus; IO, inferior oblique; MR, medial rectus; c, dorsomedial medial rectus subgroup c; E–W, Edinger-Westphal nucleus). GABA-immunoreactive staining in the adjacent section (B) demonstrates dense terminal labelling in all subdivisions *except* the ventral (a) and dorsal (b) medial rectus subgroups. GABA-immunoreactive axons are confined to the medial portion of the MLF and several GABA-immunoreactive neurons are observed in the supraoculomotor region (arrows). In the trochlear nucleus, ChAT-immunoreactive neurons (C) define the boundaries of the nucleus to which GABA-immunoreactive terminals (D) are confined. GABA-immunoreactive axons are located in the dorsal region of the MLF. In the abducens nucleus, ChAT-immunoreactive neurons (E) are uniformly distributed throughout the nucleus and define its borders. GABA-immunoreactive terminals within the abducens nucleus are sparse as are labelled axons in the MLF (F). Calibration: 500 $\mu$m.

314

with previous suggestions of functional differences between subgroups, particularly in relation to their role in vergence versus conjugate eye movements (Büttner-Ennever and Akert, 1981; Spencer and Porter, 1981; Mays and Porter, 1984). Correlated at least in part with the high density of GABA-immunoreactive terminals within the oculomotor nucleus, GABA-immunoreactive axons also are observed predominantly in the medial portion of the MLF lateral to the nucleus.

In addition to GABA-immunoreactive terminals within the oculomotor nucleus, GABA-immunoreactive neurons are observed in the supraoculomotor region dorsal and dorsolateral to the b and c medial rectus subgroups (Figs. 2B, 5E). These neurons are small in diameter (8 to 11 μm) and typically are oval in shape. In the monkey, this region has been implicated in the control of vergence eye movements (Mays, 1984; Judge and Cumming, 1986; Mays et al., 1986). In addition to those in the supraoculomotor region, some GABA-immunoreactive neurons are located within the oculomotor nucleus coexistent with superior rectus, inferior rectus, and inferior

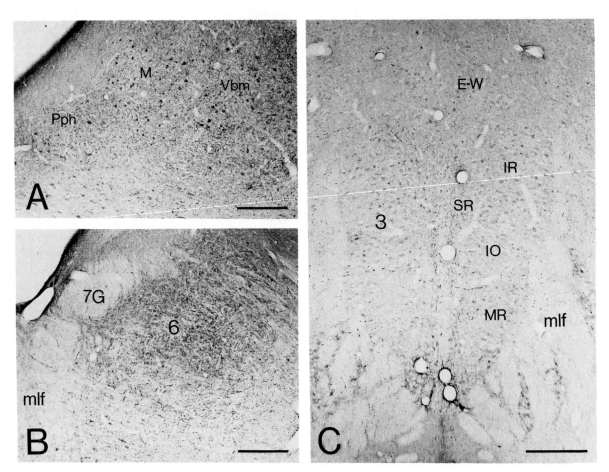

Fig. 3. Light micrographs of glycine-immunoreactive staining in the brainstem of the Rhesus monkey. In A, glycine-immunoreactive neurons are found in the prepositus hypoglossi (Pph) and the medial (Vbm) vestibular nuclei, as well as in the marginal zone (M) situated between them. In B, the abducens nucleus (6) is characterized by dense glycine-immunoreactive terminal staining. By contrast, the oculomotor nucleus (3) in C exhibits only sparse immunoreactive terminal staining that is associated specifically with the superior rectus (SR) subdivision. Calibrations: A–C, 500 μm.

oblique motoneurons. These neurons are larger in diameter (10 to 18 $\mu$m) and typically are multipolar in appearance (Fig. 5F).

The trochlear nucleus contains a dense plexus of GABA-immunoreactive terminals (Fig. 2D) that overlaps completely the distribution of ChAT-immunoreactive motoneurons (Fig. 2C). Ventral to the nucleus, GABA-immunoreactive axons are found predominantly in the dorsal half of the MLF, suggesting that the axons are segregated in the MLF according to their origin (e.g., vestibular, abducens internuclear) and/or function (i.e., inhibitory vs. excitatory).

The abducens nucleus in the monkey, defined on the basis of the distribution of ChAT-immunoreactive motoneurons (Fig. 2E), exhibits a paucity of GABA-immunoreactive terminal staining (Fig. 2F). Furthermore, only a few GABA-immunoreactive axons are observed in the MLF at this level of the brainstem.

Consistent with previous findings of the differential localization of GABA and glycine in the extraocular motor nuclei in the cat (Spencer et al., 1989), similar findings of glycine localization have been observed in the Rhesus monkey. Specifically, the abducens nucleus has a high density of glycine-immunoreactive terminals (Fig. 3B) that appears to be associated with inputs from glycine-immunoreactive neurons in known premotor areas in the posterior brainstem (e.g., prepositus hypoglossi and medial vestibular nuclei, Fig. 3A). By contrast, the oculomotor (Fig. 3C) and trochlear nuclei are characterized by a paucity or absence, respectively, of glycine-immunoreactive terminals. In the oculomotor nucleus in the monkey, however, these terminals are confined specifically to the superior rectus subdivision, whereas in the cat similar terminals appear to be distributed to the other (except medial rectus) motoneuron subdivisions as well. The source of this modest glycinergic input to the oculomotor nucleus presently is unknown. Thus, the complementary pattern of GABA and glycine localization previously observed in relation to the extraocular motor nuclei in the cat is applicable to the primate.

*Light and electron microscopic observations of GABA and GAD in the cat*

The distribution of GABA-immunoreactive terminals in the cat extraocular motor nuclei is qualitatively similar to that observed in the Rhesus monkey. Within the oculomotor nucleus, immunoreactive terminals are found within the superior rectus, inferior oblique, and inferior rectus subdivisions (Fig. 4A–C), although their density is considerably less than that seen in the same subdivisions in the monkey. Like the monkey, the medial rectus subdivision in the cat has little or no immunoreactive terminal staining (Fig. 4D).

Also like the monkey, GABA-immunoreactive neurons are found both within the oculomotor nucleus coexistent with the different motoneuron subdivisions (except medial rectus) as well as in the supraoculomotor region (Fig. 5C). In the cat, this region also contains the dendrites of oculomotor motoneurons (Fig. 5A) and is the location of many oculomotor internuclear neurons that project to the abducens nucleus (Fig. 5B; see also May et al., 1987) and other brainstem areas. Some neurons in this region also establish synaptic connections with medial rectus motoneurons (Nakao et al., 1986; May et al., 1987). Like those in the monkey, GABA-immunoreactive neurons in the supraoculomotor region in the cat are small in diameter (7 to 10 $\mu$m), and their somata are oval or circular in shape (Fig. 5D).

The densest immunoreactive terminal staining is found in the trochlear nucleus, in which immunoreactive boutons are observed adjacent to the somata of motoneurons as well as in the surrounding neuropil (Fig. 4E). By contrast, the abducens nucleus contains only a few small immunoreactive boutons interspersed in the neuropil (Fig. 4F). Occasional immunoreactive axons that presumably are of vestibular commissural origin course transversely through the nucleus.

Within the oculomotor and trochlear nuclei,

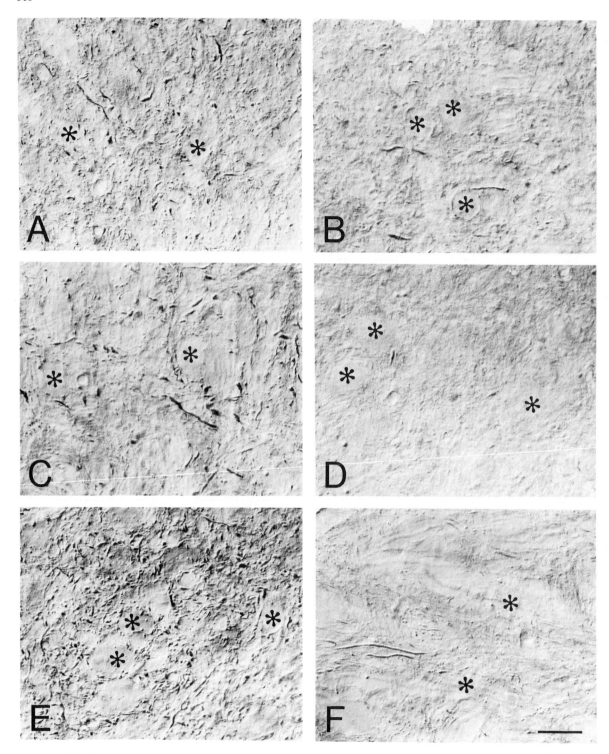

Fig. 4. Nomarski differential interference contrast photomicrographs of GABA-immunoreactive staining in the oculomotor (A–D), trochlear (E) and abducens (F) nuclei in the cat. GABA-immunoreactive boutons surround the somata of motoneurons (asterisks) and are scattered within the surrounding neuropil in the superior rectus (A), inferior oblique (B) and inferior rectus (C) subdivisions of the oculomotor nucleus and in the trochlear nucleus (E). By contrast, in the medial rectus subdivision of the oculomotor nucleus (D) and the abducens nucleus (F) few or no GABA-immunoreactive boutons are observed in particular relation to neuronal somata. Calibration: 25 μm.

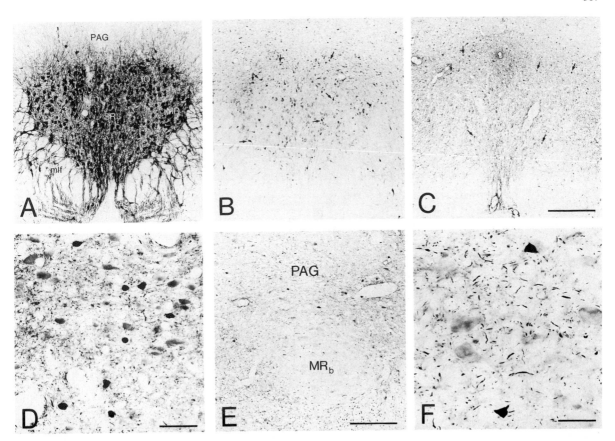

Fig. 5. Light micrographs of ChAT- (A) and GABA- (C–F) immunoreactive staining in the oculomotor nucleus. In A, ChAT-immunoreactive staining of the motoneurons defines the neuronal boundaries of the cat oculomotor nucleus and the subdivisions of superior rectus (SR), medial rectus (MR), inferior rectus (IR) and inferior oblique (IO) motoneurons. Some motoneurons are located within and ventrolateral to the MLF (mlf). Note that the dendrites of the motoneurons extend into the overlying ventral periaqueductal gray, also known as the supraoculomotor region. Neurons labelled by retrograde transport of HRP from the right abducens nucleus are shown in B. Most of these oculomotor internuclear neurons are located in the supraoculomotor region. In C, many GABA-immunoreactive neurons also are located in the supraoculomotor region. Small arrows in B and C indicate several representative labelled neurons of each type. GABA-immunoreactive neurons in the supraoculomotor region in the cat are shown at higher magnification in D. In E, GABA-immunoreactive neurons in the supraoculomotor region in the Rhesus monkey are located dorsal and lateral to the medial rectus b subgroup (MRb). Note the virtual absence of GABA-immunoreactive terminal staining within this subdivision. In F, two GABA-immunoreactive neurons within the inferior rectus subdivision of the Rhesus monkey oculomotor nucleus are shown. Calibrations: A–C, 500 $\mu$m; D and F, 50 $\mu$m; E, 250 $\mu$m.

GAD-immunoreactive boutons that by light microscopy appear to outline the somata of the motoneurons form axosomatic synaptic endings at the ultrastructural level (Fig. 6A). Many of these synaptic endings establish multiple, spatially separated synaptic contacts with postsynaptic motoneurons (Fig. 6B–C). Among superior rectus motoneurons in the oculomotor nucleus, immunoreactive synaptic endings occasionally are associated with somatic spine-like appendages

(Figs. 6C, 8F). In addition to the somatic location, GAD-immunoreactive synaptic endings also extend onto large-diameter proximal dendrites, where they more often are interspersed among other non-immunoreactive synaptic endings (Fig. 6D–E). In all instances, a single immunoreactive synaptic ending establishes synaptic contacts with only one postsynaptic profile. The distribution of many GAD-immunoreactive synaptic endings on the somata and proximal dendrites of the mo-

318

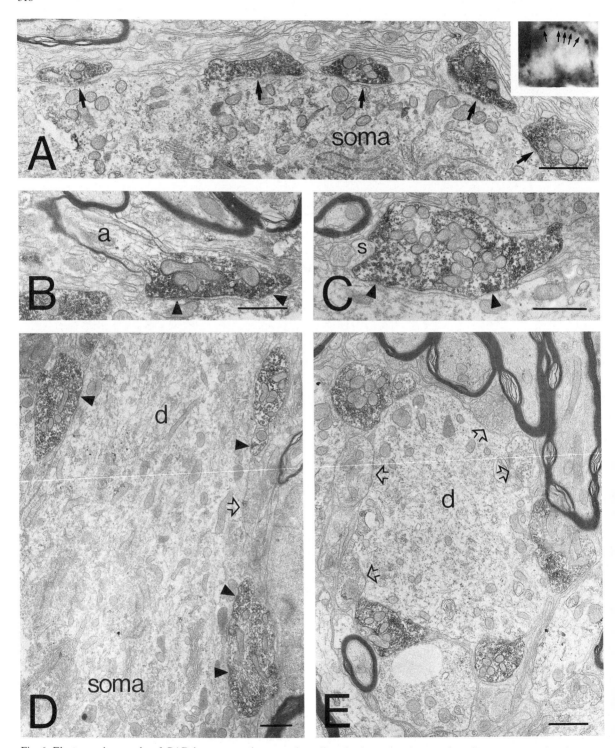

Fig. 6. Electron micrographs of GAD-immunoreactive synaptic endings in the cat oculomotor (B–D) and trochlear (A,E) nuclei. The high density of GAD-immunoreactive boutons adjacent to motoneuron somata, as observed by light microscopy (A, inset), is correlated with a large number of axosomatic synaptic endings that often are arranged in clusters (A). Like inhibitory second-order vestibular synaptic endings, GAD-immunoreactive synaptic endings on the somata (B,C) and proximal dendrites (D) exhibit multiple synaptic contact zones (arrowheads). Non-immunoreactive synaptic endings (open arrows in D and E) often are intermingled with GAD-immunoreactive synaptic endings. Calibrations: A–E, 1 $\mu$m.

toneurons, combined with the presence of multiple synaptic contact zones associated with individual synaptic endings, are features typical of the inhibitory second-order vestibular input to oculomotor and trochlear motoneurons identified previously by ultrastructural reconstructions of physiologically-identified axons stained intracellularly with HRP (Spencer and Baker, 1983).

The oculomotor and trochlear nuclei also contain many GAD-immunoreactive synaptic endings that establish synaptic contacts with medium- and small-diameter dendrites (Figs. 7A–B, 8A–D). In contrast to the presumed inhibitory vestibular synaptic endings described above, these synaptic endings typically establish synaptic contacts with two or more dendrites of similar or different sizes. Each synaptic ending furthermore exhibits only one synaptic contact zone with each postsynaptic process. The synaptic contact zones are characterized by an accumulation of pleiomorphic synaptic vesicles along the presynaptic membrane, a modest or "symmetric" postsynaptic membrane densification, and an intermediate dense line in the extracellular synaptic space (Fig. 8E).

In the abducens nucleus, GAD-immunoreactive synaptic endings are sparse and are distributed on the somata (Fig. 9A), dendrites (Fig. 9B), and dendritic spines (Fig. 9C) of abducens neurons. These synaptic endings typically have only one synaptic contact zone with a single postsynaptic profile, but their ultrastructural features generally are similar to those observed in the oculomotor and trochlear nuclei. The most likely source of this GABAergic inhibitory input to abducens neurons is a population of internuclear neurons in the oculomotor nucleus and supraoculomotor region (Graybiel, 1977; Langer et al., 1986; Maciewicz and Phipps, 1983; Maciewicz et al., 1975; Maciewicz and Spencer, 1977; May et al., 1987; Belknap and McCrea, 1988), some of which are GABA-immunoreactive (Fig. 5C). However, the overwhelming majority of synaptic endings in the abducens nucleus with similar synaptic vesicle morphology are non-immunoreactive toward GAD and most likely represent the majority of inhibitory synaptic inputs to abducens neurons that utilize glycine as a neurotransmitter (Spencer et al., 1989).

Ultrastructural findings similar to the above with GAD have been obtained with the immunohistochemical localization of GABA. In particular, both the morphology and soma-dendritic distribution of·GABA-immunoreactive synaptic endings in the oculomotor and trochlear nuclei, as visualized by both pre-embedding (Fig. 10A–D) and post-embedding (Fig. 11A–B) methods, are comparable to those of synaptic endings labelled using an antibody to the synthesizing enzyme GAD.

Differences between GAD- and GABA-immunoreactive synaptic endings in the mode (i.e., single vs. multiple synaptic contact zones), pattern (i.e., single vs. multiple postsynaptic profiles), and soma-dendritic distribution suggest that there are two inhibitory GABAergic synaptic inputs to oculomotor and trochlear motoneurons. Thus, in addition to the inhibitory second-order vestibular input that terminates proximally on the soma-dendritic tree, a second input is distributed more distally on the soma-dendritic trees of the motoneurons. One possible source of this second GABAergic inhibitory input to oculomotor and trochlear motoneurons is vertical saccade-related premotor neurons in the rostral interstitial nucleus of the MLF. Extracellular injections of the anterograde tracer biocytin into this region in the cat exquisitely label the axonal arborizations and preterminal and terminal boutons within the trochlear (Fig. 11A) and oculomotor (Fig. 11B) nuclei. Within the oculomotor nucleus, terminals are distributed exclusively among the vertical (i.e., superior rectus, inferior oblique, and inferior rectus) motoneuron populations. The projection is overwhelmingly to the ipsilateral nuclei with a small proportion of terminals targeting superior rectus motoneurons on the contralateral side. By electron microscopy using a post-embedding localization method, biocytin-labelled synaptic endings comprise two morphological types. Some

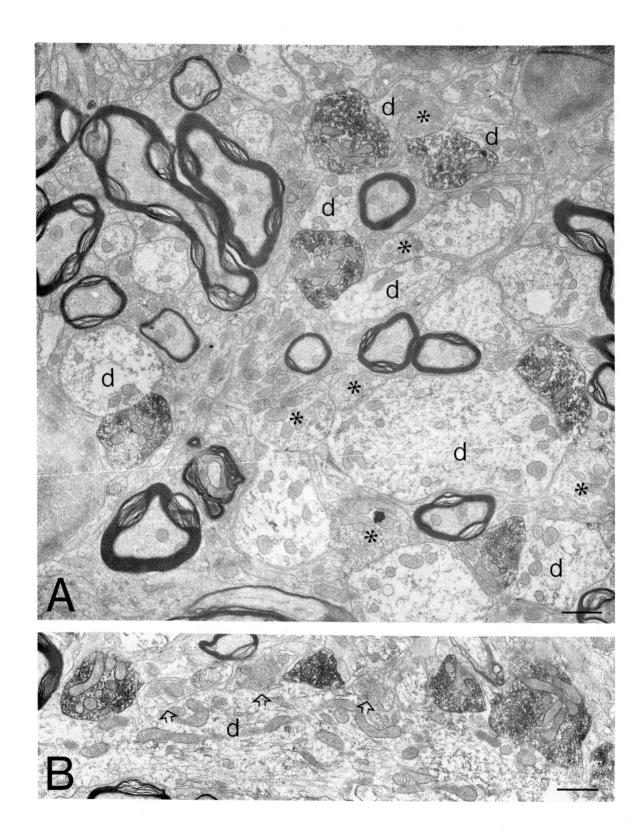

synaptic endings contain spheroidal synaptic vesicles and form asymmetric synaptic contacts, typical of a presumed excitatory input. Others contain pleiomorphic synaptic vesicles and establish symmetric synaptic contacts (Fig. 11E–F) like those labelled with GAD or GABA. Although synaptic endings of the latter type establish both axosomatic and axodendritic synaptic contacts, the majority are distributed predominantly on *distal* medium- and small-calibre dendrites, thus contrasting with the *proximal* location of inhibitory second-order vestibular inputs predominantly on the somata and proximal dendrites of oculomotor and trochlear motoneurons.

## Conclusion

It is well established that GABA is the major inhibitory neurotransmitter utilized by premotor neurons involved in vertical eye movements. By contrast, glycine is the inhibitory neurotransmitter of most premotor neurons that are related to horizontal eye movements. The significance of this dichotomy in inhibitory neurotransmitters utilized in the vertical and horizontal eye movement systems presently is unclear. On the one hand, it might reflect functional differences between different types of neurons, distinguishing, for example, between second-order vestibular neurons that participate only in *eye movement* (e.g., GABAergic inhibitory neurons in the superior vestibular nucleus that project only to the trochlear and/or oculomotor nuclei) versus those that are involved in *gaze* (e.g., glycinergic inhibitory neurons in the medial vestibular nucleus that project to both the abducens nucleus and the spinal cord). On the other hand, these differences in neurotransmitters utilized in the vertical and horizontal eye movement systems may have an embryological basis, which, in the simplest case, might reflect that the medulla, in which most of the horizontal premotor neurons are located, is a rostral extension of the spinal cord where glycine is the major inhibitory neurotransmitter, while the midbrain, which is the location or site of termination of the vertical premotor neurons, is more closely associated with the forebrain where GABA is the major inhibitory neurotransmitter. Whatever the underlying basis of this dichotomy, the postsynaptic effect of GABA or glycine acting on their respective receptors is the same, namely inhibition of the motoneurons. The secondary effects of the two neurotransmitters, however, are likely to be quite different. One example is the augmentation of the excitatory effects of glutamate activating NMDA receptors that is mediated by glycine acting on strychnine-insensitive glycine receptors. These factors, however, probably do not translate into apparent differences in the way motoneurons produce vertical or horizontal eye movements.

Inhibition clearly plays a major role in the neuronal interactions involved in the generation of all types of eye movement. In contrast to the sensory visual system, where GABAergic inhibition appears to be important in shaping the receptive field properties of neurons, inhibition of oculomotor motoneurons seems to play only a permissive role compared to the excitatory inputs that largely are responsible for the generation of eye movements. That is, while inhibition of motoneurons undoubtedly is important in providing rapid and effective relaxation of antagonistic extraocular muscles, it appears not to be involved in determining the response properties (e.g., head velocity and eye position sensitivities) and discharge patterns (e.g., burst vs. burst/tonic) of these neurons. The most dramatic example of this

Fig. 7. Electron micrographs of GAD-immunoreactive synaptic endings in the neuropil of the cat oculomotor nucleus. In A, GAD-immunoreactive synaptic endings establish synaptic contact with small-, medium- and large-diameter dendrites (d). Non-immunoreactive synaptic endings are indicated by asterisks. In B, a series of GAD-immunoreactive synaptic endings contact a medium-diameter dendrite. These labelled terminals are interspersed with several non-immunoreactive synaptic endings (open arrows). Calibrations: 1 $\mu$m.

322

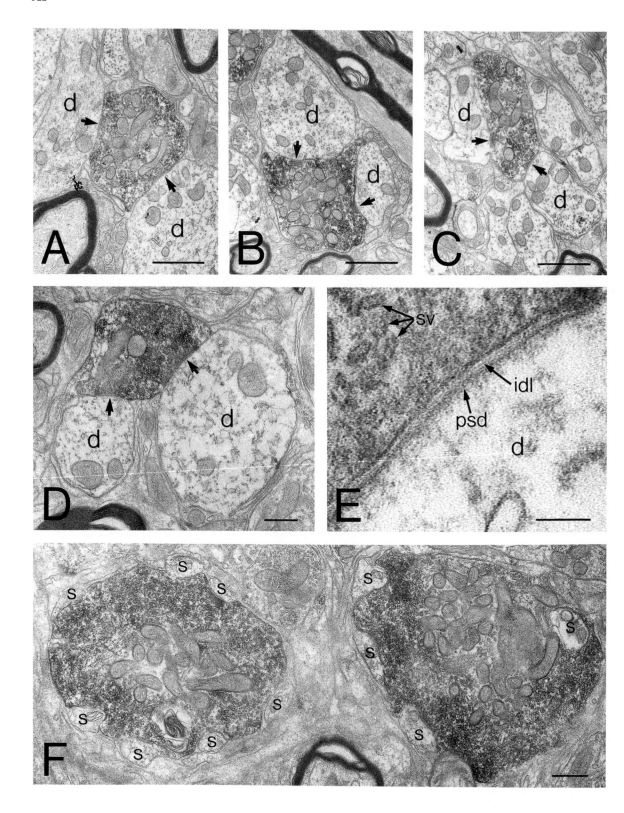

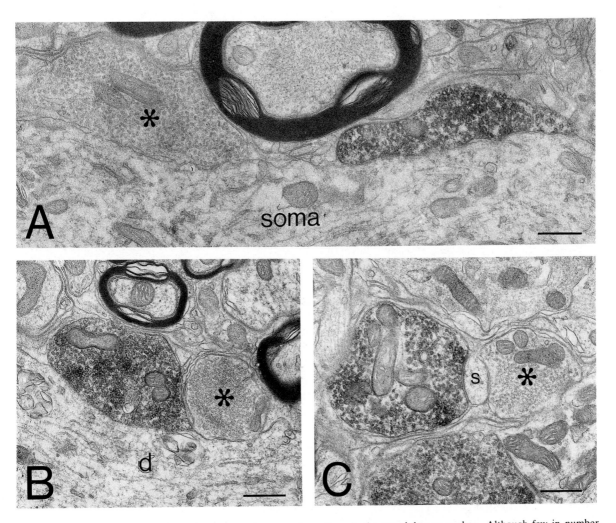

Fig. 9. Electron micrographs of GAD-immunoreactive synaptic endings in the cat abducens nucleus. Although few in number, GAD-immunoreactive synaptic endings establish synaptic contacts with somata (A), dendrites (B) and dendritic spines (C) of abducens neurons. Of greater significance, however, are the non-immunoreactive synaptic endings that contain pleiomorphic/flattened synaptic vesicles (asterisks) and presumably utilize a different inhibitory neurotransmitter (e.g., glycine). Calibrations: 0.5 µm.

Fig. 8. Electron micrographs of GAD-immunoreactive synaptic endings in the cat oculomotor (A–C ,F) and trochlear (D, E) nuclei. In contrast to identified inhibitory second-order vestibular synaptic endings, which establish multiple synaptic contacts predominantly with the somata and proximal dendrites of motoneurons, GAD-immunoreactive synaptic endings in A–D contact medium- and small-diameter dendrites. Each synaptic ending exhibits only a single synaptic contact zone with each postsynaptic process (arrows). The typical ultrastructural features of the synaptic contact zone of GAD-immunoreactive synaptic endings are demonstrated in E and include pleiomorphic synaptic vesicles (sv), an inconspicuous postsynaptic membrane densification (psd) and an intermediate dense line (idl) in the intersynaptic space. In F, two GAD-immunoreactive synaptic endings in the superior rectus subdivision establish synaptic contacts with spines (s) that were traced in serial ultrathin sections to the soma of a motoneuron. Calibrations: A–C, 1 µm; D and F, 0.5 µm; E, 0.1 µm.

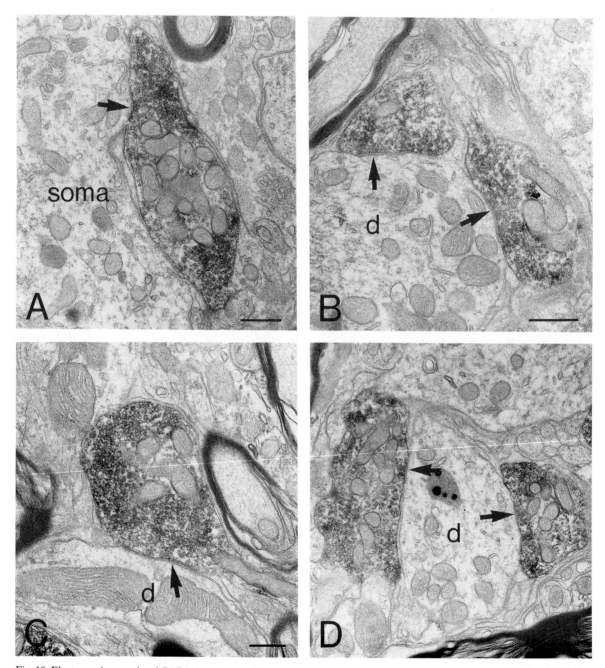

Fig. 10. Electron micrographs of GABA-immunoreactive synaptic endings in the cat oculomotor (A and B) and trochlear (C and D) nuclei. Both axosomatic (A) and axodendritic (B–D) synaptic contacts are illustrated and are representative of the population in general by their content of pleiomorphic synaptic vesicles and a modest postsynaptic membrane densification at sites of synaptic contact (arrows). Calibrations: A–D, 0.5 $\mu$m.

premise is the qualitatively similar discharge patterns of abducens motoneurons, abducens internuclear neurons, and medial rectus motoneurons (Mays and Porter, 1984; Delgado-García et al.,

1986a,b; de la Cruz et al., 1989), even though inhibitory inputs to medial rectus motoneurons are virtually absent.

Inhibition at the level of the extraocular mo-

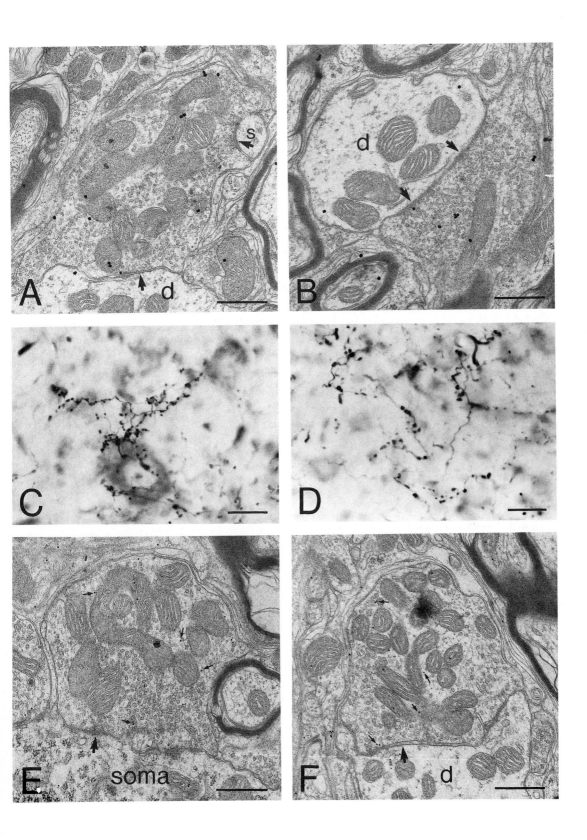

toneurons, however, is important to the extent that the reciprocal synaptic drive overlaps in respect to firing threshold. Thus, near the center of any oculomotor range (for vertical and/or horizontal eye movement) overlapping and interacting excitatory and inhibitory inputs would create more stiffness (i.e., larger dynamic response) than otherwise would be present with either input alone. This feature appears to be particularly applicable to mammals, especially primates with foveal pursuit. Second, given the peculiar relationship with direct cerebellar inhibition (via Purkinje cells), some, maybe most, aspects of eye movement must arise from inhibitory sculpting of excitatory networks. There appears to be little difference in the cerebellar control of GABAergic and/or glycinergic vestibular neurons. However, most of the inhibitory sculpting that might occur for cerebellar and/or commissural connections appears to rely much more on GABAergic than glycinergic inhibitory circuitry.

Given that baclofen has therapeutic value in the treatment of periodic alternating nystagmus (Leigh et al., 1981), apparently acting through inhibition of velocity storage mechanisms by antagonism of $GABA_B$ receptors (Cohen et al., 1987), it is clear that GABAergic inhibition has a more fundamental role in as yet poorly defined neuronal circuits in other parts of the oculomotor system that involve the cerebellum and vestibular commissural connections. The continued assessment of the pharmacology of the oculomotor system in direct relation to its neuronal and synaptic organization thus not only has important implications toward understanding neuronal interactions, but also has clinical relevance in the diagnosis and treatment of oculomotor disorders. In this regard, the identification of GABAergic inhibitory circuits and the various types of receptors with which they are associated is of paramount importance to further defining the role of such interactions in normal eye movement and the extent to which they are involved in eye movement deficits.

## Acknowledgements

The original work reported in this contribution was supported by U.S. Public Health Service MERIT Award EY02191 and Research Grant EY02007 from the National Eye Institute. We are grateful to Drs. Robert J. Wenthold and Donald E. Schmechel for generously providing the antibodies to GABA and GAD, respectively. The excellent technical assistance of Lynn Davis also is greatly appreciated.

## References

Bak, I.J. and Choi, W.B. (1974) Electron microscopic investigation of synaptic organization of the trochlear nucleus in cat. I. Normal ultrastructure. Cell Tissue Res., 150: 409–423.

Bak, I.J., Baker, R., Choi, W.B. and Precht, W. (1976) Electron microscopic investigation of the vestibular projection to the cat trochlear nuclei. Neuroscience, 1: 477–482.

Baker, R. and Berthoz, A. (1975) Is the prepositus hypoglossi nucleus the source of another vestibulo-ocular pathway? Brain Res., 86: 121–127.

Baker, R. and Highstein, S.M. (1975) Physiological identification of interneurons and motoneurons in the abducens nucleus. Brain Res., 91: 292–298.

Fig. 11. A,B. Electron micrographs of GABA-immunoreactive synaptic endings in the cat oculomotor nucleus labelled by post-embedding immunohistochemistry using 30 nm colloidal gold particles. Without the obstruction of peroxidase reaction product associated with the pre-embedding procedure, the synaptic vesicle morphology is defined clearly as pleiomorphic. Synaptic contacts (large arrows) are established with dendrites (d) and a dendritic spine (s). In C and D, preterminal and terminal boutons are labelled anterogradely in the trochlear (C) and oculomotor (D) nuclei following an extracellular injection of biocytin into the ipsilateral rostral interstitial nucleus of the MLF. Note in C the cluster of boutons that surrounds the soma of a motoneuron counterstained with cresyl violet, whereas the other boutons appear to be associated with the neuropil. E and F, electron micrographs of synaptic endings in the oculomotor nucleus labelled with biocytin localized by the post-embedding method using 15 nm gold particles (small arrows). Both axosomatic (E) and axodendritic (F) synaptic contacts (large arrows) are established and the labelled synaptic endings contain pleiomorphic synaptic vesicles like those that are immunoreactive toward GAD or GABA. Calibrations: A and B, E and F, 0.5 $\mu$m; C and D, 25 $\mu$m.

Baker, R. and Highstein, S.M. (1978) Vestibular projections to medial rectus subdivision of oculomotor nucleus. *J. Neurophysiol.*, 41: 1629–1646.

Baker, R., Berthoz, A. and Delgado-García, J. (1977) Monosynaptic excitation of trochlear motoneurons following electrical stimulation of the prepositus hypoglossi nucleus. *Brain Res.*, 121: 157–161.

Baker, R., Graf, W. and Spencer, R.F. (1982) The vertical vestibulo-ocular reflex. In: Roucoux, A. and Crommelinck, M. (Eds.), *Physiological and Pathological Aspects of Eye Movements*. The Hague: Dr P. Junk, pp. 101–116.

Baker, R., Gresty, M. and Berthoz, A. (1976) Neuronal activity in the prepositus hypoglossi nucleus correlated with vertical and horizontal eye movement in the cat. *Brain Res.*, 101: 366–371.

Baker, R.G., Mano, N. and Shimazu, H. (1969) Postsynaptic potentials in abducens motoneurons induced by vestibular stimulation. *Brain Res.*, 15: 577–1580.

Baker, R., McCrea, R.A. and Spencer, R.F. (1980) Synaptic organization of cat "accessory" abducens motoneurons. *J. Neurophysiol.*, 43: 771–790.

Belknap, D.B. and McCrea, R.A. (1988) Anatomical connections of the prepositus and abducens nuclei in the squirrel monkey. *J. Comp. Neurol.*, 268: 13–28.

Berthoz, A., Baker, R. and Precht, W. (1973) Labyrinthine control of inferior oblique motoneurons. *Exp. Brain Res.*, 18: 225–241.

Blanks, R.H.I., Volkind, R., Precht, W. and Baker, R. (1977) Responses of cat prepositus hypoglossi neurons to horizontal angular acceleration. *Neuroscience*, 2: 391–403.

Blessing, W.W., Hedger, S.C. and Oertel, W.H. (1987) Vestibulospinal pathway in rabbit includes GABA-synthesizing neurons. *Neurosci. Lett.*, 80: 158–162.

Büttner, U., Büttner-Ennever, J.A. and Henn, V. (1977) Vertical eye movement related unit activity in the rostral mesencephalic reticular formation of the alert monkey. *Brain Res.*, 130: 239–252.

Büttner-Ennever, J.A. and Akert, K. (1981) Medial rectus subgroups of the oculomotor nucleus and their abducens internuclear input in the monkey. *J. Comp. Neurol.*, 197: 17–27.

Büttner-Ennever, J.A. and Büttner, U. (1978) A cell group associated with vertical eye movements in the rostral mesencephalic reticular formation of the monkey. *Brain Res.*, 151: 31–47.

Büttner-Ennever, J.A. and Henn, V. (1976) An autoradiographic study of the pathways from the pontine reticular formation involved in horizontal eye movements. *Brain Res.*, 108: 155–164.

Büttner-Ennever, J.A., Büttner, U., Cohen, B. and Baumgartner, G. (1982) Vertical gaze paralysis and the rostral interstitial nucleus of the medial longitudinal fasciculus. *Brain*, 105: 125–149.

Cannon, S.C. and Robinson, D.A. (1987) Loss of the neural integrator of the oculomotor system from brain stem lesions in monkey. *J. Neurophysiol.*, 57: 1383–1409.

Carleton, S.C. and Carpenter, M.B. (1983) Afferent and efferent connections of the medial, inferior and lateral vestibular nuclei in the cat and monkey. *Brain Res.*, 278: 29–51.

Carpenter, M.B. and Batton, R.R., III (1980) Abducens internuclear neurons and their role in conjugate horizontal gaze. *J. Comp. Neurol.*, 189: 191–209.

Carpenter, M.B. and Carleton, S.C. (1983) Comparison of vestibular and abducens internuclear projections to the medial rectus subdivision of the oculomotor nucleus in the monkey. *Brain Res.*, 274: 144–149.

Carpenter, M.B. and Cowie, R.J. (1985) Connections and oculomotor projections of the superior vestibular nucleus and cell group "y". *Brain Res.*, 336: 265–287.

Carpenter, M.B., Harbison, J.W. and Peter, P. (1970) Accessory oculomotor nuclei in the monkey: Projections and effects of discrete lesions. *J. Comp. Neurol.*, 140: 131–154.

Cheron, G., Gillis, P. and Godaux, E. (1986a) Lesions in the cat prepositus complex: effects on the optokinetic system. *J. Physiol. (London)*, 372: 95–111.

Cheron, G., Godaux, E., Laune, J.M. and Vanderkelen, B. (1986b) Lesions in the cat prepositus complex: effects on the vestibulo-ocular reflex and saccades. *J. Physiol. (London)*, 372: 75–94.

Cohen, B., Helwig, D. and Raphan, T. (1987) Baclofen and velocity storage: a model of the effects of the drug on the vestibulo-ocular reflex in the Rhesus monkey. *J. Physiol. (London)*, 393: 703–726.

Curthoys, I.S., Nakao, S. and Markham, C.H. (1981) Cat medial pontine reticular neurons related to vestibular nystagmus: firing pattern, location and projection. *Brain Res.*, 222: 75–94.

de la Cruz, R.R., Escudero, M. and Delgado-García, J.M. (1989) Behaviour of medial rectus motoneurons in the alert cat. *Eur. J. Neurosci.*, 1: 288–295.

Delgado-García, J.M., del Pozo, F. and Baker, R. (1986a) Behavior of neurons in the abducens nucleus of the alert cat. I. Motoneurons. *Neuroscience*, 17: 929–952.

Delgado-García, J.M., del Pozo, F. and Baker, R. (1986b) Behavior of neurons in the abducens nucleus of the alert cat. II. Internuclear neurons. *Neuroscience*, 17: 953–973.

Delgado-García, J.M., Vidal, P.P., Gómez, C. and Berthoz, A. (1989) A neurophysiological study of prepositus hypoglossi neurons projecting to oculomotor and preoculomotor nuclei in the alert cat. *Neuroscience*, 29: 291–307.

Demêmes, D. and Raymond, J. (1980) Identification des terminaisons vestibulaires dans les noyaux oculomoteurs communs chez le chat par radioautographie en microscopie electronique. *Brain Res.*, 196: 381–345.

Destombes, J. and Rouvière, A. (1981) Ultrastructural study of vestibular and reticular projections to the abducens nucleus. *Exp. Brain Res.*, 43: 253–260.

Destombes, J., Gögan, P. and Rouvière, A. (1979) The fine structure of neurons and cellular relationships in the abducens nucleus in the cat. *Exp. Brain Res.*, 35: 249–267.

Escudero, M. and Delgado-García, J.M. (1988) Behavior of reticular, vestibular and prepositus neurons terminating in the abducens nucleus of the alert cat. *Exp. Brain Res.*, 71: 218–222.

Felpel, L.P. (1972) Effects of strychnine, bicuculline and picrotoxin on labyrinthine-evoked inhibition in neck motoneurons of the cat. *Exp. Brain Res.*, 14: 494–502.

Fukushima, K. (1987) The interstitial nucleus of Cajal and its

328

role in the control of movements of head and eyes. *Prog. Neurobiol.*, 29: 107–192.

Fukushima, K., Fukushima, J., Harada, C., Ohashi, T. and Kase, M. (1990) Neuronal activity related to vertical eye movement in the region of the interstitial nucleus of Cajal in alert cats. *Exp. Brain Res.*, 79: 43–64.

Furuya, N. and Markham, C.H. (1981) Arborization of axons in oculomotor nucleus identified by vestibular stimulation and intra-axonal injection of horseradish peroxidase. *Exp. Brain Res.*, 43: 289–303.

Gacek, R.R. (1971) Anatomical demonstration of the vestibulo-ocular projections in the cat. *Acta Oto-laryngol. Suppl.*, 293: 1–63.

Graf, W. and Ezure, K. (1986) Morphology of vertical canal related second order vestibular neurons in the cat. *Exp. Brain Res.*, 63: 35–48.

Graf, W., McCrea, R.A. and Baker, R. (1983) Morphology of posterior canal related secondary vestibular neurons in rabbit and cat. *Exp. Brain Res.*, 52: 125–138.

Grantyn, R., Baker, R. and Grantyn, A. (1980a) Morphological and physiological identification of excitatory pontine reticular neurons projecting to the cat abducens nucleus and spinal cord. *Brain Res.*, 198: 221–228.

Grantyn, A., Grantyn, R., Gaunitz, U. and Robiné, K.-P. (1980b) Sources of direct excitatory and inhibitory inputs from the medial rhombencephalic tegmentum to lateral and medial rectus motoneurons in the cat. *Exp. Brain Res.*, 39: 49–61.

Graybiel, A.M. (1977) Direct and indirect preoculomotor pathways of the brainstem: an autoradiographic study of the pontine reticular formation in the cat. *J. Comp. Neurol.*, 175: 37–78.

Graybiel, A.M. and Hartwieg, E.A. (1974) Some afferent connections of the oculomotor complex in the cat: an experimental study with tracer techniques. *Brain Res.*, 81: 543–551.

Gresty, M. and Baker, R. (1976) Neurons with visual receptive field, eye movement and neck displacement sensitivity within and around the nucleus prepositus hypoglossi in the alert cat. *Exp. Brain Res.*, 24: 429–433.

Highstein, S.M. (1973a) The organization of the vestibulo-oculomotor and trochlear reflex pathways in the rabbit. *Exp. Brain Res.*, 17: 285–300.

Highstein, S.M. (1973b) Synaptic linkage in the vestibulo-ocular and cerebello-vestibular pathways to the VIth nucleus in the rabbit. *Exp. Brain Res.*, 17: 301–314.

Highstein, S.M. and Ito, M. (1971) Differential localization within the vestibular nuclear complex of the inhibitory and excitatory cells innervating IIIrd nucleus oculomotor neurons in rabbit. *Brain Res.*, 29: 358–362.

Highstein, S.M., Goldberg, J.M., Moschovakis, A.K. and Fernández, C. (1987) Inputs from regularly and irregularly discharging vestibular nerve afferents to secondary neurons in the vestibular nuclei of the squirrel monkey. II. Correlation with output pathways of secondary neurons. *J. Neurophysiol.*, 58: 719–738.

Highstein, S.M., Maekawa, K., Steinacker, A. and Cohen, B. (1976) Synaptic input from the pontine reticular nuclei to abducens motoneurons and internuclear neurons in the cat. *Brain Res.*, 112: 162–167.

Hikosaka, O. and Igusa, Y. (1980) Axonal projection of prepositus hypoglossi and reticular neurons in the brainstem of the cat. *Exp. Brain Res.*, 39: 441–451.

Hikosaka, O. and Kawakami, T. (1977) Inhibitory reticular neurons related to the quick phase of vestibular nystagmus - their location and projection. *Exp. Brain Res.*, 27: 377–396.

Hikosaka, O., Igusa, Y., Nakao, S. and Shimazu, H. (1978) Direct inhibitory synaptic linkage of pontomedullary reticular burst neurons with abducens motoneurons in the cat. *Exp. Brain Res.*, 33: 337–352.

Hirai, N. and Uchino, Y. (1984) Superior vestibular nucleus neurons related to the excitatory vestibulo-ocular reflex of anterior canal origin and their ascending course in the cat. *Neurosci. Res.*, 1: 73–79.

Igusa, Y., Sasaki, S. and Shimazu, H. (1980) Excitatory premotor burst neurons in the cat pontine reticular formation related to the quick phase of vestibular nystagmus. *Brain Res.*, 182: 451–456.

Ishizuka, N., Mannen, H., Sasaki, S. and Shimazu, H. (1980) Axonal branches and terminations in the cat abducens nucleus of secondary vestibular neurons in the horizontal canal system. *Neurosci. Lett.*, 16: 143–148.

Isu, N. and Yokota, J. (1983) Morphophysiological study on the divergent projection of axon collaterals of medial vestibular nucleus neurons in the cat. *Exp. Brain Res.*, 53: 151–162.

Ito, M., Highstein, S.M. and Tsuchiya, T. (1970) The postsynaptic inhibition of rabbit oculomotor neurons by secondary vestibular impulses and its blockage by picrotoxin. *Brain Res.*, 17: 520–523.

Ito, M., Nisimaru, N. and Yamamoto, M. (1976) Postsynaptic inhibition of oculomotor neurons involved in vestibulo-ocular reflexes arising from semicircular canals of rabbits. *Exp. Brain Res.*, 24: 273–283.

Iwamoto, Y., Kitami, T. and Yoshida, K. (1990a) Vertical eye movement-related secondary vestibular neurons ascending in medial longitudinal fasciculus in cat. I. Firing properties and projection pathways. *J. Neurophysiol.*, 63: 902–917.

Iwamoto, Y., Kitami, T. and Yoshida, K. (1990b) Vertical eye movement-related secondary vestibular neurons ascending in medial longitudinal fasciculus in cat. II. Direct connections with extraocular motoneurons. *J. Neurophysiol.*, 63: 918–935.

Judge, S.J. and Cumming, B.G. (1986) Neurons in the monkey midbrain with activity related to vergence eye movement and accomodation. *J. Neurophysiol.*, 55: 915–930.

Kaneko, C.R.S., Evinger, C. and Fuchs, A.F. (1981) Role of cat pontine burst neurons in generation of saccadic eye movements. *J. Neurophysiol.*, 46: 387–408.

King, W.M. and Fuchs, A.F. (1979) Reticular control of vertical saccadic eye movements by mesencephalic burst neurons. *J. Neurophysiol.*, 42: 861–876.

King, W.M., Fuchs, A.F. and Magnin, M. (1981) Vertical eye movement-related responses of neurons in midbrain near interstitial nucleus of Cajal. *J. Neurophysiol.*, 46: 549–562.

Kumoi, K., Saito, N. and Tanaka, C. (1987) Immunohisto-chemical localization of γ-aminobutyric acid- and aspartate-containing neurons in the guinea pig vestibular nuclei. *Brain Res.*, 416: 22–33.

Labandeira-Garcia, J.L., Guerra-Seijas, M.J. and Labandeira-Garcia, J.A. (1989) Oculomotor nucleus afferents from the interstitial nucleus of Cajal and the region surrounding the fasciculus retroflexus in the rabbit. *Neurosci. Lett.*, 101: 11–16.

Lang, W., Büttner-Ennever, J.A. and Büttner, U. (1979) Vestibular projections to the monkey thalamus: an autoradiographic study. *Brain Res.*, 177: 3–17.

Langer, T., Kaneko, C.R.S., Scudder, C.A. and Fuchs, A.F. (1986) Afferents to the abducens nucleus in the monkey and cat. *J. Comp. Neurol.*, 245: 379–400.

Lanoir, J., Soghomonian, J.J. and Cadenel, G. (1982) Radioautographic study of $^3$H-GABA uptake in the oculomotor nucleus of the cat. *Exp. Brain Res.*, 48: 137–143.

Leigh, R.J., Robinson, D.A. and Zee, D.S. (1981) A hypothetical explanation for periodic alternating nystagmus: instability in the optokinetic-vestibular system. *Ann. NY Acad. Sci.*, 374: 619–635.

López-Barneo, J., Ribas, J. and Delgado-García, J.M. (1981) Identification of prepositus neurons projecting to the oculomotor nucleus in the alert cat. *Brain Res.*, 214: 174–179.

López-Barneo, J., Darlot, C., Berthoz, A. and Baker, R. (1982) Neuronal activity in prepositus nucleus correlated with eye movement in the alert cat. *J. Neurophysiol.*, 47: 329–352.

Maciewicz, R. and Phipps, B.S. (1983) The oculomotor internuclear pathway: a double retrograde labeling study. *Brain Res.*, 262: 1–8.

Maciewicz, R.J. and Spencer, R.F. (1977) Oculomotor and abducens internuclear pathways in the cat. In: R. Baker and A. Berthoz (Eds.), *Control of Gaze by Brain Stem Neurons*, Amsterdam: Elsevier/North-Holland Biomedical Press, pp. 99–108.

Maciewicz, R.J., Eagen, K., Kaneko, C.R.S. and Highstein, S.M. (1977) Vestibular and medullary brain stem afferents to the abducens nucleus in the cat. *Brain Res.*, 123: 229–240.

Maciewicz, R.J., Kaneko, C.R.S., Highstein, S.M. and Baker, R. (1975) Morphophysiological identification of interneurons in the oculomotor nucleus that project to the abducens nucleus in the cat. *Brain Res.*, 96: 60–65.

Markham, C.H., Furuya, N., Bak, I.J. and Ornitz, E.M. (1986) Synaptic connections of horizontal canal mediated ascending Deiters tract axons on medial rectus motoneurons in cat. *Auris Nasus Larynx*, 13 (Suppl. II): S1–S14.

May, P.J., Baker, H., Vidal, P.-P., Spencer, R.F. and Baker, R. (1987) Morphology and distribution of serotoninergic and oculomotor internuclear neurons in the cat midbrain. *J. Comp. Neurol.*, 266: 150–170.

Mays, L.E. (1984) Neural control of vergence eye movements: convergence and divergence neurons in midbrain. *J. Neurophysiol.*, 51: 1091–1108.

Mays, L.E. and Porter, J.D. (1984) Neural control of vergence eye movements: activity of abducens and oculomotor neurons. *J. Neurophysiol.*, 52: 743–761.

Mays, L.E., Porter, J.D., Gamlin, P.D.R. and Tello, C.A. (1986) Neural control of vergence eye movements: neurons encoding vergence velocity. *J. Neurophysiol.*, 56: 1007–1021.

McCrea, R.A. and Baker, R. (1985b) Anatomical connections of the nucleus prepositus of the cat. *J. Comp. Neurol.*, 237: 377–407.

McCrea, R.A., Strassman, A. and Highstein, S.M. (1986) Morphology and physiology of abducens motoneurons and internuclear neurons intracellularly injected with horseradish peroxidase in alert squirrel monkeys. *J. Comp. Neurol.*, 243: 291–308.

McCrea, R.A., Strassman, A. and Highstein, S.M. (1987a) Anatomical and physiological characteristics of vestibular neurons mediating the vertical vestibulo-ocular reflexes of the squirrel monkey. *J. Comp. Neurol.*, 264: 571–594.

McCrea, R.A., Strassman, A., May, E. and Highstein, S.M. (1987b) Anatomical and physiological characteristics of vestibular neurons mediating the horizontal vestibulo-ocular reflex of the squirrel monkey. *J. Comp. Neurol.*, 264: 547–570.

McCrea, R.A., Yoshida, K., Berthoz, A. and Baker, R. (1980) Eye movement related activity and morphology of second order vestibular neurons terminating in the cat abducens nucleus. *Exp. Brain Res.*, 40: 468–473.

McMasters, R.E., Weiss, A.H. and Carpenter, M.B. (1966) Vestibular projections to the nuclei of the extraocular muscles. Degeneration resulting from discrete partial lesions of the vestibular nuclei in the monkey. *Am. J. Anat.*, 118: 163–194.

Mitsacos, A., Reisine, H. and Highstein, S.M. (1983) The superior vestibular nucleus: an intracellular HRP study in the cat. I. Vestibulo- ocular neurons. *J. Comp. Neurol.*, 215: 78–91.

Moschovakis, A.K., Scudder, C.A. and Highstein, S.M. (1991a) Structure of the primate oculomotor burst generator. I. Medium-lead burst neurons with downward on-direction. *J. Neurophysiol.*, 65: 203–217.

Moschovakis, A.K., Scudder, C.A., Highstein, S.M. and Warren, J.D. (1991b) Structure of the primate oculomotor burst generator. II. Medium-lead burst neurons with upward on-direction. *J. Neurophysiol.*, 65: 218–229.

Nakao, S. and Shiraishi, Y. (1985) Direct excitatory and inhibitory synaptic inputs from the medial mesodiencephalic junction to motoneurons innervating extraocular oblique muscles in the cat. *Exp. Brain Res.*, 61: 62–72.

Nakao, S., Shiraishi, Y. and Miyara, T. (1986) Direct projection of cat midbrain tegmentum neurons to the medial rectus subdivision of the oculomotor complex. *Neurosci. Lett.*, 64: 123–128.

Nakao, S., Sasaki, S., Schor, R.H. and Shimazu, H. (1982) Functional organization of premotor neurons in the cat medial vestibular nucleus related to slow and fast phases of nystagmus. *Exp. Brain Res.*, 45: 371–385.

Nomura, I., Senba, E., Kubo, T., Shiraishi, T., Matsunaga, T., Tohyama, M., Shiotani, Y. and Wu, J.-Y. (1984) Neuropeptides and γ-aminobutyric acid in the vestibular nuclei of the rat: an immunohistochemical analysis. I. Distribution. *Brain Res.*, 311: 109–118.

Obata, K. and Highstein, S.M. (1970) Blocking by picrotoxin of both vestibular inhibition and GABA action on rabbit oculomotor neurons. *Brain Res.*, 18: 538–541.

Oertel, W.H., Schmechel, D.E., Tappaz, M.L. and Kopin, I.J. (1981) Production of a specific antiserum to rat brain glutamic acid decarboxylase by injection of an antigen-antibody complex. *Neuroscience*, 6: 2689–2700.

Ohgaki, T., Curthoys, I.S. and Markham, C.H. (1988) Morphology of physiologically identified second-order vestibular neurons in cat, with intracellularly injected HRP. *J. Comp. Neurol.*, 276: 387–411.

Porter, J.D., Guthrie, B.L. and Sparks, D.L. (1983) Innervation of monkey extraocular muscles: localization of sensory and motor neurons by retrograde transport of horseradish peroxidase. *J. Comp. Neurol.*, 218: 208–219.

Precht, W. and Baker, R. (1972) Synaptic organization of the vestibulo-trochlear pathway. *Exp. Brain Res.*, 14: 158–184.

Precht, W., Baker, R. and Okada, Y. (1973) Evidence for GABA as the synaptic transmitter of the inhibitory vestibulo-ocular pathway. *Exp. Brain Res.*, 18: 415–428.

Precht, W., Schwindt, P.C. and Baker, R. (1973) Removal of vestibular commissural inhibition by antagonists of GABA and glycine. *Brain Res.*, 62: 222–226.

Reisine, H., Strassman, A. and Highstein, S.M. (1981) Eye position and head velocity signals are conveyed to medial rectus motoneurons in the alert cat by the ascending tract of Deiters. *Brain Res.*, 211: 153–157.

Roffler-Tarlov, S. and Tarlov, E. (1975) Reduction of GABA synthesis following lesions of inhibitory vestibulo-trochlear pathway. *Brain Res.*, 91: 326–330.

Schwindt, P.C., Precht, W. and Richter, A. (1974) Monosynaptic excitatory and inhibitory pathways from medial midbrain nuclei to trochlear motoneurons. *Exp. Brain Res.*, 20: 223–238.

Scudder, C.A., Fuchs, A.F. and Langer, T.P. (1988) Characteristics and functional identification of saccadic inhibitory burst neurons in the alert monkey. *J. Neurophysiol.*, 59: 1430–1454.

Smith, P.F., Darlington, C.L. and Hubbard, J.I. (1991) Evidence for inhibitory amino acid receptors on guinea pig medial vestibular nucleus neurons in vitro. *Neurosci. Lett.*, 121: 244–246.

Soghomonian, J.-J., Pinard, R. and Lanoir, J. (1989) GABA innervation in adult rat oculomotor nucleus: a radioautographic and immunocytochemical study. *J. Neurocytol.*, 18: 319–331.

Spencer, R.F. and Baker, R. (1983) Morphology and synaptic connections of physiologically-identified second-order vestibular axonal arborizations related to cat oculomotor and trochlear motoneurons. *Soc. Neurosci. Abstr.*, 9: 1088.

Spencer, R.F. and Porter, J.D. (1981) Innervation and structure of extraocular muscles in the monkey in comparison to those of the cat. *J. Comp. Neurol.*, 198: 649–665.

Spencer, R.F. and Sterling, P. (1977) An electron microscope study of motoneurons and interneurons in the cat abducens nucleus identified by retrograde intraaxonal transport of horseradish peroxidase. *J. Comp. Neurol.*, 176: 65–86.

Spencer, R.F., Wenthold, R.J. and Baker, R. (1989) Evidence for glycine as an inhibitory neurotransmitter of vestibular, reticular, and prepositus hypoglossi neurons that project to the cat abducens nucleus. *J. Neurosci.*, 9: 2718–2736.

Steiger, H.-J. and Büttner-Ennever, J.A. (1979) Oculomotor nucleus afferents in the monkey demonstrated with horseradish peroxidase. *Brain Res.*, 160: 1–15.

Strassman, A., Highstein, S.M. and McCrea, R.A. (1986a) Anatomy and physiology of saccadic burst neurons in the alert squirrel monkey. I. Excitatory burst neurons. *J. Comp. Neurol.*, 249: 337–357.

Strassman, A., Highstein, S.M. and McCrea, R.A. (1986b) Anatomy and physiology of saccadic burst neurons in the alert squirrel monkey. II. Inhibitory burst neurons. *J. Comp. Neurol.*, 249: 358–380.

Tredici, G., Pizzini, G. and Milanesi, S. (1976) The ultrastructure of the nucleus of the oculomotor nerve (somatic efferent portion) of the cat. *Anat. Embryol.*, 149: 323–346.

Triller, A., Cluzeaud, F. and Korn, H. (1987) Gamma-aminobutyric acid-containing terminals can be apposed to glycine receptors at central synapses. *J. Cell Biol.*, 104: 947–956.

Triller, A., Cluzeaud, F., Pfeiffer, F., Betz, H. and Korn, H. (1985) Distribution of glycine receptors at central synapses: an immunoelectron microscopy study. *J. Cell Biol.*, 101: 683–688.

Uchino, Y. and Suzuki, S. (1983) Axon collaterals to the extraocular motoneuron pools of inhibitory vestibuloocular neurons activated from the anterior, posterior and horizontal semicircular canals in the cat. *Neurosci. Lett.*, 37: 129–135.

Uchino, Y., Hirai, N. and Suzuki, S. (1982) Branching pattern and properties of vertical- and horizontal-related excitatory vestibuloocular neurons in the cat. *J. Neurophysiol.*, 48: 891–903.

Uchino, Y., Hirai, N. and Watanabe, S. (1978) Vestibulo-ocular reflex from the posterior canal nerve to extraocular motoneurons in the cat. *Exp. Brain Res.*, 32: 377–388.

Uchino, Y., Hirai, N., Suzuki, S. and Watanabe, S. (1981) Properties of secondary vestibular neurons fired by stimulation of ampullary nerve of the vertical, anterior or posterior, semicircular canals in the cat. *Brain Res.*, 223: 273–286.

Uchino, Y., Ichikawa, T., Isu, N., Nakashima, H. and Watanabe, S. (1986) The commissural inhibition on secondary vestibulo-ocular neurons in the vertical semicircular canal systems in the cat. *Neurosci. Lett.*, 70: 210–216.

Vilis, T., Hepp, K., Schwarz, U. and Henn, V. (1989) On the generation of vertical and torsional rapid eye movements in the monkey. *Exp. Brain Res.*, 77: 1–11.

Walberg, F., Ottersen, O.P. and Rinvik, E. (1990) GABA, glycine, glutamate and taurine in the vestibular nuclei: an immunocytochemical investigation in the cat. *Exp. Brain Res.*, 79: 547–563.

Waxman, S.G. and Pappas, G.D. (1979) Ultrastructure of synapses and cellular relationships in the oculomotor nucleus of the Rhesus monkey. *Cell Tissue Res.*, 204: 161–169.

Wenthold, R.J., Zempel, J.M., Parakkal, M.H., Reeks, K.A.

and Altschuler, R.A. (1986) Immunocytochemical localization of GABA in the cochlear nucleus of the guinea pig. *Brain Res.*, 380: 7–18.

Yamamoto, M., Shimoyama, I. and Highstein, S.M. (1978) Vestibular nucleus neurons relaying excitation from the anterior canal to the oculomotor nucleus. *Brain Res.*, 148: 31–42.

Yoshida, K., McCrea, R., Berthoz, A. and Vidal, P.P. (1982) Morphological and physiological characteristics of inhibitory burst neurons controlling horizontal rapid eye movements in the alert cat. *J. Neurophysiol.*, 48: 761–784.

# SECTION III

# Visual cortex

R.R. Mize, R.E. Marc and A.M. Sillito (Eds.)
Progress in Brain Research, Vol. 90
© 1992 Elsevier Science Publishers B.V. All rights reserved

CHAPTER 16

# GABA$_A$- and GABA$_B$-mediated processes in visual cortex

Barry W. Connors

*Section of Neurobiology, Brown University School of Medicine, Providence, RI 02912, USA*

## GABA as a neurotransmitter in neocortex

Krnjević (1974) suggested that only 2 criteria must be satisfied in order to identify a synapse's transmitter: (1) the suspected substance must have an action on the postsynaptic cell that is identical with the action of the synapse and (2) the substance must be released in adequate amounts by activity in the presynaptic terminals. These simply stated criteria are in practice extremely difficult to achieve. Indeed, early suggestions that γ-aminobutyric acid (GABA) might be an inhibitory transmitter in neocortex were not always well-received (reviewed by Roberts, 1983), even after demonstrations that exogenous GABA profoundly inhibited cortical neurons (Krnjević and Schwartz, 1967) and that GABA was released from active cortical synapses (Jasper et al., 1969; Iversen et al., 1971). In fact, it is still true that no substance in the vertebrate brain has strictly met Krnjèvić's criteria. However, the case for GABA as a neurotransmitter in neocortex is probably as strong as for any other chemical at any synapse in the mammalian central nervous system.

Knowledge of the inhibitory transmitter's identity is not enough, however. Modern neuroscience has shown in spectacular fashion that each neurotransmitter may interact with many different types of membrane receptors, each of which may in turn operate a separate effector system. There appear to be 2 basic types of GABA receptors, termed GABA$_A$ and GABA$_B$. Both are present in high quantities in the visual cortex (Bowery et al., 1987). Moreover, the majority of endogenous inhibitory processes in the cortex can be ascribed to the actions of GABA on either GABA$_A$ or GABA$_B$ receptors. GABA$_A$ receptors belong to the family of ligand-gated ion channels, which include the nicotinic acetylcholine and glycine receptors. GABA$_B$ receptors are not directly coupled to ion channels, but instead act (in some cases at least) via G protein-coupled signal systems. These 2 basic receptor subtypes are themselves subdivided.

My goal here is to review the GABA receptor mechanisms of the visual cortex. Discussion of the functions of inhibition in the visual cortex are left to other chapters in this book. I begin by briefly and selectively summarizing recent work on GABA receptors, emphasizing their diversity and function. The cellular mechanisms of GABAergic inhibition are then described in more detail. Because of its complexity, the neocortex has never been a favorite model system for investigating the cellular and molecular mechanisms of transmitter systems, so work on other parts of the brain necessarily provides vital guidance. Nevertheless the variations of GABA receptor function are so large that ultimately only studies of the visual cortex per se can hope to define its precise mechanisms of inhibition.

### What, if anything, is the GABA$_A$ receptor?

Traditionally we have referred to *the* GABA$_A$ receptor. However GABA receptor pharmacology and, more recently, molecular biology belie that singular name. It is now clear that different neurons of the brain can, and do, synthesize a large number of $GABA_A$ receptor variants (Olsen and Tobin, 1990; Betz, 1990). Because each variant may have a distinct set of functional and pharmacologic peculiarities, we must be wary of generalizations. There are, nevertheless, some properties that still define a generic $GABA_A$ receptor and its response. First, of course, the receptor binds GABA. Second, the binding of GABA opens an integral channel with selective permeability to $Cl^-$. Third, the effects of GABA are potently antagonized by bicuculline (and its congeners) and picrotoxin. Fourth, the binding of certain benzodiazepines to a separate site on the $GABA_A$ receptor promotes the effectiveness of GABA itself. Fifth, certain barbiturates also promote GABA actions, by a mechanism separate from the benzodiazepines. Other common $GABA_A$ receptor phenomena might be added, and some of those listed might not always apply, but this inventory provides a useful benchmark.

Diversity of $GABA_A$ receptors arises primarily from the particular combination of 4 or 5 protein subunits constituting the hetero-oligomer that is the $GABA_A$ receptor-channel complex. Each subunit is about 50–60 kDa. At this writing 5 major types of subunits, $\alpha$, $\beta$, $\gamma$, $\delta$ and $\epsilon$ have been described; there are in turn at least 6 different $\alpha$ genes, 3 $\beta$ genes and 2 $\gamma$ genes (Olsen and Tobin, 1990; Betz, 1990). Further complexity is possible by alternative RNA splicing. Whiting et al. (1990) recently reported that the $\gamma 2$ subunit can exist in either a long form ($\gamma 2L$), or a form that is 8 amino acids shorter ($\gamma 2S$). The significance of this small change may be profound. The optional 8 amino acid segment contains the only consensus phosphorylation site for protein kinase C on the subunit; since the function of the $GABA_A$ receptor is known to be sensitive to phosphorylation by protein kinase C (Sigel and Baur, 1988; Stelzer et al., 1988), use of the alternative $\gamma 2$ subunits may determine the presence or absence of this modulatory mechanism.

The roots of each $GABA_A$ receptor's complex pharmacology lie in its particular subunit composition. In expression systems, it is necessary to combine both $\alpha$ and $\beta$ subunits to obtain receptors that efficiently generate large, GABA-activated $Cl^-$ currents (Verdoorn et al., 1990). The use of different types of $\alpha$ subunits confers different agonist dose-response characteristics. However, despite the fact that the $\alpha$ subunits bind benzodiazepines, receptors with only $\alpha$ and $\beta$ subunits have little or no benzodiazepine sensitivity. Addition of a $\gamma$ subunit bestows it. The presence of a $\gamma$ subunit also confers insensitivity to the otherwise potent blocking actions of $Zn^{2+}$ (Draguhn et al., 1990). To express the full range of traditional $GABA_A$ properties, including high and cooperative GABA affinity and various drug sensitivities, it seems that each receptor must at a minimum contain $\alpha$, $\beta$ and $\gamma$ subunits (Sigel et al., 1991).

There is growing evidence that much of the potential diversity implicit in the different $GABA_A$ subunits is actually used by the brain. For example, the neocortex has relatively high levels of $\alpha 3$ mRNA compared to cerebellum and hippocampus; on a more local scale, $\alpha 1$ and $\alpha 2$ mRNAs are densest in cortical layers II–IV, and $\alpha 3$ mRNA is most abundant in layers V–VI (Wisden et al., 1988). There is also laminar specificity to the expression of the 3 $\beta$ subunits in neocortex (Zhang et al., 1991). The significance of these distributions is unknown.

*Divergence, convergence and $GABA_B$ receptors*

The existence of multiple transmitter receptor subtypes suggests extensive chemical divergence: one kind of transmitter can potentially activate several different processes, depending upon the receptor types present and functioning (Nicoll et al., 1990). Compelling evidence that this is true for GABA came from the studies of Hill and Bowery (1981). They identified a new receptor they called $GABA_B$, which was insensitive to bicuculline but was activated specifically by the GABA analogue (and antispasmodic drug) baclofen. GABA$_B$ receptors are located at all levels of the neuraxis, from spinal cord to neocortex (Bowery et al., 1987). They differ distinctly from all GABA$_A$ receptors in their pharmacology, their structure, their coupling systems, and their effectors.

Evidence currently links GABA$_B$ receptors with 2 very different ionic mechanisms. The first has been studied in detail in dorsal root ganglion cells (Dunlap, 1981; Dolphin and Scott, 1986), where GABA$_B$ receptors suppress a voltage-sensitive calcium channel. This mechanism may also occur in many presynaptic terminals of the central nervous system, resulting in a GABA$_B$ receptor-mediated suppression of transmitter release (Bowery et al., 1980). The second ionic mechanism attributed to GABA$_B$ receptors is an increase in K$^+$ conductance of the somadendritic membrane, which has been observed in many central neurons (Newberry and Nicoll, 1984; Gähwiler and Brown, 1985; Stevens et al., 1985). In this way GABA$_B$ activation can generate hyperpolarizing postsynaptic inhibition. So far, I am not aware of a description of a neuron that expresses both mechanisms of GABA$_B$ action at the same site. There is thus the temptation to distinguish between *presynaptic* GABA$_B$ receptors (which inhibit transmitter release, perhaps by suppressing a calcium current) and *postsynaptic* GABA$_B$ receptors (which enhance K$^+$ conductance).

Molecular biology has yet to crack the GABA$_B$ receptor, but there is pharmacological evidence for at least 2 subtypes (Dutar and Nicoll, 1988; Scherer et al., 1988; Harrison, 1990). In hippocampus, the GABA$_B$ antagonist phaclofen blocks postsynaptic sites but not presynaptic sites (Dutar and Nicoll, 1988; Harrison, 1990). Another GABA$_B$ antagonist, 2-hydroxy saclofen, blocks both postsynaptic and presynaptic receptors, although it is less potent at the latter (Harrison et al., 1990). The second-messenger systems activated by the 2 putative receptor subtypes have not been fully characterized, however a pertussis toxin-sensitive G protein system is implicated in the postsynaptic effect (Andrade et al., 1986; Dutar and Nicoll, 1988) and the blockade of calcium currents (Dunlap et al., 1989), but not in the presynaptic effects in hippocampus (Dutar and Nicoll, 1988; Harrison, 1990). Considering the interest engendered by the GABA$_B$ receptors, it is likely that more selective ligands and gene cloning methods will soon clarify (and no doubt multiply) the diversity of receptor subtypes.

The many GABA$_A$ and GABA$_B$ receptor subtypes provide a magnificent example of neurotransmitter divergence. GABA$_B$ receptors also provide an illustration of neurotransmitter convergence. Convergence refers to the possibility that several different transmitters, binding to different receptors, can nevertheless act upon the same effector system. In hippocampal pyramidal cells, the transmitters GABA (acting via GABA$_B$ receptors), serotonin (acting via 5-HT1a receptors) and adenosine (acting via A$_1$ receptors) all evoke a similar increase in postsynaptic K$^+$ conductance (Andrade et al., 1986; Nicoll et al., 1990). The effect of one of these transmitters can occlude the action of the others, suggesting that all 3 converge on the same set of K$^+$ channel effectors. A similar form of convergence has also been demonstrated in human neocortical neurons (McCormick and Williamson, 1989).

*Where are GABA and its receptors in visual cortex?*

Aspects of this question are covered in detail elsewhere in this book (see Hendry and Carder, Chapter 22, and Barnstable et al., Chapter 23), however it is worth emphasizing certain points here. With very minor exceptions, all GABAergic terminals in the neocortex arise from intrinsic neurons. Somogyi (1990) estimates that about 20% of the neurons and 15% of the synapses in cat primary visual cortex synthesize, and presumably utilize, GABA. These numbers are similar to those from studies of other areas of neocortex. More than half of the GABAergic terminals end on dendritic shafts, about one quarter end on dendritic spines, only 13% end on somata, and 2.5% synapse upon the axon initial segments of pyramidal cells (Somogyi, 1990). All classes of neurons in the neocortex receive substantial GABAergic input.

The GABA-containing cells themselves are morphologically (Houser et al., 1984) and physiologically (Connors and Gutnick, 1990) distinct from the nonGABA-containing cells. They are recognizable by their various characteristic, almost spine-free somadendritic patterns, or by their relatively brief action potentials and ability to fire at high, sustained rates. GABAergic neurons are, nevertheless, a very diverse set of cells, and their classification has been the subject of long and controversial study (see Peters and Jones, 1984). Somogyi (1990) has concluded that there is a high degree of specificity to the pattern of connections made by different classes of GABAergic neurons. He suggests 3 basic groups: (1) *axoaxonic* (or *chandelier*) cells have the most specific targets, and each makes synapses exclusively onto the initial segments of about 200 to 400 pyramidal cells; (2) *basket* cells contact somata and (primarily) proximal dendrites and spines; (3) *neurogliaform* and *bitufted* cells preferentially contact small caliber (presumably more distal) dendritic shafts and spines. The picture that emerges is that cortical pyramidal cells are subject to selective inhibition at several levels. Axoaxonic cells are master switches, ideally positioned to abolish cell output absolutely. Some basket cells may do the same, while others might selectively inhibit the inputs from only one or more dendrites. The third group of GABA cells could exert very local control of distal excitatory inputs without affecting the rest of the cell. The hypothesis that the major inhibitory systems to neocortical neurons are highly stratified, just as the major afferent systems are (White and Keller, 1989), is appealing. However, much more data will be necessary to place the idea into the textbooks.

The wide distribution of GABAergic synapses on cortical neurons suggests that GABA receptors are also broadly distributed. Recent data confirm this, and then some. Immunocytochem-

istry of $\alpha$ and $\beta$ subunits of the $GABA_A$ receptors show staining not only at the sites of presynaptic terminals, but also in many areas of nonsynaptic membrane in all the neurons of the cortex (Somogyi et al., 1989). In fact, $GABA_A$ receptor density is apparently no higher at subsynaptic membranes than at nonsynaptic membranes. This is not so surprising considering the almost ubiquitous distribution of $GABA_A$ receptors on neuronal membranes, including many places (such as peripheral axon trunks and dorsal root ganglia) where GABA is clearly not used as a neurotransmitter (Brown et al., 1979, Dunlap, 1981). The capricious placement of $GABA_A$ receptors should make us cautious about assigning significance to receptor distribution patterns, without also assessing the patterns of functional synapses.

## The actions of GABA on neurons of neocortex

*$GABA_A$ receptor effects on neurons of neocortex*

The intracellular recordings obtained in vivo by Krnjević and Schwartz (1967) showed that GABA evoked a relatively simple hyperpolarization with an accompanying $Cl^-$ conductance increase. This mimicked the electrically evoked inhibitory postsynaptic potentials (IPSPs) in the same pyramidal cells. Some of the first hints that GABA might have more varied actions in cerebral cortex came from hippocampal pyramidal cells in vitro (Alger and Nicoll, 1979; Andersen et al., 1980), where different parts of a neuron could elicit $Cl^-$-dependent, $GABA_A$-like responses with very different reversal potentials; the soma generated the expected hyperpolarizations, but the dendrites most often depolarized in response to GABA. Mixtures of hyperpolarizing and depolarizing responses were common. Moreover, the somatic and dendritic GABA responses appeared to differ pharmacologically (Alger and Nicoll, 1982).

Complex, multiphasic responses are also seen when GABA is applied near the somata of pyramidal cells of neocortex in vitro (Weiss and Hablitz, 1984; Connors and Gutnick, 1984). Neocortical cells in slices typically have very negative resting potentials ($-75$ to $-80$ mV; Connors et al., 1982), and when the GABA responses are evoked at rest they are completely depolarizing. However, when the membrane potential is first depolarized with current injection it becomes clear that the GABA response has at least 2 or 3 components, each with a different reversal potential. At least some of this complexity arises from nonuniform spatial distribution of the components, as focal applications of GABA to the somata and dendrites reveal (Scharfman and Sarvey, 1985; Connors et al., 1988). Examples are illustrated in Fig. 1A. GABA was applied by pressure ejection through a fine micropipette, first to the region near the soma and then to several apical and basal dendritic regions. At resting potential all responses were depolarizing and simple in form, but when the potential was depolarized 2 phases of GABA-evoked hyperpolarization were disclosed. The short latency GABA hyperpolarization (GABA$_1$ for convenience; see starred response in Fig. 1A, shown expanded in B) was produced only by the perisomatic applications, while the long latency GABA hyperpolarization (GABA$_3$) was generated best by the soma and more proximal dendrites. The intermediate GABA response (GABA$_2$) was dominant, depolarizing and could be easily evoked from all but the most remote application sites. Scharfman and Sarvey (1987) have reported that this pattern of GABA responses is observed in nonpyramidal as well as pyramidal neurons of neocortex.

The complexity of the GABA responses is due to several factors (Scharfman and Sarvey, 1987; Connors et al., 1988; McCormick, 1989). First, there are at least 2 (and perhaps more) GABA receptor-effector subtypes involved, with different kinetic properties. Second, the different receptors evoke responses with different reversal potentials. Third, the different receptors are not spread uniformly across the cell. Fourth, focal application leads to large spatial and temporal gradients of GABA. Ionic and pharmacologic ex-

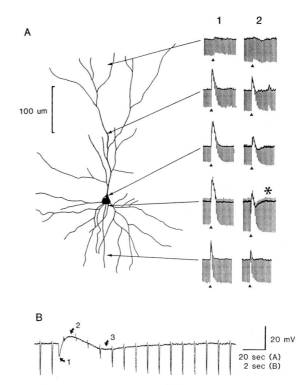

Fig. 1. Dependence of GABA responses on the site of GABA application in a single pyramidal neuron. A. Drawing of a Lucifer yellow-filled cell from layer II/III of rat neocortex, with GABA responses recorded at resting potential ($-78$ mV; A1 traces) and with membrane potential depolarized to about $-62$ mV (A2 traces). Small pressure pulses of GABA (2 mM, 80 msec duration in all but the topmost responses) were focally applied to various sites (arrows). Small hyperpolarizing current pulses were also applied at 1 Hz to monitor the input resistance of the cell. At resting potential the GABA responses were exclusively depolarizing, but at more positive potentials responses from some of the sites proved more complex. Notably, sites along the apical dendrite had late GABA$_3$ responses, and one of the somatic sites had a prominent GABA$_1$ response (starred response). B. The response with the asterisk in A is reproduced at a faster sweep speed to better resolve the components. Numbers refer to the GABA$_1$ (somatic hyperpolarization), GABA$_2$ (dendritic depolarization) and GABA$_3$ (long-latency hyperpolarization) phases. Note the extremely large increase in input conductance during the first 2 phases of the response. Modified from Connors et al. (1988).

periments are so far incomplete, but they do give some clues to the nature of neocortical inhibition. The GABA$_1$ response has a reversal potential of about $-70$ to $-80$ mV, it involves an increase in

Cl⁻ conductance, and its bicuculline and picrotoxin sensitivity indicate mediation by $GABA_A$ receptors. The $GABA_2$ response is the most prominent one in vitro; it is also $GABA_A$-mediated, bicuculline and (apparently) Cl⁻-sensitive (Thompson et al., 1988), but it has a paradoxically positive reversal potential of about $-50$ mV. The $GABA_3$ response is probably generated by $GABA_B$ receptors, as discussed in the next section.

If both the $GABA_1$ and $GABA_2$ responses are generated by increases in membrane conductance to Cl⁻, why are their reversal potentials so different? There is no direct evidence from neocortex to address this question. However a reasonable, but still surprising, hypothesis is that the intracellular Cl⁻ concentration ([Cl⁻]) in the soma is lower than it is in the dendrites. This implies that there must be a standing [Cl⁻] gradient within the cytoplasm, and that the membrane pumps responsible for maintaining intracellular [Cl⁻] are somehow different in the somatic and dendritic membranes. There is more direct evidence that such a gradient exists in the CA1 pyramidal cells of the hippocampus (Misgeld et al., 1986). Thompson et al. (1988) have demonstrated that neocortical pyramidal cells indeed have active transport systems for Cl⁻, although they did not explore the differences between soma and dendrites. More work will be necessary to clarify this problem. It must be a metabolically expensive proposition to maintain a high spatial [Cl⁻] gradient; there is no evidence for diffusion barriers between the somatic and dendritic compartments that might impede the rapid and passive redistribution of such a gradient. The obvious question is, what purpose is served by maintaining relatively high intracellular [Cl⁻] in the dendrites? One obvious answer is that it compels dendritic IPSPs to depolarize the neuron, but the advantage of this is not clear. However it is also possible that high dendritic [Cl⁻] is necessary for some other cellular process unrelated to inhibition. If that is the case, it may be the soma that is maintained, anomalously, at very low [Cl⁻] specif-

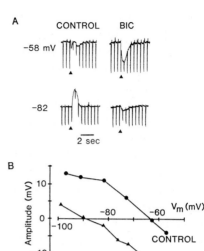

Fig. 2. Bicuculline reveals a $GABA_B$ component of the GABA response. A. Control responses to focal applications of GABA (triangles) are shown at 2 different membrane potentials (left). At $-58$ mV, the 3 phases of the response are clear, while at $-82$ mV the response is entirely depolarizing. Bath application of 10 μM bicuculline methiodide (right) blocked the more depolarizing components of the the GABA response, leaving a monophasic hyperpolarization at both membrane potentials. Downward voltage deflections are due to small current pulses (2 Hz) applied to monitor input resistance. B. Graph of data from experiment in A. Amplitudes of the GABA response were measured at a latency 1.5 s. Reversal potential shifted from about $-63$ to $-88$ mV, consistent with a relative increase in K⁺ conductance.

ically in order to maximize the inhibitory effectiveness of perisomatic IPSPs.

*GABA_B receptor effects on neurons of neocortex*

$GABA_B$ receptors mediate both postsynaptic and presynaptic effects in neocortex. This contrasts with $GABA_A$ receptors, which have not yet been implicated in presynaptic neocortical processes. Postsynaptic $GABA_B$ effects are revealed by the application of GABA itself as the $GABA_3$ response (Fig. 1B), a long-latency hyperpolarization. High doses of bicuculline suppress the $GABA_1$ and $GABA_2$ responses, leaving a larger $GABA_3$ response that has a reversal potential near $-90$ mV (Fig. 2; Connors et al., 1988). Muscimol, the specific $GABA_A$ agonist, does not generate a $GABA_3$ response phase (Connors, unpublished observations). Baclofen, the specific GABA$_B$ agonist, evokes a longer-lasting version of the GABA$_3$ response, a small hyperpolarization coinciding with a conductance increase and a reversal potential of about $-90$ mV (Howe et al., 1987a; Connors et al., 1988). The baclofen response is also barium-sensitive, as are certain K$^+$ channels, and it is suppressed by the GABA$_B$ receptor antagonist phaclofen (Kerr et al., 1989). Presumably both the GABA$_3$ and baclofen responses in neocortex are mediated by an increase in postsynaptic K$^+$ conductance.

Presynaptic GABA$_B$ receptors have been inferred from the very potent effects of the agonist baclofen (Howe et al., 1987a; Connors et al., 1988; Deisz and Prince, 1989). Low concentrations of baclofen reduce the size of all postsynaptic potentials in neocortical pyramidal cells, both EPSPs and IPSPs, by a mechanism that is independent of its effect on postsynaptic K$^+$ conductance (Howe et al., 1987a). Pharmacological evidence suggests that there may be subtypes of GABA$_B$ receptors in neocortex (Ong et al., 1990).

## Diversity of synaptic inhibition in the neocortex

Just as there are multiple types of inhibitory neurons and GABA receptors in neocortex, there are also several types of synaptic inhibition. Because of ubiquitous feed-forward and feed-back connections between pyramidal cells and GABA-ergic neurons, activity in almost any kind of afferent input will engage some inhibitory circuitry. IPSPs are most easily illustrated by stimulating within the cortex itself. Single strong shocks to the deep gray matter generate, in most pyramidal cells, a short-latency excitatory PSP (EPSP), a short-latency, fast IPSP (the f-IPSP) and a longer-latency, slow IPSP (the l-IPSP) (Fig. 3A; Connors et al., 1982). These 2 kinds of IPSPs must be considered the minimum number present, as there are hints of others.

Fast and slow types of IPSPs are probably ubiquitous features of vertebrate cerebral cortex. Similar biphasic IPSPs have been recorded in a

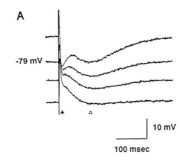

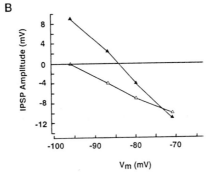

Fig. 3. IPSPs from a pyramidal neuron of layer II/III of cat primary visual cortex. A. Single shocks were delivered to layer VI below the recording site, and responses were recorded at 4 different membrane potentials. Resting membrane potential was $-79$ mV. The closed triangle marks the peak latency of the f-IPSP, and the open triangle the latency of the l-IPSP.B. The f-IPSP and l-IPSP have different reversal potentials. Amplitudes of each are plotted against membrane potential ($V_m$), using data from A. In this case the f-IPSP reversed polarity at about $-85$ mV, and the l-IPSP reversed at about $-95$ mV. Modified from Connors et al. (1988).

variety of mammalian areas, including hippocampus (Fujita, 1979; Newberry and Nicoll, 1984), olfactory cortex (Satou et al., 1982), and the sensorimotor (Connors et al., 1982), frontal (Howe et al., 1987b), visual (Connors et al., 1988) and cingulate (McCormick et al., 1985) neocortex of rodents. They are also present in the neocortex of many species, including human (Avoli and Olivier, 1989; McCormick, 1989), cat (Connors et al., 1988), mouse (Silva et al., 1991) and even the visual cerebral cortex of turtles (Kriegstein and Connors, 1986). Similar IPSPs are also seen in structures below the cerebral cortex, including the lateral geniculate nucleus (Crunelli and Leresche, 1991). It seems very likely that the 2 major forms of inhibition evolved very early, well before the mammalian radiation, and that they have been highly conserved across species and brain structures. The continuing mystery is the precise function of each.

*Fast IPSPs and GABA_A receptors*

The f-IPSP is synonymous with the classical cortical IPSP studied in vivo by many investigators. It is mediated by $GABA_A$ receptors (i.e., it is blocked by bicuculline and picrotoxin), it is generated by an increase in $Cl^-$ conductance, and it is mimicked by the perisomatic application of GABA itself (Krnjević, 1974). In experiments in vitro it is the $GABA_1$ response phase that specifically resembles the f-IPSP in conductance, reversal potential (about $-75$ mV) and pharmacology (Connors et al., 1988; McCormick, 1989). The f-IPSP has a fast activation time and reaches a peak in less than 30 msec. Because the $GABA_1$ response is apparently so restricted to somatic application sites, and because the soma and initial axonal segments of pyramidal cells are contacted exclusively by inhibitory synapses (White and Keller, 1989), we can infer that the f-IPSP is probably generated at sites on or near the soma. Extending this argument, based on anatomical considerations (Somogyi, 1990) it seems likely that either axoaxonic cells or basket cells, or both, are responsible for f-IPSPs.

We know very little about the size and time course of unitary IPSPs in neocortex. One brief report (Galvan et al., 1985) illustrates spontaneous events with the characteristics of f-IPSPs, but few details are reported. Studies involving dual intracellular recordings are needed, with at least one electrode in a presynaptic inhibitory cell. This has been achieved in parts of the hippocampus (Miles and Wong, 1984; Lacaille and Schwartzkroin, 1988), and one conclusion is that there is a large range of IPSP size and time-course from one presynaptic cell to the next. IPSPs generated by presumed axoaxonic and basket cells onto CA3 neurons varied from $-0.3$ to $-2.6$ mV in peak amplitude (Miles, 1990), and the variance

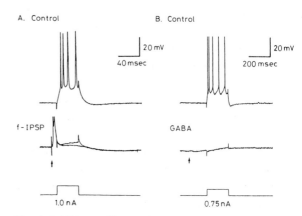

Fig. 4. Inhibitory efficacy of $GABA_A$-mediated f-IPSPs. A. Intracellular injection of a 1 nA square pulse into a pyramidal neuron evokes a train of high-frequency spikes (control). When the same current pulse is applied during the period of an evoked f-IPSP, the firing of the cell is completely abolished. Bottom traces consist of 2 superimposed sweeps: the evoked synaptic response alone (shock at arrow), and the synaptic response plus the injected current pulse. In this case the membrane potential is slightly negative to the reversal potential of the f-IPSP. B. An experiment similar to that of A, in a different neuron, substituting a $GABA_A$ response for the f-IPSP. Top trace shows the control spike train evoked by current injection, bottom trace shows complete abolition of spiking during the early phase of the GABA response (GABA pulsed at arrow). Data of L.R. Silva and B.W. Connors, unpublished.

was attributed to differences in the presynaptic cells.

The f-IPSP is impressively effective. Its peak conductance can be very large, averaging about 70 to 95 nS (Connors et al., 1988; McCormick, 1989). When maximally activated by electrical stimuli, the f-IPSP will completely prevent a neuron from generating action potentials for a period as long as about 50 msec, even in the face of depolarizing current injections that would otherwise evoke near-maximal firing rates (Fig. 4A). Activating $GABA_A$ receptors exogenously mimics this (Fig. 4B). It seems unlikely that such coherent activation of inhibition occurs naturally, but the lesson is clear: synapses generating f-IPSPs can powerfully control a neuron's firing pattern with a fine degree of temporal resolution.

We are still left with a paradox. The dominant response to focally applied GABA is the depolarizing GABA$_2$ phase, but is there a synaptic correlate of this? One interesting possibility is that dendritic GABA$_A$ receptors do not serve any synaptic function. Recordings from the soma do not reveal any obvious IPSPs with reversal potentials as positive as that of the GABA$_2$ response. However, in some cells a long-latency (peaking midway between the f-IPSP and l-IPSP), depolarizing synaptic event was revealed after applying baclofen near the soma to depress the f-IPSP and l-IPSP (Fig. 7A of Connors et al., 1988). It is possible that this PSP represents a depolarizing, GABA$_A$-mediated dendritic IPSP, which is normally obscured from our somatic view by IPSPs generated more proximally. Only further experiments will clarify this problem.

*Slow IPSPs and GABA$_B$ receptors*

The l-IPSPs of pyramidal cells in neocortex are longer than the f-IPSPs, reaching a peak in about 100–200 msec and lasting about 250–1000 msec (Connors et al., 1982, 1988; Avoli, 1986; Howe et al., 1987b; McCormick, 1989). They also tend to be smaller in peak conductance, averaging about 12 nS, and their reversal potentials are around −90 to −95 mV, which is presumed to be E$_K$ (Fig. 3B). Alterations in extracellular [K$^+$] shift the reversal potential of the l-IPSP in the manner consistent with an increase in K$^+$ conductance (Howe et al., 1987b). The l-IPSP is probably mediated by GABA$_B$ receptors, since it is mimicked by baclofen (Connors et al., 1988) and suppressed by phaclofen (McCormick, 1989). The l-IPSP has not been explicitly described in neocortical neurons in vivo. The most probable reason is that it is very difficult to make high quality intracellular recordings from cortical neurons in situ; the combination of increased shunt conductance around the electrode, increased background synaptic activity, and the usual need for general anesthesia would all decrease the likelihood of observing the l-IPSP. However some published recordings seem to show the presence of an l-IPSP (e.g., Fig. 13 of Ezure et al., 1985).

The effect of l-IPSPs on neuronal firing patterns is quite different from that of f-IPSPs, as their smaller conductance, longer time-course and more negative reversal potential might predict. While an f-IPSP can abolish all firing, an l-IPSP has a more subtle effect, slightly increasing action potential thresholds and reducing average firing rates but not preventing them (Howe et al., 1987b; Connors et al., 1988; McCormick, 1989). This was investigated quantitatively by applying baclofen to activate GABA$_B$ receptors. As shown in Fig. 5, GABA$_B$ activation simply shifted the relationship between current and steady-state firing frequency to the right, but had a more complex effect on the transient response to current stimuli. In the control state, the frequency-current relationship for the first 2 spikes was initially very steep (mean of 500 Hz/nA), but the slope abruptly fell to less than 100 Hz/nA at higher stimulus levels. Baclofen shifted the steep part of the curve to the right (i.e., increased threshold), but surprisingly the upper part of the curve was, if anything, enhanced (i.e., during strong currents the initial response frequency was higher). Thus, activation of GABA$_B$ receptors modulates tonic firing rates by increasing the amount of current necessary to reach a given steady-state frequency, but it leaves the neuron's response to strong, brief stimuli intact.

It is not known which types of inhibitory interneurons activate the l-IPSP in neocortex. Within the hippocampal CA1 area, interneurons within stratum lacunosum-moleculare generate l-IPSP-like responses in the dendrites of pyramidal cells (Lacaille and Schwartzkroin, 1988), while interneurons that make synapses onto the perisomatic regions of the CA3 cells have only been observed to generate GABA$_A$-mediated f-IPSPs (Miles, 1990). By analogy, it may be that only dendritic GABAergic synapses generate l-IPSPs in neocortical pyramidal cells; if that turns out to be true it implicates cells such as the neurogliaform and bitufted cells, and perhaps some basket cells, as likely generators (Somogyi, 1990). Pyramidal cell dendrites do show responses to

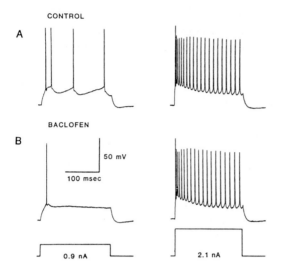

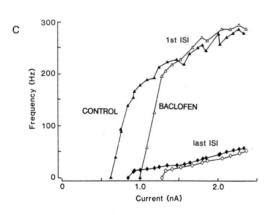

Fig. 5. Effects of GABA$_B$ receptor activation on firing properties of pyramidal cells. A. Control responses of a layer II/III pyramidal neuron of rat neocortex to 2 intensities of current injection (200 msec pulses). Note the characteristically strong adaptation of these cells. B. In the presence of a saturating dose of the GABA$_B$ agonist baclofen, firing of the neuron is strongly curtailed during the lower current intensity but only the adapted rate of firing is diminished during the stronger current. C. Graphical display of baclofen effects; data from the cell shown in A and B. Instantaneous firing frequency (calculated from the reciprocal of the interspike interval) plotted against injected current amplitude for the first 2 spikes (1st ISI) and the last 2 spikes (last ISI). In control cells (closed triangles) the initial firing rate changes steeply with just-suprathreshold currents, then more slowly above about 1 nA. Baclofen strongly affects only the low-current part of the curve. The adapted firing rate (last ISI) is shifted to higher currents at all tested levels. Modified from Connors et al. (1988).

baclofen (Connors et al., 1988), although cable properties probably reduce their visibility from the soma (cf. Koch et al., 1990).

There is still one major loose end to tie up regarding the GABA$_B$ receptors. As noted above, GABA$_B$ agonists cause profound depression of synaptic potentials, apparently via a presynaptic effect. Nevertheless, there is no ultrastructural evidence in neocortex for specific GABAergic synapses onto presynaptic terminals, as there are in many subcortical areas (Peters et al., 1976). Is this just another example of capricious placement of GABA receptors, serving only to incite the imaginations of physiologists and autoradiographers? Perhaps not. Stimulation faster than about 0.1 Hz causes depression of the l-IPSP (Connors

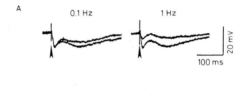

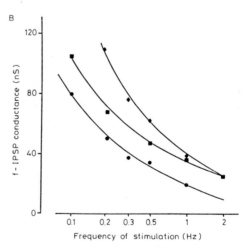

Fig. 6. Frequency sensitivity of neocortical IPSPs. A. f-IPSP and l-IPSP were evoked by single shocks at different frequencies. First and third responses are superimposed at 0.1 Hz and 1.0 Hz. Resting potential was −68 mV. B. Frequency sensitivity of f-IPSP conductance. Peak conductance of f-IPSP was measured during tetanic stimulation at various frequencies; data from 3 different cells are shown. Modified from Deisz and Prince (1989).

et al., 1982); after about 20 stimuli at 1 Hz, the l-IPSP may be strongly fatigued and require minutes to recover (Howe et al., 1987b). Deisz and Prince (1989) showed that both the f-IPSP and the l-IPSP, but not the EPSPs, are depressed by activation at 0.5 to 2 Hz (Fig. 6), and they presented evidence that the depressions are mediated by actions of GABA on presynaptic GABA$_B$ receptors. This implies that GABAergic synapses regulate their own transmitter release in a frequency-sensitive way, with released GABA itself feeding back upon presynaptic GABA$_B$ receptors.

## Conclusions

*"It is still early to venture any definite view of the intimate nature of 'central inhibition'."*
(**C.S. Sherrington**, Nobel Lecture, 1932)

We are still far from a satisfactory understanding of inhibition. One secure conclusion is that GABA-mediated function in neocortex is not a single phenomenon. Rather, inhibition is diverse at all levels: the cells that mediate it, the locations and numbers of its synapses, the types of GABA receptors it utilizes, the ionic changes it induces, the processes that regulate it, and the means by which it finally shapes the output of each postsynaptic neuron. Figure 7 summarizes some of the salient findings described in this review.

As we recognize greater diversity of inhibitory mechansimss, we also raise more questions. One of the large problems is to identify which type of interneuron generates which type of IPSP. It is not even clear yet whether f-IPSPs and l-IPSPs are necessarily evoked by separate interneurons, or whether single interneurons (and perhaps single synapses) can activate both kinds of GABA receptors and thus both kinds of IPSP. In other words, just how specifically can the different types of inhibition be activated? And what of dendritic inhibition? What purpose is served by maintaining an energetically costly gradient of intracellu-

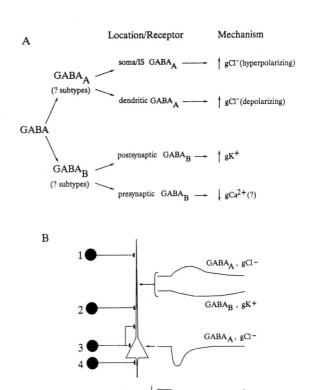

Fig. 7. Hypothesized mechanisms of GABA-mediated inhibition in neocortex. A. GABA can activate both GABA$_A$ and GABA$_B$ receptors (and presumably their various subtypes). GABA$_A$ receptors are widely distributed along the initial segment (IS), soma and dendrites, where they are coupled directly to Cl$^-$ channels. Opening Cl$^-$ channels on the soma or IS causes relative hyperpolarization, while increased Cl$^-$ conductance in the dendrites causes depolarization. GABA$_A$-generated dendritic depolarization may still be very inhibitory because of the substantial shunting effects of the high conductance, and because of the relatively negative reversal potential of the response. The precise distribution of GABA$_B$ receptors is not clear, but there are both pre- and postsynaptic versions. Activation of postsynaptic GABA$_B$ receptors opens a K$^+$ conductance; presynaptic GABA$_B$ activation suppresses the release of neurotransmitter, perhaps because of a suppression of Ca$^{2+}$ channels. B. As described by Somogyi (1990), GABAergic interneurons (solid circles) can make synaptic contacts with pyramidal cells (open triangle) with spatial specificity; e.g., axoaxonic cells (cell 4) contact only initial segments, and basket cells (cell 3) tend to contact somata and proximal dendrites. Postsynaptic inhibitory responses from dendritic and somatic locations are schematized at right. The sum of these IPSPs is a multiphasic response (lower right traces) that is frequency sensitive due to feedback activation of presynaptic GABA$_B$ receptors.

lar $[Cl^-]$ between soma and dendrites? Do dendrites have both hyperpolarizing, $GABA_B$-mediated l-IPSPs as well as depolarizing ($GABA_2$-like), $GABA_A$-mediated IPSPs? What is the precise distribution of $GABA_A$ and $GABA_B$ receptor subtypes; which cells are they on, and which parts of each cell, and what is the significance of receptor subtype diversity? What is the nature of GABA-mediated inhibition onto GABAergic neurons themselves? How is inhibition modulated?

The molecular and cellular peculiarities of inhibition are of great intrinsic interest. However the most fundamental question is, what are the various functions of inhibition in the visual cortex? Discussions of this question have been frequent and stimulating (see Sillito, 1985; Martin, 1988; other chapters in this book), but most have assumed the existence of only unitary, generic forms of $GABA_A$-mediated IPSPs. The functions of other forms of neocortical inhibition have been neglected in vivo, but they now deserve serious attention.

## Acknowledgments

Research from the author's laboratory was supported by the NIH, the Klingenstein Fund and the ONR.

## References

Alger, B.E. and Nicoll, R.A. (1979) GABA-mediated biphasic inhibitory responses in hippocampus. *Nature* 281: 315–317.

Alger, B.E. and Nicoll, R.A. (1982) Pharmacological evidence for two kinds of GABA receptor on rat hippocampal pyramidal cells studied in vitro. *J. Physiol. (London),* 328: 125–141.

Andersen, P., Dingledine, R., Gjerstad, L., Langmoen, I.A. and Laursen, A. (1980) Two different responses of hippocampal pyramidal cells to application of gamma-aminobutyric acid. *J. Physiol. (London),* 305: 279–296.

Andrade, R., Malenka, R.C. and Nicoll, R.A. (1986) A G protein couples serotonin and $GABA_B$ receptors to the same channels in hippocampus. *Science,* 234: 1261–1265.

Avoli, M. (1986) Inhibitory potentials in neurons of the deep layers of the in vitro neocortical slice. *Brain Res.,* 370: 165–170.

Avoli, M. and Olivier, A. (1989) Electrophysiological properties and synaptic responses in the deep layers of the human epileptogenic neocortex in vitro. *J. Neurophysiol.,* 61: 589–606.

Betz, H. (1990) Ligand-gated ion channels in the brain: The amino acid receptor superfamily. *Neuron,* 5: 383–392.

Bowery, N.G, Hill, D.R., Hudson, A.L., Doble, A., Middlemiss, D.N., Shaw, J. and Turnbull, M. (1980) (−)Baclofen decreases transmitter release in the mammalian CNS by an action at a novel GABA receptor. *Nature,* 283: 92–94.

Bowery, N.G., Hudson, A.L. and Price, G.W. (1987) $GABA_A$ and $GABA_B$ receptor site distribution in the rat central nervous system. *Neuroscience,* 20: 365–383.

Brown, D.A., Adams, P.R., Higgins, A.J. and Marsh, S. (1979) Distribution of GABA receptors and GABA carriers in the mammalian nervous system. *J. Physiol. (Paris),* 75: 667–671.

Connors, B.W. and Gutnick, M.J. (1984) Neocortex: Cellular properties and intrinsic circuitry. In: R. Dingledine (Ed.), *Brain Slices,* New York: Plenum Press, pp. 313–339.

Connors, B.W. and Gutnick, M.J. (1990) Intrinsic firing patterns of diverse neocortical neurons. *Trends Neurosci.,* 13: 99–104.

Connors, B.W., Gutnick, M.J. and Prince, D.A. (1982). Electrophysiological properties of neocortical neurons in vitro. *J. Neurophysiol.,* 48: 1302–1320.

Connors, B.W., Malenka, R.C. and Silva, L.R. (1988). Two inhibitory postsynaptic potentials, and $GABA_A$ and $GABA_B$ receptor-mediated responses in neocortex of rat and cat. *J. Physiol. (London),* 406: 443–468.

Crunelli, V. and Leresche, N. (1991) A role for $GABA_B$ receptors in excitation and inhibition of thalamocortical cells. *Trends Neurosci.,* 14: 16–21.

Deisz, R.A. and Prince, D.A. (1989) Frequency-dependent depression of inhibition in guinea-pig neocortex in vitro by $GABA_B$ receptor feed-back on GABA release. *J. Physiol. (London),* 412: 513–41.

Dolphin, A.C. and Scott, R.H. (1986) Inhibition of calcium currents in dorsal root ganglion neurones by baclofen. *Br. J. Pharmacol.,* 88: 213–220.

Draguhn, A., Verdoorn, T.A., Ewert, M., Seeburg, P.H. and Sakmann, B. (1990) Functional and molecular distinction between recombinant rat $GABA_A$ receptor subtypes by $Zn^{2+}$. *Neuron,* 5: 781–788.

Dunlap, K. (1981) Two types of γ-aminobutyric acid receptor on embryonic sensory neurons. *Br. J. Pharmacol.,* 74: 579–585.

Dunlap, K., Holz, G.G., Lindgren, C.A., Moore, J.W. (1989) Calcium channels that regulate neurosecretion. *Soc. Gen. Physiol. Ser.,* 44:239–50

Dutar, P. and Nicoll, R.A. (1988) Pre- and postsynaptic $GABA_B$ receptors in the hippocampus have different pharmacological properties. *Neuron,* 1: 585–591.

Ezure, K., Oguri, M., Oshima, T. (1985) Vertical spread of neuronal activity within the cat motor cortex investigated with epicortical stimulation and intracellular recording. *Jpn. J. Physiol.*, 35: 193–221.

Fujita, Y. (1979) Evidence for the existence of inhibitory postsynaptic potentials in dendrites and their functional significance in hippocampal pyramidal cells of adult rabbits. *Brain Res.*, 175: 59–69.

Gähwiler, B. and Brown, D.A. (1985) GABA$_B$ receptor-activated K$^+$ current in voltage-clamped CA3 pyramidal cells in rat hippocampal cultures. *Proc. Natl. Acad. Sci. USA*, 82: 1558–1562.

Galvan, M., Franz, P. and Constanti, A. (1985) Spontaneous inhibitory postsynaptic potentials in guinea pig neocortex and olfactory cortex neurones. *Neurosci. Lett.*, 57: 131–135.

Harrison, N.L. (1990) On the presynaptic action of baclofen at inhibitory synapses between cultured rat hippocampal neurons. *J. Physiol. (London)*, 422: 433–446.

Harrison, N.L., Lovinger, D.M, Lambert, N.A., Teyler, T.J., Prager, R., Ong, J. and Kerr, D.I.B. (1990) The actions of 2-hydroxysaclofen at presynaptic GABA$_B$ receptors in the rat hippocampus. *Neurosci. Lett.*, 119: 272–276.

Hill, D.R. and Bowery, N.G. (1981) $^3$H-baclofen and $^3$H-GABA bind to bicuculline-insensitive GABA$_B$ sites in rat brain. *Nature*, 290: 149–152.

Houser, C.R., Vaughn, J.E., Hendry, S.H.C., Jones, E.G. and Peters, A. (1984) GABA neurons in the cerebral cortex. In: E.G. Jones and A. Peters (Eds.), *Cerebral Cortex, Vol. 2, Functional Properties of Cortical Cells*, New York: Plenum Press, pp. 63–90.

Howe, J.R., Sutor, B. and Zieglgänsberger, W. (1987a) Baclofen reduces postsynaptic potentials of rat neocortical neurones by actions other than its hyperpolarizing action. *J. Physiol. (London)*, 384: 539–569.

Howe, J.R., Sutor, B. and Zieglgänsberger, W. (1987b) Characteristics of long-duration inhibitory postsynaptic potentials in rat neocortical neuron *Cell. Mol. Neurobiol.*, 7: 1–18.

Iversen, L.L., Mitchell, J.F. and Srinivasan, V. (1971) The release of γ-aminobutyric acid during inhibition in the cat visual cortex. *J. Physiol. (London)*, 212: 519–534.

Jasper, H.H. and Koyama, I. (1969) Rate of release of amino acids from the cerebral cortex in the cat as affected by brainstem and thalamic stimulation. *Can. J. Physiol. Pharmacol.*, 47: 889–905.

Kerr, D.I.B., Ong, J., Johnston, G.A.R. and Prager, R.H. (1989) GABA$_B$ receptor mediated actions of baclofen in the rat isolated cortical slice preparation: antagonism by phosphono-analogues of GABA. *Brain Res.*, 480: 312–316.

Koch, C., Douglas, R. and Wehmeier, U. (1990) Visibility of synaptically induced conductance changes: Theory and simulations of anatomically characterized cortical pyramidal cells. *J. Neurosci.*, 1728–1744.

Kriegstein, A.R. and Connors, B.W. (1986) Cellular physiology of the turtle visual cortex: Synaptic properties and intrinsic circuitry. *J. Neurosci.*, 6: 178–191.

Krnjević, K. (1974) Chemical nature of synaptic transmission in vertebrates. *Physiol. Rev.*, 54: 418–540.

Krnjević, K. and Schwartz, S. (1967) The action of γ-

aminobutyric acid on cortical neurones. *Exp. Brain Res.* 3: 320–336.

Lacaille, J.-C. and Schwartzkroin, P.A. (1988) Stratum lacunosum-moleculare interneurons of hippocampal CA1 region. II. Intrasomatic and intradendritic recordings of local circuit synaptic interactions. *J. Neurosci.*, 8: 1411–1424.

Martin, K.A.C. (1988) The Wellcome Prize Lecture: From single cells to simple circuits in the cerebral cortex. *Q.J. Exp. Physiol.*, 73: 637–702.

McCormick, D.A. (1989) GABA as in inhibitory neurotransmitter in human cerebral cortex. *J. Neurophysiol.*, 62, 1018–1027.

McCormick, D.A., Connors, B.W., Lighthall, J.W. and Prince, D.A. (1985). Comparative electrophysiology of pyramidal and sparsely spiny stellate neurons of the neocortex. *J. Neurophysiol.* 54, 782–806.

McCormick, D.A. and Williamson, A. (1989) Convergence and divergence of neurotransmitter action in human cerebral cortex. *Proc. Natl. Acad. Sci. USA* 86: 8098–8102.

Miles, R. (1990) Variation in strength of inhibitory synapses in the CA3 region of guinea-pig hippocampus in vitro. *J. Physiol. (London)* 431: 659–676.

Miles, R. and Wong, R.K.S. (1984) Unitary inhibitory synaptic potentials in the guinea-pig hippocampus in vitro. *J. Physiol. (London)*, 356: 97–113.

Misgeld, U., Deisz, R.A., Dodt, H.U. and Lux, H.D. (1986) The role of chloride transport in postsynaptic inhibition of hippocampal neurones. *Science*, 232: 1413–1415.

Newberry, N.R. and Nicoll, R.A. (1984a) Direct hyperpolarizing action of baclofen on hippocampal pyramidal cells. *Nature*, 308: 450–452.

Newberry, N.R. and R.A. Nicoll (1984b) A bicuculline-resistant inhibitory post-synaptic potential in rat hippocampal pyramidal cells in vitro. *J. Physiol. (London)*, 348: 239–254.

Nicoll, R.A., Malenka, R.C and Kauer, J. (1990). Functional comparison of neurotransmitter receptor subtypes in mammalian central nervous system. *Physiol. Rev.*, 70, 513–565.

Olsen, R.W. and Tobin, A.J. (1990) Molecular biology of GABA$_A$ receptors. *FASEB J.*, 4: 1469–1480.

Ong, J., Kerr, D.I.B., Johnston, G.A.R. and Hall, R.G. (1990) Differing actions of baclofen and 3-aminopropylphosphonic acid in rat neocortical slices. *Neurosci. Lett.*, 109: 169–173.

Peters, A. and Jones, E.G. (Eds.) (1984) *Cerebral Cortex, Vol. 1, Cellular Components of the Cerebral Cortex*, New York: Plenum Press, 565 pp.

Peters, A., Palay, S.L. and Webster, H. (1976) *The Fine Structure of the Nervous System: The Neurons and Supporting Cells*, Philadelphia: W.B. Saunders Co., 406 pp.

Roberts, E. (1983) γ-Aminobutyric acid (GABA): From discovery to visualization of GABAergic neurons in the vertebrate nervous system. In: N.G. Bowery (Ed.), *Actions and Interactions of GABA and Benzodiazepines*, New York: Raven Press, pp. 1–26.

Satou, M., Mori, K., Tazawa, Y. and Takagi, S.F. (1982) Two

types of postsynaptic inhibition in pyriform cortex of the rabbit: Fast and slow inhibitory postsynaptic potentials. *J. Neurophysiol.*, 48: 1142–1156.

Scharfman, H.E. and Sarvey, J.M. (1985) Responses to γ-aminobutyric acid applied to cell bodies and dendrites of rat visual cortical neurons. *Brain Res.*, 358: 385–389.

Scharfman, H.E. and Sarvey, J.M. (1987) Responses to GABA recorded from identified rat visual cortical neurons. *Neuroscience*, 23: 407–422.

Scherer, R.W., Ferkany, J.W. and Enna, S.J. (1988) Evidence for pharmacologically distinct subsets of GABA$_B$ receptors. *Brain Res. Bull.*, 21: 439–443.

Sigel, E. and Baur, R. (1988) Activation of protein kinase C differentially modulates neuronal Na$^+$, Ca$^{++}$, and γ-aminobutyrate type A channels. *Proc. Natl. Acad. Sci. USA,* 85, 6192–6196.

Sigel, E., Baur, R., Trube, G., Möhler, H. and Malherbe, P. (1991) The effect of subunit composition of rat brain GABA$_A$ receptors on channel function. *Neuron*.

Silva, L.R., Gutnick, M.J. and Connors, B.W. (1991) Laminar distribution of neuronal membrane properties in neocortex of normal and reeler mouse. *J. Neurosci.*, in press.

Sillito, A. (1984) Functional considerations of the operation of GABAergic inhibitory processes in the visual cortex. In: E.G. Jones and A. Peters (Eds.), *Cerebral Cortex, Vol. 2, Functional Properties of Cortical Cells,* New York: Plenum Press, pp. 91–118.

Somogyi, P. (1990) Synaptic organization of GABAergic neurons and GABA$_A$ receptors in the lateral geniculate nucleus and the visual cortex. In: D.M. Lam and C.D. Gilbert (Eds.), *Neural Mechanisms of Visual Perception*, Houston: Gulf Publishing, pp. 35–62.

Somogyi, P., Roberts, J.D.B., Gulyas, A., Richards, J.G. and DeBlas, A.L. (1989) GABA and the synaptic or nonsynaptic localization of benzodiazepine/GABA$_A$ receptor/Cl$^-$ channel complex in visual cortex of cat. *Soc. Neurosci. Abstr.*, 15: 1397.

Stelzer, A., Kay, A.R. and Wong, R.K.S. (1988) GABA$_A$-receptor function in hippocampal cells is maintained by phosphorylation factors. *Science*, 242, 339–341.

Stevens, D.R., Gallagher, J.P. and Shinnick-Gallagher, P. (1985) Further studies on the actions of baclofen on neurons of the dorsolateral septal nucleus of the rat. *Brain Res.*, 358: 360–363.

Thompson, S.M., Deisz, R.A. and Prince, D.A. (1988) Relative contributions of passive equilibrium and active transport to the distribution of chloride in mammalian cortical neurons. *J. Neurophysiol.*, 60: 105–124.

Verdoorn, T.A., Draguhn, A., Ymer, S. Seeburg, P. and Sakmann, B. (1990) Functional properties of recombinant rat GABA$_A$ receptors depend on subunit composition. *Neuron*, 4: 919–928.

Weiss, D.S. and Hablitz, J.J. (1984) Interaction of penicillin and pentobarbital on inhibitory synaptic mechanisms in neocortex. *Cell. Mol. Neurobiol.*, 4: 301–317.

White, E.L. and Keller, A. (1989) *Cortical Circuits: Synaptic Organization of the Cerebral Cortex: Structure, Function and Theory,* Boston: Birkhauser.

Whiting, P., McKernan, R.M. and Iversen, L.L. (1990) Another mechanism for creating diversity in γ-aminobutyrate type A receptors: RNA splicing directs expression of two forms of γ2 subunit, one of which contains ·a protein kinase C phosphorylation site. *Proc. Natl. Acad. Sci. USA* 87: 9966–9970.

Wisden, S., Morris, B.J., Darlison, M.G., Hunt, S.P. and Barnard, E.A. (1988) Distinct GABA$_A$ receptor α subunit mRNAs show differential patterns of expression in bovine brain. *Neuron*, 1: 937–947.

Zhang, J.-H., Sato, M. and Tohyama, M. (1991) Region-specific expression of the mRNAs encoding β subunits (β$_1$, β$_2$ and β$_3$) of GABA$_A$ receptor in the rat brain. *J. Comp. Neurol.*, 303: 637–657.

R.R. Mize, R.E. Marc and A.M. Sillito (Eds.)
Progress in Brain Research, Vol. 90

CHAPTER 17

# GABA mediated inhibitory processes in the function of the geniculo-striate system

A.M. Sillito

*Department of Visual Science, Institute of Ophthalmology, Judd Street, London WC1H 9QS, England, UK*

## Introduction

Despite the clarity of the insight provided by the early models of the synaptic circuitry underlying the transformation of receptive field properties from retina to cortex, subsequent work has revealed an increasingly complex and subtle synaptic substrate to the function of the central visual system. The primary difficulty at present lies in bringing together the many pieces of the jigsaw into an intelligible pattern. The object of this review is to provide an overview of our knowledge regarding the way inhibitory mechanisms are utilised in the synaptic circuits determining the response properties of cells at both geniculate and cortical levels in the visual system. The circuitry and function at these two levels are strongly interlinked by the subcortical and cortical interconnections of layer VI cells in the visual cortex and it is no longer logically acceptable to treat them as entirely separate processing stages in a hierarchical sequence. This account will centre around a discussion of the feline visual system, but where appropriate reference will be made to the primate visual system. A major concern in presenting this account has been to place the action of the GABAergic interneurons in the perspective of that of other elements of the circuitry and our knowledge of the system function as addressed by analysis of receptive field organisation. The inhibitory circuitry at both geniculate and thalamic levels is strongly influenced by neu-

romodulatory inputs. These establish the pattern of operation linked to the waking state. The cholinergic system has potent and rather different effects on inhibitory interneurons and circuitry at the two levels considered here, and its action and pattern of connectivity will be used as an example of the way the modulatory systems can influence GABAergic mechanisms in the central visual system.

## Basic synaptic circuit in the dLGN

The main elements of the circuitry in the dorsal lateral geniculate nucleus are summarised in Fig. 1. The retinal afferents make synaptic contact with both the proximal dendrites of relay cells and the presynaptic dendrites of the intrinsic inhibitory interneurons of the dLGN. These interneurons are GABAergic (Sterling and Davis, 1980; Sillito and Kemp, 1983; Fitzpatrick et al., 1984; Montero, 1986; Montero and Singer, 1984, 1985; Montero and Zempel, 1985; Uhlrich and Cucchiaro, Chapter 9) and their presynaptic dendrites, referred to as F2 terminals, form triadic synaptic arrangements with the retinal afferents and the relay cell dendrite. This synaptic structure, encapsulated by a glial sheet, is called a glomerulus. The essential logic of this arrangement seems to be that a retinal terminal would both directly excite the relay cell and initiate a short latency inhibitory input to it via the contact

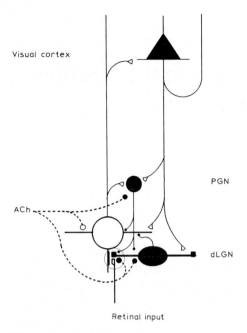

Visual cortex

PGN

ACh

dLGN

Retinal input

Fig. 1. Synopsis of the basic circuit for the dorsal lateral geniculate nucleus (dLGN) and its feedback from the visual cortex. Open terminals correspond to excitatory synapses and closed terminals to inhibitory synapses. The cholinergic input is shown by the dashed line and the different pattern of its effect signalled by the variation from closed to filled terminals. The components linked to the triadic synapses in the synaptic glomeruli are highlighted by the faint circle. Here the dendrite of the relay cell is thickened to indicate a dendritic spine and the retinal afferent is presynaptic to both the relay cell and the presynaptic dendrite of the inhibitory interneuron. The cholinergic terminal in this arrangement is shown as hatched to indicate the question regarding its pattern of action here (see text for further discussion). Conventional presynaptic contacts from axons are made by both the intrinsic inhibitory interneuron and the perigeniculate cells (PGN). Both these cell groups are GABAergic. The details of the circuitry and variations for different cell types are discussed in the text.

on the presynaptic dendrite. The axons of these same inhibitory interneurons make extraglomerular synaptic contact via "F1" terminals on the dendrites of relay cells (Montero, 1987). A second level of inhibitory input derives from another group of GABAergic cells, the perigeniculate cells. These provide extraglomerular axonal synaptic input via "F1" terminals to the dendrites and cell body of relay cells and intrageniculate inhibitory interneurons. They also make contact

via F1 terminals, with presynaptic dendrites in the synaptic glomeruli (Montero, 1987). In addition the perigeniculate cells inhibit other perigeniculate cells and it seems that the presynaptic dendrites of the intrinsic inhibitory interneurons may also make contact with each other. The perigeniculate cells receive input from collaterals of the relay cells projecting to the visual cortex. Layer VI cells in the visual cortex provide a corticofugal projection which makes synaptic contacts on perigeniculate cells, the extraglomerular dendrites of relay cells and intrageniculate inhibitory interneurons and to a lesser extent, presynaptic dendrites (Weber et al., 1989).

Further inputs reach the dLGN from the cholinergic, noradrenergic and serotinergic brain stem modulatory systems. These interact with the synaptic circuitry in the dLGN and seem to be concerned particularly with shifts in functional organisation linked with behavioural state. As summarised in Fig. 1, the cholinergic system provides synaptic input to perigeniculate cells, relay cells, intrinsic inhibitory interneurons and their presynaptic dendrites within glomeruli (De Lima et al., 1985).

## Variations in the basic circuit

Whilst the above description provides a broad overview of the type of synaptic mechanisms within the dLGN it is important to identify the way this applies to the relay cells associated with the different categories of input. In the cat, three groups of retinal ganglion cell project to the dLGN, the X, Y and W cells. The basic circuit as defined here most closely applies to X cells where the triadic synapses are associated with the inputs on their dendritic spines. Y cells have far fewer spines and few if any glomeruli and this also appears to apply to W cells. The primary inhibitory control for Y cells derives from synaptic input from F1 terminals of both perigeniculate and intrageniculate inhibitory interneurons. The density of F1 type synapses on or close to the Y cell soma is greater than for X cells and this may enhance their influence (Hamos et al., 1987; Somogyi, 1989). It is to be noted that there is anatomical evidence favouring the subdivision of the intrinsic interneurons into two groups, a small diameter (8–13 $\mu$) beta group constituting the majority (86%) and a larger diameter (14–19 $\mu$) alpha group (14%) (Montero and Singer, 1985; Montero and Zempel, 1985). This is matched by electrophysiological evidence showing that the IPSPs in Y cells seem to be driven by Y type axons and those in X cells by X type axons, suggesting private inhibitory channels for the two groups (Lindstrom and Wrobel, 1990a). An earlier suggestion indicating that inhibitory interneurons are only driven by X cell afferents from the retina (Sherman and Friedlander, 1988) seems to be incorrect. The pattern of retinal input to relay cells seems to vary within the X and Y categories. The most detailed evidence so far refers to X cells (Hamos et al., 1987) and suggests that whilst some cells are dominated by input from a single retinal ganglion cell, others receive convergent input from up to five. Other evidence has led to the view that the X cell population can be subdivided into so called "lagged" and "non-lagged" groups following from the presence and absence of synaptic glomeruli on their dendrites (Mastronarde, 1987a,b; Humphrey and Weller, 1988a,b). A further suggestion is that there are some "lagged" Y cells (Saul and Humphrey, 1990). These observations are at variance with the broad consensus regarding the anatomical characteristics distinguishing X and Y cells and the issues are yet to be fully resolved. Some of the likely functional implications are discussed later.

## Functional pharmacology of the dLGN and the role of GABAergic inhibitory circuits

Testing cells in the dLGN with simple visual stimuli reveals response properties that are superficially very similar to those seen in retinal ganglion cells. Thus dLGN cells have concentrically organised "on" or "off" centre receptive fields with centre-surround antagonism (Hubel

and Wiesel, 1961). Examining the situation more closely reveals that the degree of surround antagonism of centre responses is significantly higher in dLGN cells than retinal ganglion cells. This can be linked to IPSPs generated by stimuli overlying the surround and centre surround border (Singer et al., 1972; Singer and Creutzfeldt, 1970). It would seem that this inhibitory input must follow from inhibitory interneurons with receptive fields overlying the centre-surround border and surround of the recipient cell field. However the interneurons are organised, a significant component of their influence on receptive field structure seems to follow $GABA_A$ receptor mediated effects as illustrated in Fig. 2 with data from Sillito and Kemp (1983). These data document the effect of microiontophoretic application of the $GABA_A$ antagonist $N$-methyl bicuculline (Nmb) on the response curves of dLGN cells to variation in the diameter of a stationary flashing stimulus. The records in the middle of Fig. 2 show an example of the test used to demonstrate the effectiveness of Nmb application on the fast GABA mediated blockade of a visual response produced by an iontophoretic pulse of GABA synchronised to overlap one of a pair of two flash stimuli delivered to the receptive field centre of a dLGN cell. The short 10 nA GABA pulse completely suppresses the response to the first of the two flashes but leaves the second unaffected, this suppression is then eliminated by Nmb application. The PSTHs at the bottom of Fig. 2 illustrate the effect of the level of inhibitory blockade shown above during Nmb application, on the surround attenuation of the centre response. Under control conditions, increasing stimulus diameter so that it expands within the centre and then crosses into the surround, results in a rise then a sharp fall in response magnitude. A component of this fall reflects centre-surround interaction at retinal levels, but there is also a significant contribution from intrageniculate mechanisms as indicated by the responses during Nmb application. In the presence of the GABA blockade responses to the larger diameter stimuli are notably increased in magnitude relative to those elicited from the centre. This point is further emphasised by the curves plotted at the top of the figure. During Nmb application the cell's responses reflect the level of surround antagonism associated with retinal ganglion cells. Comparing the responses of X and Y

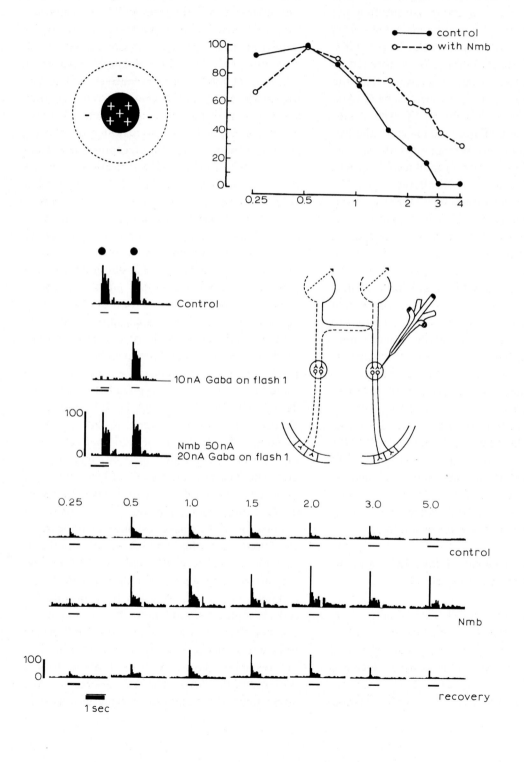

cells it is clear that although the absolute degree of surround antagonism of centre responses is lower in Y cells than X cells, it is still enhanced by GABAergic inhibitory mechanisms in the dLGN (Sillito and Kemp, 1983). Another way of analysing the synaptic processing of the visual input at the level of the dLGN is to explore the spatial and temporal frequency tuning curves of cells. When constructing spatial frequency tuning curves from sinusoidal gratings of varying contrast and spatial frequency the results define an upper limit for the spatial resolution of the field and a lower frequency cut off point. In X cells, blockade of GABAergic inhibitory mechanisms reduces the lower frequency cut off point. This would seem to follow logically from the reduction in the effectiveness of the surround driven inhibitory mechanisms (Berardi and Morrone, 1984).

## Influence of corticofugal feedback on inhibitory processes in the dLGN

We know that anatomically the corticofugal system provides the dominant input to the dLGN and that GABAergic inhibitory interneurons are apparently its major target (Weber et al., 1989). In accord with this recent physiological studies have emphasised corticofugal contributions to inhibitory processes (Murphy and Sillito, 1987). Surprisingly there is little general reference to its functional contribution to visual processing in the dLGN. In part this follows from the fact that dLGN cells, when tested by methods routinely used to examine retinal ganglion cell fields, exhibit a very similar concentric receptive field structure and have thus been seen to reflect an intrageniculate elaboration of retinal processing. On reflection, given that we know layer VI cells in the visual cortex have orientation tuned receptive fields that are not well activated by small stationary flashing stimuli, it is clear that any attempt to examine their contribution to dLGN function requires the use of stimuli that best activate them. In short, we need to consider stimulus configurations that drive the visual cortex and provoke output from the corticofugal system. In this way we may establish at least some elements of the functional influence of the corticofugal system.

With respect to the functional organisation of the corticofugal projection to the dLGN there are several issues that need to be stressed in relation to the present account. Firstly, the projection which derives primarily from areas 17 and 18 is broadly retinotopically organised so that there are reciprocal projections between dLGN and cortical locations subserving the same region of visual space (Hollander, 1970; Kawamura et al., 1974; Updyke, 1975). Secondly, there is a fairly coherent body of evidence favouring the view that the projection comprises axons of several conduction velocities. Three groups seem likely, with respective conduction velocities in the range 13–

Fig. 2. The effect of inhibitory blockade induced by iontophoretic application of the GABA antagonist *N*-methylbicuculline (Nmb) on centre surround antagonism in the dLGN. The line diagrams summarise the centre-surround receptive field organisation classically associated with dLGN cells and the method for inducing inhibitory blockade and recording single cell activity with a multibarreled microiontophoretic pipette. GABA exerts a very potent inhibitory effect on dLGN cells. The middle peristimulus time histograms (PSTHs) show that a 10 nA pulse of GABA (marked by bar under flash time marker) will completely suppress the response to one of a pair of flashed stimuli (1 sec flashes as indicated by two short bars under records). Application of Nmb (50 nA) completely blocks this action of GABA. Lower PSTHs document for an on centre Y cell, the variation in response magnitude as the diameter of a flashing spot of light (0.5 sec duration), centred over the receptive field, is increased from 0.25° to 5.0°. Under control conditions there is marked response attenuation beyond 1.5°, but this is greatly reduced during Nmb application (80 nA). This is documented for an on centre X cell by the response curves at the top right of the figure. The response magnitude on these curves is expressed as a percentage of the maximum control response and the range of stimulus diameters used extends from 0.25–4.0°. For all PSTHs the bin size is 50 msec and vertical calibration indicates range corresponding to 0–100 counts/bin. See text for further details.

32 m/sec, 3.2–12 m/sec and 0.3–1.6 m/sec (Tsumoto et al., 1978; Tsumoto and Suda, 1980; Boyapati and Henry, 1987). The larger and smaller diameter fibres go to PGN and dLGN and some individual axons seem to innervate both (Robson, 1983; Boyapati and Henry, 1984). The fast and intermediate groups seem to correlate with cells with complex and simple receptive field properties respectively whilst those with the lowest conduction velocity appear to be largely unresponsive to visual stimuli in the experimental situations used for these studies (Tsumoto et al., 1978; Tsumoto and Suda, 1980).

The detail of the visual response properties of the corticofugally projecting complex and simple cells identifies the type of stimuli which will exert maximal influence on dLGN mechanisms. The complex cells are spontaneously active and are strongly binocular, directional, broadly orientation tuned and capable of responding at high stimulus velocities (Gilbert, 1977; Tsumoto et al., 1978; Tsumoto and Suda, 1980; Harvey, 1980). The simple cells on the other hand have little or no spontaneous activity, are sharply orientation tuned and include cells strongly or exclusively dominated by one eye. One factor stands out from all the available evidence and that is that both the simple and complex cells projecting to the dLGN tend to be strongly directionally sensitive. Another issue that is less clear concerns the length tuning of the receptive fields (Gilbert, 1977; Tsumoto et al., 1978; Tsumoto and Suda, 1980; Harvey, 1980). Following the study of Gilbert, who first identified in layer VI cells with the longest receptive fields seen in the visual cortex, there has been a general assumption that the corticofugal projection originates from cells with long fields (generally 8° or more). Recent work for layer VI in general questions the extent to which it is dominated by cells with very long receptive fields. Whilst Gilbert's original definition of such cells in layer VI is clearly correct, there is a substantial population of cells with much shorter receptive fields (Grieve and Sillito, 1989, 1991). This is of importance, because as is

discussed later, a number of observations require at least some layer VI corticofugal cells to have short rapidly summating receptive fields.

In summary, it seems that the major visually driven feedback to the dLGN comes from two channels of output: a fast conducting binocularly driven system with significant background activity, broad orientation tuning but high directionality, and a slower system with little background activity, sharp orientation tuning and directionality but less binocularity. The fast conducting system also appeared to respond to higher stimulus velocities than the slower conducting system. The functional impact of the fast system may be more prominent than that of the slower system. Tsumoto et al. (1978) using cross correlation techniques to explore links between layer VI cells and dLGN cells noted that all the cells exhibiting an excitatory or inhibitory interaction in the cross correlogram were complex cells. They also explored the influence of retinotopic alignment between cortex and dLGN on the type of effect elicited from the cortex. Excitatory effects were observed when the field centres of the cortical and geniculate cells were within 1.7° of each other. Inhibitory effects were also seen for cells within this domain of retinotopic register, but in addition were found for separations up to 3°. Thus it seems that for a given retinotopic location in the dLGN there is a broad overlying field of corticofugal inhibitory influence with a more closely aligned or focussed corticofugal facilitatory field.

The effects of the corticofugal inhibitory influence do show when geniculate cells are tested with stimuli appropriate for activating cortical cells. When tested with moving bars of varying length dLGN cells exhibit a high degree of length tuning (Schiller et al., 1976; Cleland et al., 1983; Jones and Sillito, 1987, 1991). Thus cells are best activated by a short bar and with increasing length the response declines dramatically. This is illustrated in Fig. 3 for an on-centre X cell (see also Fig. 4). This response property was first reported by Hubel and Wiesel (1965, 1968) for the so-called

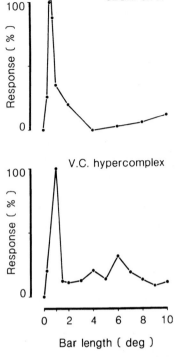

Fig. 3. Comparison of the length tuning curves of an "on" centre dLGN cell tested with moving bars of varying length and a cortical hypercomplex cell. Responses expressed as a percentage of the maximum response seen for an optimal length stimulus. See text for further details.

level of the dLGN raises a number of issues which question some of the background assumptions regarding the mechanisms underlying receptive field organisation at both cortical and geniculate levels. Considering here the implications for the geniculate, the primary issue is whether there is a cortical contribution to the processes generating length tuning in the dLGN cell field. The surround antagonism of centre responses in the dLGN cell field discussed above with respect to stationary flashing stimuli, implies that a moving bar extended in length so that it encroaches on cell surround as well as centre will provoke a reduction in response. There should be two components to this, one following from centre-surround interactions at the retinal level and the other from interactions at geniculate level. A brief consideration of the comparative geometry of the stimulus configuration for moving bars, as opposed to a flashing circle of light, makes it clear that a bar will activate a smaller component of the surround and hence a lower degree of centre-surround antagonism. However, feedback from cortical cells well activated by moving bars, to inhibitory interneurons contributing to centre-surround antagonism at the level of the dLGN, could reinforce the surround inhibition elicited by bars. These ideas are summarised by the diagram in Fig. 4.

This issue has been explored in experiments comparing the length tuning of dLGN cells with and without corticofugal feedback (Murphy and Sillito, 1987). Removing the corticofugal feedback caused a substantial reduction in the length tuning of both X and Y cells in the dLGN under circumstances where centre-surround antagonism as tested by flashing spots of varying diameter was unaffected. This is illustrated in Fig. 4 which compares the length tuning curves of two on-centre Y cells recorded in left and right dLGNs of a preparation with areas 17 and 18 of the visual cortex removed on one side. Although the cell lacking corticofugal feedback showed a much reduced response attenuation with increasing stimulus length the response attenuation caused

"hypercomplex" cells in the visual cortex, a group of cells at that time considered to follow from complex cells in a hierarchical processing sequence. In the cortex the response reduction has been attributed to inhibitory zones, lying to either end of the receptive field centre, the so-called "inhibitory end-zones". A response attenuation of 50% with increasing stimulus length has been considered to be a criterion for placing cortical cells in the hypercomplex category (Yamane et al., 1985). In the cat dLGN, for X and Y cells with clear centre-surround antagonism, the mean response reduction with increasing stimulus length is 71% ($n = 186$, Jones and Sillito, 1987, 1991). For comparison, a highly length tuned cortical hypercomplex cell is illustrated together with the dLGN X cell in Fig. 3. The presence of this apparently cortical response property at the

356

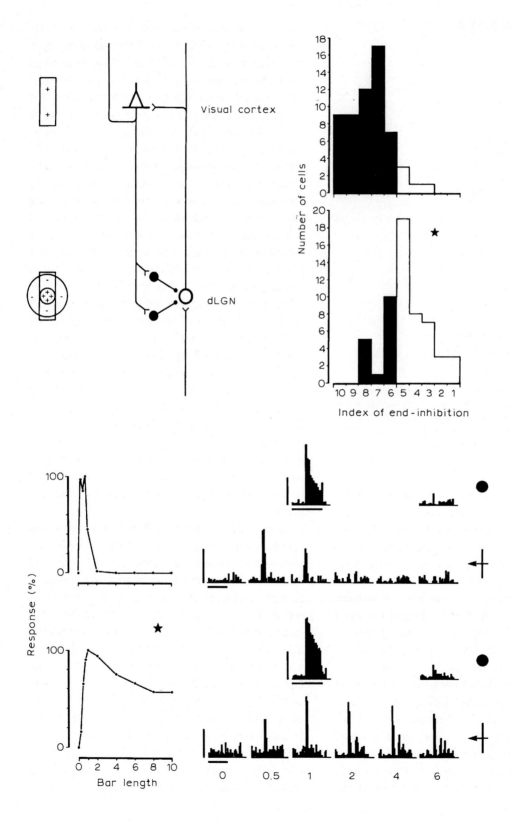

Visual cortex

dLGN

Number of cells

Index of end-inhibition

Response (%)

Bar length

by increasing the diameter of a stationary flashing spot from 1° to 6° was similar in both cases. Taking the population of dLGN cells, subdivided into categories on the basis of an index of end-inhibition, there is a very significant difference in the distribution of length tuning in groups with and without feedback (Fig. 4 Index of end-inhibition histograms). The mean response reduction shifts from 71 to 43%. The cortical feed back does seem to facilitate the drive from GABAergic inhibitory interneurons as bar lengths increase beyond the dimensions of the dLGN cell receptive field centre. The effect of surround inhibition effectively enhances the resolution of the receptive field to a discontinuity in contrast between field centre and surround. The corticofugal feedback driving the intrageniculate inhibitory mechanisms, would seem to optimise this effect for thin contrast contours, so that the resolution of the field for a discontinuity over the field centre is retained despite the reduced area of surround activated by the stimulus.

The presence of a corticofugal influence on inhibitory mechanisms in the dLGN raises the question of orientation bias in their operation. Layer VI cells are orientation tuned and hence either each location in the dLGN effectively receives feedback from a complete subset of cortical orientation columns or there must be a degree of orientation bias to the feedback affecting any

given cell (Fig. 5). The problem has been examined recently (Sillito et al., 1991) by a series of experiments utilising a visual stimulus subdivided into an inner window located over the receptive field centre, and an outer window. The diameter of the inner window was chosen to match the value for the optimal length assessed from a length tuning curve constructed for the cell. The motion of the inner and outer stimuli were phase locked so that when both were at the same alignment they appeared as a single bar or grating moving over the receptive field. The effect of varying the orientation alignment of the two components of the stimulus was then documented. For dLGN cells the overall circular symmetry of the receptive field might be expected to result in similar magnitude inhibitory effects from the surround, irrespective of the orientation alignment of the two components of the stimulus. On the other hand, layer VI cortical cells with non-end-stopped orientation tuned fields respond best to the aligned condition (Fig. 5). Thus the corticofugal influence driving the inhibitory processes enhancing length tuning in dLGN cells should be most effective for the aligned condition of this stimulus. Furthermore, if such an influence derives from a complete subset of orientation columns, this should apply for the alignment condition at any absolute orientation of the overall stimulus. The data from dLGN cells show that

Fig. 4. The corticofugal contribution to length tuning in the dLGN. Diagram summarises the logic of the suggestions. The data is taken from Murphy and Sillito, 1987. The lower records document the responses of two on-centre Y cells, with fields at the same eccentricity in the same preparation, one recorded in the left dLGN with corticofugal feedback and the other in the right dLGN without corticofugal feedback (Areas 17 and 18 of the visual cortex removed by aspiration). The length tuning curves showing responses expressed as a percentage of the maximum are illustrated to the left and samples of the peristimulus histograms for the actual response shown to the right. Immediately above these there are two PSTHs documenting the cells response to a 1° and 6° diameter flashing spot. The cell with corticofugal feedback shows a high level of length tuning to the drifting bar stimuli, and strong centre-surround antagonism as revealed by the flashing spots. The cell without corticofugal feedback (*) shows equally strong centre-surround antagonism to the flashing spots, but poor length tuning to the moving bars. The histograms in the upper right of the figure summarize the distribution of length tuning in the population of cells (59) studied with corticofugal feedback and those (56) without (*). This is expressed as an index of end-inhibition, where cells with the strongest end-inhibition (total suppression of resting discharge at longer lengths) are in group 10 (left side of histogram) and those with none in group 1 (right side). The shaded portion of the PSTHs identifies those cells that if studied in the cortex, would have been classified as hypercomplex. There is a strong shift to the right in the population without feedback. Scale bars under PSTHs show 2 sec period and those to the left range for 0–50 impulses per second. All PSTHs averaged for 20 trials. Figures modified from Murphy and Sillito, 1987. See text for further details.

maximal suppression of the response to the inner stimulus is seen for the stimulus alignment condition (Fig. 5) and that for a given cell this alignment effect obtains at a range of different overall

orientations for the alignment condition. The plots in Fig. 5 for a dLGN cell show the response elicited at varying orientations of the inner stimulus for three different orientations of the outer

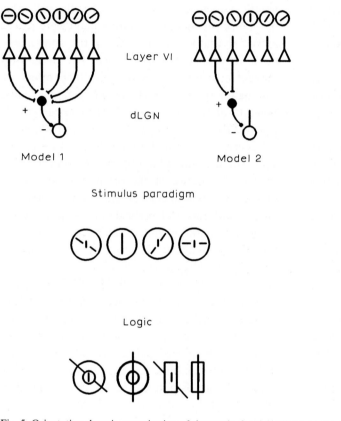

Cortical orientation columns

Layer VI

dLGN

Model 1        Model 2

Stimulus paradigm

Logic

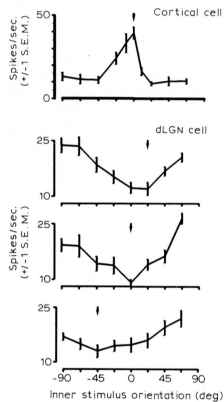

INFLUENCE OF ORIENTATION ALIGNMENT
Arrows indicate alignment condition

Spikes/sec. (+/-1 S.E.M.)

Cortical cell

dLGN cell

Spikes/sec. (+/-1 S.E.M.)

Inner stimulus orientation (deg)

Fig. 5. Orientation domain organisation of the corticofugal feedback to the inhibitory interneurons enhancing length tuning in the dLGN (see Fig. 4 also). Diagrams to the left summarise two possible models for the way the feedback to the inhibitory interneurons might be organised. To test this a bipartite stimulus was used to examine dLGN cell fields as shown in the stimulus paradigm. The inner component of the stimulus was located over the receptive field centre, and the orientation of the inner and outer components could be varied. The motion of the inner and outer components was phase locked so that when in alignment they appeared as a single stimulus moving over the receptive field. Inner and outer stimulus orientation were varied on a randomised interleaved sequence. The essential logic of the experiment is that the inhibitory effect elicited from the surround of the dLGN cell receptive field should not be sensitive to the relative alignment of the two components of the stimulus, because of the circular concentric arrangement. Conversely the fields of the visual cortical cells driving the corticofugal feedback should be optimally activated by the orientation aligned condition of the stimulus. This is shown by the tuning curve for a cortical cell at the top right of the figure. The arrow above the curve indicates the alignment condition. As the orientation alignment of the stimulus is varied it is clear that maximal responses are obtained as the inner and outer stimuli approach and reach alignment. Thus the corticofugal contribution to length tuning should be maximal when the inner and outer components of the stimulus are in alignment. If model 1 applies, this should be true for alignment at any given overall orientation. The curves for the dLGN cell in the lower three records on the right show the effect of varying the inner stimulus orientation for three different orientations of the outer stimulus as indicated by the arrows above the records. Maximum suppression is clearly seen as the stimuli approach and reach the alignment condition. This is seen for each of three different alignment conditions illustrated. Thus the effect seems to occur at any given orientation supporting model 1.

stimulus. The essential point is that there is a clear shift in the focus of the smallest response to follow the orientation of the outer stimulus.

The orientation alignment effects demonstrated by these procedures might be argued to follow from receptive field elongation of the type described by several laboratories for retinal ganglion cells and considered to underly the orientation bias seen in some cells at retinal and geniculate levels (Hammond, 1974; Levick and Thibos, 1980, 1982; Vidyasagar, 1984; Shou and Zhou, 1986; but note Soodak et al., 1987). There are several arguments against this, the main being that elongation in a particular plane cannot account for an alignment effect that follows the overall orientation of the alignment condition around the "clock", as suggested by the data in Fig. 5. It is also not clear that a simple elongation of the field could account for the alignment effect even at a single orientation. In essence the data requires an inhibitory influence sensitive to the orientation alignment of a contour crossing centre and surround at any given orientation. Whilst a subcortical contribution to such an effect cannot be excluded, the simplest explanation is that the effect follows from the cortex, and that an entire subset of orientation columns from the visual cortex generate the feedback effects influencing any given dLGN cell. This feedback ensures that cells are sensitive to the orientation alignment of contours crossing their receptive field centre and surround mechanisms. The outcome of this would seem to be that the output from the dLGN would be sensitive to discontinuities in the orientation domain for contours moving through visual space. A perfectly straight contour would produce a relatively uniform output from the rows of dLGN cell fields it engaged, with peaks at either end. Discontinuities in the orientation along the length of the contour would result in peaks in the output from those cells with fields crossed by the discontinuity, because the corticofugal feedback driving the inhibition would be reduced at these points.

## Binocular inhibition in the dLGN and corticofugal feedback

Although the retinal input to the dLGN is segregated into eye specific laminae, dLGN cells frequently exhibit weak responses to stimulation of corresponding receptive field locations in the other "non-dominant" eye. For stimulation of the non-dominant eye field alone, these responses are most commonly inhibitory, but facilitatory and mixed responses are also seen (Sandersen et al., 1971; Kato et al., 1981; Guido et al., 1989). Similarly, in binocular stimulation paradigms there is evidence for both inhibitory and facilitatory effects of non-dominant eye field stimulation on dominant eye field responses (Schmeilau and Singer, 1977; Varela and Singer, 1987; Xue et al., 1987). Schmeilau and Singer (1977) found that cooling the visual cortex eliminated facilitatory influences from the non-dominant eye but left some inhibitory effects. The presence of these binocular interactions are hardly surprising given that many of the corticofugal cells in layer VI have strong binocular fields (Gilbert, 1977; Tsumoto et al., 1978; Tsumoto and Suda, 1980) and hence should provide both direct excitatory input to dLGN cells and indirect inhibitory input via synapses on GABAergic inhibitory interneurons. This point is further emphasised by the observation that individual corticofugal axons do not seem to be restricted in their termination pattern to dLGN laminae subserving a given eye (Robson, 1983). Accepting the magnitude of the corticofugal projection to the dLGN one might ask why the binocular responses of dLGN cells are not stronger. One possibility is that they are organised in a way which is sensitive to the disparity of the retinal image, a property normally associated with cortical neurons concerned with depth perception. This does not seem to be the case (Xue et al., 1987) but the inhibitory effects do seem to be stronger when the stimuli influencing the dominant and non-dominant eye fields differ in orientation, direction of motion or con-

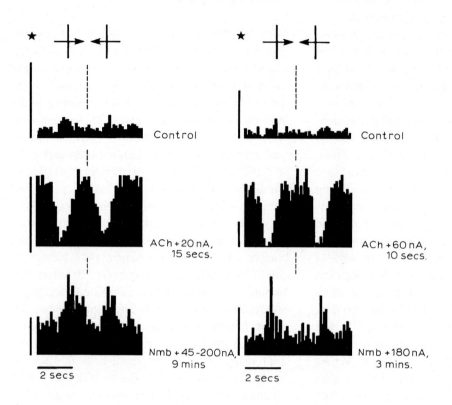

2 secs        2 secs

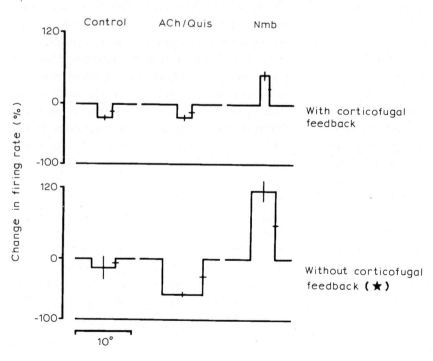

trast (Varela and Singer, 1987). If the cortex is removed these "feature" dependent effects are lost. This observation stands in contrast to that made by Schmielau and Singer (1977) who found facilitatory effects in the dLGN to be dependent on the corticofugal influence.

The non-dominant eye responses of dLGN cells to stimuli that will drive layer VI cells should in principle provide the most direct access to the direct corticofugal excitatory influence on dLGN relay cells. In the early studies assessment of this would have been complicated by the presence of the corticofugal drive to inhibitory interneurons. Blockade of the inhibitory input with Nmb offers the possibility of dissecting out the corticofugal excitatory influence and exploring the stimulus conditions that optimize it. In an attempt to achieve this Murphy and Sillito (1989) examined the responses of X and Y cells in the A laminae of the dLGN to bars moving over their non-dominant eye fields during inhibitory blockade. In the absence of any pharmacological manipulation the cells studied showed weak inhibitory responses. Increasing background discharge by iontophoretically applying either an excitatory amino acid or acetylcholine (ACh) revealed potent inhibitory dips against the elevated discharge of the cells. Iontophoretic application of Nmb revealed the anticipated excitatory responses to the stimuli. These responses, if from the cortificofugal fibres, should be eliminated by removal of the corticofugal drive. This turned out not to be the case; the duration and the magnitude of both the inhibitory and the excitatory responses were in-

creased by removal of areas 17 and 18 of the visual cortex. These results are summarised in Fig. 6. The upper part of this figure shows the response of two dLGN cells to non-dominant eye stimulation in preparations where both areas 17 and 18 had been removed to eliminate the feedback. The control responses of these cells showed just detectable excitatory effects. Raising background discharge with iontophoretically applied ACh revealed a very potent inhibition of the induced discharge by the visual stimulus. Inhibitory blockade with Nmb conversely unmasked strong excitatory responses. The lower part of this figure provides a comparison for the population, of the magnitude and duration of the inhibitory and excitatory responses to non-dominant eye stimulation in the presence and absence of feedback. Both duration and magnitude of the effects revealed by drug application seem to be greater in the absence of feedback. It seems that dLGN cells receive subcortically mediated binocular inhibitory and facilitatory inputs. Judged from this data in the monocular stimulus paradigm, the corticofugal system seems to diminish the expression of both excitatory and inhibitory responses to the non-dominant eye. Others have also reported what appears to be an increase in such binocular inhibition after loss of corticofugal feedback (Pape and Eysel, 1986).

## Interaction between inhibitory, excitatory and neuromodulatory mechanisms in the dLGN

In attempting to identify GABA circuitry functions in the dLGN it is important to consider the

Fig. 6. Responses of dLGN cells to stimulation of the non-dominant eye (see text) in the absence of corticofugal feedback. The PSTHs document the responses of an off-centre (left records) and on-centre (right records) Y cell to a bar of light drifting over the field in the non-dominant eye. In both cases the stimuli seem to elicit very weak excitatory responses. Increasing background discharge with iontophoretically applied ACh reveals a potent inhibitory input as the stimulus passes over the field. Conversely iontophoretic application of the GABA antagonist Nmb revealed excitatory responses. Vertical calibrations show range corresponding to 0–20 (off Y cell) and 0–6 (on Y cell) impulses/sec. Records averaged from 50 trials with a bin size of 100 msec. The lower diagram summarises the non-dominant eye responses seen with and without corticofugal feedback, under control conditions and when background activity was raised (iontophoretic application of ACh or quisqualate) or inhibition blocked (Nmb application). Response width and percentage change with respect to background discharge level were calculated for each condition, by averaging the data obtained from all the tested cells. These figures were then used to calculate the composite pictures above, with error bars showing standard errors of the mean. See text for further details. Data from Murphy and Sillito, 1989.

overall pharmacological organisation linked to the various neurotransmitter systems operating at this level. Both $GABA_A$ and $GABA_B$ receptor mediated effects are seen in dLGN cells. In the in vitro preparation these appear respectively as early, 5 msec or less, and longer latency (35–45 msec) events following electrical stimulation of the optic tract. The $GABA_A$ receptor mediated effects are linked to a short duration, chloride dependent (25–35 msec) IPSP (Hirsch and Burnod, 1987; Crunelli et al., 1988) and a marked (75%) decrease in input resistance. Effects mediated by $GABA_B$ receptors in dLGN cells are much longer in duration (250–300 msec) and relate to an influence on a potassium conductance (Soltesz et al., 1988) with a smaller (45%) overall decrease in input resistance. Recent immunohistochemical evidence regarding the detailed distribution of the $GABA_A$/benzodiazepine receptor/$Cl^-$ channnel complex in the dLGN is interesting because it suggests that whilst present on the cell bodies and proximal dendrites of relay cells, they are not present on intrinisic inhibitory interneurons (Somogyi, 1989). If this is true, and some doubt must persist regarding the global effectiveness of the antibody used for tagging the receptor complex, it would seem that inhibitory interneurons are not themselves regulated by $GABA_A$ receptor mediated IPSPs. This is supported by the limited electrophysiological evidence available which indicates that in contrast to relay cells, interneurons in the dLGN do not show short duration IPSPs in response to optic tract stimulation (Bloomfield and Sherman, 1988). Thus there might not be a short latency disinhibition of GABAergic interneurons within the dLGN either from the dendro-dendritic (F2) or axonal inputs from other GABA cells. These connections between GABA cells nonetheless exist (Montero, 1987; Somogyi, 1989) and at the moment it is tempting to consider the possibility that their functional import should be sought in the postsynaptic effects wrought by $GABA_B$ receptor activation.

Recent advances in our understanding of the excitatory mechanisms responsible for the translation of the retinal input through the dLGN have a bearing on our understanding of the likely impact of the GABAergic inhibitory processes reviewed here. The excitatory input to the dLGN from both retina and cortex seems to involve excitatory amino acid receptors (Kemp and Sillito, 1982; Crunelli et al., 1987; Sillito et al., 1990a,b). At present, within the central nervous system, these are generally subdivided into $N$-methyl-D-aspartate (NMDA), $\alpha$-amino-3-hydroxy-5-methyl-4-isoxazole-propionic acid (AMPA) and kainate receptors. The AMPA and kainate receptors are frequently grouped and referred to as non-NMDA receptors. The response of dLGN cells to visual stimulation is dependent on both NMDA and non-NMDA receptors. Selective blockade of either category of excitatory amino acid receptor can greatly reduce or eliminate the visual response of dLGN cells. The voltage dependence of effects mediated via the NMDA receptor following from the $Mg^{2+}$ blockade of its ionophore (Nowak et al., 1984) suggests the potential at the retino-geniculate synapse for a relatively complex pattern of interaction between the excitatory, inhibitory and neuromodulatory inputs. When a cell is hyperpolarised the $Mg^{2+}$ blockade of the NMDA ionophore could be regarded as effectively negating its contribution to the postsynaptic impact of neurotransmitter release from the terminals of retinal ganglion cells. As the cell depolarizes the $Mg^{2+}$ block of the NMDA ionophore is progressively disenabled. Thus a level of background depolarization is required for events mediated via the NMDA receptor to contribute to the transfer of visual information. This issue is of particular importance to our understanding of the dynamics of the visual response to moving and complex visual stimuli where there is an interplay between both inhibitory and excitatory inputs to the cell.

The influence of time linked excitatory and inhibitory feedback from the corticofugal system into this equation will be a significant factor in shaping the transfer of the visual input through the dLGN. The duration of NMDA mediated EPSPs allows time for integration with excitatory signals from the cortex. It seems likely that the corticofugal effects involve NMDA receptors (De Curtis et al., 1989; Deschenes and Hu, 1990; Scharfman et al., 1990) and presumably non-NMDA receptors. The effects of the cholinergic

modulatory input is very important to these processes underlying the transfer of retinal information. Acetylcholine depolarizes relay cells via a nicotinic mechanism (Sillito et al., 1983; McCormick and Prince, 1987, 1990; McCormick and Pape, 1988, 1990) and hyperpolarizes perigeniculate cells (Sillito et al., 1983; McCormick and

Action of ACh in dLNG

Action of ACh in visual cortex

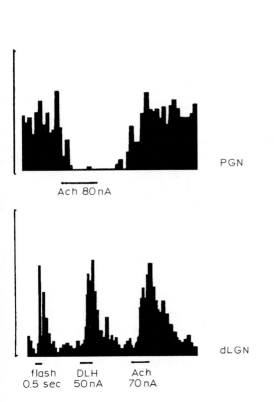

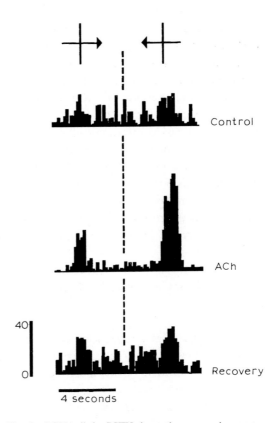

Fig. 7. Actions of acetylcholine (ACh) in PGN, dLGN and visual cortex. For the PGN cell the PSTH shows the averaged response (10 trials) to a 2 sec 80 nA pulse of iontophoretically applied ACh. The spontaneous activity of the cell is absolutely suppressed by the ACh application. Bin size is 200 msec and vertical calibration indicates range corresponding to 0–100 counts/bin. The record for the dLGN cell (on-centre Y cell) shows by contrast the powerful excitatory action of ACh (70 nA ejecting current) which is similar in impact to the response to an iontophoretic pulse of the excitatory amino acid D,L-homocysteate (50 nA) and a visually elicited input (0.5 sec flash located to the receptive field centre). Bin size is 400 msec and number of trials 2, vertical calibration as for PGN cell. The records for the visual cortex show the effect of ACh on the visual response of a layer IV simple cell to an optimally oriented bar passing forwards and backwards over the receptive field. Under control conditions this cell gave weak bidirectional responses to the stimulus. Iontophoretic application of ACh (20 nA) reduced the background activity and greatly increased the visual responses, but in particular enhanced the directional selectivity. This is likely to reflect two different components of action of ACh. Firstly, a direct excitation of adjacent inhibitory interneurons influencing background discharge and directional selectivity, and secondly, an action on the voltage dependent and calcium dependent potassium channels underlying the after hyperpolarization of the cell recorded from (see text for further discussion). The records are averaged for trials and plotted with 150 msec bins.

Prince, 1987, 1990) and intrinsic inhibitory interneurons via a muscarinic mechanism (McCormick and Pape, 1988). Examples of the effect of ACh on a perigeniculate cell and a dLGN relay cell are given in Fig. 7. The increased activity of the cholinergic input in the waking state will thus result in disinhibition and direct excitation of relay cells, consequently helping to enable NMDA receptor mediated effects. There are some contradictions in this. Although the cholinergic input may hyperpolarize inhibitory interneurons, the inhibitory mechanisms are not nullified by ACh or the enhanced cholinergic input in the waking state. In particular, short range inhibitory interactions appear to be very effective in the presence of ACh although long range processes are diminished (Sillito et al., 1983; Eysel et al., 1986; Murphy and Sillito, 1989). The potent non-dominant eye inhibition seen in Fig. 6 in the presence of continuous ACh application exemplifies this point. Clearly it would be surprising if the stimulus dependent inhibitory effects that shape visual responses were lost in the waking state, they are hardly likely to be significant during sleep.

### Triadic synapses and functional interactions in the dLGN

It is worth questioning our assumptions regarding the interactions that may take place at the triadic synapses on X cells. Firstly there is a puzzling feature regarding the organisation of the inhibitory events mediated by triadic synapses in the context of the receptive field properties of dLGN cells. A retinally driven feedforward inhibition at the triadic synapse would have the same spatial distribution in the field as the excitatory mechanism because it is driven by the excitatory mechanism. In short, it could not easily mediate the enhanced surround antagonism that seems to be one of the main features distinguishing the field of dLGN cells from retinal ganglion cells. This point is most clearly enunciated for those X cells that seem to be dominated by the input from

one retinal ganglion cell (Hamos et al., 1987). One is thus led to the view that surround mediated inhibition in these cells must come from the extraglomerular F1 terminals. The retinal afferent induced depolarization of the presynaptic dendrite might actually constitute a presynaptic inhibitory input serving to reduce a tonic inhibitory influence. The retinal drive to a relay cell would in this context enable its own disinhibition of an inhibitory control that might amongst other things, limit responses to descending corticofugal excitation. One consequence of this view would be that the short latency IPSP following the retinally mediated EPSP would have to be linked to an F1 terminal mediated input from the intrinsic inhibitory interneurons. Following through these arguments the interpretation of the hyperpolarizing influence of the cholinergic terminals on the presynaptic dendrites might not be disinhibitory in the most simple sense. There are several other issues that need to be placed in perspective. One concerns the evidence for lagged X cells (Mastronade, 1987a,b; Humphrey and Weller, 1988a,b). The case presented for these is that their visual responses to a contrast step (of a polarity that is excitatory) over their receptive field centre are lagged, so that instead of an early onset transient there may even be an inhibitory pause followed by a slow rise to a plateau in the response profile. This has been linked to the triadic synapses where the feedforward inhibition evoked by the high frequencies in the initial onset transient of the retinal input masks the excitatory response. Logically this is attractive because it fits the anatomical situation whereby the terminals driving the excitation drive the inhibition. As discussed earlier, it is difficult to equate effects mediated by these synapses with the enhanced surround antagonism seen in dLGN cell fields. The implication of this interpretation is that all the triad dominated cells have lagged fields, and that the dendrites of non-lagged X cells lack triadic synapses. This stands much of the earlier work linking X cells to triads on its head. If the triadic synapses evoke an inhibitory effect capable of suppressing the onset transient of the excitatory input from the retinal afferents, one would anticipate that the feedforward inhibitory input from these synapses would be faster or more potent than that seen in Y cells. It may turn out that the lagged response properties reflect a particular functional state of the geniculate circuitry. Taking up the issue that there is a cholinergic disinhibitory influence on the dLGN from the pedunculopontine tegmental nucleus, work from Sherman's laboratory has recently shown that activation of this system by electrical stimulation can "unlag" cells that seem to have a lagged type response profile. Certainly, if the cells were hyperpolarized initially, the NMDA receptor mediated component of the response might be very vulnerable to the feedforward inhibition and this could severely diminish the visual response (Sillito et al., 1990).

## Primary elements of the synaptic circuit in the visual cortex

The main neuronal types in the visual cortex are summarised in Fig. 8. The excitatory cells have spiny dendrites and are made up of pyramidal cells and spiny stellates, with the spiny stellates only occurring in layer IV. The inhibitory interneurons either lack dendritic spines or are sparsely spined, they can be broadly subdivided into basket cells, chandelier cells, neurogliaform cells and bitufted cells. The target distribution of inhibitory axon terminals varies with the type of inhibitory interneuron. For example, chandelier cells make synaptic contacts that appear to be restricted to the initial segment of pyramidal cells, whilst basket cells make contacts on the cell body and proximal dendrites. The neurogliaform and bitufted cells make contact only on dendritic shafts and spines with a bias to what appears to be small diameter distal dendritic processes (Somogyi, 1989). This suggests a discrete functional role for the different groups of inhibitory interneuron. Although it once seemed that inhibitory synapses were concentrated in the region

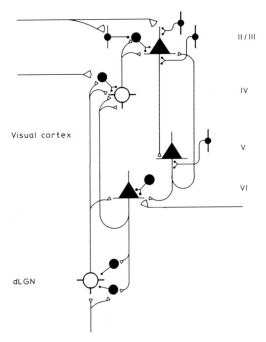

Fig. 8. Summary diagram to illustrate the nature of the pattern of connectivity seen in the visual cortex and its interactions with the dLGN. Pyramidal cells are shown as filled pyramids and other excitatory cells as open circles with three dendrites, all excitatory connections shown by open terminals. Inhibitory interneurons are shown as filled circles only or filled circles with two dendrites. All inhibitory contacts are shown by filled terminals. Long distance horizontal excitatory connections (e.g., between columns of similar orientation selectivity) are shown by large open terminals. Patterns of inhibitory contact include specific axo-axonic input from chandelier cells to pyramidal cells, basket cell type input to proximal dendrites and cell body and input from bitufted and neurogliaform cells to dendrites only. Note the presence of contacts between inhibitory interneurons and the circuit linking all layers of the cortex and the dLGN. Notional laminar locations are indicated to the right of the figure.

of the cell body, it is now clear (Somogyi, 1989) that the majority are directed to dendritic shafts (58%) and spines (26%) with smaller numbers on the cell body (13%) and initial segment (2.5%). Despite the substantial advances in our knowledge of the morphology of the circuitry and the place of inhibitory interneurons in it, the functional significance of much of the detail still eludes us. There is no simple linear sequence in the pattern of connections relaying information through the visual cortex. This point is made in

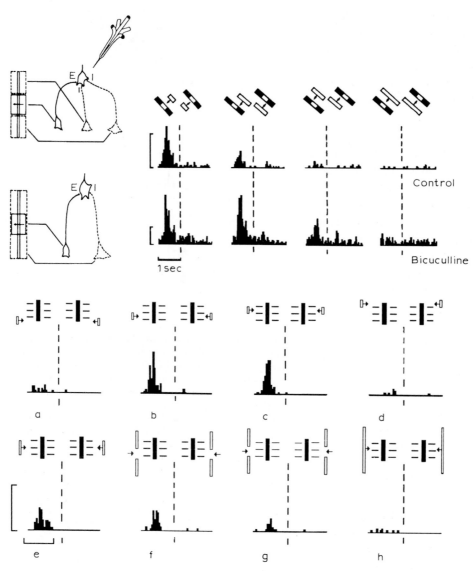

Fig. 9. Organisation of the hypercomplex cell receptive field and the role of inhibitory mechanisms. Concept diagram to the left of the figure summarises Hubel and Wiesel's original suggestions regarding the synaptic connections generating hypercomplex cell orientation tuning. The PSTHs to the right of this show a test of the model, by utilising iontophoretic application of bicuculline to block the inhibitory inputs to the cell. The hypercomplex cell receptive field is shown schematically above these records, with central excitatory region (open rectangle) and inhibitory end-zones (closed rectangles). The visual stimulus used to test this field is shown by the open bar and arrow. Bicuculline application (50 nA) reduces the strength of the end-inhibition, particularly to one side of the field, but does not block the length tuning. The cell still fails to respond to the bar extended to either side of the field, suggesting a length tuned excitatory input. Records averaged for 25 trials. Bin size is 50 msec and vertical calibrations indicate range corresponding to 0–25 counts/bin. The lower records attempt to dissect out the organisation of the inhibitory and excitatory zones in the hypercomplex cell field with a sequence of different moving stimuli as depicted by the schematic outlines above each PSTH. The receptive field is shown as a solid rectangle. Whilst short stimuli elicit excitatory responses from two central locations in the field (b,c), stimulation of both these together fails to reveal summation and produces a response smaller than that seen to stimulation of either alone (e). A stimulus which extends to cover putative end-zones, but excludes the primary excitatory discharge centre of the field (f,g) actually produces an excitatory response, maximum inhibition is only seen when the stimulus actually drives the field centre mechanism as well (h). Details as for PSTHs above. Records adapted from Sillito and Versiani, 1977, and Sillito, 1977a. For further discussion see text.

Fig. 8 for the excitatory connections between the cortical laminae and between visual cortex and dorsal lateral geniculate nucleus (dLGN). The representation here is highly simplified but it draws attention to the multiple connections between laminae and the mixture of feedforward and feedback interactions. These broad patterns of connectivity involve both excitatory and inhibitory elements. For example the connections made by layer VI cell axons are to both inhibitory and excitatory cells in layer IV and to both relay cells and inhibitory interneurons in the dLGN. The possible function of these connections will be considered in some detail here.

## The contribution of inhibitory mechanisms and connections from layer VI cells in the generation of length tuning

The hypercomplex or endstopped receptive field was the first attribute of visual cortical cell response properties to be clearly linked to a model involving inhibitory interneurons in the original work of Hubel and Wiesel (1965, 1968). In their hierarchical scheme these cells were seen as a processing step beyond the level of complex cells. They suggested two possible synaptic mechanisms and these are summarised in Fig. 9. These involve a cell with a short excitatory receptive field receiving inhibitory input from either a single cell with an overlapping but longer receptive field, or two cells with receptive fields displaced to either side of the excitatory field. In both cases elongation of a stimulus beyond the excitatory field would increase the magnitude of the inhibitory input converging on the hypercomplex cell. The first direct test of this hypothesis came from iontophoretic experiments examining the effect of bicuculline on the responses of hypercomplex cells in layers II and III of area 17 (Sillito and Versiani, 1977). The data from these experiments was interesting because hypercomplex cell length tuning was reduced by inhibitory blockade, but was not eliminated, suggesting the presence of a length tuned excitatory input. An example of the

effects of inhibitory blockade on one of the cells examined in this work is given in Fig. 9. Inspection of this figure also reveals marked asymmetries in the strength of the two inhibitory end zones (Hubel and Wiesel, 1965: Sillito and Versiani, 1977; Orban et al., 1979a,b). It is clear in Fig. 9 that extension of the bar to one side of the excitatory zone provokes a much bigger response reduction than extension to the other. In many cases these data certainly cannot be simply accounted for by spatially discrete inhibitory fields of differing strength. In the majority of superficial layer hypercomplex cells the inhibitory and excitatory mechanisms overlap (Sillito, 1977a). This is illustrated in the lower section of Fig. 9 which shows the results of an experiment which dissects the field of a hypercomplex cell by first mapping its responses with short stimuli and then exploring the responses to longer stimuli. The records trace the responses to a short, optimally oriented bar through four locations covering the apparent extent of the excitatory field. Each produce some excitatory response, but the main excitatory responses are obtained from the two central locations. Stimulating both these central locations together however, does not produce response summation, in fact there is a reduction in response magnitude. A bar gap stimulus, with the gap centred over two successive locations in the two central zones, produces excitatory responses in both cases. The maximum "end-zone" effect only being obtained when the centre as well as the end-zones of the field are stimulated with an uninterrupted bar. These observations seem best explained by an inhibitory field overlying the excitatory field with a slightly shallower length summation curve than the excitatory field. The cell generating the inhibitory field would give a maximal response only when the centre of its field is stimulated, hence the effects shown in records f–h. As the inhibitory blockade reduced but did not eliminate the length tuning of these cells (Sillito and Versiani, 1977) it seems that the field must be constructed from a length tuned excitatory input reinforced by an additional inhibitory mechanism in the superficial layers. The effects in Fig. 9 would reflect synaptic processes operating at two levels.

The presence of a length tuned excitatory input to superficial layer hypercomplex cells is in accord with the demonstration that many layer IV simple family cells also have "hypercomplex fields". Although at variance with the Hubel and Wiesel's suggested location of hypercomplex cells at a stage beyond complex cells in their proposed serial processing sequence, simple type cells in layers II/III, IV and VI can have strongly length tuned fields. In layer IV, which receives the major component of the input from the dLGN, the length tuning of simple cells might be considered to follow at least in part from the length tuning of dLGN cells. Interestingly, recent work has laid emphasis on intracortical circuitry involving layer VI cells. These cells sit in a critical location regulating both the transfer of visual information through the dLGN and the access of that information to the cortex (see summary, Fig. 8). Examples of their subcortical effects have already been discussed. It is known from intracellular electrophysiological studies that layer VI cells can exert both excitatory and inhibitory effects in layer IV cells (Ferster and Lindstrom, 1984a,b). However, in terms of a contribution to visual processing, considerable emphasis has been given to the capacity for layer VI cells to drive inhibitory interneurons in layer IV. In particular Bolz and Gilbert (1986) reported results suggesting that layer VI cells may establish the end-inhibition generating the length tuning layer IV hypercomplex cells. The logic for this view lay in the original surmise of McGuire et al. (1984) that layer VI cell collaterals arborising in layer IV terminated primarily on the smooth dendritic processes of what seemed likely to be inhibitory interneurons. This, linked to Gilbert's (1977) finding that layer VI cells have the longest receptive fields found in the striate cortex, led to the conclusion that cells with long receptive fields provided a predominantly inhibitory influence on layer IV. This connection from VI to IV seemed

to be the realisation of the circuit illustrated in Fig. 9. To test this issue, Bolz and Gilbert used microinjection of GABA to block the activity of layer VI cells whilst studying the response properties of length tuned layer IV cells. They observed that layer IV cells lost their length tuning during the blockade of layer VI. This appeared to reflect the loss of an inhibitory input generating the hypercomplex cell end-zone inhibition because the excitatory responses to short bars were unchanged. Similar effects were seen for length tuned layer III cells and they proposed that these received their excitatory drive from length tuned layer IV cells. This view is in accord with the data obtained from inhibitory blockade (Sillito and Versiani, 1977).

Although this link of cortical circuitry to visual response properties seems compelling it raises a number of questions. One immediate problem is whether the $8°$ or more long receptive fields of layer VI cells, proposed by Bolz and Gilbert to drive the inhibitory mechanism in the hypercomplex cell receptive field, are in fact appropriate to the task. Careful quantitative study of simple type hypercomplex cells (Kato et al., 1978; Yamane et al., 1985) suggests that the spatial extent of the inhibitory end zone region is much more restricted than that which would derive from an input summing to $8°$ or more. Specifically, the central excitatory region is on average $1.5°$ in length (Kato et al., 1978) and the maximum response reduction occurs when the stimulus is increased in length by a further $1.3°$ (Yamane et al., 1985). This implies a very steep slope in the curve for the decrement in response with length. Thus the inhibitory input would appear to be driven by a mechanism exhibiting its primary rise in response magnitude for stimulus lengths in the range $1.5-2.8°$. Alternatively, if the end inhibition were derived from the summed action of separate inhibitory fields, offset to either end of a central excitatory zone (Fig. 9), the mechanisms driving these two inhibitory fields would need to show an even more rapid rise in response magnitude. In this latter case, the major change in response magnitude should occur for lengths up to 0.7°, or slightly more according to the degree of overlap of the two zones with the central excitatory field. Thus the logical link between hypercomplex cell inhibitory fields and layer VI cells with long receptive fields is not compelling. If layer VI cells do provide a contribution to the inhibitory fields of layer IV hypercomplex cells, one would expect them to have short receptive fields appropriate to the mechanisms identified by Yamane et al. (1985). Interestingly, a recent quantitative study suggests that many do indeed have such short fields (Grieve and Sillito, 1990a, 1991) with 61% of the population showing summation to 4° or less. Thus there is a capacity in layer VI to generate the necessary drive for end-zone inhibition.

One of the puzzling features of the layer VI blockade data reported by Bolz and Gilbert is that it only revealed effects on inhibitory mechanisms in layer IV. It is clear from anatomical (Somogyi, 1989) and electrophysiological studies (Ferster and Lindstrom, 1984a,b) that there is the potential for significant excitatory drive. The anatomical data suggest that only 14% of layer VI cell terminals contact GABAergic cells suggesting a strong bias towards connections on excitatory interneurons. Indeed, in contradistinction to Bolz and Gilbert, further work indicates that localised blockade of layer VI cells does reveal changes commensurate with the loss of an excitatory drive to cells in the overlying layer IV (Grieve and Sillito, 1990b, 1991). In these experiments, blockade of layer VI was produced by localised iontophoretic application of either GABA or the potent $GABA_A$ receptor agonist, muscimol. A multibarreled iontophoretic electrode and a tungsten in glass recording electrode were carefully aligned so that they sampled cells in layers VI and IV with receptive fields of the same orientation selectivity and location in visual space. During blockade of layer VI two patterns of effect were observed on length tuned cells in the overlying layers III and IV. Either the visual responses to all stimuli were reduced in a non-specific man-

ner, or the responses to the short optimal length stimuli were selectively reduced with respect to those to the longer non-optimal stimuli. None of the cells studied revealed a selective increase in the responses to longer length non-optimal stimuli commensurate with a loss of end-zone inhibition. This applied even in cases where the blockade of layer VI was continued until there were direct effects on layer IV cell excitability. Where the responses to the shorter stimuli were selectively reduced, the length tuning was in turn reduced, but this followed from the relative reduction of short as opposed to long bar responses (Fig. 10). This suggests the loss of an excitatory influence from layer VI cells with short receptive fields and the ideas are summarised in the diagram of Fig. 10. The data would thus seem to be explained by a facilitatory input from layer VI cells to hypercomplex cells in the immediately overlying layer IV with overlapping receptive fields. The relative "resistance" of the responses to longer length stimuli may well reflect the presence of horizontally directed facilitatory inputs from more remote regions of layer VI or IV. These could be activated by the ends of the elongated stimulus driving cells in laterally displaced columns of similar orientation selectivity. It is already known that there are horizontal facilitatory connections between columns of similar orientation selectivity (Tso et al., 1986; Gilbert and Wiesel, 1989; Engel et al., 1990). The cases where the responses to both the optimal short stimuli and the long stimuli declined together could reflect cells that lack longer distance facilitatory inputs.

Although many of the available findings seem to present contradictory views of the inhibitory processes underlying the generation of length tuned receptive fields, there are many common themes which begin to generate a coherent overview. A major component of the excitatory input from the dLGN to the cortex seems to be length tuned (Schiller et al., 1976; Rose, 1979; Cleland et al., 1983; Jones and Sillito, 1987, 1991), thus there is no need to identify a special mecha-

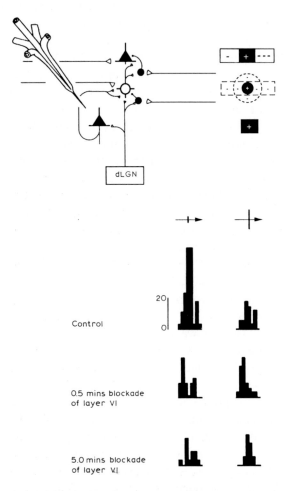

Fig. 10. Exploration of the effect of blocking layer VI cells on the length tuning of a hypercomplex cell in layer IV. Schematic diagram at the top of the figure summarises some of the connections that may be involved. PSTHs document the responses to a short optimal length bar and a long bar crossing the receptive field. Blockade of layer VI by iontophoretic application of the GABA$_A$ agonist muscimol (25 nA) for 0.5 minutes reduces the response to the short bar but has no significant effect on the response to the long bar. Continued application of muscimol to 5.0 minutes causes a further reduction in the short bar response and a slight reduction of the long bar response. Schematic receptive fields to the right of the circuit diagram summarise some of the influences that may underlie these effects. The primary suggestion is that an excitatory drive from layer VI cells with receptive fields showing rapid spatial summation provide the critical stimulus locked facilitation to enable the layer IV cell to overcome feedforward inhibitory influences. See the text and discussion of Fig. 11 for further explanation. PSTHs averaged for 5 trials and bin size is 150 msec.

nism to establish length tuning in cortical cells. Indeed, the converse really applies, the problem is how it may be eliminated. Hypercomplex cells outside layer IV seem to receive a length tuned excitatory input (Sillito and Versiani, 1977) and this could derive either from layer IV hypercomplex cells or a direct input from length tuned dLGN cells. There is strong evidence for the view that intracortical inhibitory mechanisms contribute to the inhibitory influences in cortical hypercomplex cell receptive fields (Sillito and Versiani, 1977; Sillito, 1977; Kato et al., 1978; Orban et al., 1979a,b). The length selectivity of layer IV cells could be enhanced in the cortex by any inhibitory mechanism that decreased the excitability of layer IV hypercomplex cells, so that only the maximal response point in the length tuning curve of the geniculate input drove them to threshold. The available data suggest that intracortical excitatory interactions are important here (Ferster and Lindstrom, 1984a,b; Grieve and Sillito, 1991). The geniculate input would drive both layer IV cells and layer VI cells. The stimulus locked nature of the facilitatory input from layer VI to layer IV seems to be a critical factor in establishing the level of summation necessary for the expression of the full excitatory response in layer IV hypercomplex type simple cells. It is important to note that the corticofugal projection from layer VI to the dLGN seems to enhance the length tuning of the input dLGN cells by increasing the gain of inhibitory mechanisms acting on them (Murphy and Sillito, 1987). These same layer VI cells provide the recurrent projection to layer IV, and their apical dendrites pass up to layer IV where they can collect input from both geniculate afferents and the terminals of intracortical cells. They also receive input from geniculate afferents to layer VI. From this viewpoint it is apparent that we are looking at the function of a circuit with interlinked elements. In this circuit, the layer VI cells seem to play a crucial role in regulating the access of visual information to the cortex by their subcortical influence on the responses of dLGN cells and their cortical influence at the primary site of termination of dLGN cell axons in layer IV. The stress here on a facilitatory influence in layer IV and an inhibitory influence in the dLGN is consistent with biases suggested by the anatomical evidence and much of the recent physiological data. The overall balance of the two patterns of effect would seem to be complementary and clearly has interesting functional consequences. The suggestions discussed here are summarised in Fig. 11.

In the cortex, cells with hypercomplex fields are not in reality a sharply defined subgroup, but one end of a spectrum of cells extending from those with very powerful end-stopped fields to those with none (e.g., Rose, 1979; Yamane et al., 1985). Consideration of the mechanisms underlying the generation of their response properties is possibly better placed in the perspective of those processes that may contribute to the fields of cells showing little or no end stopping in their fields. The end stopping of dLGN cells poses an interesting problem for models of the synaptic convergence underlying non-length tuned fields. Were the input to a simple cell to derive from a single geniculate cell or a group of geniculate cells with strongly overlapping fields, it is immediately apparent that it would have an end-stopped receptive field. However, the geniculate input to layer IV spiny cells forms only a small part of their excitatory input, the rest derives from intracortical sources. In the orientation domain, the primary long distance excitatory connections occur between columns of similar orientation selectivity (Tso et al., 1986; Gilbert and Wiesel, 1989; Engel et al., 1990). Thus extending the length of a bar along the axis of the optimal orientation of a cell will elicit facilitatory effects from columns of similar orientation. Clearly this type of connection would serve to offset the decrement in response from the primary geniculate input. Thus varying the strength of these laterally directed excitatory influences gives the capability of varying degrees of reduction in the length tuning of cortical cells. An alternative view is that the input to a layer IV spiny cell derives

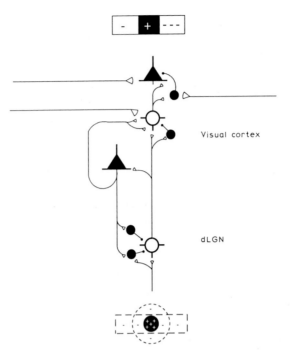

Fig. 11. Schematic diagram summarising some of the factors that may contribute to length tuning. Centre-surround antagonism in the dLGN cell receptive field following from both the retinal input characteristics and intrageniculate GABAergic inhibitory mechanisms establishes the first stage of length tuning. Feedback from layer VI cells in the visual cortex to the GABAergic inhibitory interneurons enhances the inhibitory drive attenuating the response to longer bars. This is summarised by the circular (subcortical) and rectangular (cortically derived) inhibitory fields in the receptive field schematic at the bottom of the figure. The input from dLGN to cortex carries these influences forward and provides direct excitatory input to layer IV simple cells and a disynaptic inhibitory drive via GABAergic cells. The collateral excitatory input from layer VI to IV reinforces excitatory responses to short bar lengths. Thus length tuning is established at the level of the dLGN and modulated by an intracortical thresholding inhibition and selective facilitation at short bar lengths. Longer distance excitatory connections from columns of similar orientation selectivity may provide either facilitatory or inhibitory drive strengthening or weakening the end-zone influences to one or the other side of the field. See text for further discussion.

from a group of dLGN cells with receptive fields forming a row through visual space along the axis of the optimal orientation. This type of arrangement is frequently considered to account for the mechanisms establishing orientation tuned fields in layer IV (Hubel and Wiesel, 1962). A short bar moving over the centre of the receptive field of the input dLGN cell contributing to the centre of the simple cell field, would evoke a maximal response from the input cell. Increasing stimulus length would cause a decline in the response from the central input cell but start to recruit input from adjacent input cells, however their input in turn would decline as bar length further increased. To avoid response decline at longer bar lengths it is necessary to increase the number of input cells or synaptic weighting for locations displaced from the simple cell receptive field centre. This has the corollary that two short bars spatially displaced from the centre and moved over the ends of the field would evoke strong responses; this does not appear to happen. Mapping the field of a simple cell with small stationary flashing stimuli shows that the primary excitatory effects are elicited from the central region of the field and are not balanced by strong inputs from the ends (e.g., Creutzfeldt et al., 1974b; Jones and Palmer, 1987). Thus from the geniculate data one would predict length tuning in these cells because the drive from their input will fall as stimulus length increases. Many of such cells do not show length tuned fields. The conclusion here must be that a long stimulus provokes effects in the circuitry that are not revealed by short stimuli. Time locked facilitatory inputs from columns of similar orientation selectivity, such that there is optimal summation between the events elicited from these and those from the reduced drive from the receptive field centre, may be the issue here (see Fig. 11).

## Orientation specific inhibition

Possibly the greatest controversy regarding the function of GABAergic mechanisms in the visual cortex centres around their role in the generation of orientation tuned receptive fields. The classical model of Hubel and Wiesel (1962) suggested that orientation selectivity was established by the alignment of the receptive fields of the dLGN cells providing the convergent excitatory input to individual simple cells in layer IV of the cortex. In one way or another this view has held to the present day. It was first challenged by the intracellular and electrophysiological analysis carried out by Creutzfeldt's laboratory (Creutzfeldt and Ito, 1968; Creutzfeldt et al., 1974a,b). These experiments emphasised the importance of inhibitory mechanisms to the responses of visual cortical cells and provided evidence indicating that the receptive fields of some cortical cells were virtually circular despite their orientation tuning. The latter led to the suggestion that intracortical inhibition was structuring the response of these cells in the orientation domain with the logical consequence that the inhibition would be maximal at 90° to the cells optimal orientation. However, this interpretation, based largely on an appraisal of receptive field shape, had to be balanced by their intracellular observations. They noted "....in most cells, inhibition as well as excitation appeared to be less marked during stimulation in the non-optimal orientation......" (Creutzfedlt et al., 1974b). A simplistic interpretation of Hubel and Wiesel's early model would predict just this observation. This paradox has been central to much of the subsequent debate in the field. The focus of the debate was sharpened by experiments using iontophoretic application of the GABA antagonist bicuculline to produce a localised block of GABA mediated inhibitory processes acting on visual cortical cells (Sillito, 1974, 1975, 1977a,b, 1979, 1984; Sillito et al., 1980; Tsumoto et al., 1979). As in the dLGN this approach allowed the possibility of reversibly ascertaining the effect of inhibitory blockade on orientation tuning. GABA exerts a very potent inhibitory effect on the responses of visual cortical cells as the example given on the top right section of Fig. 12 illustrates. This action is reversed by iontophoretic application of Nmb. During such inhibitory blockade the data showed that orientation selectivity in virtually all cortical cells could be reduced and in some it could be eliminated. For complex cells about half the population showed a broadening of the orientation

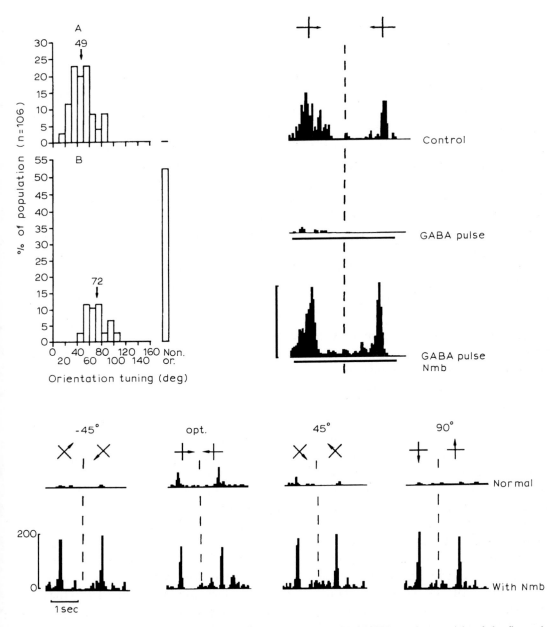

Fig. 12. Influence of GABAergic mechanisms on orientation tuning. The PSTHs to the top right of the figure document the powerful suppressive effect that GABA (15 nA pulse as marked by bar under middle record) has on the excitatory response of cortical cells to an optimal stimulus and the effectiveness of iontophoretically applied Nmb in blocking this (70 nA ejecting current). PSTHs averaged for 25 trials and plotted with 20 msec bins. Vertical calibration indicates range corresponding to 0–100 counts/bin. The histogram to the left of the figure shows the distribution of orientation tuning in a population of 106 complex cells before (A) and during inhibitory blockade (B). The orientation tuning of the cells is derived from the width of the tuning curve at half height. Cells losing orientation tuning during bicuculline application are shown in the "Non or" column to the right of the figure (B). Arrows show median orientation tuning for those cells showing selectivity. The lower set of PSTHs show responses of a simple cell to a moving bar of varying orientation before and during inhibitory blockade. Vertical calibration indicates range for 0–200 counts/50 msec bin. See text for discussion of the effect.

tuning and half changes that essentially eliminated the original bias (Sillito, 1979). This is summarised by the histograms in the top left section of Fig. 12. In the case of simple cells their orientation tuning seemed to be more resistant to inhibitory blockade and early experiments showed only a broadening of the orientation tuning curve (Sillito, 1974, 1975). However more potent blockade of their inhibitory inputs (Tsumoto et al., 1979; Sillito et al., 1980) clearly eliminated orientation tuning. In many cases the response profiles observed during the blockade resembled those of a dLGN cell (Sillito et al., 1980). An example of the effect of inhibitory blockade on a simple cell is given in the lower part of Fig. 12. This data supported the view that inhibitory mechanisms played a crucial role in establishing the orientation tuning of cells in the visual cortex.

The next major contribution to the debate came from the work of Ferster (1986, 1987, see also Chapter 20) who extended the original intracellular techniques of Creutzfeldt's laboratory and showed essentially the same point, stimuli crossing the receptive field at orientations orthogonal to the optimal elicited few EPSPs and IPSPs. If intracortical inhibition were shaping orientation tuning in the simple manner envisaged, it is logical to anticipate both EPSPs and IPSPs in response to this stimulus. One of the paradoxes is that various studies (Sillito, 1979; Ramoa et al., 1986; Morrone et al., 1982, 1986) have demonstrated a cross-orientation suppression of elevated background discharge levels produced either by conditioning visual stimuli or iontophoretic application of an excitatory amino acid. Nonetheless, Ferster's data in conjunction with that of Creutzfeldt underline the inability of anyone so far to detect effective cross-orientation inhibition from intracellular recordings (see also Berman et al., Chapter 21). One possibility is that the inhibition is primarily of a shunting type on remote dendritic locations and not easily detectable at the cell body. This does not seem to be the case (Douglas et al., 1988). Were cross-orientation inhibition to occur it would require

connections between columns of differing or even orthogonal orientation. The bulk of the available evidence, from cross correlation studies (Tso et al., 1986; Gilbert and Wiesel, 1989; Engel et al., 1990) and anatomical reconstruction of patterns of connectivity, has suggested that the major connections are made between columns of like orientation and end on spiny not smooth cells (Martin, 1988). There are two points here, one concerns the dominance of connections between columns of like orientation and the other the fact that these connections favour excitatory not inhibitory interneurons. The only major exception is a paper by Matsubara et al. in area 18 (1985) which presents evidence consistent with cross-orientation connections between columns, but this pattern has not been seen in area 17, at least for the long distance interactions between columns. On balance, the anatomical evidence, and that from cross correlation studies, would seem superficially to support the evidence obtained from the intracellular investigations in area 17. As always the situation is more complex, and in attempting to isolate the likely role of inhibitory mechanisms in orientation selectivity it is necessary to consider a number of other observations including recent work from Eysel's laboratory reported in detail in this volume (Eysel et al., 1990; Eysel, Chapter 19). In one group of these experiments the iontophoretic application of GABA at a series of locations surrounding a cell produces marked changes in the orientation tuning of that cell. In particular this local inactivation of adjacent groups of cortical cells reveals excitatory responses in the cell under study to orientations that were previously ineffective. It is difficult to avoid the conclusion that the GABA application is switching off a neural influence on the cell studied that is suppressing responses to some orientations. A simple interpretation here is that it is a cross-orientation inhibitory influence. To back up this possibility, anatomical data from the same laboratory provides evidence for inhibitory connections between cells/columns of differing orientation selectivity (see Kisvarday, Chapter 18).

Whilst this may seem to contradict the anatomical and electrophysiological evidence referred to above, it addresses a level of analysis that the previous work overlooked. In essence, the major documentation available previously from both the correllograms (Tso et al., 1986) and the anatomical studies (Gilbert and Wiesel, 1989) looked at connections that extended beyond the domain of the patch of orientation columns concerned with a given location in visual space. The new anatomical data from Eysel's laboratory addresses the local connections that appear to fall within the domain of the orientation columns subserving one location in visual space. Here it seems there may be the morphological basis for cross-orientation inhibition. These findings are in many ways complementary to those obtained by the use of iontophoretically applied GABA. They do not seem to match the intracellular observations.

There are several other issues that need to be highlighted. Firstly, emphasis should be given to that fact that orientation selectivity does not depend on mechanisms operating in layer IV of the visual cortex. Experiments from Malpeli's laboratory (Malpeli et al., 1981, 1986; Malpeli, 1983) have shown that selective blockade of the geniculate input driving layer IV and VI cells, leaves many cells in layers II,III and V with apparently normal orientation tuned fields. Thus the mechanism for generating orientation selectivity would seem to be expressed independently in several laminar locations, a view which matches conclusions drawn from the earlier data obtained with GABA blockade (Sillito, 1979, 1984; Sillito et al., 1980). Is the conjectured pattern of dLGN cell convergence on simple cells, with input fields staggered in a row through visual space (Hubel and Wiesel, 1962) necessary to the generation of orientation tuning? The link between the spatial alignment of the convergent geniculate input fields and the orientation selectivity of a cortical cell is not as clearly defined as is sometimes suggested. This issue was first raised by the data from Creutzfeldt's laboratory. Certainly the excitatory fields of simple cells can be elongated, but

the excitatory effects elicited from the portions of the field extending away from the centre along the axis of the optimal orientation are much weaker than those from the centre (e.g., Jones and Palmer, 1987). This point has been discussed above with respect to length tuned and non-length tuned cells in the cortex and has implications to the mechanisms generating orientation selectivity. For example, where there is considerable overlap of a number of geniculate input fields driving the central zone of a simple cell field, one would expect a short orthogonally oriented bar moving over the field to evoke a geniculate input of similar magnitude to that seen from a longer but optimally oriented stimulus. During inhibitory blockade causing an elimination of orientation tuning, the excitatory discharge profiles of simple cell fields revealed by moving bars of differing orientation frequently appear similar to that for single dLGN cells (Sillito et al., 1980). This conclusion is interesting because a small spot moving over the receptive field of simple and complex cells can elicit excitatory responses for a direction of motion that is orthogonal to that of an optimally oriented bar, and the magnitude of these approaches that of the optimal bar response (Worgotter and Eysel, 1989).

Considering the profile of output from the dLGN to cortex, it is apparent that the length tuning of dLGN cells will result in a minimal output to cortex from those dLGN cells covered by the centre of the bar and with the strongest output from fields at the ends of the bar where only part of the surround mechanism is covered by the stimulus. These end inputs should be driving the central regions of the fields of cortical cells with similar orientation, but a location spatially shifted along the axis of the optimal orientation. It is at this point that the intracortical connections from columns of like orientation selectivity may be critical. The time locked facilitation from the intracortical connections interacting with the reduced drive from the dLGN cells at a level that enables the cell response. A stimulus rotated away from the optimal orientation loses this facilitation and the cell responds little if at all. An orthogonally oriented bar, reduced in length until it is a spot, will evoke a powerfully excitatory input from the input dLGN cells and drive the cortical cell (Worgotter and Eysel, 1989). Increasing its length will radically reduce the magnitude of the dLGN input cell responses because of their length tuning, and will not bring in any compensatory intracortical facilitation because the ends of the bar are not activating the correct columns. At this point it is clear that the excitatory input from an incorrectly oriented bar would be low, much as the intracellular studies show. The critical issue is the intracortical facilitation and the threshold for the effectiveness of this may be modulated by feedforward inhibitory effects driven by dLGN terminals which also contact non-spiny GABAergic cells. The input from these, for the same reasons, could be greater for optimal orientations. In this argument the two critical issues are the length tuning of dLGN cells and the intracortical facilitatory connections be-

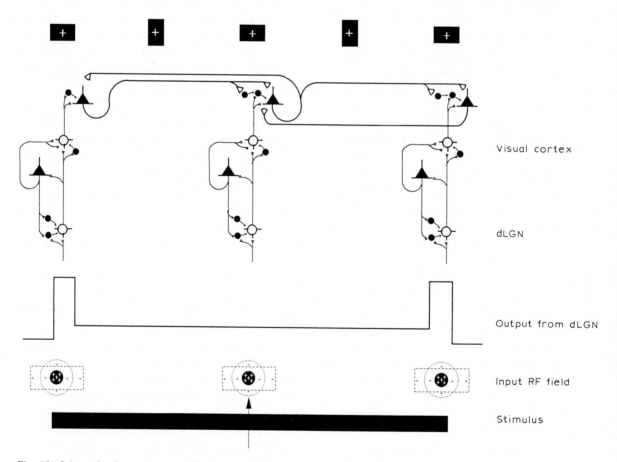

Fig. 13. Schematic diagram summarising some of the connections that might influence orientation tuning, but excluding connections underlying cross-orientation inhibition. The primary suggestion that feedforward inhibition depresses the response to the input from the dLGN and that full excitatory response to a long bar depend on time locked facilitation and disinhibition from columns of similar orientation preference (determined by the pattern of connectivity in the cortical map of visual space). The input to the cortex driven by a moving bar will involve a low profile of dLGN cell activity elicited from fields underlying the middle portion of the bar (because of the cells length tuning) and a peak from those fields at the end of the bar. Cells in these columns activated by the ends of the stimulus interact in a network effect with those receiving the time locked but lower level drive from the dLGN fields under the middle of the bar. See text for further discussion. Conventions and details of the figure as for earlier schematics in the review.

tween columns of like orientation. Although this may seem to require orientation selectivity to be set up in other columns to achieve the facilitation, in the first instance one need not regard the columns as orientation tuned, but simply strongly connected points on a map of visual space in the cortex which are simultaneously activated by a bar of particular orientation. The orientation follows from this pattern of excitatory connection across the cortex, the length tuning of the dLGN input and local thresholding feedforward inhibition. These interactions involve the corticofugal feedback to the geniculate inhibitory circuitry enhancing length tuning as well as the intracortical connections. They are summarised in Fig. 13. Other patterns of influence need to be considered in this and, for example, particularly the mechanisms influencing directional selectivity. The directional selectivity that cortical cells exhibit for an optimally oriented bar could derive either from inhibitory or facilitatory influences feeding forward through visual space. There are theoretical arguments for both of these (Barlow and Levick, 1965) and intracellular and pharmacological evidence to support them (Creutzfeldt et al., 1974; Sillito, 1977b; Sato et al., 1990; see work from Eysel discussed in this volume). The tuning of the directional influences and the orientation dependent interactions are not necessarily matched (Hammond et al., 1975; Hammond and Pomfret, 1990) so that the final response profile of a cell to a moving bar will reflect several sets of mechanisms with an optimum response compromised by both.

### Interaction between inhibitory, excitatory and neuromodulatory mechanisms in the visual cortex

As in the dLGN, both $GABA_A$ and $GABA_B$ receptor mediated effects are seen in visual cortical cells. The $GABA_A$ receptor mediates a rapid and large increase in chloride conductance (Connors et al., 1990; Avoli, 1986, see also Connors, Chapter 16). This can produce both hyperpolariz-

ing and depolarizing effects. The balance of the evidence favours the view that hyperpolarizing effects are elicited from the soma whilst depolarizing effects are associated with the dendritic membrane (Scharfman and Sarvey, 1985, 1987, 1988; Connors et al., 1990). A number of explanations have been offered for this, but the most economical is the suggestion that the intracellular chloride concentration is substantially higher in the dendrites than in the soma. The $GABA_B$ receptor is linked to a slow longer lasting hyperpolarization thought to reflect a small selective increase in potassium conductance (Avoli, 1986; Howe et al., 1987; Connors et al., 1990). The functional implications of these GABA mediated effects are likely to be different. The fast hyperpolarizing action can be logically linked to precisely timed inhibitory processes controlling cell responsiveness to excitatory inputs. This would be important in the mechanisms associated with the fast ongoing processing of visual information (Sillito, 1984). By contrast, the slower time course of the $GABA_B$ receptor mediated hyperpolarization would not seem to be compatible with the time linked dynamics of sensory processing. However it may influence a cell's transfer properties by virtue of its impact on resting membrane potential and input conductance (Connors et al., 1990). It has been suggested by Connors et al. (1990) that for neocortical pyramidal cells it would tend to reduce background firing rates and responses to weak excitatory stimuli, whilst leaving responses to strong transient stimuli unimpaired. The $GABA_A$ mediated dendritic depolarization would exert a localised shunting inhibition at the location of the GABA synapses on the dendrites, but might facilitate inputs from more remote dendritic locations.

The details of these different actions of GABA need to be placed in the perspective of both the patterns of axonal termination characterising each class of inhibitory interneuron and of potential differences in the distribution of $GABA_A$ and $GABA_B$ receptors over the target neurons. The chandelier cells contacting initial segments of pyramidal cells might be presumed to evoke the strongest clamp over neuronal responses of any type of inhibitory interneuron in the visual cortex. Interestingly, the evidence so far available suggests that whilst $GABA_A$ receptors are present on dendrites, dendritic spines and cell bodies of pyramidal cells, they are not found on the initial segments (Somogyi, 1989). The same constraints apply to this latter point as discussed above for the apparent absence of $GABA_A$ receptors on intrageniculate inhibitory interneurons. Nonetheless, if there is a lack of $GABA_A$ receptors on the initial segment, the nature of the inhibitory control at this location may be more concerned with level setting of transfer properties than with a fast pre-emptive regulation of neuronal output. Following from this it is not clear on theoretical grounds, even assuming the existence of $GABA_A$ receptor mediated effects on the initial segment, that the inhibition here would be effective against strong excitation (Douglas and Martin, 1990). Similar comments apply to $GABA_A$ receptor mediated effects on the cell body and proximal dendrites. This is interesting because it requires GABA mediated inhibitory effects to exert their influence via the control of weak excitatory effects in the neocortical circuitry, which in the absence of such control would develop in an interactive sense through the circuit to precipitate a strong excitatory response (Douglas et al., 1989). The distribution of $GABA_A$ receptors surprisingly reveals a higher proportion on GABA-ergic neurons than pyramidal cells (Somogyi, 1989). If this is any indication of the functional strength of inhibitory influences it would seem to imply that GABA mediated disinhibition is a very important component of the cortical circuitry. Of course the presence of excitatory synapses on the soma of GABA cells might in itself necessitate a higher density of inhibitory terminals for effective control of the cell's activity.

The excitatory interactions in the neocortex and visual cortex involve NMDA and non-NMDA receptors (Tsumoto et al., 1986; Tsumoto, 1990; Kisvarday et al., 1988; Jones and Baughman, 1988;

Shirokawa et al., 1989; Fox et al., 1989, 1990). However, it seems likely that in the adult, NMDA receptor mediated effects play a small role in the visually driven responses of layer IV cells, although they are an important component of visually driven excitatory events outside layer IV. Where NMDA receptors do play a role in visual responses the duration of the EPSP provides a broader window of excitation for the correlation of effects from several inputs to a cell. Their voltage dependency introduces a further facet to our understanding of the potential impact of inhibitory inputs in terms of suppressing the regenerative development of an excitatory response that can follow the initiation of effects via NMDA receptors. The pattern of influence of the cholinergic system on the cortical circuitry is somewhat different to that seen in the dLGN. There is a direct depolarising influence on inhibitory interneurons which can drive a discharge and will contribute to their normal background activity (McCormick and Prince, 1985). In addition pyramidal cell responses are modulated via an action on the voltage dependent potassium channel underlying the M current and the calcium dependent potassium channel (Halliwell and Adams, 1982; Benardo and Prince, 1982; McCormick and Prince, 1985, 1990; McCormick et al., 1985). In both cases the effectiveness of these currents is diminished by ACh. The impact on pyramidal cells will be to facilitate their responses to an existing excitatory input, allowing higher frequency discharge because of the reduction of the after hyperpolarization linked to the two potassium channels. This contrasts with the strong excitatory and at least partial disinhibitory effects on the geniculate circuitry. The gain of the intracortical inhibitory mechanisms should be enhanced by activity in the cholinergic system. This is exemplified by the action of ACh on the stimulus specific responses of visual cortical cells. Responses to optimal stimuli are enhanced, and selectivity in a significant number of cases is increased commensurate with facilitatory effects on the inhibitory circuitry generating response selectivity (Sillito and Kemp, 1983; Sillito and Murphy, 1986; Murphy and Sillito, 1991). An example of the action of ACh on the responses of a visual cortical cell is given in Fig. 6.

The interpretation of the effects of application of the GABA$_A$ antagonist bicuculline (Sillito, 1984) and Eysel's multi point GABA applications needs to be considered in the context of some of the issues raised in this section and the arguments presented in the previous one. Inhibitory blockade will release a cell from local feedforward inhibition and other inhibitory inputs converging on all but the far distal dendrites of pyramidal cells. Where NMDA receptors are involved the loss of the hyperpolarizing influence may enable their effect at lower levels of excitatory drive to the cell and because of the duration of the EPSPs so generated open a wider temporal window for the summation of visually driven excitatory inputs. This alone may generate enough facilitation to enable cells to respond to direct geniculate input without the permissive influence of the iso-orientation intracortical facilitation. This effect does not require cross-orientation inhibition. In the case of the data from Eysel's group it could be argued that the high density of GABA$_A$ receptors on GABA cells makes them more susceptible than the pyramidal cells to the inwardly diffusing field of GABA. Thus there would be a time window where this simply causes general disinhibition in the manner of bicuculline. However, their most recent work (Crook and Eysel, 1991) has shown that the reduction in orientation tuning seems only to occur when the inactivation electrodes are located to columns of dissimilar orientation. It seems that the arguments favouring cross-orientation inhibition, at least for some cells, cannot be easily discarded. The complexity of the circuitry however, argues for caution in building our models of the mechanisms underlying particular effects. For example, some visual cortical cells can utilise excitatory inputs from a range of different inputs to express the same overt receptive field properties. Thus layer III complex cells seem to respond similarly

whether driven by inputs originating in the A laminae of the dLGN via layer IV, the C laminae of the dLGN, area 18 or all of these (Malpeli, 1983; Malpeli et al., 1986; Schwark et al., 1986). This multiple sourcing of inputs poses problems for gain control, and it may be that particular inputs are regulated by the bitufted and neurogliaform GABAergic cells synapsing at specific locations on dendrites. Lifting this type of inhibitory control may bring a massive barrage of facilitatory influence to bear on cells and generate significant non-linearities in the way the effects of the inputs sum.

Whilst we are still far from bringing the individual elements of the inhibitory circuitry in the visual cortex into a detailed model of the mechanisms underlying receptive field properties, the convergent anatomical, electrophysiological and neuropharmacological data should leave no one in doubt as to its importance. The issue is not if, but how, GABAergic mechanisms underpin the functional organization of the visual cortex. For example, the absence of detectable cross-orientation inhibition in the intracellular studies does not negate the contribution of inhibitory mechanisms to orientation tuning, but merely indicates that we have not understood the way inhibitory and excitatory influences interact in establishing this pattern of response selectivity (see Berman et al., Chapter 21). Part of the problem lies with the fact that we are looking at the function of multiple embedded circuits (consider the connections of layer VI cells alone) that would seem to be doing much more than generating the narrow profile of response properties routinely assessed in studies of cortical mechanisms. The appreciation of this will be very important to establishing the next level of our understanding of the role of GABAergic mechanisms in the system.

## References

Avoli, M. (1986) Inhibitory potentials in neurons of the deep layers of the in vitro neocortical slice. *Brain Res.*, 370: 165–170.

Barlow, H.B. and Levick, W.R. (1965) The mechanism of directionally selective units in the rabbit's retina. *J. Physiol.*, 178: 477–504.

Benardo, L.S. and Prince, D.A. (1982) Cholinergic excitation of mammalian hippocampal pyramidal cells. *Brain Res.*, 249: 315–331.

Berardi, N. and Morrone, M.C. (1984a) Development of γ-aminobutyric acid mediated inhibition of X cells of the cat lateral geniculate nucleus. *J. Physiol.*, 357: 525–537.

Berardi, N. and Morrone, M.C. (1984b) The role of γ-aminobutyric acid mediated inhibition in the response properties of cat lateral geniculate nucleus neurons. *J. Physiol.*, 357: 505–523.

Bloomfield, S.A. and Murray, S.M. (1988) Postsynaptic potentials recorded in neurons of the cat's lateral geniculate nucleus following electrical stimulation of the optic chiasm. *J. Neurophysiol.*, 60: 1924–1945.

Bolz, J. and Gilbert, C.D. (1986) Generation of end-inhibition in the visual cortex via interlaminar connections. *Nature*, 320: 362–365.

Boyapati, J. and Henry, G.H. (1984) Corticofugal axons in the lateral geniculate nucleus of the cat. *Exp. Brain Res.*, 53: 335–340.

Boyapati, J. and Henry, G.H. (1987) The duplex character of the corticofugal pathway from the striate cortex to the lateral geniculate complex of the cat. *Vision Res.*, 27: 723–726.

Cleland, B.G. and Lee, B.B., Vidyasagar, T.R. (1983) Response of neurons in the cat's lateral geniculate nucleus to moving bars of different length. *J. Neurosci.*, 3: 108–116.

Connors, B.W., Malenka, R.C. and Silva, L.R. (1990) Two inhibitory postsynaptic potentials, and GABAa and GABAb receptor-mediated responses in neocortex of rat and cat. *J. Physiol.*, 406: 443–468.

Creutzfeldt, O.D. and Ito, M. (1968) Functional synaptic organisation of primary visual cortex neurons in the cat. *Exp. Brain Res.*, 6: 324–352.

Creutzfeldt, O.D., Innocenti, G.M. and Brooks, D. (1974a) Vertical organisation in the visual cortex (area 17) in the cat. *Exp. Brain Res.*, 21: 315–336.

Creutzfeldt, O.D., Kuhnt, U. and Benevento, L.A. (1974b) An intracellular analysis of visual cortical neurons to moving stimuli: responses in a co-operative neuronal network. *Exp. Brain Res.*, 21: 251–274.

Crook, J.M. and Eysel, U.T. (1991) Modulation of cortical orientation tuning by iontophoretic application of GABA at functionally characterized sites. In: N. Elsner and H. Penin (Eds.), *Proceedings of the 19th Gottingen Neurobiology Conference*, Stuttgart, New York: Thieme Verlag..

Crunelli, V., Kelly, J.S., Leresche, N. and Pirchio, M. (1987) On the excitatory post-synaptic potential evoked by stimulation of the optic tract in the rat lateral geniculate nucleus. *J. Physiol.*, 384: 603–618.

Crunelli, V., Haby, M., Jassik-Gerschenfeld, D., Leresche, N. and Pirchio, M (1988) Cl⁻ and K⁺ dependent inhibitory postsynaptic potentials evoked by interneurons of the rat lateral geniculate nucleus. *J. Physiol.*, 399: 153–176.

De Curtis, M., Spreafico, R. and Avanzino, G.L. (1989) Exci-

tatory amino acids mediate responses elicited in vitro by stimulation of cortical afferents to reticularis thalami neurons of the rat. *Neuroscience*, 33: 275–283.

De Lima, A.D., Montero, V.M. and Singer, W. (1985) The cholingergic innervation of the visual thalamus: an EM immunocytochemical study. *Exp. Brain Res.*, 59: 206–212.

Deschenes, M. and Hu, B. (1990) Electrophysiology and pharmacology of the corticothalamic input to lateral thalamic nuclei: an intracellular study in the cat. *Eur. J Neurosci.*, 2: 140–152.

Douglas, R.J., Martin, K.A.C. and Whitteridge, D. (1988) Selective responses of visual cortical cells do not depend on shunting inhibition. *Nature*, 332: 642–644.

Douglas, R.J., Martin, K.A.C. and Whitteridge, D. (1989) A canonical microcircuit for neocortex. *Neural Computation*, 1: 480–488.

Douglas, R.J. and Martin, K.A.C. (1990) Control of neuronal output by inhibition at the axon initial segment. *Neural Computation*, 2: 283–292.

Engel, A.K., König, P., Gray, C.M. and Singer, W. (1990) Stimulus-dependent neuronal oscillations in cat visual cortex: Inter-columnar interaction as determined by cross-correlation analysis. *Eur. J Neurosci.*, 2: 588–606.

Eysel, U.T., Pape, H.C. and Van Schayck, R. (1986) Excitatory and differential disinhibitory actions of acetylcholine in the lateral geniculate nucleus of the cat. *J. Physiol.*, 370: 233–254.

Eysel, U.T., Crook, J.M. and Machemer, H.F. (1990) GABA-induced remote inactivation reveals cross-orientation inhibition in the cat striate cortex. *Exp. Brain Res.*, 80: 626–630.

Ferster, D. and Lindstrom, S. (1984a) Synaptic excitation of neurons in area 17 of the cat by intracortical axon collaterals of cortico-geniculate cells. *J. Physiol.*, 367: 233–252.

Ferster, D. and Lindstrom, S. (1984b) Augmenting responses evoked in area 17 of the cat by intracortical axon collaterals of cortico-geniculate cells. *J. Physiol.*, 367: 217–232.

Ferster, D. (1986) Orientation selectivity of synaptic potentials in neurons of cat primary visual cortex. *J. Neurosci.*, 6: 1264–1301.

Ferster, D. (1987) Origin of orientation-selective EPSPs in simple cells of cat visual cortex. *J. Neurosci.*, 7: 1780–1791.

Fitzpatrick, D., Penny, G.R. and Schmechel, D.E. (1984) Glutamic acid decarboxylase-immunoreactive neurons and terminals in the lateral geniculate nucleus of the cat. *J. Neurosci.*, 4: 1809–1829.

Fox, K., Sato, H. and Daw, N. (1989) The location and function of NMDA receptors in cat and kitten visual cortex. *J. Neurosci.*, 9: 2443–2454.

Fox, K., Sato, H. and Daw, N. (1990) The effect of varying stimulus intensity on NMDA-receptor activity in cat visual cortex. *J. Neurophysiol.*, 64: 1413–1428.

Gilbert, C.D. (1977) Laminar differences in receptive field properties of cells in cat primary visual cortex. *J. Physiol. (London)*, 268: 391–421.

Gilbert, C.D. and Wiesel, T.N. (1989) Columnar specificity of intrinsic horizonal and corticocortical connections in cat visual cortex. *J. Neurosci.*, 9/7: 2432–2442.

Grieve, K.L. and Sillito, A.M. (1989) Length summation in

layer VI cells of cat visual cortex and hypercomplex cell inhibitory end zones in the anaesthetised cat. *J. Physiol. (London)*, 416: 21P.

Grieve, K.L. and Sillito, A.M. (1990a) The role of feedback from layer VI to IV in the generation of length tuning in the visual cortex of the anaesthetised cat. *J. Physiol.*, 429: 48P.

Grieve, K.L. and Sillito, A.M. (1990b) The length summation properties of layer VI cells in the visual cortex and hypercomplex cell end zone inhibition. *Exp. Brain Res.*, in press.

Grieve, K.L. and Sillito, A.M. (1991) A re-appraisal of the role of of layer VI of the visual cortex in the generation of cortical end-inhibition. *Exp. Brain Res.,*: In press.

Guido, W., Salinger, W.L. and Schroeder, C.E. (1989) Binocular interactions in the dorsal lateral geniculate nucleus of monocularly paralyzed cats: extraretinal and retinal influences. *Exp. Brain Res.*, 70: 417–428.

Halliwell, J.V. and Adams, P.R. (1982) Voltage-clamp analysis of muscarinic excitation in hippocampal neurons. *Brain Res.*, 250: 71–92.

Hammond, P. (1974) Cat retinal ganglion cells: size and shape of receptive field centres. *J. Physiol.*, 242: 99–118.

Hammond, P., Andrews, D.P. and James, C.R. (1975) Invariance of orientational and directional tuning in visual cortical cells of the adult cat. *Brain Res.*, 96: 56–59.

Hammond, P. and Pomfrett, C.J.D. (1990) Influence of spatial frequency on tuning and bias for orientation and direction in the cat's striate cortex. *Vision Res.*, 30: 359–369.

Hamos, J.E., Van Horn, S.C., Raczkowski, D. and Sherman, S.M. (1987) Synaptic circuits involving an individual retinogeniculate axon in the cat. *J. Comp. Neurol*, 259: 165–192.

Harvey, A.R. (1980) A physiological analysis of subcortical and commissural projections of areas 17 and 18 of the cat. *J. Physiol.*, 302: 507–534.

Hirsch, J. and Burnod, Y. (1987) A synaptically evoked late hyperpolarization in the rat dorsolateral geniculate neurons in vitro. *Neuroscience*, 23: 457–468.

Hollander, H. (1970) The projection from the visual cortex to the lateral geniculate body (LGB). An experimental study with silver impregnation methods in the cat. *Exp. Brain Res.*, 21: 430–440.

Howe, J.R., Sutor, B. and Zieglgansberger, W. (1987) Characteristics of long duration inhibitory postsynaptic potentials in rat neocortical neurons. *Cell Mol. Neurobiol.*, 7: 1–18.

Hubel, D.H. and Wiesel, T.N. (1961) Integrative activity in the cat's lateral geniculate body. *J. Physiol.*, 155: 385–398.

Hubel, D.H. and Wiesel, T.N. (1962) Receptive fields binocular interaction and functional architecture in the cat's visual cortex. *J. Physiol.*, 160: 106–154.

Hubel, D. and Wiesel, T.N. (1965) Receptive fields and functional architecture in two nonstriate visual areas (18 and, 19) of the cat. *J. Neurophysiol.*, 28: 229–289.

Hubel, D. and Wiesel, T.N. (1968) Receptive fields and functional architecture of monkey striate cortex. *J. Physiol.*, 195: 215–243.

Humphrey, A.L. and Weller, R.E. (1988a) Structural correlates of functionally distinct X-cells in the lateral geniculate nucleus of the cat. *J. Comp. Neurol*, 268: 448–468.

Humphrey, A.L. and Weller, R.E. (1988b) Functionally distinct groups of X-cells in the lateral geniculate nucleus of the cat. *J. Comp. Neurol.*, 268: 429–447.

Jones, H.E. and Sillito, A.M. (1987) The length tuning of cells in the feline dorsal lateral geniculate nucleus (dLGN). *J. Physiol. (London)*, 390: 32P.

Jones, H.E. and Sillito, A.M. (1991) The length response properties of cells in the feline dorsal lateral geniculate nucleus (dLGN). *J. Physiol.*, in press.

Jones, J. and Palmer, L.A. (1987) The two-dimensional spatial structure of simple receptive fields in cat striate cortex. *J. Neurophysiol.*, 5: 86–1187–1211.

Jones, K.A. and Baughman, R.W. (1988) NMDA- and non-NMDA-receptor components of excitatory synaptic potentials recorded from cells in layer V of rat visual cortex. *J. Neurosci.*, 8: 3522–3534.

Kato, H., Bishop, P.O. and Orban, G.A. (1978) Hypercomplex and simple/complex cell classifications in cat striate cortex. *J. Neurophysiol.*, 14: 1071–1095.

Kato, H., Bishop, P.O. and Orban, G.A. (1981) Binocular interaction on monocularly discharged lateral geniculate and striate neurons in the cat. *J. Neurophysiol.*, 46: 932–951.

Kawamura, S., Sprague, J. and Nimi, K. (1974) Corticofugal projections from the visual cortices to the thalamus, pretectum and superior colliculus in the cat. *J. Comp. Neurol*, 158: 339–362.

Kemp, J.A. and Sillito, A.M. (1982) The nature of the excitatory transmitter mediating X and Y cell inputs to the cat dorsal lateral geniculate nucleus. *J. Physiol.*, 323: 377–391.

Kisvarday, Z.F., Cowey, A., Smith, A D. and Somogyi, P. (1988) Interlaminar and lateral excitatory amino acid connections in the striate cortex of monkey. *J. Neurosci.*, 9: 667–682.

Levick, W.R. and Thibos, L.N. (1980) Orientation bias of cat retinal ganglion cells. *Nature*, 286: 389–390.

Levick, W.R. and Thibos, L.N. (1982) Analysis of orientation bias in cat retina. *J. Physiol.*, 329: 243–261.

Lindström, S. and Wróbel, A. (1990a) Frequency dependent corticofugal excitation of principal cells in the cat's dorsal lateral geniculate nucleus. *Exp. Brain Res.*, 79: 313–318.

Lindström, S. and Wróbel, A. (1990b) Private inhibitory systems for the X and Y pathways in the dorsal lateral geniculate nucleus of the cat. *J. Physiol. (London)*, 429: 259–280.

Malpeli, J.G., Schiller, H. and Colby, C. (1981) Response properties of single cells in monkey striate cortex during reversible inactivation of individual lateral geniculate laminae. *J. Neurophysiol.*, 46: 1102–1119.

Malpeli, J.G. (1983) Activity of cells in area 17 of the cat in absence of input from layer A of lateral geniculate nucleus. *J. Neurophysiol.*, 49: 595–610.

Malpeli, J.G., Lee, C., Schwark, H.D. and Weyand, T.G. (1986) Cat area 17 I pattern of thalamic control of cortical layers. *J. Neurophysiol.*, 56: 1062–1073.

Martin, K.A.C. (1990) From single cells to simple circuits in the cerebral cortex. *QJ Exp. Physiol.*, 73: 637–637.

Mastronarde, D.N. (1987a) Two classes of single-input X-cells in cat lateral geniculate nucleus II retinal inputs and the

382

generations of receptive-field properties. *J. Neurophysiol.*, 57: 2–381–413.

Mastronarde, D.N. (1987b) Two classes of single-input X-cells in cat lateral geniculate nucleus I receptive-field properties and classification of cells. *J. Neurophysiol.*, 57: 2–357–380.

Matsubara, J., Cynader, M., Swindale, N.V. and Stryker, M. (1985) Intrinsic projections within visual cortex: Evidence for orientation-specific local connections. *Proc. Natl. Acad. Sci. USA*, 82: 935–939.

McCormick, D.A., Connors, B.W., Lighthall, J.W. and Prince, D.A. (1985) Comparative electrophysiology of pyramidal and sparsely spiny stellate neurons of the neocortex. *J. Neurophysiol.*, 54: 782–806.

McCormick, D.A. and Prince, D.A. (1985) Two types of muscarinic response to acetylcholine in mammalian cortical neurons. *Proc. Natl. Acad. Sci. USA*, 82: 6344–6348.

McCormick, D.A. and Prince, D.A. (1987) Actions of acetylcholine in the guinea pig and cat medial and dorsal lateral geniculate nucleus, in vitro. *J. Physiol.*, 3920: 147–165.

McCormick, D.A. and Pape, H.-C. (1988) Acetylcholine inhibits identified interneurons in the cat lateral geniculate nucleus. *Nature*, 334: 246–248.

McCormick, D.A. and Pape, H.-C. (1990) Properties of a hyperpolarization-activated cation current and its role in rhythmic oscillation in thalamic relay neurons. *J. Physiol. (London)*, 431: 291–318.

McCormick, D.A. and Prince, D.A. (1990) Pirenzepine discriminates among ionic responses to acetylcholine in guinea-pig cerebral cortex and reticular nucleus of thalamus. *TIPS*, 1986–1986.

McGuire, B.A., Hornung, J P., Gilbert, C.D. and Wiesel, T.N. (1984) Patterns of synaptic input to layer 4 of cat striate cortex. *J. Neurosci.*, 4: 3021–3033.

Montero, V.M. and Singer, W. (1984) Ultrastructure and synaptic relations of neural elements containing glutamic acid decarboxylase (GAD) in the perigeniculate nucleus of the cat. *Exp. Brain Res.*, 56: 115–125.

Montero, V.M. and Singer, W. (1985) Ultrastructural identification of somata and neural processes immunoreactive to antibodies against glutamic acid decarboxylase (GAD) in the dorsal lateral geniculate nucleus of the cat. *Exp. Brain Res.*, 59: 151–165.

Montero, V.M. and Zempel, J. (1985) Evidence for two types of GABA-containing interneurons in the A-laminae of the cat lateral geniculate nucleus: a double-label HRP and GABA-immunocytochemical study. *Exp. Brain Res.*, 60: 603–609.

Montero, V.M. (1986) Localization of γ-aminobutyric Acid (GABA) in Type 3 Cells and demonstration of their source to F2 terminals in the cat lateral geniculate nucleus: a golgi-electron-microscopic GABA-immunocytochemical study. *J. Comp. Neurol.*, 254: 228–245.

Montero, V.M. (1987) Ultrastructural identification of synaptic terminals from the axon of Type 3 interneurons in the cat lateral geniculate nucleus. *J. Comp. Neurol.*, 264: 268–283.

Morrone, M.C., Burr, D.C. and Maffei, L. (1982) Functional implications of cross-orientation inhibition of cortical visual cells. I. Neurophysiological evidence. *Proc. R. Soc. London*, B216: 335–354.

Morrone, M.C. and Burr, D.C. (1986) Evidence for the existence and development of visual inhibition in humans. *Nature*, 321: 235–237.

Murphy, P.C. and Sillito, A.M. (1987) Corticofugal feedback influences the generation of length tuning in the visual pathway. *Nature*, 329(6141): 727–729.

Murphy, P.C. and Sillito, A.M. (1989) The binocular input to cells in the feline dorsal lateral geniculate nucleus. *J. Physiol. (London)*, 415: 393–409.

Murphy, P.C. and Sillito, A.M. (1991) Cholinergic enhancement of direction selectivity in the visual cortex of the cat. *Neuroscience*, 40 13–20.

Nowak, L., Bregestovski, P., Ascher, P., Herbet, A. and Prochiantz, A. (1984) Magnesium gates glutamate-activated channels in mouse central neurons. *Nature*, 307: 460–462.

Orban, G.A., Kato, H. and Bishop, P.O. (1979a) End-zone region in receptive fields of hypercomplex and other striate neurons in the cat. *J. Neurophysiol.*, 42: 818–832.

Orban, G.A., Kato, H. and Bishop, P.O. (1979b) Dimensions and properties of end-zone inhibitory areas in receptive fields of hypercomplex cells in cat striate cortex. *J. Neurophysiol.*, 42: 833–849.

Pape, H.C. and Eysel, U.T. (1986) Binocular interactions in the lateral geniculate nucleus of the cat: GABAergic inhibition reduced by dominant afferent activity. *Exp. Brain Res.*, 61: 265–271.

Ramoa, A.S., Shadlen, M., Skottun, B.C. and Freeman, R.D. (1986) A comparison of inhibition in orientation and spatial frequency selectivity of cat visual cortex. *Nature*, 321: 237–239.

Robson, J.A. (1983) The morphology of corticofugal axons to the dorsal lateral geniculate nucleus in the cat. *J. Comp. Neurol.*, 216: 89–103.

Rose, D. (1979) Mechanisms underlying the receptive field properties of neurons in cat visual cortex. *Vision Res.*, 19: 533–544.

Sanderson, K.J., Bishop, P.O. and Darian-Smith, I. (1971) The properties of the binocular receptive fields of lateral geniculate neurons. *Exp. Brain Res.*, 13: 178–207.

Sato, H., Daw, N. and Fox, K. (1990) Intracellular recording study of stimulus specific response properties in the cat visual cortex. *Soc. Neurosci.*, 16:.

Saul, A.B. and Humphrey, A.L. (1990) Spatial and temporal response properties of lagged and nonlagged cells in cat lateral geniculate nucleus. *J. Neurophysiol.*, 64: 206–224.

Scharfman, H.E. and Sarvey, J.M. (1985) Responses to γ-aminobutyric acid applied to cell bodies and dendrites of rat visual cortical neurons. *Brain Res.*, 358: 385–389.

Scharfman, H.E. and Sarvey, J.M. (1987) Responses to GABA recorded from identified rat visual cortical neurons. *Neuroscience*, 23: 407–422.

Scharfman, H.E. and Sarvey, J.M. (1988) Physiological correlates of responses to gamma-aminobutyric acid (GABA) recorded from rat visual cortical neurons in vitro. *Synapse*, 2: 619–626.

Scharfman, H.E., Lu, S-M., Guido, W., Adams, P.R. and Sherman, S.M. (1990) N-Methyl-D-aspartate receptors contribute to excitatory postsynaptic potentials of cat lateral geniculate neurons recorded in thalamic slices. Proc. Natl Acad. Sci. USA, 87: 4548–4552.

Schiller, P.H., Finlay, B.L. and Volman, S. (1976) Quantitative studies of single-cell properties in monkey striate cortex I spatiotemporal organization of receptive fields. J. Neurophysiol., 39: 1288–1319.

Schmielau, F. and Singer, W. (1977) The role of visual cortex for binocular interactions in the cat lateral geniculate nucleus. Brain Res., 120: 354–361.

Schwark, H.D., Malpeli, J.G., Weyand, T.G. and Lee, C. (1986) Cat area 17 II response properties of infragranular layer neurons in the absence of supragranular layer activity. J. Neurophysiol., 56: 1074–1087.

Sherman, S.M. and Friedlander, M.J. (1988) Identification of X versus Y properties for interneurons in the A-laminae of the cat's lateral geniculate nucleus. Exp. Brain Res., 73: 364–392.

Shirokawa, T., Nishigori, A., Kimura, F. and Tsumoto, T. (1989) Actions of excitatory amino acid antagonists on synaptic potentials of layer II/III neurons of the cat's visual cortex. Exp. Brain Res., 78: 489–500.

Shou, T. and Zhou, Y. (1986) The orientation bias of LGN neurons shows topographic relation to area centralis in the cat retina. Exp. Brain Res., 64: 233–236.

Sillito, A.M. (1974) The effectiveness of bicuculline as an antagonist of GABA and visually evoked inhibition in the cat's striate cortex. J. Physiol., 250: 287–304.

Sillito, A.M. (1975) The contribution of inhibitory mechanisms to the receptive field properties of neurons in the striate cortex of the cat. J. Physiol. (London), 250: 305–329.

Sillito, A.M. (1977a) The spatial extent of excitatory and inhibitory zones in the receptive field of superficial layer hypercomplex cells. J. Physiol. (London), 273: 791–803.

Sillito, A.M. (1977b) Inhibitory processes underlying the directional specificity of simple complex and hypercomplex cells in the cat's visual cortex. J. Physiol., 271: 699–720.

Sillito, A.M. and Versiani, V. (1977) The contribution of excitatory and inhibitory inputs to the length preference of hypercomplex cells in layers II and III of the cat's striate cortex. J. Physiol. (London), 273: 775–790.

Sillito, A.M. (1979) Inhibitory mechanisms influencing complex cell orientation selectivity and their modification at high resting discharge levels. J. Physiol., 289: 33–53.

Sillito, A.M., Kemp, J.A., Milson, J.A. and Berardi, N. (1980) A re-evaluation of the mechanisms underlying simple cell orientation selectivity. Brain Res., 194: 517–520.

Sillito, A.M., Kemp, J.A. and Berardi, N. (1983) The cholinergic influence on the function of the cat dorsal lateral geniculate nucleus (dLGN). Brain Res., 280: 299–307.

Sillito, A.M. and Kemp, J.A. (1983) The influence of GABAergic inhibitory processes on the receptive field structure of X and Y cells in the cat dorsal lateral geniculate nucleus (dLGN). Brain Res., 277: 63–77.

Sillito, A.M. (1984) Functional considerations of the operation of GABAergic inhibitory processes in the visual cortex. Cerebral Cortex, 2A: 91–172.

Sillito, A.M., Murphy, P.C. and Salt, T.E. (1990a) The contribution of the non-N-methyl-D-aspartate group of excitatory amino acid receptors to retinogeniculate transmission in the cat. Neuroscience, 34: 273–280.

Sillito, A.M., Murphy, P.C., Salt, T.E. and Moody, C.I. (1990b) Dependence of retinogeniculate transmission in cat on NMDA receptors. J. Neurophysiol., 63: 347–355.

Sillito, A.M., Murphy, P.C. and Cudeiro, J. (1991) Orientation domain substructure to centre surround interactions in the dorsal lateral geniculate nucleus (dLGN) of the anaesthetized cat. J. Physiol., in press.

Singer, W., Poppel, E. and Creutzfeldt, O.D. (1972) Inhibitory interaction in the cat's lateral geniculate nucleus. Exp. Brain Res., 14: 210–226.

Singer, W. and Bedworth, N. (1973) Inhibitory interaction between X and Y units in the cat lateral geniculate nucleus. Brain Res., 49: 291–307.

Singer, W. and Creutzfeldt, O.D. (1970) Reciprocal lateral inhibition of on- and off-center neurons in the lateral geniculate body of the cat. Exp. Brain Res., 10: 311–330.

Soltesz, I., Haby, M., Leresche, N. and Crunelli, V. (1988) The GABA antagonist phaclofen inhibits the late $K^+$-dependent IPSP in cat and rat thalamic and hippocampal neurons. Brain Res., 448: 351–354.

Somogyi, P. (1989) Synaptic organisation of GABAergic neurons and $GABA_A$ receptors in the lateral geniculate nucleus and visual cortex. In: D.K.T. Lam and CD Gilbert (Eds.), Neural Mechanisms of Visual Perception, Portfolio Pub Co. pp. 35–62.

Soodak, R.E., Shapley, R. and Kaplan, E. (1987) Linear mechanism of orientation tuning in the retina and lateral geniculate nucleus of the cat. J. Neurophysiol., 58: 267–275.

Sterling, P. and Davis, T.L. (1980) Neurons in cat lateral geniculate nucleus that concentrate exogenous [$^3$H]-γ-aminobutyric acid (Gaba). J. Comp. Neurol., 192: 737–749.

Ts'o, D.Y., Gilbert, C.D. and Wiesel, T.N. (1986) Relations between horizontal interactions and functional architecture in cat striate cortex as revealed by cross-correlation analysis. J. Neurosci., 6: 1160–1170.

Tsumoto, T., Creutzfeldt, O.D. and Legendy, C.R. (1978) Functional organisation of the corticofugal system from visual cortex to lateral geniculate nucleus in the cat (with an appendix on geniculo-cortical mono-synaptic connections). Brain Res., 345: 364.

Tsumoto, T., Eckart, W. and Creutzfeldt, O.D. (1979) Modification of orientation sensitivity of cat visual cortex neurons by removal of GABA-mediated inhibition. Exp. Brain Res., 34: 351–363.

Tsumoto, T. and Suda, K. (1980) Three groups of corticogeniculate neurons and their distribution in binocular and monocular segments of cat striate cortex. J. Comp. Neurol., 193: 223–236.

Tsumoto, T., Masui, H. and Sato, H. (1986) Excitatory amino acid transmitters in neuronal circuits of cat visual cortex. J. Neurophysiol., 55: 469–483.

Tsumoto, T. (1990) Excitatory amino acid transmitters and their receptors in neural circuits of the cerebral neocortex. Neurosci Res., 9: 79–102.

Updyke, B.V. (1975) The patterns of projection of cortical

areas 17, 18 and, 19 onto the laminae of the dorsal lateral geniculate nucleus in the cat. *J. Comp. Neurol.*, 163: 377–396.

Varela, F.J. and Singer, W. (1987) Neuronal dynamics in the visual corticothalamic pathway revealed through binocular rivalry. *Exp. Brain Res.*, 66: 10–20.

Vidyasagar, T.R. (1984) Contribution of inhibitory mechanisms to the orientation sensitivity of cat dLGN neurons. *Exp. Brain Res.*, 55: 192–195.

Weber, A.J., Kalil, R.E. and Behan, M. (1989) Synaptic connections between corticogeniculate axons and interneu-rons in the dorsal lateral geniculate nucleus of the cat. *J. Comp. Neurol.*, 289: 156–164.

Worgotter, F. and Eysel, U.T. (1989) Axis of preferred motion is a function of bar length in visual cortical receptive fields. *Exp. Brain Res.*,.

Xue, J.T., Ramoa, A.S., Carney, T. and Freeman, R.D. (1987) Binocular interaction in the dorsal lateral geniculate nucleus of the cat. *Exp. Brain Res.*, 68: 305–310.

Yamane, S., Maske, R. and Bishop, P.O. (1985) Properties of end-zone inhibition of hypercomplex cells in cat striate cortex. *Exp. Brain Res.*, 60: 200–203.

R.R. Mize, R.E. Marc and A.M. Sillito (Eds.)
Progress in Brain Research, Vol. 90

CHAPTER 18

# GABAergic networks of basket cells in the visual cortex

## Zoltán F. Kisvárday

*Department of Neurophysiology, Ruhr-Universität Bochum, Universitätsstrasse 150, MA 4 / 149, D-4630 Bochum 1, FRG*

## Introduction

GABA is the major inhibitory neurotransmitter in the cerebral cortex (Krnjevic and Schwartz, 1966). It has been associated with several neuronal types (Somogyi, 1986) showing morphological features radically different from those of pyramidal cells which are considered to be excitatory in function (Baughman and Gilbert, 1981). Of the GABA cell types, the so-called cortical basket cells are very characteristic in that their axons, when viewed under the light microscope, terminate on somata and proximal dendrites of other cells, mainly pyramidal and spiny stellate cells. Such a distribution pattern of basket cell terminals strongly suggests a very significant influence on the output characteristics of their target cells. In the following discussion, my purpose is to give an updated briefing about the varieties and distribution pattern of basket cells in the feline visual cortex, and to highlight some of their intriguing connectivity rules which may be related to their particular functional tasks.

## Background

Although cortical basket cells have appeared in a number of studies since Ramón y Cajal (1899) discovered them in Golgi preparations of human infant motorcortex, it was Szentágothai (1965, 1973) and Marin-Padilla (1969) who first elaborated much of their basic structural constraints. A major impetus to their work was probably given by contemporary electrophysiological findings such as those of Andersen and Eccles (1963a,b), reporting on the functional significance of somatic inhibition in the cerebellum and the hippocampus. With the invention of the chronically isolated slab method, Szentágothai (1965) was able to find that axo-somatic contacts could be contributed by local interneurons with axons up to 1–2 mm in length. With fortuitous Golgi-staining, Marin-Padilla (1969) gave detailed descriptions about the distribution and spatial characteristics of the so-called large basket cells in the motor cortex of human infants. In ensuing years a large number of Golgi-impregnated basket cells were described providing more and more bits of information about their anatomy. By the 1980s a general picture about cortical basket cells had gradually emerged (for review, see Jones and Hendry, 1984), that is: (i) they are prevalent in many cortical areas of various mammalian species, including rabbit, cat, and primate; (ii) they are heterogeneous with respect to their axonal distribution; (iii) a single basket cell can influence large cortical regions via its long oriented axons; (iv) basket cells can directly influence more than one layer; (v) the pericellular baskets around pyramidal cells are probably formed by axons of more than one basket cell.

## GABA is the transmitter of basket cells

The strategic location of basket cell axons has long suggested that they subserve inhibitory mechanisms on the somata of their target cells. It is thus not surprising that ever since GABA was proposed to act as depressing cortical neuronal activity, the GABAergic nature of basket cells had become generally acknowledged well before there was clearcut evidence for this. Direct proof became available with the employment of immunocytochemical techniques using antisera raised against glutamic acid decarboxylase (GAD), the rate limiting enzyme of GABA, and directly against GABA. A number of subsequent studies have shown that the somata and dendrites of virtually all pyramidal as well as non-pyramidal cells receive dense input from GABAergic axon terminals (Ribak, 1978; Freund et al., 1983; Hendry et al., 1983). Eventually, with the combination of immunoelectron microscopy and intracellular HRP-labelling (Somogyi and Soltész, 1986; Kisvárday et al., 1987) it was directly proven that basket cells invariably contain GABA as is shown in Fig. 1 for the axon terminals of a layer V large basket cell.

## Morphological heterogeneity of basket cells

As mentioned above, former anatomical descriptions about basket cells relied entirely on Golgi impregnation techniques which provide an incomplete picture of the impregnated cell. This technical pitfall was overcome with the application of numerous extracellular and intracellular labelling techniques, allowing, for the first time, complete visualization of the axonal and dendritic fields of virtually any neuronal type. Consequently, it was possible to give very detailed descriptions about the types and subtypes of intracellularly HRP-labelled basket cells, which can be summarized as follows.

The first type is the so-called large basket cell. This name refers to the large soma size of this type of basket cell, often reaching 30 $\mu$m in diameter. Characteristically their axonal fields extend laterally at least three times farther than the strongly beaded smooth dendrites (Somogyi et al., 1983). Although large basket cells were originally

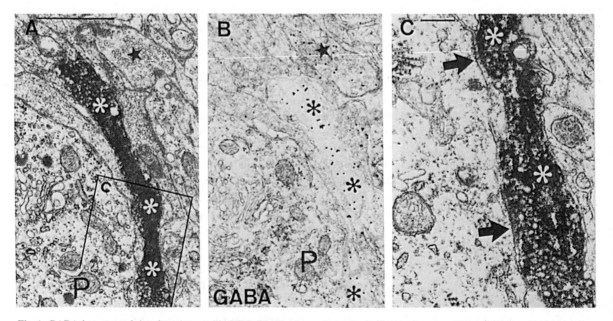

Fig. 1. GABA-immunostaining demonstrated in HRP-filled basket cell terminals. Soma of a pyramidal cell (P) is contacted by three basket cell terminals (asterisks) in A, two of which in the framed area are shown at higher magnification in C, establishing type II synaptic contacts (arrows). The section in B is reacted for GABA with the postembedding gold method. Selective accumulation of gold particles over the basket cell terminals indicates that they contain GABA. A nearby terminal (stars in A and B) of unknown origin is also labelled for GABA. Modified from Kisvárday et al., 1987. Bars: A and B, 1 $\mu$m; C, 0.2 $\mu$m.

described in layer III of area 17, similar basket cells were later found in layers IV (area 18, Fig. 2) and V (area 17, Kisvárday et al., 1987) as well. Large basket cells can thus be subdivided into layer specific subtypes as schematically illustrated in Fig. 4.

The second major type is a medium-sized basket cell with axonal fields confined predominantly to layer IV. Its soma is smaller than that of large basket cells, rarely exceeding 20 $\mu$m in diameter. Characteristically, the dense axonal field is composed of thin collaterals studded with bulbous boutons which often "clutch" somata of neighbouring cells (Fig. 3A–C); hence the name, clutch cell (Kisvárday et al., 1985).

The third type is a small basket cell type because it has the smallest soma (8–12 $\mu$m in diameter) of all basket cell types. It is distinct from clutch cells in that its main location is in the superficial layers, chiefly in layers II and upper III. In contrast to the other two basket cell types, this type of basket cell has not been encountered in any of the intracellular studies, so that information concerning the extent of its axonal arborization is quite limited. Nonetheless, on the basis of Golgi studies (Szentágothai, 1973, 1975; Meyer, 1983) and recent immunocytochemical work (Freund et al., 1986; Meyer and Wahle, 1988), it is well established that they form a separate population of basket cells with a laterally restricted axonal field up to about a few hundred $\mu$m in the superficial layers.

Novel information on the complexity of basket cells was provided by computer aided reconstructions, whereby their axons could be rotated and viewed from their most informative planes. For example, looking from the surface of the cortex, large basket cells have 2–5 major axonal arms, each of which can extend up to 1 mm from the dendritic field (e.g., Fig. 2). Many of these axonal arms run in many directions parallel with the cortical surface and, along their course, emit radially aligned secondary collaterals at certain intervals which ultimately give off bouton-laden fine axons to contact somata and proximal dendrites

of neighbouring cells or terminate in the neuropile. The axonal field of intracellularly HRP-labelled clutch cells (Kisvárday et al., 1985) showed a different kind of anisotropy, as is shown in Fig. 5A. Viewed from the cortical surface, the clutch cell axon occupies an area of about 300 × 500 $\mu$m in layer IV just about the size of a single ocular dominance column or the axonal territory of a thalamic afferent. Based on analogous anatomical features, clutch cells have been identified in the monkey primary visual cortex (Kisvárday et al., 1986a). They differ however from those of the cat in that their axon termination field is considerably smaller, 100–150 $\mu$m in diameter and restricted to the sublamina of layer IVC$\beta$ (Fig. 5B).

A prominent and common feature of each basket cell type is that, in addition to their main axonal field, they give off radially running axon bundles which provide inputs to cells in a column some few hundred $\mu$m in width, as is shown schematically in Fig. 4A,C. These axonal columns usually lie in register with the column of the dendritic field of the parent basket cell and they are often, but not always, centered about the main axonal field. Another interesting phenomenon of these interlaminar projections is that they can selectively skip over certain layers as shown in Fig. 2 for the descending axonal tuft of a layer IV large basket cell which provides its main termination zone in layer VI leaving layer V largely unaffected.

## Efferent connections of basket cells

The very nature of basket cells is that they make multiple contacts with somata of pyramidal and spiny stellate cells as an example is shown in Fig. 3D and E. This has long been recognized and has constituted the basic structural phenomenon in distinguishing basket cells from other smooth or sparsely spiny dendritic cell types. Although it was noted in a number of Golgi studies that each of the so-called "pericellular nest" is probably composed of more than one basket cell axon, the

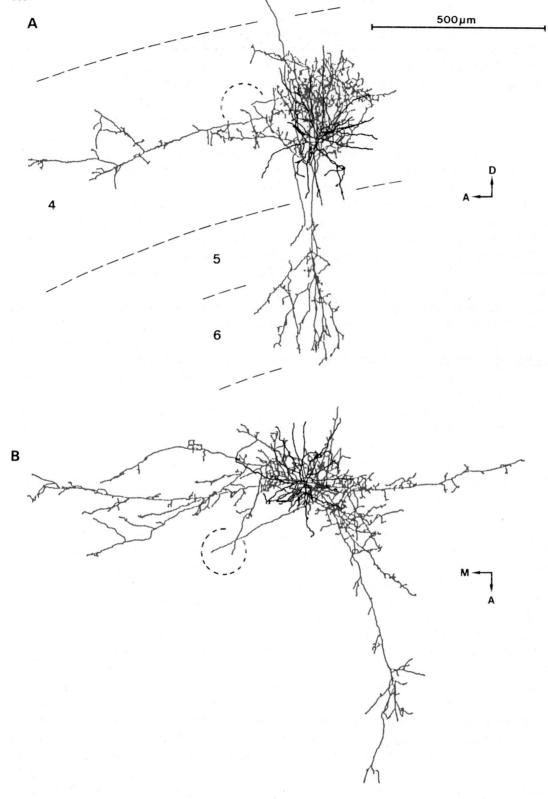

A

500μm

4

5

6

D
A

B

M
A

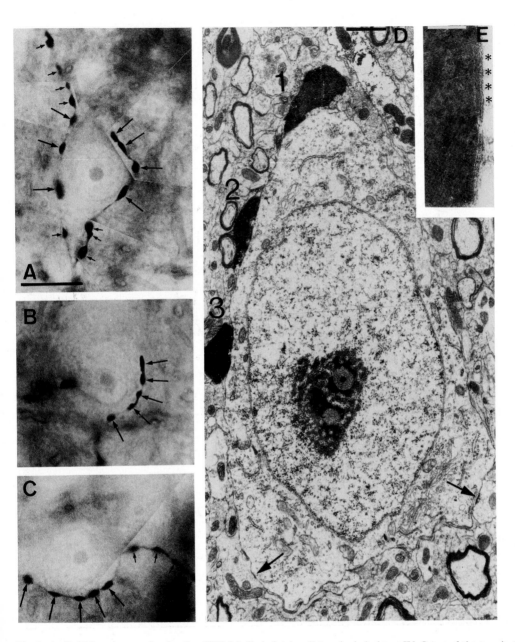

Fig. 3. A–C. Light micrographs showing HRP-labelled clutch cell terminals in layer IV. Some of the terminals surround somata (long arrows), others are in the neuropile (short arrows). D. Electron micrograph of a pyramidal shaped cell in layer IV receiving three axo-somatic contacts (Nos. 1–3) from the axon collateral of a HRP-filled clutch cell. Type II or symmetrical synapse (asterisks) made by bouton No. 3 is shown in a serial section in E. Modified from Kisvárday et al., 1985. Bars: A–C, 10 μm; D, 1 μm; E, 0.1 μm.

Fig. 2. Computer-assisted reconstructions of the axonal (in red) and dendritic (in black) fields of a large basket cell that was labelled with *Phaseolus vulgaris* leucoagglutinin (PHA-L) deposited with extracellular iontophoresis in layer IV of area 18 of cat. A. Parasagittal view showing that the soma, and the majority of the dendrites and axons are in layer IV. Note the descending axonal tuft which profusely branches in layer VI but ignores layer V. B. Viewed from the cortical surface the basket cell has long axonal arms in many directions in layer IV extending up to 1 mm from the parent soma. PHA-L injection site is indicated by broken lines. Reconstruction courtesy of A. Gulyás. A, anterior; D, dorsal; M, medial.

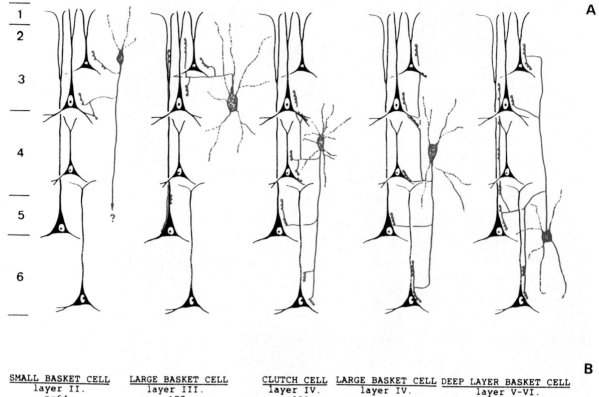

**A**

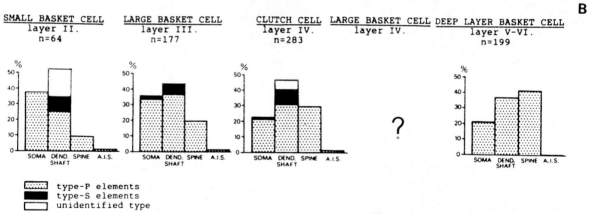

**B**

SMALL BASKET CELL
layer II.
n=64

LARGE BASKET CELL
layer III.
n=177

CLUTCH CELL
layer IV.
n=283

LARGE BASKET CELL
layer IV.

DEEP LAYER BASKET CELL
layer V-VI.
n=199

type-P elements
type-S elements
unidentified type

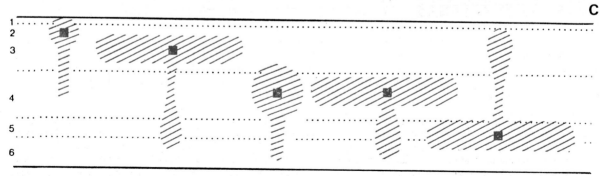

**C**

1 mm

real contribution of basket cells in the total inhibitory inputs of their target cells could only be revealed by quantitative electron microscopic analyses (Somogyi et al., 1983; Kisvárday et al., 1985, 1986a, 1987; Freund et al., 1986). These studies led to the unexpected result that a single basket cell can provide only a small proportion of type II contacts onto its target somata, implying strong inhibitory convergence of other basket cells (see below). From the same studies an even more striking feature emerged, notably, contrary to earlier assumptions, many of the basket cell terminals established synaptic contacts on dendritic shafts and dendritic spines. Furthermore, the quantitative results showed that basket cells make no more than 20–40% of their synaptic contacts onto somata of other cells (Fig. 4B). Most of their targets are dendritic shafts (44–55%) and dendritic spines (10–44%), many of which are located proximal to the soma of the target cell. In the perspective of quantitative data for the main basket cell types, it is noteworthy that the more superficially located basket cells establish a relatively larger proportion of axo-somatic contacts on their target cells (Fig. 4B). Conversely, basket cells in the deeper layers contact substantially more dendritic shafts and dendritic spines (Fig. 4B). At present there is no adequate explanation for this apparently systematic shift in the proportion of the postsynaptic targets as a function of laminar position.

### Identified targets

Pyramidal cells and spiny stellate cells are heterogeneous with respect to their afferent and efferent connections (Gilbert and Wiesel, 1979;

Martin and Whitteridge, 1984). Many of them are true intrinsic neurons with local axons only, others project to different cortical and/or subcortical regions. Since they are the chief targets of basket cells it is essential to determine whether different basket cell types contact different types of pyramidal cells. Due to the difficulty of such an analysis, which requires a combination of techniques, as yet there are only three studies providing direct evidence for the character of the target pyramidal cells. In one study, a layer IV clutch cell was shown to contact the basal dendrite of an intracellularly HRP-labelled layer III pyramidal cell (Kisvárday et al., 1985). The axonal distribution of the same pyramidal cell was analyzed in a different study and was shown to provide long horizontal patchy axons extending over 1 mm in layers III and V (Kisvárday et al., 1986a). In another study, the apical dendrite of a layer V pyramidal cell, retrogradely labelled with HRP from the superior colliculus, was shown to receive synaptic contacts from two axon terminals of an intracellularly HRP-labelled clutch cell (Gabbott et al., 1988). Finally, the ascending axonal tuft of a large layer V basket cell is shown here to terminate on somata of transcallosally HRP-labelled layer III pyramidal cells (Fig. 6). Since many of the pyramidal cells in both supra- and infragranular layers have axonal fields extending up to 5 mm (Gilbert and Wiesel, 1979, 1983; Gabbott et al., 1987; Kisvárday and Eysel, 1990), the implication of these results is that the inhibitory influence of basket cells can actually be conveyed far beyond their axonal field, to regions where the receptive fields are, perhaps, no longer overlapping with that of the basket cell.

Fig. 4. A. Schematic representation of the type of pyramidal cells (in black) targeted by the axons (in red) of small basket cells, large basket cells, and clutch cells in cat visual cortex. Note that each basket cell type provide input as well to somata as to apical and basal dendrites. B. Summary chart of the quantitative distribution of postsynaptic elements of the main basket cell types. Quantitative electron microscopic data for layer IV large basket cells are not available. Type-P and type-S elements represent postsynaptic structures characteristic to pyramidal and smooth dendritic cells, respectively. C. Schematic representation of the radial and horizontal extent of the axonal fields (hatched in red) for the main basket cell types shown in A. Somata are indicated by filled patterns. Data based on several studies: Somogyi et al., 1983; Kisvárday et al., 1985, 1987; Freund et al., 1986.

*Convergence*

One of the major findings of electron microscopic studies carried out on intracellularly HRP-filled basket cells is that each basket cell provides only a fraction of the total inhibitory input converging onto a single target neuron. It was estimated that a total of 10–25 large basket cells would be needed to provide all the type II contacts on the soma of a layer III pyramidal cell (Somogyi et al., 1983). This is in good agreement with the convergence value obtained with cross-correlation analysis, suggesting that about 10 cells may account for certain inhibitory interactions (Toyama et al., 1981). Therefore the early view derived largely from Golgi studies of human material that pericellular basket formations around pyramidal cells are the product of single basket cell axons should be considered with some reservations (Marin-Padilla, 1969). In the monkey and cat, the lack of such a heavy input from a basket cell onto its target pyramidal cells may reflect inter-species differences. Nonetheless it has to be admitted that strong somatic and proximal dendritic inputs of certain pyramidal cells have occasionally been observed in the latter species. An example for this is shown in Fig. 6 demonstrating 22 terminals of the same basket cell axon embracing a pyramidal cell soma in layer III that was retrogradely labelled from the contralateral visual cortex. Further examples were obtained for large layer V basket cells, one of which was shown to establish 34 contacts onto the soma and apical dendrite of a large pyramidal cell in the same layer (neuron $P_3$ in Fig. 3 of Kisvárday et al., 1987). Of those axo-somatic and axo-dendritic contacts, 15 were subsequently verified by electron microscopy. These findings indicate that basket cells can, though infrequently, provide heavy input to some of their targets.

Pyramidal and spiny stellate cells are apparently the main targets of basket cells. Does this mean that basket cells can account for all inhibitory synapses on somata or, alternatively, axon terminals from other sources share the same soma targets with basket cells? Recent electron microscopic studies on Golgi-impregnated and cholecystokinin-immunoreactive double bouquet cells (Somogyi and Cowey, 1981; Freund et al., 1986), and on a Golgi-impregnated fusiform cell with axonal arcade in layers II–III (DeFelipe and Fairen, 1988) showed that up to 9 and 1%, respectively, of their synaptic contacts are directed to somata of pyramidal and non-pyramidal cells. Recent immunocytochemical and tract tracing studies examining the axon termination sites of "non-specific" ascending pathways from subcortical structures such as the brain stem nuclei and the basal forebrain have led to some surprising results. It was observed that serotonergic axons most likely originating from the raphe nuclei formed pericellular baskets in the superficial layers in various cortical areas (Mulligan and Törk, 1988). Moreover preliminary studies indicate that extracortical sources such as those of cholinergic and particularly some GABAergic afferents from the nuclei of the basal forebrain can establish axo-somatic contacts with cortical cells invariably with the GABAergic types, containing somatostatin and parvalbumin (Freund and Meshkenajte, 1989).

The above findings suggest that intracortical GABAergic cell types other than basket cells and GABAergic axons originating from extracortical sources can also contribute to axo-somatic contacts. Notwithstanding, the axo-somatic contacts of these "non-basket cells" represent a much smaller proportion of their total postsynaptic structures than that of any of the genuine basket cell types.

*Divergence*

The spatial extent and density of basket cell axons suggest that the same basket cell may provide axo-somatic input to hundreds of neighbouring cells. Direct counts of the total number of cells contacted by the same basket cell have been carried out only for two clutch cells in layer IV (cells CC1 and CC2 in Kisvárday et al, 1985), showing that their axons contact as many as 454 and 345 somata, respectively. Considering that clutch cells represent a medium size basket cell type with a fairly restricted axonal field of some 500–300 $\mu$m in layer IV (Kisvárday et al., 1985), it would be interesting to know whether large basket cells with axons occupying at least 10–20-times larger areas would actually influence a considerably larger population of neurons. An estimate* based upon available quantitative data shows that the layer III large basket cell shown in Fig. 8 may contact as many as 222 other cells, a minimum value that is unexpectedly smaller than those obtained for clutch cells. The reason for this may be that the neuronal packing density in layer III is smaller than in layer IV or that some of the axonal collaterals of the large basket cell could not be recovered. Nevertheless it is reasonable to postulate that basket cells, irrespective of the spatial extent of their axons, can ultimately target an approximately equal number of cells.

Another important issue is the extent to which basket cells participate in inhibitory connections, in other words what proportion of GABAergic cells are of the basket cell type? A conservative estimate** conducted for cat visual cortex area 17 indicates that about 17% of all GABAergic cells actually belong to the family of basket cells. Although this figure seems to be high it leaves no doubt that basket cells are likely to be one of the most common non-pyramidal cell types, at least in cat visual cortex. Considering that in other species, for example primates, a much larger variety of neuronal types have developed, in those species, basket cells may represent a less significant population of GABAergic cells, though per-

haps with even more sophisticated subtypes (see Lund et al., 1988). The most important implication here is that basket cells, probably due to the high physiological impact of somatic inhibition, by evolution became one of the most significantly represented inhibitory cell types in cat.

## Input to basket cells

### Thalamic input

The functional role(s) of basket cells cannot be conceived without determining their input drive. The limited information that is available at present derives from combined electrophysiological and anatomical works. So far only five intracellularly HRP-filled basket cells have been tested for a battery of electrophysiological tests (Martin et al., 1983; Gabbott et al., 1988). They included three large basket cells in layer III and two clutch cells in layer IV. It was reported that four of them could be monosynaptically activated by either X- or Y-type geniculate afferents, the remaining one received polysynaptic visual thalamic input (Table 1 in Martin et al., 1983; Gabbott et al., 1988). Additionally, two of the basket cells could be monosynaptically activated via the corpus callosum (Martin et al., 1983).

Subsequent anatomical evidence for the relationship between basket cells and specific thalamic afferents was brought about by the study of intracellularly HRP-filled X- and Y-type geniculate axons whose axonal termination fields were

---

* The estimation for layer III large basket cells is as follows. They establish an average of 1.13 synapses per bouton, and a total of 35.6% of their postsynaptic elements are neuronal somata each of which receive, on average, five boutons from the same basket cell (Somogyi et al., 1983). Furthermore, in a separate study, a total of 2755 boutons were counted for a large basket cell in layer III (Kisvárday and Eysel, 1991b). Taken together, it can be calculated that the above large basket cell would establish $1.13 \times 2755$ synapses of which 35.6%, that is 1108 contacts, would be on somata of a total of 222 other cells.

---

** Recent electron microscopic data suggest that, of the 278.5 million synapses per mm$^3$, 16% are the so-called flat symmetrical type (Beaulieu and Colonnier, 1985) of which 97% are GABAergic (Beaulieu and Somogyi, 1990). Of the latter 13.1%, that is 5.66 million per mm$^3$, contact somata of pyramidal as well as non-pyramidal cells. Since every basket cell establishes approximately 1000 axo-somatic contacts it can be calculated that about 1900 basket cells are present in every mm$^3$ of visual cortex. Taken these values together with the notion that there are about 11 000 GABAergic cells in the same unit volume of cortex (Gabbott and Somogyi, 1986) it is just conceivable that about 17% of all GABAergic cells are basket cells.

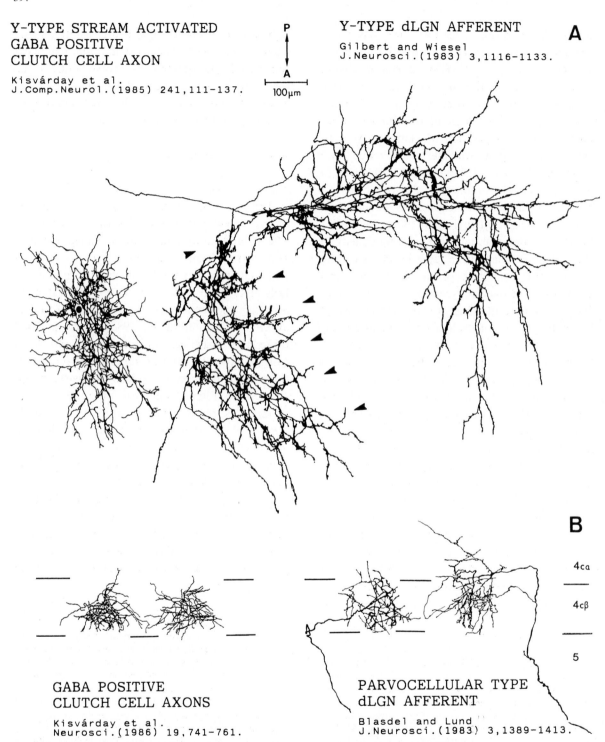

Y-TYPE STREAM ACTIVATED
GABA POSITIVE
CLUTCH CELL AXON

Kisvárday et al.
J.Comp.Neurol.(1985) 241,111-137.

P
A
100μm

Y-TYPE dLGN AFFERENT

A

Gilbert and Wiesel
J.Neurosci.(1983) 3,1116-1133.

B

4cα

4cβ

5

GABA POSITIVE
CLUTCH CELL AXONS

Kisvárday et al.
Neurosci.(1986) 19,741-761.

PARVOCELLULAR TYPE
dLGN AFFERENT

Blasdel and Lund
J.Neurosci.(1983) 3,1389-1413.

Fig. 5. Resemblance between the axon termination patterns of GABAergic clutch cells and dLGN afferents in layer IV of cat (A) and monkey (B) visual cortex (area 17). A. Computer reconstructions in a plane parallel with the pia, showing that both the clutch axon and each of the Y-axonal clumps occupy an area of about $500 \times 300$ μm elongated in anterior-posterior direction. Notice the small repeat in both axonal types at about 100 μm intervals (arrowheads). B. Drawings of two Golgi-impregnated clutch cell axons (on the left) and two intracellularly HRP-labelled parvocellular-type geniculate afferents (on the right). Note that both axonal types are confined to layer IVCβ and have similar size and density of fine collaterals. A and B are at the same scale.

subjected to quantitative electron microscopic analysis (Freund et al., 1985). The results showed that, in areas 17 and 18, X- and Y-type geniculate axons occasionally terminate on somata of layer IV neurons, each of which showed immunopositivity for GABA, and their ultrastructure was very similar to identified basket cells. Area measurements of the targeted GABA neurons revealed that X-type geniculate axons synapse predominantly on smaller somata than do Y-type axons (see Fig. 10 in Freund et al., 1985). It was then concluded that the smaller GABA-immunopositive cells might represent clutch cells while the large GABA cells probably represent large basket cells. This assumption is supported by previous ultrastructural data obtained for the somatic input of identified large basket cells and clutch cells (Somogyi et al., 1983; Kisvárday et al., 1985). They were shown to receive dense synaptic input from large horseshoe shaped terminals containing large, round vesicles and forming type I synapses with the soma membrane; all these features are characteristic for the terminals of the specific thalamic afferents (Freund et al., 1985).

Another positive indication for an interaction between the basket cells and the specific thalamic afferents is based upon comparisons between their axon termination patterns. In this respect it is informative to compare the axon of a layer IV clutch cell that was monosynaptically activated via Y-type geniculate afferents with a Y-type axon terminating in the same layer (Fig. 5A). The Y axon established two clumps of terminals each about the size of the clutch cell. Furthermore both axons composed dense axonal stripes at about 100 $\mu$m intervals (Fig. 5A). Similar comparison is made in the monkey striate cortex as shown in Fig. 5B. The high level of correspondence between the clutch axons and the thalamic afferents in cat and monkey supports the notion that they may have common targets in layer IV, presumably leading to feed forward type of inhibition (see Sillito, Chapter 17).

*Intracortical input*

One of the weakest points in the otherwise large body of data on basket cells is the almost complete lack of knowledge concerning the intracortical input to their dendritic shafts. Although electron microscopy of basket cells' dendrites showed that they are, in general, abundantly supplied with type I and II contacts (Somogyi et al., 1983; Kisvárday et al., 1985), hardly any anatomical data is available as yet on their precise origin. In view of recent observations of the target distribution of identified pyramidal cells providing sparse input to any of their targeted cells, it can be argued that basket cells receive strongly converging input from intracortical excitatory sources, including the long-range patchy axonal system of certain pyramidal cells (Kisvárday et al., 1986b; Kisvárday and Eysel, 1991).

As far as the somatic input to basket cells is concerned, a clear picture is emerging. Immunocytochemical studies using antisera against GAD and GABA have demonstrated that, in addition to pyramidal cells, GABAergic neurons also receive dense axo-somatic input from GABAergic terminals (Ribak, 1978; Hendry et al., 1983; Freund et al., 1983). Undoubtedly these observations are comparable with the view that basket cells contact other inhibitory neurons. Electron microscopic evidence for the type of GABAergic cells postsynaptic to an HRP-filled large basket cell showed that they have ultrastructural features of identified large basket cells (Fig. 7, Somogyi et al., 1983). Further evidence was recently obtained using a combination of extracellular labelling with biocytin and immunocytochemical detection of the calcium binding protein, parvalbumin, in the same sections (Kisvárday and Eysel, 1991). The neuronal tracer, biocytin, labelled large basket cells in their entire morphology in layers III and V while parvalbumin was used to reveal somata of a subpopulation of GABAergic cells including basket cells. It was found that the axon of the biocytin labelled large basket cells established

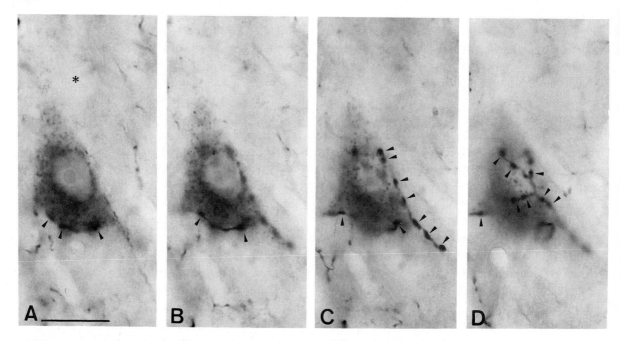

Fig. 6. A–D. A callosally projecting pyramidal cell receives basket cell input in layer III. The pyramidal cell was retrogradely labelled with HRP (dark intracellular deposit) from contralateral area 18. For comparison an unlabelled soma is marked by asterisk in A. At different focal depths the same cell is shown to receive 22 contacts (arrowheads) onto its soma and proximal dendrites from an ascending collateral of a large basket cell labelled with extracellularly deposited PHA-L in layer V. Bar: A–D, 20 μm.

multiple contacts, usually 2–5, with the somata of many PV-immunopositive neurons (Fig. 8, Kisvárday and Eysel, 1991b). By visual estimation, the distribution of the basket recipient PV-immunopositive cells show a quasi-regular distribution with an average of 100 μm intervals (Fig. 8). Remarkably, most of them had medium-to-large soma similar in size to those of identified large basket cells (Fig. 9C and D), suggesting that large basket cells, apart from their well-known pyramidal targets, selectively contact each other. This hypothesis was confirmed by quantitative soma size measurements carried out for the target PV-immunopositive neurons and for basket cells that were labelled in their entire morphology by extracellularly deposited *Phaseolus vulgaris* leucoagglutinin and biocytin (Fig. 9A, B). The direct interpretation of the results is that the axons of large basket cells contact somata of other large basket cells up to 1.5 mm from their parent soma (Fig. 8). A straightforward functional consequence of such a specific wiring would be a kind

of double duty of large basket cells; inhibiting remote inhibitory cells in a cascade-like manner whose targets would thus be disinhibited while, on the other hand, directly inhibiting cells in a simple feed-forward manner (see below).

## Chemical heterogeneity of basket cells

Basket cells comprise a heterogeneous population with respect to their anatomical features. It is therefore entirely logical to assume that their diversity seen at the anatomical level may represent heterogeneity in their overall chemical content other than GABA. Indeed, more recent immunocytochemical experiments have revealed that several of the brain-gut peptides co-exist in cortical GABAergic cells (for review, see Jones and Hendry, 1986; Demeulemeester et al., 1988). At present at least two neuropeptides, cholecystokinin (CCK) and neuropeptide-Y (NPY), have been shown to co-localize with GABA in certain cells showing similar soma size, shape and dendritic morphology to identified basket cells

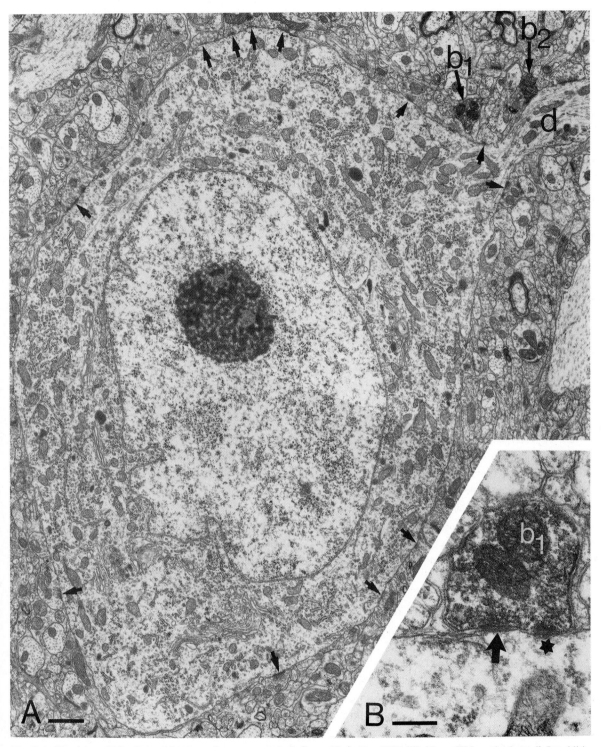

Fig. 7. A. Non-pyramidal cell receiving input from two terminals ($b_1$ and $b_2$) of an HRP-filled layer III large basket cell. In addition to these terminals the non-pyramidal soma receives a large number of type I and type II contacts (arrows) of unknown origin. Bouton $b_1$ is shown in a serial section in B to establish a type II contact (arrow) and a punctum adherens (star) with the soma. Note the difference in the somatic input, the density of mitochondria and ribosomes between this neuron and the pyramidal shaped cell shown in Fig. 3D. With permission from Somogyi et al., 1983. Bars: A, 1 $\mu$m; B, 0.2 $\mu$m.

(Freund et al., 1986; Wahle et al, 1986; Meyer and Wahle, 1988). Other immunocytochemical findings indicate that large basket cells and clutch cells contain intracellular calcium-binding proteins, e.g., parvalbumin (Celio, 1986; Hendry et al., 1989), and on the basis of their medium-to-large soma size and predominantly vertically oriented dendritic field they are likely to express cell surface antigens for monoclonal antibodies Cat-301, VC.1.1 and VC5.1, and for the lectin extracted from plant seeds of hairy vetch (*Vicia villosa*, for review see Barnstable and Naegele, 1989).

Thus it is just conceivable that subsets of basket cell types, such as large basket cells, in addition to their main inhibitory transmitter GABA, express different "cocktails" of intra- and extracellular matrix molecules, perhaps in relation to their target specificity or some of their functional roles that is unknown yet.

## What do basket cells do?

There is now overwhelming evidence that many of the receptive field properties in the visual cortex are strongly, if not entirely dependent upon inhibitory mechanisms mediated by GABAergic interneurons (for review, see Sillito and Murphy, 1988). It is well established that GABAergic interneurons constitute a heterogeneous population with respect to their anatomical, chemical and physiological properties, suggesting that different types of GABAergic cells underlie different receptive field transformation tasks. Of the many GABAergic cell types basket cells are unique in that they provide the major source of perisomatic inhibitory input to virtually all cortical neurons, implying their distinguished functional role(s). Indeed there is a large body of theoretical evidence suggesting that perisomatic inhibition, as opposed to inhibition on the distal dendrites and spines, is divisive, that is, very efficient in preventing incoming excitatory signals to bring the cell to its firing treshold (Blomfield, 1974; Koch and Poggio, 1985). Experimental data for orientation tuning (Rose, 1977; Morrone et al., 1982), direction

selectivity (Dean et al., 1980), and suppression of foreground bar responses by moving noise background (Crook, 1990) have been shown to depend, at least partially, upon divisive inhibition, suggesting the involvement of basket cells. Evidence for the type of basket cells involved in these mechanisms derives from experiments using iontophoretic application of GABA and simultaneous recordings of single units at remote locations. It was found that orientation selectivity can be influenced effectively from lateral distances of 500–600 $\mu$m (Eysel et al., 1990; Crook et al., 1991), and direction tuning from about 1 mm up to an overall distance of 2.5 mm (Eysel et al., 1988) of the recorded cell. Thus, orientation and direction tuning would seem to involve long-range lateral inhibition, suggesting that the type of GABAergic cells taking part in these mechanisms must have extensive axonal collaterals over a range of 0.5–2.5 mm from their somata. It has to be admitted, however, that while the distance of lateral inhibition involved in orientation tuning could fit to the axonal extent of a number of GABAergic cell types, including basket cells with short-range axons, the very large distance observed in the generation of direction tuning meets only with the axonal extent of the type of large basket cell. Since much of this issue is extensively discussed by Eysel (Chapter 19), I would like to highlight only some very recent anatomical findings concerning the cell-to-cell interactions supposedly involved in direction tuning. Notably, as is shown here, in addition to their well-known pyramidal cell targets, large basket cells selectively contact each other along their elongated axonal fields (Fig. 8). The following wiring is proposed to account for direction preference (Fig. 10). Firstly, the local axonal collaterals of the large basket cell contact pyramidal cells with like direction preference, as opposed to the remote collaterals which terminate on pyramidal cells with opposite direction preference to that of the large basket cell. Secondly, in addition to their pyramidal targets, the remote collaterals of the large basket cell inhibit other large basket cells

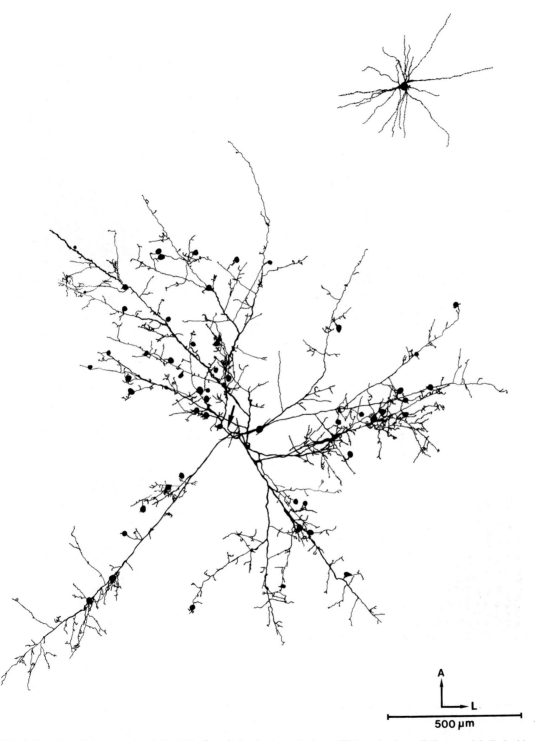

Fig. 8. Drawing of the axonal and dendritic (inset) distribution of a layer III large basket cell that was labelled with extracellular deposit of biocytin into the same layer and reconstructed from 7 consecutive 80 μm thick horizontal sections. The axon established contacts with the somata (dots) of 58 cells that showed positive immunoreaction for parvalbumin, presumably representing other large basket cells. Arrow indicates the soma location of the basket cell. A, anterior; L, lateral.

400

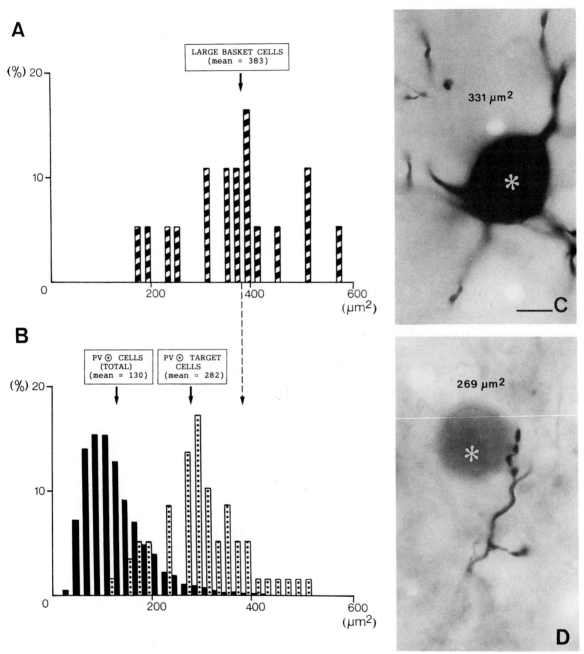

Fig. 9. Area distribution of the somata of identified layer III large basket cells (hatched bars in A, *n* = 18), the total population of parvalbumin-immunopositive cells in layer III (filled bars in B, *n* = 4552), and parvalbumin-immunopositive cells (dotted bars in B, *n* = 58) which are targeted by the layer III large basket cell shown in Fig. 8. Arrows indicate mean values for each group. Note that values in A were not corrected for soma size increase caused by the strong labelling of the tracer. In C and D, somata of a biocytin labelled large basket cell, and a parvalbumin-immunopositive cell targeted by four terminals of the biocytin labelled basket cell shown in Fig. 8, respectively, are seen. Note that the soma size of cells in C and D are above the average value shown for the total population of parvalbumin positive neurons in B. Bar: C and D, 10 $\mu$m.

whose local axons provide input only to those pyramidal cells which do not receive input from axons of the remote large basket cell. Thus the latter pyramidal cells would show like direction preference to that of the large basket cell. This connectivity pattern implies that pyramidal cells receiving direct feed-forward inhibition have opposite direction preference, and pyramidal cells receiving feed-forward disinhibition, since their large basket cell input is inhibited, have like direction preference to that of the large basket cell (Fig. 10). Considering that a large basket cell can contact a number of other large basket cells, a more general picture about an extensive network underlying direction specificity can be conjectured. That is, when a visual stimulus moves across the visual field it would result in widespread inhibition as well as disinhibition sweeping ahead of the stimulus. Only those cells can respond to the stimulus whose inhibitory input is sufficiently supressed by feed-forward inhibition (disinhibition) mediated by large basket cells' interaction. When the stimulus moves in the opposite direction the same cells would receive feed-forward and local inhibition from a different set of large basket cells. The present anatomical findings of specific basket cell-to-basket cell interactions strongly support such an hypothesis although in attempting to resolve many of the details it would be particularly important to know the exact relationship between the axonal fields of interconnected large basket cells, and the complete pattern of large basket cell axons supplying each pyramidal cell.

*Interlaminar inhibition*

A prominent feature of the structural organization of the cerebral cortex is that each layer has extensive reciprocal connections with virtually any other layer in the same column. This organization scheme applies for the axonal distribution of basket cells with regard to their different morphological types invariably providing descending and ascending collaterals to contact cells in layers other than that of their parent somata. These radially running collaterals usually form narrow axonal cylinders of approximately a few hundred $\mu$m in diameter as illustrated schematically in Fig. 4C. Pertinent to this are the findings that the basket cell cylinders often lie in precise register with the somata and dendritic field of their parent cells. This precise topographical arrangement indicates that their target cells belong to the very same functional column. Surprisingly, however, contrary to their horizontally running collateral systems, no particular functional role has yet been associated to the interlaminar connections of basket cells. It may be an important clue to determine the type of cells on which these interlaminar basket axons terminate. Based on light- and electron microscopic observations, it is probably fair to say that most of the cells targeted by the interlaminar projections of basket cells are pyramidal cells in the three major output laminae, layers III, V and VI. Thus one of the likely roles of the radial collateral system of basket cells is to influence certain output streams projecting to other cortical and/or subcortical structures. Indeed, this line of thought is affirmed by the fact that the ascending axonal tuft of a large layer V basket cell is shown here to contact pyramidal neurons in layer III projecting to other cortical areas via the corpus callosum (see Fig. 6). Because callosal connections have been assumed to play a special role in mechanisms underlying binocularity of visual cortical cells, certain basket cells thus may be functionally related to processing involved in stereopsis (Payne et al., 1984).

Another set of anatomical data indicates that the same interlaminar basket cell projections are involved in the control of corticofugal pathways originating in layer V. Somata and apical dendrites of giant layer V pyramidal cells similar to those projecting to the optic tectum (Garey, 1971; Gilbert and Kelly, 1975) were demonstrated to receive a mixture of dense inhibitory input from each of the three main tiers of the cortex, namely, from the interlaminar collaterals of large basket cells in layers III (Somogyi et al., 1983) and of clutch cells in layer IV (Kisvárday et al., 1985;

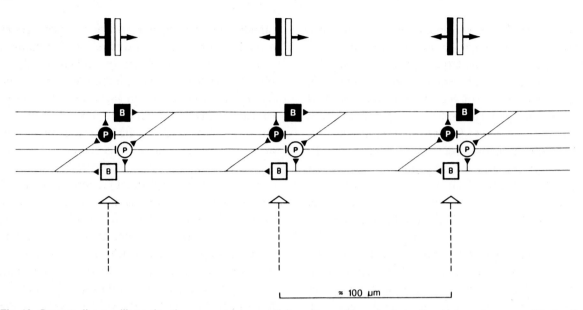

Fig. 10. Concept diagram illustrating the asymmetric connectivity pattern of large basket cells which maybe responsible for the generation of direction selectivity in cat visual cortex. [B], GABAergic large basket cell; P, excitatory pyramidal cell. Neurons with direction preferences towards left and right are indicated by filled and unfilled symbols, respectively. Input from the dLGN (broken lines) reaches both inhibitory and excitatory neurons. Connections of each basket cell is shown only to its closest targeted basket cell, at about 100 $\mu$m. See further details in the text.

Gabbott et al., 1988) and from the local and interlaminar collaterals of large basket cells in layer V (Kisvárday et al., 1987). Since layer V pyramidal cells have been assumed to convey information concerning motion analysis, at present, the most straightforward functional implication for their intracolumnar basket inputs is the involvement in their control of visual guidance processing.

Layer VI pyramidal cells have been demonstrated as the main source of corticogeniculate input (Baughman and Gilbert, 1981) and, via their recurrent collaterals, intracortical input to layer IV (Gilbert and Wiesel, 1979). It was recently shown by local application of GABA in layer VI that silencing layer VI, length tuning of overlying layer IV cells is eliminated (Bolz and Gilbert, 1986). In a separate experiment, Murphy and Sillito (1987, see also Sillito, Chapter 17) have shown that removal of striate cortex causes marked reduction of length tuning characteristics of cells in the dLGN. These studies indicate that any inhibitory action on the perisomatic region of

layer VI neurons can influence the length tuning properties of their target cells both at cortical and thalamic levels. However, no suggestion for the origin of such an inhibitory input has been made. At present there are two types of large basket cell which, by the distribution pattern of their axonal fields, can directly inhibit layer VI cells; firstly, large layer V basket cells occasionally contact the somadendrites of layer VI cells (Kisvárday et al., 1987); secondly, and it is proposed for the first time here, that the descending collaterals of large layer IV basket cells impinge upon the somadendrites of layer VI pyramidal cells (Fig. 2). While the projections of large layer V basket cells are mainly concerned with the output control of pyramidal cells in layers III and V, as shown above, the descending axonal tuft of large layer IV basket cells is engaged in providing dense input to layer VI. Accordingly, the latter basket cells can account for a powerful inhibitory control of layer VI pyramidal cells, suggesting that information concerning the generation of length tuning in layer IV is under a supervision by feed-back projections of layer IV inhibitory neurons transmitted most likely via large basket cells (see Fig. 2). This wiring scheme is further complicated if one considers that layer IV basket cells are themselves exposed to direct thalamic input which is itself probably length tuned (see Sillito, Chapter 17). Thus it is conceivable that the generation of length tuning is an integrative phenomenon of all those feed-forward and feed-back interactions, taking place between layers IV and VI, and the dLGN rather than the product of a single pathway.

## Acknowledgment

The author wishes to thank Dr. U.T. Eysel for stimulating discussions throughout the course of this work, Dr. J.M. Crook for critically reading the manuscript, Ms. Eva Tóth for excellent technical assistance, and Ms. Dorothy Strehler and Mr. Ernst Steven for high quality photography. Z.F.K. is supported by the Alexander von Humboldt Foundation and the Hungarian Academy of Sciences.

## References

Albus, K. (1975) A quantitative study of the projection area of the central and the paracentral visual field in area 17 of the cat. I. The precision of the topography. *Exp. Brain Res.*, 24: 159–179.

Andersen, P., Eccles, J.C. and Loyning, Y. (1963a) Recurrent inhibition in the hippocampus with identification of the inhibitory cell and its synapses. *Nature*, 198: 540–542.

Andersen, P., Eccles, J.C. and Voorhoeve, P.E. (1963b) Inhibitory synapses on somata of Purkinje cells in the cerebellum. *Nature*, 199: 540–542.

Baughman, R.W. and Gilbert, C.D. (1981) Aspartate and glutamate as possible neurotransmitters in the visual cortex. *J. Neurosci.*, 1: 427–439.

Beaulieu, C. and Colonnier, M. (1985) A laminar analysis of the number of round-asymmetrical and flat-symmetrical synapses on spines, dendritic trunks, and cell bodies in area 17 of the cat. *J. Comp. Neurol.*, 231: 180–189.

Beaulieu, C. and Somogyi, P (1990) Targets and quantitative distribution of GABAergic synapses in the visual cortex of the cat. *Eur. J. Neurosci.*, 2: 296–303.

Benevento, L.A., Creutzfeldt, Benevento, L.A., Creutzfeldt, O.D. and Kuhnt, U. (1972) Significance of intracortical inhibition in the visual cortex. *Nature*, 238: 124–126.

Blasdel, G.G. and Lund, J.S. (1983) Termination of afferent axons in macaque striate cortex. *J. Neurosci.*, 3: 1389–1413.

Blomfield, S. (1974) Arithmetical operations performed by nerve cells. *Brain Res.*, 69: 115–124.

Bolz, J. and Gilbert, C.D. (1986) Generation of end-inhibition in the visual cortex via interlaminar connections. *Nature*, 320: 362–365.

Celio, M.R. (1986) Parvalbumin in most γ-aminobutyric acid-containing neurons of the rat cerebral cortex. *Science*, 231: 995–996.

Crook, J.M. (1990) Modulatory influences of a moving visual noise background on bar-evoked responses of cells in area 18 of the feline visual cortex. *Exp. Brain Res.*, 80: 562–576.

Crook, J.M., Eysel, U.T. and Machemer, H.F. (1991) Influence of GABA-induced remote inactivation on the orientation tuning of cells in area 18 of feline visual cortex: a comparison with area 17. *Neuroscience*, 40: 1–12.

Dean, A.F., Hess, R.F. and Tolhurst, D.J. (1980) Divisive inhibition involved in directional selectivity. *Proc. J. Physiol. Soc.*, 84–85PP.

DeFelipe, J. and Fairen, A. (1988) Synaptic connections of an interneuron with axonal arcades in the cat visual cortex. *J. Neurocytol.*, 17: 313–323.

Demeulemeester, H., Vandesande, F., Orban, G.A., Brandon, C. and Vanderhaeghen, J.J. (1988) Heterogeneity of GABAergic cells in cat visual cortex. *J. Neurosci.*, 8: 988–1000.

Eysel, U., Muche, T. and Wörgötter, F. (1988) Lateral interactions at direction-selective striate neurones in the cat demonstrated by local cortical inactivation. *J. Physiol. (London)*, 399: 657–675.

Eysel, U.T., Crook, J.M. and Machemer, H.F. (1990) GABA-induced remote inactivation reveals cross-orientation inhibition in the cat striate cortex. *Exp. Brain Res.*, 80: 626–630.

Freund, T.F. and Meshkenajte, V. (1990) Termination pattern of GABAergic basal forebrain afferents in the cat neocortex: innervation of somatostatin- and parvalbumin-immunoreactive interneurons. *Eur. J. Neurosci.*, Suppl. 3, 1113.

Freund, T.F., Maglóczky, Zs, Soltész, I. and Somogyi, P. (1986) Synaptic connections, axonal and dendritic patterns of neurons immunoreactive for cholecystokinin in the visual cortex of the cat. *Neuroscience*, 19: 1133–1159.

Freund, T.F., Martin, K.A.C., Smith, A.D. and Somogyi, P. (1983) Glutamate decarboxylase-immunoreactive terminals of Golgi-impregnated axoaxonic cells and of presumed basket cells in synaptic contact with pyramidal neurons of the cat's visual cortex. *J. Comp. Neurol.*, 221: 263–278.

Freund, T.F., Martin, K.A.C., Somogyi, P. and Whitteridge, D. (1985) Innervation of cat visual areas 17 and 18 by physiologically identified X- and Y-type thalamic afferents. II. Identification of postsynaptic targets by GABA immunocytochemistry and Golgi impregnation. *J. Comp. Neurol.*, 242: 275–291.

Gabbott, P.L.A. and Somogyi, P. (1986) Quantitative distribution of GABA-immunoreactive neurons in the visual cortex (area 17) of the cat. *Exp. Brain Res.*, 61: 323–331.

Gabbott, P.L., Martin, K.C.A. and Whitteridge, D. (1987)

Connections between pyramidal neurons in layer 5 of cat visual cortex (area 17). *J. Comp. Neurol.*, 259: 364–381.

Gabbott, P.L.A., Martin, K.A.C. and Whitteridge, D. (1988) Evidence for the connections between a clutch cell and a corticotectal neuron in area 17 of the cat visual cortex. *Proc. R. Soc. London B.*, 233: 385–391.

Garey, L.J. (1971) A light and electron microscopic study of the visual cortex of the cat and monkey. *Proc. R. Soc. London B.*, 179: 21–40.

Gilbert, C.D. and Kelly, J.P. (1975) The projections of cells in different layers of the cat's visual cortex. *J. Comp. Neurol.*, 163: 81–106.

Gilbert, C.D. and Wiesel, T.N. (1979) Morphology and intracortical projections of functionally characterized neurones in the cat visual cortex. *Nature*, 280: 120–125.

Gilbert, C.D. and Wiesel, T.N. (1983) Clustered intrinsic connections in cat visual cortex. *J. Neurosci.*, 3: 1116–1133.

Hendry, S.C.H., Jones, E.G., Emson, P.C., Lawson, D.E.M., Heizmann, C.W. and Streit, P. (1989) Two classes of cortical GABA neurons defined by differential calcium binding protein immunoreactivities. *Exp. Brain Res.*, 76: 467–472.

Hendry, S.H.C., Houser, C.R., Jones, E.J. and Vaughn, J.E. (1983) Synaptic organization of immunocytochemically identified GABA neurons in the monkey sensory-motor cortex. *J. Neurocytol.*, 12: 639–660.

Hubel, D.H. and Wiesel, T.N. (1962) Receptive fields binocular interaction and functional architecture in the cat's visual cortex. *J. Physiol.*, 160: 106–154.

Jones, E.G. and Hendry, S.H.C. (1986) Co-localization of GABA and neuropeptides in neocortical neurons. *TINS*, 71–76.

Jones, E.G. and Hendry, S.H.C. (1984) Basket cells. In: A. Peters and E.G. Jones (Eds.), *Cerebral Cortex. Vol. 1. Cellular Components of the Cerebral Cortex*, New York and London: Plenum Press, pp. 309–336.

Kisvárday, Z.F. and Eysel, U.T. (1991a) Cellular organization of reciprocal patchy networks in Layer III of cat visual cortex (area 17). *Neuroscience*, in press.

Kisvárday, Z.F. and Eysel, U.T. (1991b) Basket cells receive long-range inhibition from other basket cells in cat visual cortex (area 18). *Eur. J. Neurosci.*, Suppl. 4: 1228.

Kisvárday, Z.F. and Eysel, U.T. (1990) Relationship between excitatory and inhibitory long range connections in the cat visual cortex. *Soc. Neurosci. Abstr.*, 16: 523.9.

Kisvárday, Z.F., Martin, K.A.C., Friedlander, M.J. and Somogyi, P. (1987) Evidence for interlaminar inhibitory circuits in the striate cortex of the cat. *J. Comp. Neurol.*, 260: 1–19.

Kisvárday, Z.F., Cowey, A. and Somogyi, P. (1986a) Dendritic and axonal patterns of a type of GABA-immunoreactive neuron and its synaptic relationship to spiny stellate cells in layer IVC of the monkey striate cortex. *Neuroscience*, 19: 741–761.

Kisvárday, Z.F., Martin, K.A.C., Freund, T.F., Maglóczky, Zs., Whitteridge, D. and Somogyi, P. (1986b) Synaptic targets of HRP-filled layer III pyramidal cells in the cat striate cortex. *Exp. Brain Res.*, 64: 541–552.

Kisvárday, Z.F., Martin, K.A.C., Whitteridge, D. and Somogyi, P. (1985) Synaptic connections of intracellularly filled clutch cells: a type of small basket cell in the visual cortex of the cat. *J. Comp. Neurol.*, 241: 111–137.

Koch, C. and Poggio, T. (1985) The synaptic veto mechanism: does it underlie direction and orientation selectivity in the visual cortex? In: D. Rose and V.G. Dobson (Eds.), *Models of the Visual Cortex*, New York: John Wiley, pp. 408–419.

Krnjevic, K. and Schwartz, S. (1966) The action of $\gamma$-aminobutyric acid on cortical neurons. *Exp. Brain Res.*, 3: 320–336.

Lund, J.S., Hawken, M.J. and Parker, A.J. (1988) Local circuit neurons of macaque monkey striate cortex. II. Neurons of laminae 5B and 6. *J. Comp. Neurol.*, 276: 1–29.

Marin-Padilla, M. (1969) Origin of the pericellular baskets of the pyramidal cells of the human motor cortex: a Golgi study. *Brain Res.*, 14: 633–646.

Martin, K.A.C. and Whitteridge, D. (1984) Form, function and intracortical projections of spiny neurones in the striate visual cortex of the cat. *J. Physiol.*, 353: 463–504.

Martin, K.A.C., Somogyi, P. and Whitteridge, D. (1983) Physiological and morphological properties of identified basket cells in the cat's visual cortex. *Exp. Brain Res.*, 50: 193–200.

Meyer, G. (1983) Axonal patterns and topography of short-axon neurons in visual areas 17, 18, and 19 of the cat. *J. Comp. Neurol.*, 220: 405–438.

Meyer, G. and Wahle, P. (1988) Early postnatal development of cholecystokinin-immunoreactive structures in the visual cortex of the cat. *J. Comp. Neurol.*, 276: 360–386.

Morrone, M.C., Burr, D.C. and Maffei, L. (1982) Functional implications of cross-orientation inhibition of cortical visual cells. I. Neurophysiological evidence. *Proc. R. Soc. London B.*, 216: 335–354.

Mulligan, K.A. and Törk, I. (1988) Serotonergic innervation of the cat cerebral cortex. *J. Comp. Neurol.*, 270: 86–110.

Murphy, P.C. and Sillito, A.M. (1987) Corticofugal feedback influences the generation of length tuning in the visual pathway. *Nature*, 329: 727–729.

Naegele, J.R. and Barnstable, C.J. (1989) Molecular determinants of GABAergic local-circuit neurons in the visual cortex. *TINS*, 12: 28–34.

Payne, B.R., Pearson, H.E. and Berman, N. (1984) Role of corpus callosum in functional organization of cat striate cortex. *J. Neurophysiol.*, 52: 570–594.

Ramón y Cajal, S. (1899) Estudios sobre la corteza cerebral humana. Corteza visual. *Rev. Trim. Microgr.*, 4: 1–63.

Ribak, C.E. (1978) Aspinous and sparsely-spinous stellate neurons in the visual cortex of rats contain glutamic acid decarboxylase. *J. Neurocytol.*, 7: 461–478.

Rose, D. (1977) On the arithmetical operation performed by inhibitory synapses onto the neuronal soma. *Exp. Brain Res.*, 28: 221–223.

Sillito, A.M. and Murphy, P.C. (1988) GABAergic processes in the central visual system. In: M. Avoli, R.W. Dykes, T.A. Reader and P. Gloor (Eds.), *Neurotransmitters and Cortical Function From Molecules to Mind*, New York: Plenum, pp. 167–186.

Somogyi, P. (1986) Seven distinct types of GABA-immunoreactive neuron in the visual cortex of cat. *Soc. Neurosci. Abstr.*, 12: 583.

Somogyi, P. and Cowey, A. (1981) Combined Golgi and electron microscopic study on the synapses formed by double bouquet cells in the visual cortex of the cat and monkey. *J. Comp. Neurol.*, 195: 547–566.

Somogyi, P. and Soltész, I. (1986) Immunogold demonstration of GABA in synaptic terminals of intracellularly recorded, horseradish peroxidase-filled basket cells and clutch cells in the cat's visual cortex. *Neuroscience*, 19: 1051–1065.

Somogyi, P., Kisvárday, Z.F., Martin, K.A.C. and Whitteridge, D. (1983) Synaptic connections of morphologically identified and physiologically characterized large basket cells in the striate cortex of the cat. *Neuroscience*, 10: 261–294.

Szentágothai, J. (1975) The "module-concept" in cerebral cortex architecture. *Brain Res.*, 95: 475–496.

Szentágothai, J. (1973) Synaptology of the visual cortex. In: R. Jung (Ed.), *Handbook of Sensory Physiology. Vol. 7. Part 3B, Central Processing of Visual Information*, Heidelberg: Springer Verlag, pp. 269–324.

Szentágothai, J. (1965) The use of degeneration methods in the investigation of short neuronal connexions. In: W. Singer and J.P. Schadé (Eds.), *Progress in Brain Research, Vol. 14*, Amsterdam: Elsevier, pp. 1–32.

Toyama, K., Kimura, M. and Tanaka, K. (1981) Cross-correlation analysis of interneuronal connectivity in cat visual cortex. *J. Neurophysiol.*, 46: 191–201.

Wahle, P., Meyer, G. and Albus, K. (1986) Localization of NPY-immunoreactivity in the cat's visual cortex. *Exp. Brain Res.*, 61: 364–374.

R.R. Mize, R.E. Marc and A.M. Sillito (Eds.)
Progress in Brain Research, Vol. 90

CHAPTER 19

# Lateral inhibitory interactions in areas 17 and 18 of the cat visual cortex

Ulf T. Eysel

*Department of Neurophysiology, Ruhr-Universität Bochum, Universitätsstrasse 150, MA 4 / 149, D-4630 Bochum 1, FRG*

## Introduction

About 20% of visual cortical cells are GABAergic (Ribak, 1978; Hendrickson et al., 1981; Gabbott and Somogyi, 1986; Fitzpatrick et al., 1987; Hendry et al., 1987). This heterogeneous group of nonpyramidal cells displays quite distinct morphological specializations which allow to distinguish seven different types (Somogyi, 1986). Many aspects of structure, function and connectivity of these cells are dealt with in other chapters of this book and the functional significance of GABAergic inhibition in relation to visual cortical response specialization has been discussed in recent reviews (Sillito, 1984; Sillito and Murphy, 1988). This contribution concentrates on the topographical aspects of horizontal connections and the possible functions of GABAergic lateral inhibitory processes in areas 17 and 18 of the feline visual cortex.

Orientation selectivity and direction selectivity (Hubel and Wiesel, 1962) as well as length tuning (Hubel and Wiesel, 1965; Rose, 1977; Gilbert, 1977) have been originally described as typical properties of visual cortical cells in response to moving bar shaped stimuli. Ever since Sillito and others demonstrated the loss of all three specificities in many cells during blockade of GABAergic transmission with the $GABA_A$ an-

tagonist bicuculline (Sillito, 1975, 1977, 1979; Sillito et al., 1980; Tsumoto et al., 1979; Wolf et al., 1986), the possible contributions of GABA-mediated inhibitory interactions to such cortical response specificities have remained a matter of continuous and controversial debate. End-inhibition (Bishop and Henry, 1972; Rose, 1977) has been ascribed to interlaminar connections mediating inhibition from layer 6 cells predominantly to cells in layer 4 (Gilbert, 1977). In a study applying local inactivation in layer 6, cells in layer 4 have been shown to selectively loose end-inhibition while the other response properties remained unaffected (Bolz and Gilbert, 1986). The involvement of lateral inhibition as shown by intracellular recordings (Benevento et al., 1972; Innocenti and Fiore, 1974) in direction selectivity has been supported by a number of detailed studies of that specific property (Goodwin et al., 1975; Emerson and Gerstein, 1977; Ganz and Felder, 1984). Several models have assumed that inhibition generates direction selectivity in the visual cortex (Sillito, 1977; Barlow, 1981), however, excitatory convergence has also been considered to contribute to direction selectivity in complex cells (Movshon et al., 1978). Using intracortical local inactivation we have shown a loss of direction selectivity in cells of layers 2–6 when laterally remote areas were silenced by GABA microiontophoresis (Eysel et al., 1988). This loss of directional selectivity was indeed linked to reduction of inhibitory drive in many simple cells while the majority of complex cells responded with losses of excitation. Orientation specificity was originally ascribed to spatially oriented subcortical inputs (Hubel and Wiesel, 1962) but the above mentioned effects of bicuculline led to the assumption that intracortical cross-orientation inhibition might be involved (Sillito, 1979; Sillito et al., 1980). However, intracellular recordings failed to demonstrate the corresponding inhibitory potentials and disclosed merely iso-orientation excitation and inhibition (Ferster, 1986, 1987). On the other hand, several studies demonstrated inhibition from a broader range of orientations with respect to a target cell (Blakemore and Tobin, 1972; Morrone et al., 1982; Ramoa et al., 1986; Matsubara et al., 1987a; Hata et al., 1988). Such interactions imply lateral connections between columns of different orientation preferences.

The presence of laterally directed axons as morphological substratum for lateral signal processing in the visual cortex was initially shown by degeneration methods in monkey (Fisken et al., 1975) and cat (Creutzfeldt et al., 1977). Following the demonstration of clusters of terminals emitted at regular intervals by intracellularly labelled pyramidal cell axons spanning several mm of horizontal distance (Gilbert and Wiesel, 1979, 1983; Martin and Whitteridge, 1984; Kisvárday et al., 1986) and the observation of periodic patchy labelling in the visual cortex of monkey (Rockland and Lund, 1982; 1983) and cat (Matsubara et al., 1985; Luhmann et al., 1986; LeVay, 1988; Gilbert and Wiesel, 1989) increasing interest was directed towards horizontal interactions within areas 17 and 18. This interest was focussed on the long-range axonal systems of pyramidal cells and predominantly on excitatory functions (Nelson and Frost, 1985) as shown with cross-correlation analysis of recordings from pairs of cells with similar orientation specificity (T'so et al., 1986). More details about the lateral excitatory network were

disclosed by 2-deoxyglucose labelling combined with local injections of rhodamine latex beads (Gilbert and Wiesel, 1989) which revealed connections between iso-orientation domains in area 17. However, patches of retrogradely transported horseradish peroxidase (HRP) were observed in area 18 of the cat in regions with cross-orientation preferences as seen with microelectrode mapping (Matsubara et al., 1985, 1987a). This finding was discussed with respect to possible inhibitory functions. In fact, inhibitory lateral interactions have been observed between cells with dissimilar orientation preferences in cross-correlation histograms obtained from pairs of cells in the cat visual cortex (Hata et al., 1988). To connect orientation columns of all different preferred orientations, connections have to travel laterally over at least 1 mm which is the average distance between iso-orientation bands (Löwel et al., 1987). Excitatory as well as inhibitory connections can bridge this distance although their maximal possible horizontal spread is markedly different: axons of pyramidal cells span up to about 3 mm in the neonatal (Luhmann et al., 1990) and 5 mm in the adult cat visual cortex (Kisvárday and Eysel, 1991) while the axons of GABAergic cells give rise to axons over distances of 0.5–2 mm (Somogyi et al., 1983; Matsubara et al., 1987b).

Lateral inhibitory interactions could play a significant role in generating or sharpening specific response properties of visual cortical neurons. Lateral iso-orientation inhibition can cause direction selectivity (Bishop et al., 1971; Creutzfeldt et al., 1974; Innocenti and Fiore, 1974). An orientation bias might be primarily introduced by aligned geniculate inputs (Hubel and Wiesel, 1962), an orientational bias already present in retina (Levick and Thibos, 1982; Leventhal and Schall, 1983; Thibos and Levick, 1985) and LGN (Daniels et al., 1977; Vidyasagar and Urbas, 1982; Soodak et al., 1987; Shou and Leventhal, 1989), or inhibition between non-oriented cells with laterally displaced receptive fields (Heggelund, 1981). Inhibition between cells with different preferred orientations ("cross-orientation inhibition") can further refine the orientation tuning (Ferster and Koch, 1987).

## Remote local cortical inactivation with GABA

The bicuculline blockade of GABAergic transmission (Sillito, 1975, 1977, 1979; Tsumoto et al., 1979; Wolf et al., 1986) succeeded in ascribing various specific cortical functions to GABA-mechanisms. However, the method does not allow directly to address questions of topography and lateral interaction. To achieve this one has to apply simultaneous double recordings (T'so et al., 1986; Hata et al., 1988) or to record and manipulate cortical cells simultaneously at different locations. By the latter method lateral inhibition over 400 $\mu$m was shown by local application of the excitatory transmitter L-glutamate lateral to cortical recording sites (Hess et al., 1975). Later studies tried to disclose the origins of length tuning

(Bolz and Gilbert, 1986) and direction selectivity (Eysel and Wörgötter, 1986) by first applying locally restricted cortical inactivation by GABA microiontophoresis, local cooling and small thermolesions (Eysel et al., 1987, 1988).

The method of local remote inactivation by GABA microiontophoresis has been further elaborated in our laboratory over the years as the method of choice which combines local restriction with reversibility (Figs. 1, 5). All experiments described in this report were performed under standard conditions in lightly anaesthetized cats (Eysel et al., 1987, 1988, 1990; Crook et al., 1991). Single cell recordings were made with glass-coated tungsten electrodes (Wörgötter and Eysel, 1988) or with single or multi-barrel glass pipettes. During continuous recording of a single cell remote cortical cell clusters were locally inactivated by GABA microiontophoresis from a multibarrel pipette (Fig. 1) or a circular array of such pipettes (Fig. 5). The tips of the inactivation pipettes were

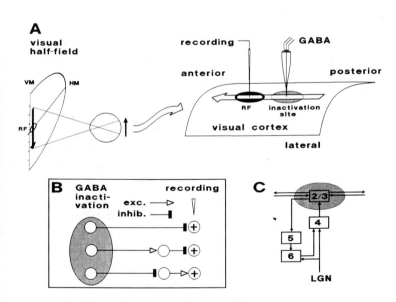

Fig. 1. Schematic drawings of the projection of a visual half-field to the visual cortex with recording and local inactivation (A), simple connection schemes leading to increased responses during inactivation (B), and diagram showing the key position of the inactivated layers 2/3 in vertical and horizontal processing. A. The right visual hemi-field (HM, horizontal meridian, VM, vertical meridian) is projected to the contralateral visual cortex in a way that the response wave to a downwards moving stimulus (black arrow) travels from posterior to anterior across the cortex (white arrow). The inactivation site (hatched region) is close to the projection of the classic receptive field (RF). B. Increased responses (+) at the recording site are observed, when inactivation (hatched) silences inhibitory cells or chains of connections including an inhibitory cell. C. Inactivation in layers 2/3 (hatched) takes place in region with horizontal connections as well as projections to all deeper cortical layers.

always placed in the supragranular layers (2/3) of area 17 or 18. The supragranular layers occupy a key position for horizontal and vertical processing (Fig. 1) since they combine extensive horizontal connections with a strategic location as switch between the upward and downward streams of signal flow. Light bars were presented as visual stimuli on a computer controlled display moving across the receptive field or stationary flashing within the receptive field. Responses to visual stimulation with different stimulus orientations were stored and peri-stimulus-time histograms (PSTHs) computed as controls prior to remote GABA application and continuously during local inactivation and recovery. Polar diagrams with the response peaks in impulses per second represented as vector length and the direction of stimulus motion (or the stimulus orientation for stationary stimuli) as vector angle were derived from the PSTHs. The cells were conventionally classified as belonging to the S- or C-family (Henry et al., 1979; Orban, 1984).

Local remote inactivation can disclose horizontal interactions in the visual cortex, if connections are specifically arranged with respect to topographical origin and synaptic action at the target cell, i.e., when given projections of the visual field with certain response specificities interact with others according to spatio-temporal rules. Inactivation of a cluster of cortical cells horizontally displaced from a target cell should then result in specific losses of functions normally dependent on contributions of the silenced cortical cells.

A specific advantage of the GABA inactivation method is that it silences cells by activation of $GABA_A$ and/or $GABA_B$ receptors but does not affect axons of passage. This keeps the inactivation locally restricted to the radius of GABA diffusion which can be assumed to be proportional to the ejected amount of GABA, which in turn depends on current and time of iontophoresis (see Hicks, 1984). It can further be assumed that the GABA effects decline with increasing distance and that they are limited by metabolism

and uptake so that in most cases the affected cortical volume remains rather close to the tip of the inactivation pipette. Using small ejection currents and short application times the effect can be kept very local (within a few hundred microns) but it can also directly reach cells over distances as large as 1.4 mm when high ejection currents (160 nA) and long durations (30 minutes) are chosen (Eysel and Wörgötter, 1991).

For the interpretation of effects of GABA inactivation on responses of remotely recorded cells it is important to discriminate between effects due to silencing of lateral inputs to a given cell on the one hand and direct effects of GABA at the cell under study on the other hand (Fig. 1, inset). Loss of inhibition as underlying mechanism is quite likely if the response increases during GABA iontophoresis. Decreased responses, however, can be due to a reduced excitatory input as well as to a direct inhibitory action of the applied transmitter at the investigated cell. Effects of inactivation of lateral excitation are discussed elsewhere (for reviews, see Bolz et al., 1989; Eysel and Wörgötter, 1991). This chapter will be restricted to lateral inhibitory effects as revealed by inactivation methods.

On the basis of single unit recordings combined with local remote inactivation and anatomical tracer techniques we arrive at a tentative picture of the functional contributions of medium to long range inhibitory horizontal interactions (0.5–2 mm) in visual cortical areas 17 and 18.

## Effects of laterally remote local cortical inactivation

### Lateral inhibition involved in directional specificity

It is well established that GABAergic mechanisms underlie direction selectivity of visual cortical cells because microiontophoretic blockade of $GABA_A$ receptors with bicuculline reversibly abolishes this response property (Sillito, 1975, 1977). With remote inactivation of cells some 700–1000 $\mu$m away we were able to selectively disinhibit the response to motion in the non-pre-

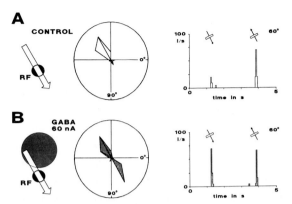

Fig. 2. Direction selective cell in area 17 with inactivation posterior to the recording site. Influence of remote inactivation on direction selectivity. A. Control recording with strong direction selectivity upwards. B. Loss of direction selectivity within 12 minutes of GABA application 700 μm posterior to the recording site. The hatched region symbolizes inactivation along the course of the cortical response wave during downwards motion of the stimulus. The histograms to the right show the specifically increased response to downwards motion. The effect was completely reversible after termination of GABA microiontophoresis.

different and independent method our approach disclosed new information about the involved cortical connectivity (Eysel et al., 1988). Thirty-six percent of 143 simple and complex cells in area 17 showed increases of response during local remote inactivation (7% remained totally unaffected and 57% reacted with reduced responses in the preferred direction). Increased responses during inactivation were only seen when the inactivation site was placed close to the course of the response wave elicited in the visual cortex by stimulation of the RF along the preferred axis of motion (Fig. 2), i.e., anterior or posterior to cells with upwards or downwards preferred directions of motion. Furthermore, increased responses could only be observed when the elicited cortical response wave moved from the inactivation site towards the recorded cell. Given these prerequisites responses could increase to the non-preferred as well as the preferred direction of motion. Such increased responses during remote GABA application were interpreted as release from lateral inhibition. This type of lateral inhibition was more frequently seen in simple cells (61% of 66 cells) than in complex cells (38% of 29

ferred direction without any side effect on orientation tuning (Fig. 2). In addition to supporting the results of the bicuculline experiments with a

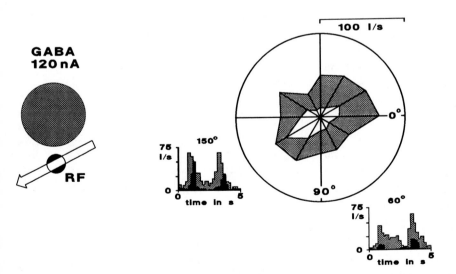

Fig. 3. Orientation selectivity changes during remote cortical inactivation. Complex cell in area 17 with inactivation at a distance of 700 μm posterior to the recording site. The region of inactivation (hatched circle) is situated away from the track of the preferred response across the cortex. Although responses increase to all orientations (hatched polar diagrams and histogram peaks) facilitation is stronger in the originally non-optimal orientations and leads to reduced orientation tuning.

cells). The remaining cells in each class showed reduced responses during remote inactivation. Such increases of response leading to reduced or increased direction selectivity led us to the conclusion that lateral inhibition is controlling the cells in area 17 from both sides along the axis of preferred motion and that an imbalance in this inhibition might be involved exclusively in direction selectivity since orientation tuning could remain completely unaltered.

### Lateral inhibition involved in orientation tuning

Orientation tuning was reduced or abolished in many cells during bicuculline application (Sillito, 1975, 1979; Sillito et al., 1980) indicating participation of cortical GABAergic inhibition. With remote GABA-induced inactivation we were able to broaden orientation tuning (Fig. 3). Similar to bicuculline experiments this could be accompanied by an increase of responses to all orientations and directions of motion like in the selected complex cell, which showed the strongest increase in responses to non-optimal orientations and thus lost most of its orientation selectivity. The effect was observed independent of the localization of the inactivation site within or outside the projection of the preferred axis of motion. Among 145 cells studied with inactivation at a single remote site 45% displayed no effect on orientation tuning. The majority of the remaining cells (36%) displayed broadening of tuning width due to increased responses to non-optimal orientations, while 19% showed reductions of orientation tuning due to decreased response to the optimal orientation. A broadening of orientation tuning width by more than 25% (twice the standard deviation of spontaneously occurring changes observed in 50 cells; Eysel and Wörgötter, 1991) was considered to be a significant effect of remote GABA application. Such significant effects were due to a net increase of responses in 63% of 48 simple cells and 69% of 32 complex cells. Thus the majority of both cell types showed changes in orientation tuning during remote lateral inactiva-

tion that might be interpreted as losses of lateral inhibition.

### Topography of lateral inhibition

In addition to the topographical rule derived above for direction specificity, distance appears to play a crucial role with respect to whether an effect is evoked at all and which type of inhibition is exerted at a given target cell. We analyzed the influence of distance between recorded cell and inactivation site on the effects most easily evoked by remote GABA iontophoresis (Eysel and Wörgötter, 1991). The amount of ejected GABA is proportional to current and time of iontophoresis (Hicks, 1984), accordingly we defined it in terms of "GABA units" (ejection current multiplied by ejecting time, $I \cdot t$). For different distances between inactivation and recording sites we determined the value of GABA units that were necessary to elicit broadening of orientation tuning by increased responses to non-optimal orientations or to change directionality by increased responses along the axis of preferred motion (Fig. 4). The latter was most easily possible from a distance of 1 mm while increased responses to non-optimal orientations leading to a reduction in orientation tuning were obtained with similarly

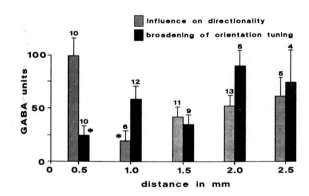

Fig. 4. Influence of distance on predominant inactivation effects. GABA units (ordinate, $I \cdot t$) leading to a given effect at a given distance (abscissa) are shown as histogram bars. Filled bars indicate number of cells showing loss of orientation tuning, hatched bars changes in directionality both due to losses of inhibition. Lateral inhibition involved in orientation tuning is most effective from 500 $\mu$m, direction selectivity is most easily affected by inactivation at a distance of 1.0 mm.

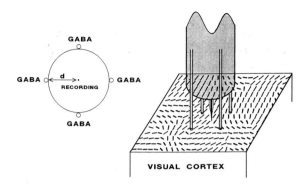

Fig. 5. Four inactivation pipettes arranged in a circular array with average distance d (500 μm in area 17 and 600 μm in area 18) between inactivation and recording sites. While the GABA pipettes remained in layers 2/3 the recording electrode could be freely moved. The right part of the figure schematically demonstrates the central recording electrode and the inactivation pipettes in regions of similar or different orientation selectivity. (Map modified from Swindale et al., 1987).

low amounts of GABA from a distance of about 0.5 mm. The optimum to reduce excitatory inputs was again around 1 mm (Eysel and Wörgötter, 1991).

To further investigate the effects of inhibition possibly involved in orientation tuning we therefore constructed an array of 4 GABA pipettes surrounding the recording electrode at average distances of 0.5 mm for area 17 and 0.6 mm for area 18 (Fig. 5, Eysel et al., 1990; Crook et al., 1991). With this configuration of recording and inactivation sites very strong effects on orientation tuning could be exerted both in area 17 and 18 (Eysel et al., 1990; Crook et al., 1991) and with comparable effects on responses to moving or stationary flash-presented bars (Crook et al., 1991). A strongly direction and orientation selective simple cell (Fig. 6A) lost most of its direction and orientation tuning within 5 minutes without any change in spontaneous activity (not shown) when only 20 nA GABA ejection currents were applied at all four pipettes, the effect being maximal at 20 minutes when also background activity began to rise (Fig. 6B). Some of the inactivation induced responses even surpassed in peak rate the response to the originally optimal orientation.

Complete recovery was seen only 10 minutes after termination of GABA microiontophoresis (Fig. 6C). An important question is whether motion is necessary to invoke the type of intracortical lateral inhibition described so far. When stationary flash-presented bars were used in area 18 (Crook et al., 1991) we observed equally strong effects on orientation tuning (Fig. 6D–F). Moreover, among the cells with significant effects the broadening of orientation tuning, which was on the average narrower in the controls when tested with the stationary flashing bars as opposed to moving bars, was more pronounced during remote inactivation with GABA. In 3 area 18 cells, the significant changes induced by remote GABA inactivation have been directly compared. The tuning width for the moving bar increased by 55% during GABA application, while a nearly threefold broadening of tuning width (by 147%) was observed for the stationary flash-presented bar (Crook et al., 1991).

*Comparison of area 17 and area 18*

In normal cells the differences between the tuning widths of comparable cell classes in area 17 and 18 of the cat roughly confirmed the results of Crook (1990). However, changes in orientation tuning induced by inactivation of remote regions of either area were not significantly different (Fig. 7; Crook et al., 1991).

Applying the significance level defined above, 61% of 74 cells in area 18 showed a significant broadening of orientation tuning (half-width at half height) due to increased responses in non-optimal orientations. In area 17, 66% of 54 cells showed a significant broadening of orientation tuning due to increased responses in the non-optimal orientations. Among the cells with significant effects, the average increase was slightly larger in area 17 than in area 18 (90 and 79%, respectively). Area 18 cells always retained a residual orientation bias while about 6% of the area 17 cells completely lost their orientation tuning. However, the differences between effects observed in area 17 and area 18 were not statistically significant. Importantly, in individual cells the changes in orientation tuning were in no way correlated to changes in spontaneous activity (Crook et al., 1991) which clearly demonstrated that the observed effects were not merely due to unspecific disinhibition.

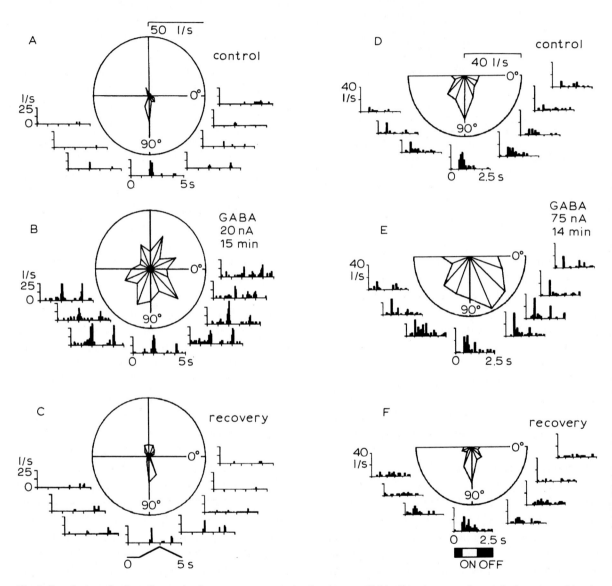

Fig. 6. Broadening of orientation tuning in response to a moving bar in area 17 (A–C) and to a stationary flash presented bar in area 18 (D–F). A. S-cell in area 17 before remote inactivation. Peri-stimulus time histograms are shown for each orientation and both directions of motion, respectively. The cell was sharply tuned for horizontal orientation and downwards movement. B. After 15 minutes of GABA release from all four surrounding pipettes some previously non-optimal orientations evoked responses larger than the original optimum, the cell had lost most of its direction selectivity and spontaneous activity had slightly increased. C. Recovery was nearly complete 12 minutes after termination of GABA microiontophoresis. D. On response of an area 18 simple cell to a stationary flash presented bar centered to the on subregion of the receptive field. E. Broadening of orientation tuning during GABA release from all four surrounding pipettes with minute increase in spontaneous activity (from 0.6 to 1.3 I/sec). F. Recovery was complete within 8 minutes after termination of GABA application.

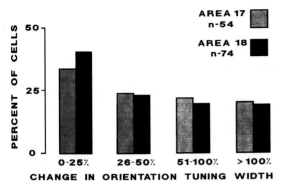

Fig. 7. Percentage change in orientation tuning width of cells in area 17 (hatched bars) and area 18 (black bars). Very similar percentages of cells were found in areas 17 and 18 for the different degrees of loss of tuning. (Modified from Crook et al., 1991).

## Functional specificity of lateral interactions

According to the topographical maps of orientation specificity in the cat visual cortex (Albus, 1975; Löwel et al., 1988) and the spatial auto-correlation function obtained from area 18 (Swindale et al., 1987) we could estimate the statistical probability of similar or dissimilar orientation specificity at inactivation sites as a function of distance. An important additional improvement of the method was recording of clusters of cells through the multibarrel pipettes at the different inactivation sites (Crook and Eysel, 1990, 1991a,b). This finally enabled us to show that "cross-orientation" inhibition (inhibition from clusters of cells with radically different orientation preference compared to the target cell) is involved in sharpening orientation tuning and iso-orientation inhibition is participating in shaping the (directional) response along the axis of preferred motion (Fig. 8). A complex cell in area 18 showed very effective orientation tuning. Two of the inactivation sites (anterior and posterior) silenced clusters of cells with orientations similar to that of the single cell recorded from the center of the array. Inactivation of these cell clusters (Fig. 8A) selectively led to increased responses along the preferred axis of motion. The two other inactivation sites, medially and laterally of the cell under study contained cells with orientation

selectivities approximately orthogonal to that of the recorded cell. Inactivation at these sites induced a tremendous broadening of orientation tuning (Fig. 8B) leading to a complete loss of the original orientation specificity. This example im-

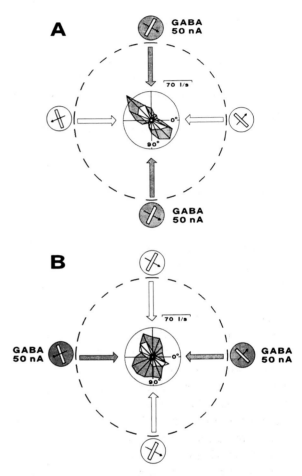

Fig. 8. Influence of orientation specificity of cells at the inactivation sites on the effects of remote inactivation. A. Inactivation of two sites (hatched) containing clusters of cells with iso-orientation tuning relative to the cell at the recording site in the center. The empty polar plot in the center represents the control recording prior to remote inactivation. The hatched polar plot demonstrates the change during remote inactivation due to a loss of iso-orientation inhibition. B. Inactivation of two sites (hatched) which contain cells with orientation tuning perpendicular to that of the cell in the center. The circles with broken lines indicate the 600 $\mu$m distance between inactivation and recording sites. The control is shown as empty polar plot in the center; the hatched polar plot depicts broadening of orientation tuning specifically by loss of cross-orientation inhibition. (Modified from Crook and Eysel, 1991b).

pressively shows that the increase of responses to non-optimal orientations (Fig. 8B) is not due to saturation of the response to optimal stimuli, since inactivation of other cell clusters induced as strong increases of responses to optimally oriented stimuli (Fig. 8A). On the other hand it is also clearly demonstrated that the broadening of tuning is not due to an unspecific release of inhibition that merely affects null oriented inputs more because they operate close to threshold in a range of higher non-linearity of responses. Quite differently, the effects of inactivation prove to be highly specific and completely dependent on the orientation specificity at the inactivation sites.

## Horizontal distribution of pyramidal and large basket cells

Localized extracellular injections of horseradish peroxidase as a neuronal tracer have been used to show horizontal patterns of intracortical connections (Rockland and Lund, 1982; Matsubara et al., 1985; Luhmann et al., 1986; LeVay, 1988; Gilbert and Wiesel, 1989). Such injections have shown characteristic patterns of patchy labelling which were generally ascribed to excitatory connections but in one study to inhibitory connections as well (Matsubara et al., 1985). Specific patterns of excitatory and inhibitory connections could not be discriminated with this method. The new neuronal tracer biocytin (King et al., 1989) has the fortunate property to be taken up by several classes of excitatory cells including pyramidal cells and selectively by only one type of inhibitory cells in cat visual cortex (Kisvárday and Eysel, 1990a,b). A small microiontophoretic deposit of the tracer biocytin restricted to a small orientational domain (diameter $< 150$ $\mu$m) reveals a very detailed picture of excitatory and inhibitory connections. Golgi-like staining of pyramidal cells with their dendrites and axons allows the reconstruction of the patchy network of excitatory connections (Kisvárday and Eysel, 1990a, 1991). In addition to the excitatory cells

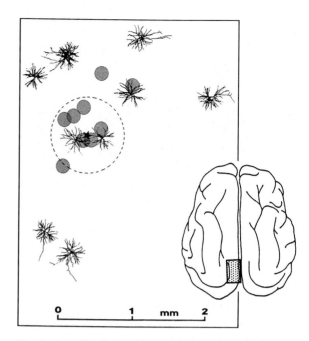

Fig. 9. A small volume of the tracer biocytin was microiontophoretically deposited in area 17 (black star). Ten completely filled pyramidal cells are shown with their reconstructed dendritic fields. The soma and dendritic field position of the strongly labelled basket cells ($n = 9$) is indicated by hatched circles. The broken circle has the radius of 500 $\mu$m which was the typical distance for the inactivation pipettes to influence orientation tuning in area 17.

large basket cells with characteristic smooth dendrites and perisomatic axons take up the tracer. These cells form an irregular mosaic, only partially overlapping with the excitatory network (Kisvárday and Eysel, 1990b). All cells, excitatory and inhibitory, when strongly labelled by the tracer are assumed to have in common the uptake from the small injection site (star in Fig. 9). Thus one can interpret the reconstructed distribution as an approximation of the connections converging on a target cell in the orientation column injected with the tracer. The example shows data from the reconstruction of a $6.5 \times 3.5$ mm part of area 17 (Kisvárday and Eysel, 1990a,b, 1991). The reconstructed dendritic trees of 10 completely labelled pyramidal cells in area 17 are distributed within 2 mm from the injection site and as a rule not much closer than 1 mm to their target cells. Conversely, the somata of 9 basket cells surround the uptake site at maximum distances below 1 mm and the majority is encountered within a radius of 500 $\mu$m (Fig. 9). About half of the basket cells in this case are situated so that they partially overlap the dendritic territories of the pyramidal cells; the other half were irregularly spaced but avoided the regions occupied by the pyramidal cells and their patchy axonal network. Pyramidal and basket cells thus seem to form two distinctly different connection patterns, a periodic horizontal excitatory system of longer spatial range, and a more irregularly distributed inhibitory system with shorter range and only partially overlap the territory of the excitatory network.

## Conclusions

At this stage our results seem to show several links between anatomy and function of the inhibitory horizontal cortical network and with some caution conclusions can now be drawn concerning the connections that might underlie the effects observed during laterally remote inactivation.

All observations made so far with remote inactivation are summarized in a model of intracortical inhibitory lateral interactions which is schematically drawn in Fig. 10. The central core with a radius of about 250 $\mu$m (containing the orientation column with the recorded cell) cannot be assessed with the inactivation method because

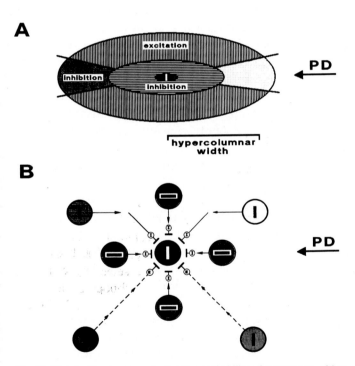

Fig. 10. Simple diagrams summarize the probability of occurrence of lateral inhibition and excitation (A) and possible horizontal connections (B) derived from the experimental results of our studies. A cell with vertical orientation preference and preferred direction of motion (PD) to the right is shown in the center in A and B. The close vicinity of the cell (black) cannot be investigated with our method (see text). Clusters of cells contributing broadly tuned cross-orientation inhibition (horizontal hatching) surround the cell and sharpen orientational tuning. The long-range iso-orientation inhibition shown in sectors of the outer ring (stippled) in A and in the upper half of the diagram in B, is stronger from the left leading to a preferred direction of motion from the right. Iso-orientation excitation is indicated by vertical hatching (A,B) and broken lines in the lower part of the diagram (B). The interrupted pathways and arrows in B indicate the uncertainty concerning the anatomical substrate for the functional mechanisms (i.e., direct connections vs. interneuronal chains).

once this region is affected during GABA microiontophoresis the cell under study is silenced concomitantly.

Inhibitory connections, directly or indirectly acting via interneurons, seem predominantly to originate from intermediate distances between 250–1000 $\mu$m. This ring of inhibitory cells within a radius of about one half hypercolumn around the cell in the center (Fig. 10A) is formed by cells with orientation preferences predominantly different from that of the center cell (Fig. 10B). This follows from the spatial organization of the orientation domain in the cat striate cortex (Albus, 1975) and can be directly shown by the spatial autocorrelation computed from mapping experiments. Accordingly, the highest statistical probability to meet cross-orientation tuning is found at a distance of 600 $\mu$m in area 18 of the cat (Swindale et al., 1987). Inactivation of these cells in our experiments leads to significant broadening or complete loss of orientation tuning clearly indicating that the inhibitory effects from the surrounding of a cell do sharpen orientation selectivity.

Another type of lateral inhibition from cells with orientations predominantly similar to that of the center cell and on the average about one hypercolumn away was found restricted to a sector of cortical tissue close to the axis of preferred direction of motion (Figs. 2, 10A). That type of lateral inhibition was derived from inactivation experiments that showed changes of direction selectivity due to loss of inhibition (Fig. 2) only when the GABA pipette was placed along the projection of the preferred axis of motion in area 17 of the cat (Eysel et al., 1988). This inhibition seems exclusively to contribute to directional mechanisms since influences on directionality elicited by remote inactivation from those regions were not contaminated with effects on orientation tuning (Eysel et al., 1988). This seems to support the hypothesis that directional and orientational tuning in the visual cortex might depend on different mechanisms (Hammond, 1978). From our data it seems that direction specificity is probably added to orientation specificity in a hierarchical manner. However, a statistical analysis of the dependence of orientation and direction tuning in a large number of cat visual cortical cells showed that the two properties are not completely independent. A low but significant correlation was found between direction and orientation tuning (Wörgötter et al., 1991a). This might be explained by a partial overlap of the populations of cells subserving the two different functions. Those cells that are involved in sharpening of orientational tuning seem to be predominantly situated in the vicinity of their target cells and are tuned to dissimilar orientations. In terms of topography these cells are partially intermingled with the population of cells contributing to direction specificity which are tuned to orientations similar to that of the target cell. It cannot be ruled out that a part of both cell groups is involved in shaping both specificities; this might apply to broadly tuned cells and could explain the weak correlation of tuning strengths for direction and orientation (Wörgötter et al., 1991a). This view is supported by our finding, that inactivation of the inhibitory elements at distances around 500 $\mu$m from the target cell decreased orientation tuning and concomitantly eliminated directionality in area 17 (Fig. 6A–C, Eysel et al., 1990). Alternatively, the short range inhibitory cells situated close to the column of the target cell might represent a common final path for inhibition involved in both properties. The inhibition observed in direction selectivity could be elicited by excitation of a subpopulation of the inhibitory cells close to the target cell. Direct inactivation of these inhibitory cells would consequently result in a loss of both properties as actually observed with inactivation with the array of inactivation pipettes at 500–600 $\mu$m distances.

Excitatory convergence was predominantly found by inactivation at longer horizontal distances (Eysel and Wörgötter, 1991), mainly from about 1 mm and above. The underlying excitatory connections seem to be made with cells possessing iso-orientation properties (Gilbert and Wiesel,

1989). The patchy network of excitatory connections is more extensively discussed elsewhere (LeVay, 1988; Gilbert and Wiesel, 1989; Kisvárday and Eysel, 1991).

In the light of the most recent data summarized in Fig. 8, the actual orientation specificity of the laterally inhibiting cells (Fig. 10) is functionally crucial (Crook and Eysel, 1991a,b) and more relevant than the distance which merely reflects probability as evident from the autocorrelation function of orientation specificities. Similar or dissimilar orientation with respect to the target cell determines whether orientational or directional components of the response are affected. From this and the above considerations it follows that, although inhibition from non-iso- as well as iso-orientation columns can be found at one and the same cell (Fig. 8), there is a quantitatively greater overall convergence of inhibition from cells with different orientations. Activation of these cells does sharpen orientation specificity in visual cortex.

Our anatomical data (Fig. 9) are in good agreement with the above picture that has emerged from the inactivation studies. They support a predominance of inhibitory cells with short range lateral connections in the direct vicinity of a given visual cortical cell and a differently organized, longer range excitatory system. Apart from showing for the first time the inhibitory and excitatory connections at the same time in a large scale horizontal reconstruction (Kisvárday and Eysel, 1990a,b), our results match to the connectivity pattern and the known axonal lengths of excitatory and inhibitory cell types in the visual cortex. Extracellular tracer injections have revealed a periodic, patchy system of connections (Gilbert and Wiesel, 1983; Rockland and Lund, 1982, 1983) with a periodicity around 1 mm. Similar experiments in area 18 of the cat, however, suggested horizontal connections over shorter distances with non-isooriented cells, including cross-orientation columns (Matsubara et al., 1985, 1987a). In fact, the different spatial scale of excitatory and inhibitory horizontal connections has

been shown for single identified excitatory and inhibitory cell types by intracellular injections (Gilbert and Wiesel, 1979, 1983; Somogyi et al., 1983; Martin and Whitteridge, 1984; Kisvárday et al., 1985, 1986, 1987). It has been further demonstrated that the horizontally long-ranging connections are made by axons of pyramidal cells; (Gilbert and Wiesel, 1983; Martin and Whitteridge, 1984; Kisvárday et al., 1986) with a high percentage of synapses at other excitatory and a comparatively low percentage at inhibitory cells (Kisvárday et al., 1986; LeVay, 1988). The longest axons of this system reach up to 5 mm (Kisvárday and Eysel, 1991) while the far reaching horizontal connections of the inhibitory system are made by large basket cell axons (Somogyi et al., 1983) and are restricted to distances of about 2 mm. The involvement of long-range GABAergic connections between iso-orientation columns is indicated by the lower threshold to influence directionality by remote inactivation from 1 mm than closer to the cell and by the direct evidence provided by inactivation of clusters of cells with iso-orientation tuning (Fig. 8A). The anatomical substrate for this function could be those basket cells sharing the patches of the excitatory system (Fig. 9).

Quite recently a model of inhibitory connectivity in the visual cortex was independently developed that closely relates to our findings (Wörgötter et al., 1991b). In this model circular inhibition with a broad non-iso-orientation tuning in a way similar to that derived from our inactivation results and tracer injections was shown to create directionality and strengthened orientational tuning in computer simulations of visual cortical circuitry when slightly orientation biased subcortical inputs were used.

### Acknowledgements

I would like to thank Dr. J.M. Crook for providing valuable comments on the manuscript. I am indebted to my coworkers Drs. J.M. Crook, Z.F. Kisvárday and F. Wörgötter for their important

420

contributions to this work which was made possible by the generous financial support of the Deutsche Forschungsgemeinschaft (SFB200/A4; Ey 8/17-1), the European Communities (SC1 * 0329-C (MB)) and the Alexander von Humboldt Stiftung (fellowship to Z.F. Kisvárday).

## References

Albus, K. (1975) A quantitative study of the projection area of the central and the paracentral visual field in area 17 of the cat. II. The spatial organization of the orientation domain. *Exp. Brain. Res.*, 24: 181–202

Barlow, H.B. (1981) Critical limiting factors in the design of the eye and visual cortex. *Proc. R. Soc. London B.*, 212: 1–34.

Benevento, L.A., Creutzfeldt, O.D. and Kuhnt, U. (1972) Significance of intracortical inhibition in the visual cortex. *Nature*, 238: 124–126.

Bishop, P.O., Coombs, J.S. and Henry, G.H. (1971) Interaction effects of visual contours on the discharge frequency of simple striate neurones. *J. Physiol.*, 219: 659–687.

Blakemore, C. and Tobin, E.A. (1972) Lateral inhibition between orientation detectors in the cat's visual cortex. *Exp. Brain. Res.*, 15: 439–440.

Bolz, J. and Gilbert, C.D. (1986) Generation of end-inhibition in the visual cortex via interlaminar connections. *Nature*, 320: 362–365.

Bolz, J., Gilbert, C.D. and Wiesel, T.N. (1989) Pharmacological analysis of cortical circuitry. *TINS*, 12(8): 292–296.

Bishop, P.O. and Henry, G.H. (1972) Striate neurones: receptive field concepts. *Invest. Ophthalmol.*, 11: 346–354.

Creutzfeldt, O.D., Kuhnt U. and Benevento, L.A. (1974) An intracellular analysis of visual cortical neurones to moving stimuli: Responses in a cooperative neuronal network. *Exp. Brain. Res.*, 21: 251–274.

Creutzfeldt, O.D., Garey, L.J., Kuroda, R. and Wolff, J.R. (1977) The distribution of degenerating axons after small lesions in the intact and isolated visual cortex of the cat. *Exp. Brain Res.*, 27: 419–440.

Crook, J.M. (1990) Directional tuning of cells in area 18 of the feline visual cortex for visual noise, bar and spot stimuli: a comparison with area 17. *Exp. Brain Res.*, 80: 545–561.

Crook, J.M. and Eysel, U.T. (1990) GABA-induced local inactivation and cross-orientation inhibition in area 18 of the feline visual cortex. *Soc. Neurosci. Abstr.*, 16: 1270.

Crook, J.M. and Eysel, U.T. (1991a) Evidence for cross-orientation inhibition in the visual cortex of the anaesthetized cat. *J. Physiol.*, 438: 38P.

Crook, J.M. and Eysel, U.T. (1991b) Modulation of cortical orientation tuning by iontophoretic application of GABA at functionally characterized sites. In: N. Elsner and H.

Penin (Eds.), *Proceedings of the 19th Göttingen Neurobiology Conference*, Stuttgart, New York: Thieme Verlag.

Crook J.M., Eysel. U.T. and Machemer, H.F. (1991) Influence of GABA-induced remote inactivation on the orientation tuning of cells in area 18 of feline visual cortex: a comparison with area 17. *Neuroscience*, 40: 1–12.

Daniels, J.D., Norman, J.L, and Pettigrew, J.D. (1977) Biases for oriented moving bars in lateral geniculate nucleus neurons of normal and stripe-reared cats. *Exp. Brain Res.*, 29: 155–172.

Emerson, R.C. and Gerstein, G.L. (1977) Simple striate neurons in the cat. II. Mechanisms underlying directional asymmetry and directional selectivity. *J. Neurophysiol.*, 40: 136–155.

Eysel, U.T., Crook, J.M. and Machemer, H.F. (1990) GABA-induced remote inactivation reveals cross-orientation inhibition in the cat striate cortex. *Exp. Brain Res.*, 80: 626–630.

Eysel, U.T. and Wörgötter, F. (1986) Specific cortical lesions abolish direction selectivity of cortical visual cells in the cat. *Soc. Neurosci. Abstr.*, 12: 583.

Eysel, U.Th. and Wörgötter, F. (1988) Analysis of a neuronal network with local inactivation. *Eur. J. Neurosci. Suppl.*, 1: 334.

Eysel, U.Th. and Wörgötter, F. (1991) Intracortical horizontal cortical connections and functional specificity of single cells in cat visual cortex. In: A. Aertsen and V. Braitenberg (Eds.), *Proceedings Schloss Ringberg Meeting*, Heidelberg: Springer, in press.

Eysel, U.T., Muche, T. and Wörgötter, F. (1988) Lateral interactions at direction selective striate neurones in the cat demonstrated by local cortical inactivation. *J. Physiol.*, 399: 657–675.

Eysel, U.T., Wörgötter, F. and Pape, H.C. (1987) Local cortical lesions abolish lateral inhibition at direction selective cells in cat visual cortex. *Exp. Brain Res.*, 68: 606–612.

Ferster, D. (1986) Orientation selectivity of synaptic potentials in neurons of cat primary visual cortex. *J. Neurosci.*, 6: 1284–1301.

Ferster, D. (1987) Origin of orientation-selective EPSPs in simple cells of cat visual cortex. *J. Neurosci.*, 7: 1780–1791.

Ferster, D. and Koch, C. (1987) Neuronal connections underlying orientation selectivity in cat visual cortex. *TINS*, 10: 487–492.

Fisken, R.A., Garey, L.J. and Powell, T.P.S. (1975) The intrinsic, association and commissural connections of area 17 of the visual cortex. *Phil. Trans. R. Soc. London B*, 272: 487–536.

FitzPatrick, D., Lund, J.S., Schmechel, D.E. and Towles, A.C. (1987) Distribution of GABAergic neurons and axon terminals in the macaque striate cortex. *J. Comp. Neurol.*, 264: 3–91.

Gabbott, P.L.A. and Somogyi, P. (1986) Quantitative distribution of GABA-immunoreactive neurons in the visual cortex (area 17) of the cat. *Exp. Brain Res.*, 61: 323–331.

Ganz, L. and Felder, R. (1984) Mechanism of directional selectivity in simple neurons of the cat's visual cortex analyzed with stationary flash sequences. *J. Neurophysiol.*, 51: 294–324.

Gilbert, C.D. (1977) Laminar differences in receptive field properties of cells in cat primary visual cortex. *J. Physiol.*, 268: 391–421.

Gilbert, C.D. and Wiesel, T.N. (1979) Morphology and intracortical projections of functionally characterized neurones in the cat visual cortex. *Nature*, 280: 120–125.

Gilbert, C.D. and Wiesel, T.N. (1983) Clustered intrinsic connections in cat visual cortex. *J. Neurosci.*, 3: 1116–1133.

Gilbert, C.D. and Wiesel, T.N. (1989) Columnar specificity of intrinsic horizontal and corticocortical connections in cat visual cortex. *J. Neurosci.*, 9: 2432–2442.

Goodwin, A.W., Henry, G.H. and Bishop, P.O. (1975) Direction selectivity of simple striate cells: properties and mechanism. *J. Neurophysiol.*, 38: 1500–1523.

Hammond, P. (1978) Directional tuning of complex cells in area 17 of the feline visual cortex. *J. Physiol.*, 285: 479–491.

Hata, Y., Tsumoto, T., Sato, H., Hagihara, K. and Tamura, H. (1988) Inhibition contributes to orientation selectivity in visual cortex of cat. *Nature*, 335: 815–817.

Heggelund, P. (1981) Receptive field organization of simple cells in cat striate cortex. *Exp. Brain Res.*, 42: 89–98.

Hendrickson, A.E., Hunt, S.P. and Wu, J.-Y. (1981) Immunocytochemical localization of glutamic acid decarboxylase in monkey striate cortex. *Nature*, 292: 605–607.

Hendry, S.H.C., Schwark, H.D., Jones, E.G. and Yan, J. (1987) Numbers and proportions of GABA-immunoreactive neurons in different areas of monkey cerebral cortex. *J. Neurosci.*, 7: 1503–1519.

Henry, G.H., Harvey, A.R. and Lund, J.S. (1979) The afferent connections and laminar distributions of cells in the cat striate cortex. *J. Comp. Neurol.*, 187: 725–744.

Hess, R., Negishi, K. and Creutzfeldt, O. (1975) The horizontal spread of intracortical inhibition in the visual cortex. *Exp. Brain Res.*, 22: 415–419.

Hubel, D.H. and Wiesel, T.N. (1962) Receptive fields, binocular interaction and functional architecture in the cat's visual cortex. *J. Physiol.*, 160: 106–154.

Innocenti, G.M. and Fiore, L. (1974) Post-synaptic inhibitory components of the responses to moving stimuli in area 17. *Brain Res.*, 80: 122–126.

King, M.A., Louis, P.M. Hunter, B.E. and Walker, D.W. (1989) Biocytin: a versatile anterograde neuroanatomical tract-tracing alternative. *Brain Res.*, 497: 361–367.

Kisvárday, Z.F., Cowey, A.C. and Somogyi, P. (1986) Synaptic relationships of a type of GABA-immunoreactive neuron (clutch cell), spiny stellate cells and lateral geniculate nucleus afferents in layer IVC of the monkey striate cortex. *Neuroscience*, 19: 741–761.

Kisvárday, Z.F. and Eysel, U.T. (1990a) Evidence for reciprocal patchy connections in cat visual cortex. *Eur. J. Neurosci., Suppl.*, 3: 303.

Kisvárday, Z.F. and Eysel, U.T. (1990b) Relationship between excitatory and inhibitory long range connections in the cat visual cortex. *Soc. Neurosci. Abstr.*, 1271.

Kisvárday, Z.F. and Eysel, U.T. (1991) Cellular organization of reciprocal patchy networks in Layer III of cat visual cortex (Area 17). *Neuroscience*, in press.

Kisvárday, Z.F., Martin, K.A.C., Freund, T.F., Maglóczky, Zs., Whitteridge,D. and Somogyi, P. (1986) Synaptic targets of HRP-filled layer III pyramidal cell in the cat striate cortex. *Exp. Brain Res.*, 64: 541–552.

Kisvárday, Z.F., Martin, K.A.C., Friedlander, M.J. and Somogyi,P. (1987) Evidence for interlaminar inhibitory circuits in the striate cortex of the cat. *J. Comp. Neurol.*, 260: 1–19.

Kisvárday, Z.F., Martin, K.A.C., Whitteridge, D. and Somogyi, P. (1985) Synaptic connections of intracellularly filled clutch cells: a type of small basket cell in the visual cortex of the cat. *J. Comp. Neurol.*, 241: 111–137.

LeVay, S. (1988) Patchy intrinsic projections in visual cortex, area 18, of the cat: Morphological and immunocytochemical evidence for an excitatory function. *J. Comp. Neurol.*, 269: 265–274.

Leventhal, A.G. and Schall, J.D. (1983) Structural basis of orientation sensitivity of cat retinal ganglion cells. *J. Comp. Neurol.*, 220: 465–475.

Levick, W.R. and Thibos, L.N. (1982) Analysis of orientation bias in cat retina. *J. Physiol.*, 237: 49–74.

Löwel, S., Bischof, H.-J., Leutenecker, B. and Singer, W. (1988) Topographic relations between ocular dominance and orientation columns in the cat striate cortex. *Exp. Brain Res.*, 71: 33–46.

Löwel, S., Freeman, B. and Singer, W. (1987) Topographic organization of the orientation column system in large flat-mounts of the cat visual cortex: a 2-deoxyglucose study. *J. Comp. Neurol.*, 255: 401–415.

Luhmann, H.J., Martinez Millan, L. and Singer, W. (1986) Development of horizontal intrinsic connections in cat striate cortex. *Exp. Brain Res.*, 63: 443–448.

Luhmann, H.J., Singer, W. and Martinez-Millán, L. (1990) Horizontal interactions in cat striate cortex: I. Anatomical substrate and postnatal development. *Eur. J. Neurosci.*, 2: 344–357.

Martin, K.A.C. and Whitteridge, D. (1984) Form, function and intracortical projections of spiny neurones in the striate visual cortex of the cat. *J. Physiol.*, 353: 463–504.

Matsubara, J.A., Cynader, M.S. and Swindale, N.V. (1987a) Anatomical properties and physiological correlates of the intrinsic connections in cat area 18. *J. Neurosci.*, 7: 1428–1446

Matsubara, J., Cynader, M., Swindale, N.V. and Stryker, M.P. (1985) Intrinsic projections within visual cortex: Evidence for orientation-specific local connections. *Proc. Natl. Acad. Sci. USA*, 82: 935–939.

Matsubara, J.A., Nance, D.M. and Cynader, M.S. (1987b) Laminar distribution of GABA-immunoreactive neurons and processes in area 18 of the cat. *Brain. Res. Bull.*, 18: 121–126.

Morrone, M.C., Burr, D.C. and Maffei, L. (1982) Functional implications of cross-orientation inhibition of cortical visual cells. I. Neurophysiological evidence. *Proc. R. Soc. London*, 216: 335–354.

Movshon, J.A., Thompson, I.D. and Tolhurst, D.J. (1978) Receptive field organization of complex cells in the cat's striate cortex. *J. Physiol.*, 283: 79–99.

Nelson, J.I. and Frost, B.J. (1985) Intracortical facilitation among cooriented, coaxially aligned simple cells in cat striate cortex. *Exp. Brain Res.*, 61: 54–61.

422

Orban, G.A. (1984) Neuronal operations in the visual cortex. In: *Studies in Brain Function, Vol. 11*, Heidelberg: Springer.

Ramoa, A.S., Shadlen, M., Skottun, B.C. and Freeman, R.D. (1986) A comparison of inhibition in orientation and spatial frequency selectivity of cat visual cortex. *Nature*, 321: 237–239.

Ribak, C.E. (1978) Aspinous and sparsely-spinous stellate neurons in the visual cortex of rats contain glutamic acid decarboxylase. *J. Neurocytol.*, 7: 461–478.

Rockland, K. and Lund, J.S. (1982) Widespread periodic intrinsic connections in the tree shrew visual cortex. *Science*, 215: 1532–1534.

Rockland, K. and Lund, J.S. (1983) Intrinsic laminar lattice connections in primate visual cortex. *J. Comp. Neurol.*, 216: 303–318.

Rose, D. (1977) Responses of single units in cat visual cortex to moving bars of light as a function of bar length. *J. Physiol.*, 271: 1–23.

Shou, T. and Leventhal, A.G. (1989) Organized arrangement of orientation-sensitive relay cells in the cat's dorsal lateral geniculate nucleus. *J. Neurosci.*, 9: 4287–4302.

Sillito, A.M. (1975) The contribution of inhibitory mechanisms to the receptive field properties of neurones in the striate cortex of the cat. *J. Physiol.*, 250: 305–329.

Sillito, A.M. (1977) Inhibitory processes underlying the directional specificity of simple, complex and hypercomplex cells in the cat's visual cortex. *J. Physiol.*, 271: 699–720.

Sillito, A.M. (1979) Inhibitory mechanisms influencing complex cells orientation selectivity and their modification at high resting discharge levels. *J. Physiol.*, 289: 33–53.

Sillito, A.M., Kemp, J.A., Milson, J.A. and Berardi, N. (1980) A reevaluation of the mechanisms underlying simple cell orientation selectivity. *Brain Res.*, 194: 517–520.

Sillito, A.M. (1984) Functional considerations of the operation of GABAergic inhibitory processes in the visual cortex. *Cerebral Cortex*, 2: 91–117.

Sillito, A.M. and Murphy, P.C. (1988) GABAergic processes in the central visual system. *Neurotransmitters Cortical Function*, 11: 167–185.

Somogyi, P. (1986) Seven distinct types of GABA-immunoreactive neurons in the visual cortex of cat. *Soc. Neurosci. Abstr.*, 12: 583.

Somogyi, P., Kisvárday, Z.F., Martin, K.A.C. and Whitteridge, D. (1983) Synaptic connexions of morphologically identified and physiologically characterized large basket cells in the striate cortex of the cat. *Neuroscience*, 10: 261–294.

Soodak, R.E., Shapley, R.M. and Kaplan, E. (1987) Linear mechanisms of orientation tuning in the retina and lateral geniculate nucleus of the cat. *J. Neurophysiol.*, 58: 267–275.

Swindale, N.V., Matsubara, J.A. and Cynader, M.S. (1987) Surface organization of orientation and direction selectivity in cat area 18. *J. Neurosci.*, 7: 1414–1427.

Thibos, L.N. and Levick, W.R. (1985) Orientation bias of brisk transient Y-cells of the cat retina for drifting and alternating gratings. *Exp. Brain Res.*, 58: 1–10.

Ts'o, D.Y., Gilbert, C.D. and Wiesel, T.N. (1986) Relationships between horizontal interactions and functional architecture in cat striate cortex as revealed by cross correlation analysis. *J. Neurosci.*, 6: 1160–1170.

Tsumoto, T., Eckart, W. and Creutzfeldt, O.D. (1979) Modification of orientation sensitivity of cat visual cortex neurons by removal of GABA-mediated inhibition. *Exp Brain Res.*, 34: 351–363.

Vidyasagar, T.R. and Urbas, J.V. (1982) Orientation sensitivity of cat lgn neurones with and without inputs from visual cortical areas 17 and 18. *Exp. Brain Res.*, 46: 157–169.

Wolf, W., Hicks, T.P. and Albus, K. (1986) The contribution of GABA-mediated inhibitory mechanisms to visual response properties of neurones in the kitten's striate cortex. *J. Neurosci.*, 6: 2779–2795.

Wörgötter, F. and Eysel, U.T. (1988) A simple glass-coated, fire-polished tungsten electrode with conductance adjustment using hydrofluoric acid. *J. Neurosci. Methods*, 25: 135–138.

Wörgötter, F., Muche, T. and Eysel, U.T. (1991a) Correlations between directional and orientational tuning of cells in cat striate cortex. *Exp. Brain Res.*, 83: 665–669.

Wörgötter, F., Niebur, E. and Koch, C. (1991b) Isotropic connections generate functional asymmetrical behavior in visual cortical cells. *J. Neurophysiol.*, in press.

R.R. Mize, R.E. Marc and A.M. Sillito (Eds.)
Progress in Brain Research, Vol. 90

CHAPTER 20

# The synaptic inputs to simple cells of the cat visual cortex

David Ferster

*Department of Neurobiology and Physiology, Northwestern University, Evanston, IL 60208, USA*

## Introduction

The mammalian visual cortex seems an almost ideal place to study the contribution of inhibitory mechanisms to sensory processing. The receptive field properties of cortical neurons though complex, are not so complex as to be daunting, and they have been precisely described in many elegant receptive field studies. Cortical receptive field properties are also of interest in that they clearly relate to high-level perceptual processes such as form vision, or motion and depth perception. That the anatomy of the cortical circuit is so well described also makes it an ideal subject for physiological study. The precise projections of thalamic and cortical inputs, of intracortical collaterals of cortical neurons, and of extracortical projections have all been well characterized. But what has perhaps drawn the most attention to the visual cortex is that the receptive field properties there are novel: the neurons that bring visual information to the cortex have very much simpler receptive field properties than do cortical neurons, making it possible to identify down to a single set of synapses, the point at which complex receptive field properties appear for the first time in the visual pathways. As a result, the cortex is a favorite subject for models of how complex receptive field properties, such as orientation and direction selectivity, are created. The cortical circuit provides an approachable system in which to address the problem of how complex computa-

tions are performed by the synaptic hardware that is available to the nervous system.

For testing models of cortical function, and for probing the machinery of the cortex in general, one of the most direct approaches (and one of the oldest) is to record intracellularly from cortical neurons. The method currently provides the only access to the membrane potential of a cell, and to the synaptic potentials, both excitatory and inhibitory, that a neuron integrates in the process of deciding when to fire, which stimuli to respond to and which to ignore. Intracellular recording has the potential to determine the specific contributions of individual synaptic inputs to the origins of neuronal stimulus specificity.

Intracellular recording has been employed in two types of experiment, either with electrical stimulation of the visual pathways, or with visual stimulation. In combination with electrical stimulation, the technique provides important information about synaptic connections: who is connected to whom, whether by excitatory or inhibitory pathways, by how powerful a synapse, with what degree of convergence. These are questions that are not easily answered precisely by other physiological or anatomical experiments. They are approachable, however, with intracellular circuit-tracing techniques that have been refined, beginning with Eccles and his colleagues, in over 30 years of work in the spinal cord and elsewhere in the central nervous system. It is in combination with visual stimulation, however, that

424

intracellular recording provides a window into the normal functioning of the neuron as it processes visual signals.

The focus of this chapter will be on a subset of cortical neurons, the simple cells of layer 4 in the visual cortex of the cat. Simple cells are the primary (though not the sole) recipient of the major visual input from the thalamus, the relay cells of the lateral geniculate nucleus (LGN). Simple cells are highly sensitive to the orientation, direction and speed of motion, retinal disparity (depth) and spatial frequency (size) of a visual stimulus, while geniculate relay cells are largely insensitive to these stimulus features. The synapse between geniculocortical axons and the simple cells of layer 4 is therefore the point at which many of the interesting features of cortical neurons are generated for the first time. As a result, simple cells have been the focus of many models of cortical organization and function, some of which can be tested with intracellular methods.

Classical simple cells were first defined by Hubel and Wiesel (Hubel and Wiesel, 1962) as those cortical neurons whose receptive fields could be divided into 2 or more elongated, adjacent ON and OFF regions. ON regions are those parts of the receptive field in which the onset of a bright stimulus excites the cell, OFF regions being defined as those in which the offset of a stimulus excites the cell. In addition, the offset of light in an ON region, or the onset of light in an OFF region are inhibitory to the cell and antagonize the response to an excitatory stimulus delivered simultaneously in any other part of the receptive field. Like all neurons in the cat visual cortex, simple cells are highly selective for the orientation of a stimulus. They respond best to an elongated bar or edge of light with an orientation within about 30° of the optimal, which for any given simple cell lies parallel to the orientation of the subregions.

Since the temporal pattern of a simple cell's responses to flashing stimuli in its ON and OFF subregions resembles that of ON-and OFF-center

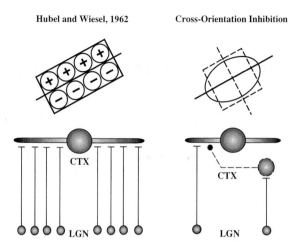

Fig. 1. Two models for the establishment of orientation selectivity in cells of the visual cortex. A. The mechanism proposed by Hubel and Wiesel (1962) in which geniculate neurons whose receptive fields are arranged in parallel rows excite a simple cell. Above is the arrangement of the receptive field centers of the presynaptic geniculate neurons. Below is a circuit diagram showing the geniculate neurons exciting the simple cell. B. The cross orientation inhibition model in which one cortical neuron inhibits another with a different preferred orientation. The receptive field of the inhibitory interneuron is shown in dashed lines, the postsynaptic cell in solid lines. A circuit diagram is shown below in which both cortical neurons receive excitation from relay cells of the LGN.

geniculate relay cells, Hubel and Wiesel proposed that simple cells receive direct monosynaptic excitation from relay cells. They explained the orientation selectivity of simple cells by proposing that ON-center relay cells, whose receptive field centers are aligned in a row, excite the simple cell and provide the basis for each ON region (Fig. 1). Similarly, a set of OFF-center cells with their receptive field centers in a row could generate a simple cell's OFF region. Orientation selectivity in the simple cell would result from a simple threshold process. Only when all the relay cells in at least one row were excited simultaneously by a moving or flashing stimulus of the appropriate orientation could the combined excitation in the simple cell reach threshold and cause a discharge of action potentials. A stimulus of the inappropriate orientation would excite only a small subset of the presynaptic geniculate neurons, which by themselves would fail to muster enough excitation in the simple cell to fire it. The essence of the model is the elongated rows of geniculate receptive fields. Because geniculate neurons are largely orientation insensitive, the total number of spikes evoked in each presynaptic geniculate cell by a bar sweeping across at any orientation is always the same. So, then, the total amount of excitation delivered to the simple cell must be from geniculate inputs. What changes with orientation is the relative timing of the excitation from the many presynaptic cells, occurring in a massive burst in response to a properly oriented stimulus, and in a long, low-amplitude sequence in response to a stimulus of the non-preferred orientation.

Several more quantitative versions of this general scheme laid out by Hubel and Wiesel have been evaluated, each of which indicates that strong orientation selectivity could in theory be established in this manner (Daugman, 1980; Ferster, 1987; Rose, 1979; Soodak, 1986). Experimental tests have also suggested that the organization of excitatory input from the LGN is sufficient to explain the orientation tuning of simple cells. Jones and Palmer (Jones and Palmer, 1987; Jones et al., 1987), for example, probed the receptive field structure of simple cells with small flashing spots of light. By using an extremely sensitive method of averaging (reverse correlation) they obtained detailed receptive field maps of the excitatory inputs to each cell. In many cases, the spatial organization of these inputs could be used to predict accurately the orientation tuning of the cell's responses to drifting gratings, using only a linear summation of the inputs from each part of the receptive field. Assuming that the spatial map of the receptive field obtained from flashing spots largely reflects the input from geniculate relay cells, the experiment gives strong evidence that the geniculate input by itself can account for much of the orientation selectivity of some simple cells.

The appeal of Hubel and Wiesel's model lies in large part in its simplicity. But while the basic plan of a simple cell's receptive field may be laid down by geniculate input in a manner similar to that described in the model, some experiments suggest that the model is inadequate in itself to explain all the behavior of simple cells. They indicate that intracortical inhibitory mechanisms may also contribute to orientation selectivity. Synaptic inhibition is ordinarily difficult to detect directly in extracellular experiments, particularly since cortical neurons are usually silent in the absence of a stimulus. To detect it, the activity of the cell must be elevated in some way, either with a visual conditioning stimulus (Bishop et al., 1971; Morrone et al., 1982) or with excitatory amino acids (Ramoa et al., 1986), and the inhibitory effects of a stimulus measured as a suppression of this background activity. It is not always possible to determine whether stimulus-evoked decreases in activity result from synaptic inhibition or from a withdrawal of excitation. When the background activity of a cortical neuron is elevated, however, in some cases it has been observed that test stimuli oriented away from the optimal orientation can suppress the background activity.

These observations have given rise to a class of models (cross orientation inhibition models) in which inhibition between cortical neurons with different orientations sharpens the orientation bias established by the geniculate excitatory inputs, a bias which in the model is rather weak compared to the orientation selectivity of cortical cells (Fig. 1). This bias may arise either from a scheme similar to that proposed by Hubel and Wiesel (1962), or from some intrinsic orientation bias that some have observed in individual geniculate relay cells (Vidyasagar and Heide, 1984). The inhibition of one cortical cell by another with a different preferred orientation would prevent the postsynaptic cell from responding to stimuli of the nonpreferred orientation. The argument for the contribution of inhibitory mechanisms to orientation selectivity is supported by pharmacological experiments. When $GABA_A$-mediated inhibition is blocked by cortical iontophoresis or systemic injection of $GABA_A$ antagonists, orientation selectivity is reduced or even abolished in some simple cells (Sillito et al., 1980; Tsumoto et al., 1979; Wolf et al., 1986).

One way to evaluate these models is to record intracellularly the inhibitory and excitatory synaptic potentials evoked in simple cells by visual stimuli of different orientations, and to compare the potentials found with the predictions of the models. Before examining records of this kind, however, it is useful to look briefly at the synaptic circuitry of simple cells, and the various neuronal sources that provide excitation and inhibition.

## Three major synaptic inputs to simple cells

Electrical stimulation of the visual pathways reveals three major synaptic inputs to simple cells, excitation from geniculate relay cells, excitation from the corticogeniculate neurons of layer 6, and inhibition from cortical interneurons, some of which are themselves simple cells in layer 4. No doubt there are other inputs, but a diagram of the layer 4 circuitry as revealed by the intracellular experiments is shown in Fig. 2.

### Monosynaptic geniculate excitation

Intracellular experiments confirm Hubel and Wiesel's prediction that all simple cells receive strong monosynaptic excitation from relay cells of the LGN (Ferster and Lindström, 1983). Stimulation of the LGN evokes in simple cells an EPSP of approximately 1.4 msec latency (Fig. 3a, upper traces). That this potential is actually mediated by geniculocortical relay cells is shown by stimulation of the optic nerves, which gives rise to a potential nearly identical to the one evoked from the LGN, but with a longer latency accounted for by the conduction time of the optic nerve axons and the synaptic delay in the LGN (Fig. 3c, upper traces).

That the EPSP evoked by stimulation of the LGN is actually mediated by a monosynaptic connection can be shown by an extrapolation procedure (Ferster and Lindström, 1983). The total latency from the LGN is the sum of the spike initiation time at the site of stimulation (0.2

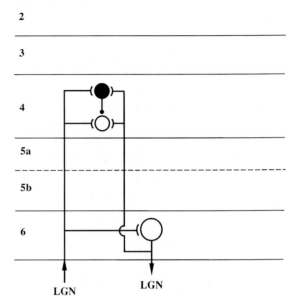

Fig. 2. A schematic diagram of the major synaptic inputs to simple cells identifiable with current physiological and anatomical methods. Included are (1) excitation from geniculate relay cells, (2) inhibition from cortical interneurons which themselves receive geniculate excitation and (3) excitation from corticogeniculate neurons of layer 6.

msec), the axon conduction time, and the synaptic delay within the cortex. The conduction time is estimated by stimulating the geniculate axons at a point nearer the cortex, in the optic radiations about 2/3 of the way to the cortex from the LGN. The EPSP latency in response to optic radiation stimulation is approximately 0.5 msec shorter than the EPSP evoked by LGN stimulation. Assuming a constant conduction velocity along the axons, the total conduction time is approximately 0.7 msec. Subtract the spike initiation time, and the 0.5 msec remaining of the total latency is the synaptic delay, and as short as it is, it can only be monosynaptic.

In every identified simple cell in layer 4, electrical stimulation of the optic tract, LGN and optic radiations revealed an EPSP of similar latency. While a significant monosynaptic input to layer 4 was expected from anatomical studies showing the termination of geniculocortical fibers

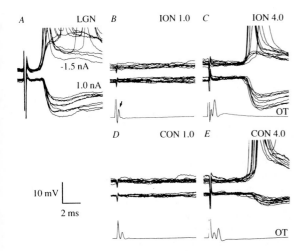

Fig. 3. Intracellular potentials recorded from a cortical neuron (area 17) with exclusive input from X cells of the LGN. A. Monosynaptic EPSPs (upper records) and disynaptic IPSPs (lower records) evoked by electrical stimulation of the LGN. EPSPs and IPSPs were recorded separately by polarizing the neuron with the injected DC currents indicated by each set of traces. B. Potentials from the same neuron evoked by stimulation of Y axons of the ipsilateral optic nerve. EPSPs and IPSPs (upper and middle records) were recorded with the same injected current indicated for the corresponding records in A. The bottom record (OT) is an average of the optic tract traces recorded simultaneously with the individual cortical records above. The field potential contains only a single positive component which represents activity in fast-conducting Y-axons. C. EPSPs and IPSPs from the same neuron evoked by stimulation of the optic nerve at 4.0 times the threshold for the X component in the optic tract. A second component is now visible in the field potential recorded in the optic tract, which represents activity in slowly-conducting X axons. D and E. Comparable records for the contralateral eye. Stimulus strengths in B–E are expressed as a multiples of the threshold of the X-component in optic tract potentials.

on many layer 4 cells (Davis and Sterling, 1979; Hornung and Garey, 1981; LeVay and Gilbert, 1976), the intracellular results indicate that every layer 4 cell receives a large direct input from these terminals.

There is a large degree of convergence in the geniculocortical pathway, as would be required by Hubel and Wiesel's model. This was shown in an experiment in which the electrical stimulus to the LGN was increased gradually in amplitude from 0 while the response of a simple cell was being recorded intracellularly (Ferster, 1987). As the stimulus amplitude increased, the stimulus be-

came suprathreshold for each of the presynaptic axons in turn. As each successive axon was recruited, the EPSP evoked in the simple cell increased slightly in amplitude. The number of such increases provides an indication of the number of presynaptic axons, and where tested, the increases in amplitude were small compared to the noise in the response and therefore difficult to measure accurately. But it was clear that the number of presynaptic axons was greater than 10 or 20. Anatomical experiments also indicate a high degree of convergence (Freund et al., 1985).

In area 17, intracellular experiments show that the monosynaptic geniculocortical EPSP is mediated largely by relay cells of the X type (Ferster, 1990a). The indicator of whether potentials are mediated by X or Y cells used in intracellular experiments was the threshold of the potentials evoked by stimulation of the optic nerves. Y axons of the optic nerve, having larger diameters than X axons, have uniformly lower thresholds to electrical stimulation (Bishop and McLeod, 1954; Lindström and Wrobel, 1984). It is possible, therefore, to stimulate nearly all of the Y axons and none of the X axons of the optic nerve by carefully adjusting the intensity of an electrical stimulus. Any synaptic potentials evoked in the LGN or in the cortex by such a stimulus must therefore be mediated exclusively by Y retinal ganglion cells. Synaptic potentials with higher thresholds are X-mediated.

Examples of X- and Y-mediated monosynaptic input from geniculate relay cells are shown in Figs. 3 and 4. Simple cells with X-mediated input were confined to area 17. Those with Y-mediated input were largely confined to area 18, with some mixing of inputs near the 17/18 border (Ferster, 1990a). Current source density analysis of field potentials, which reflects the synaptic activity of all the neurons in a small region of cortex, shows the same picture: Stimulation of the Y axons in the nerve evoked no obvious synaptic activity in area 17 and ample activity in area 18. Only when the stimulus amplitude is adjusted to activate X and Y cells together do synaptic currents appear in area 17 (Ferster, 1990b). These results have yet to be reconciled with previous evidence for a projection of Y axons to area 17 (Ferster and LeVay, 1978; Freund et al., 1985a,b; Gilbert and Wiesel, 1979; Humphrey et al., 1985; Martin and Whitteridge, 1984; Singer et al., 1975; Tanaka, 1983).

The monosynaptic geniculate input is partly responsible for the binocularity of simple cells. Figure 3 shows that the latency of the EPSPs evoked from the two optic nerves in each of the two neurons are nearly equal. This means that the synaptic pathway from each eye is identical. In other words, if a neuron receives monosynaptic geniculate excitation from the left eye, it also receives it from the right, rather than from other simple cells dominated by the right eye. The mechanisms by which the receptive field is constructed from geniculate input are duplicated for each eye (Ferster, 1990c).

*Intracortical excitation*

In addition to the monosynaptic geniculocortical EPSP, stimulation of the LGN gives rise in

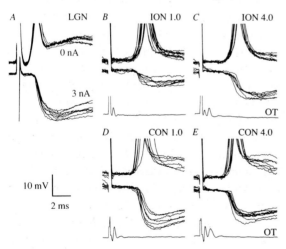

Fig. 4. Records from a cortical neuron (area 18) with exclusive input from Y cells of the LGN. The organization of the figure is identical to that of Fig. 3. The major difference to note is that in this cell, large potentials were evoked from both nerves when only Y axons were stimulated (B and D). These potentials were little altered when the stimulus strength was increased to activate X cells (C and E). Note also that the EPSPs and IPSPs evoked from the LGN and optic nerves have much shorter latencies than those in Fig. 3.

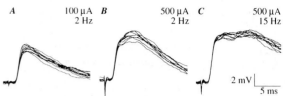

Fig. 5. Synaptic potentials arising from the excitation of a layer 4 simple cell by axon collaterals of cortico-geniculate neurons. A. EPSPs evoked by 100 $\mu$A stimulation of the LGN at 2 Hz. This early EPSP (1.5 msec latency) reflects the monosynaptic input from geniculate relay cells. B. When the stimulus strength is increased to 500 $\mu$A, the early EPSP is unaffected, but a second EPSP appears rising from the peak of the first with a latency of approximately 3 msec. C. When the stimulus frequency is increased to 15 Hz, the late EPSP is enhanced and is longer lasting. This late EPSP reflects the antidromic activation of corticogeniculate neurons.

layer 4 simple cells to an EPSP with very different properties (Fig. 5). The figure shows that this second input has a much longer latency than the geniculate input (3.5–4 msec). It has a higher threshold (compare Fig. 5a and b). And it shows strong temporal facilitation or augmentation. In Fig. 5c, the stimulation frequency was raised to 16 Hz, and the late EPSP can be seen to grow with each successive stimulus, while the geniculate EPSP is virtually unchanged in amplitude.

Like the geniculocortical EPSP, this late augmenting potential reflects a monosynaptic input, but it arises from the antidromic activation of geniculocortical neurons in layer 6 (Fig. 2). These neurons send rich axon collaterals to layer 4 (Gilbert and Wiesel, 1979), where they make contact with every cell in the layer. The augmenting potential (or more precisely, the extracellular field potential associated with the intracellular synaptic potential) can be evoked from the LGN even after the relay cells of the LGN have been completely destroyed by injections of kainic acid (Ferster and Lindström, 1985a,b). The long latency of the augmenting potential derives from the slowly conducting axons of the corticogeniculate neurons, whose antidromic latencies after stimulation of the LGN range from 3 to 40 msec.

Bolz and Gilbert (1986) have suggested a role for the layer 6–layer 4 connections in end-stopping. They found that when a small region of layer 6 is inactivated by injections of GABA, simple cells in layer 4 above the injection site lose their end-stopping. Many of the cells in layer 6 have very long narrow receptive fields, and were they inhibitory to layer 4 cells might produce end-inhibition. The projection from layer 6 to layer 4 appears in intracellular records to be exclusively excitatory, however: Every layer 4 cell tested shows strong augmenting EPSPs when the LGN is stimulated at 10–15 Hz. For layer 6 cells to mediate end-inhibition, they would have to do so through an interneuron, perhaps those located within layer 4 itself. The purpose of the direct excitation from layer 6 to layer 4 cells is still unclear.

*Intracortical inhibition*

When an intracellularly penetrated neuron is depolarized by current injected through the recording electrode, the driving force on excitatory synaptic currents is decreased while the driving force on inhibitory synaptic currents is increased. With sufficient depolarization, EPSP amplitudes are reduced almost to zero, and IPSP amplitudes are increased. Under these conditions, stimulation of the LGN invariably evokes large IPSPs in simple cells. Compare, for example, the response of the simple cell in Fig. 3a to electrical stimulation of the LGN during the injection of 1.0 nA of depolarizing current (lower traces), with the response recorded during the injection of 1.5 nA of hyperpolarizing current (upper traces). As previously discussed, the upper traces contain a monosynaptic EPSP. The depolarizing current, however, suppresses the EPSP and reveals an IPSP with a latency of approximately 0.7–1.0 msec longer than the monosynaptic EPSP. IPSPs with correspondingly longer latencies are evoked from the optic nerves (Fig. 3c, middle traces), indicating that the IPSP is mediated by axons of geniculate relay cells and not, for example, the antidromic activation of corticogeniculate neurons.

The IPSP might have a longer latency than the EPSP for one of two reasons. The first is that some geniculate relay cells directly inhibit simple cells, but that the axons mediating the inhibition have longer conduction times than those mediating the EPSP. The second is that the same type of axon mediates both potentials, but that the IPSP is disynaptic (Fig. 2). If an intracortical interneuron, which in turn receives monosynaptic excitation from geniculate axons, is the source of the inhibition, then the longer latency will arise from the extra synaptic delay. An extrapolation procedure, similar to the one described above to show that the EPSP was monosynaptic, also shows that the IPSP's longer latency arises from intracortical synaptic delays and not from longer axonal conduction delays (Ferster and Lindström, 1983). Therefore, the IPSP is disynaptic (Fig. 2). Evidence will be presented below that at least some of the inhibitory interneurons are likely to be other simple cells.

In vivo, the electrically-evoked IPSP can last as long as 200 msec (Fig. 6). These IPSPs were obtained in vivo with the whole cell patch recording technique (Blanton et al., 1989). The long duration of the IPSP could in part be due to the high input resistance and long time-constants of cells recorded with this technique. The non-exponential decay of the IPSP, however, suggests that it does not depend solely on the time constant of the cell. Pharmacological experiments in neocortical and hippocampal pyramidal cells in the neuronal slice preparation indicate that the electrically-evoked IPSP is made up of at least two components, a fast component arising from

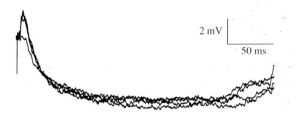

Fig. 6. Long-duration IPSPs recorded from a cortical cell in vivo using the whole-cell patch technique.

430

the action of $GABA_A$ receptors, and a slower component arising from the action of $GABA_B$ receptors. The $GABA_A$ receptors open a chloride channel and the $GABA_B$ receptors a potassium channel (Dutar and Nicoll, 1988). The $GABA_A$ receptors are widely distributed in the neuron, while the $GABA_B$ receptors are concentrated in the distal dendrites (Connors et al., 1988; Newberry and Nicoll, 1985).

## The receptive field properties of synaptic inputs to layer 4 simple cells

To determine how these identified synaptic inputs, and perhaps other unknown inputs, drive a simple cell during visual stimulation, it is possible to record the synaptic potentials that are evoked by visual stimuli. One of the aims of such an experiment is to evaluate the separate contribution of EPSPs and IPSPs to stimulus specificity in a neuron's responses. It is therefore necessary to distinguish inhibitory and excitatory inputs in the records of visually evoked changes in membrane potential. This is not as simple, however, as looking for depolarizations and hyperpolarizations since, for example, a withdrawal of excitation and an increase in inhibition could each produce a hyperpolarization. The solution to the problem is to record responses to each visual stimulus twice, with the membrane held at two different base potentials by the injection of polarizing DC current through the recording electrode.

As shown in Fig. 3, current injection easily distinguishes between EPSPs and IPSPs evoked by electrical stimulation of the LGN and optic tract. By virtue of the different reversal potentials for EPSPs (near 0 mV) and for IPSPs (near rest), the injection of depolarizing current decreases the amplitude of the former and increases the amplitude of the latter. Hyperpolarizing current does just the opposite. The same principle may be applied to visually-evoked responses. Depolarizing current will enhance the components of the response that are generated by synaptic inhibition. Hyperpolarization will enhance the effects

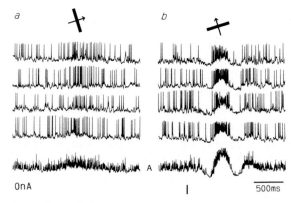

Fig. 7. Intracellular records from a simple cell in layer 4 of area 17 showing the response of the cell's excitatory inputs to a bar of light swept across its receptive field at two different orientations. a. Null orientation for the EPSPs. b. Preferred orientation. The top four traces of each panel show responses to four different stimulus sweeps (calibration bar = 10 mV); the bottom trace (A) shows an average of eight individual responses, including the four shown above. The averaged traces are shown at twice the gain of the individual traces (calibration bar = 5 mV). The resting potential of the cell was 60 mV. The velocity of motion of the bar was 2°/sec.

of excitatory inputs. By comparing two sets of records evoked by the same stimuli but with different injected currents, it is possible to distinguish excitatory from inhibitory components of the response. Note that the visual stimuli in each case activate the same synapses, and the same synaptic ion channels are opened or closed. In one case, however, few ions flow through the inhibitory channels since the membrane potential is near their equilibrium potential. In the other case, little current flows through the excitatory channels.

### Visually-evoked excitatory postsynaptic potentials

EPSPs evoked in a simple cell by visual stimulation, that is responses to a bar swept through the receptive field of a simple cell, are shown in Fig. 7. The responses to four repeated sweeps of the stimulus bar at two different orientations are shown above averages of 10 similar records. These changes in membrane potential visible in the records arise largely from excitatory inputs, and little from inhibitory inputs. As shown in Fig. 8a, without any current injected into the cell, re-

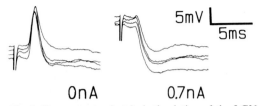

Fig. 8. Responses to electrical stimulation of the LGN in the neuron illustrated in Figs. 7 and 11 showing the presence of EPSPs when no current is injected through the electrode (left), and the presence of IPSPs when the cell is depolarized with 0.7 nA (right).

sponses to electrical stimulation of the LGN are dominated by EPSPs. IPSPs are barely visible; the membrane potential is presumably near the reversal potential for inhibitory synapses. The same is presumably true for the visually-evoked records, assuming that visually and electrically-evoked responses arise from the same or similar synapses. Only when the membrane is depolarized with injected DC current do IPSPs appear in the electrically-evoked records (Fig. 8b).

Note that individual or unitary EPSPs evoked by single action potentials in presynaptic neurons are not visible in these records. The relatively slow waves of depolarization and hyperpolarization reflect the increase and decrease in the activity of many excitatory inputs, the effects of each of which are too small to resolve. This is another indication of the high degree of convergence of excitatory inputs onto simple cells.

From the records of Fig. 7b, it appears that the receptive field of the excitatory input to this cell is made up of three subfields, two flanking OFF regions and a central ON region. The response to the optimally oriented bar is made up of four components: four different waves of alternating hyperpolarization and depolarization. The first wave of hyperpolarization likely represents the withdrawal of excitation evoked by the bar entering the centers of the geniculate OFF-center receptive fields that underlie the first OFF region of the simple cell. The following depolarization reflects an excitation caused by the bar entering the receptive field centers of the ON-center geniculate cells that underlie the central ON re-

gion, while at the same time the bar is leaving the receptive field centers of the OFF-center geniculate neurons making up the first OFF region. The third phase, another wave of hyperpolarization, represents the second OFF region (and the second underlying row of OFF center geniculate neurons). Finally, weak depolarization occurs as the bar leaves the second OFF region. In each of the four phases of the response, the changes in excitation are interpreted as coming from relay cells since relay cells constitute a major excitatory input to simple cells evoked by electrical stimulation of the LGN. In addition, the excitatory drive is modulated both above and slightly below the baseline indicating that there is both an increase and a withdrawal of ongoing excitatory activity. Since cortical neurons have little spontaneous spike activity, they are not likely responsible for such a pattern of synaptic excitation.

When the bar is turned 90°, it encounters all three subfields end-on simultaneously. The simultaneous increase in activity from the ON-center geniculate cells will be partially offset by the decrease in activity from the OFF-center geniculate cells. In addition, as outlined above the bar passes over the receptive fields of each row in sequence instead of simultaneously. As can be seen in the responses of Fig. 7a, the result is a long, low-amplitude, single wave of depolarization, rather than the larger, short duration multiphased response to the optimally oriented bar.

Figure 9 represents an attempt to model the excitatory input observed in the neuron of Fig. 7 (Ferster, 1987). In the model it was assumed that each of the three subfields arises from the excitatory input from six geniculate neurons in a row, one row for each subfield. The response of each geniculate ON-center cell is taken from the actual response of the geniculate relay cell (Fig. 9a,b). These are post-stimulus time histograms generated by moving and flashing bars, and it is assumed that the response of each individual relay cell is independent of the stimulus orientation. Similarly the response of each modeled OFF-center cell is taken from the response of an

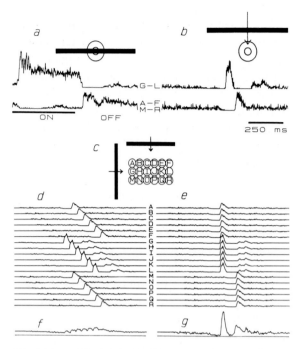

Fig. 9. A model of the excitatory connections between neurons in the lateral geniculate nucleus and a simple cell in the visual cortex. a. The responses of two geniculate neurons to a bar of light flashed in their receptive field centers. An ON-center cell is above, an OFF-center cell below. Each histogram is the averaged response to 100 stimulus presentations. The two neurons were recorded close together within lamina A. b. The responses of the same two cells to a bar swept across their receptive fields at 5°/sec. c. The postulated arrangement of eighteen neurons in the LGN, all of which monosynaptically excite the simple cell whose responses are to be calculated. A–F and M–N are OFF-center cells; G–L are ON-center cells. d. The synaptic input to the modeled simple cell from each of the eighteen geniculate neurons, evoked when a vertical slit is swept across the receptive field. The letters labelling the curves correspond to the letters labelling the geniculate receptive fields in c. The input from each ON-center cell is proportional to the upper curve in a; the input from each OFF-center cell is proportional to the lower curve. The relative displacement of the curves was calculated from the relative position of the receptive fields in c and from the initial position and orientation of the stimulus. e. Same as d, but for a horizontal stimulus. f and g. The point-by-point sums of the curves in d and e. These sums are taken to be the total excitation from the LGN to the simple cell for the vertical and horizontal stimuli. A high degree of orientation selectivity for the total geniculate excitation is predicted.

actual geniculate OFF-center cell. As the bar sweeps across the receptive fields of each of the 18 relay cells, they will respond in a sequence

dependent upon the speed and direction of motion of the bar and upon the relative placement of the 18 receptive fields. The relative timing of each of the responses is shown in d and e for two orientations of the bar. Assuming for simplicity's sake, that the excitation to the modeled simple cell is proportional to the rate of firing of the presynaptic inputs (and that the connection from each input has equal strength), the excitatory drive to the simple cell will be proportional to the sum of the activity in the 18 presynaptic geniculate cells. These sums for the two stimulus orientations are shown in Fig. 7f and g.

The model is based on as few assumptions as possible: each connection has the same strength; all inputs combine linearly; the responses of individual inputs are independent of stimulus orientation and are taken from real geniculate cells. Yet the accuracy with which the inputs to the modeled simple cell mimic the synaptic potentials recorded in the simple cell of Fig. 7 is striking. Many of the features of the records fall out of the model, including the four phases of the optimal response, the single phase of the null response, and the relative durations and amplitudes of the optimal and null responses.

Figure 10 shows an orientation tuning curve for the modeled simple cell, the maximum amplitude of the calculated input plotted at 1° increments in stimulus orientation. Here again the model accounts well for the properties of real simple cells. By applying a simple threshold to the modeled cell, it can be seen that spikes would be evoked only by stimuli in a narrow range of orientations.

*Visually-evoked inhibitory postsynaptic potentials*

The visually-evoked EPSPs of Fig. 7 indicate that a large measure of orientation selectivity can be established as early in the visual pathway as the excitatory synapse between LGN relay cells and layer 4 simple cells. As outlined above, however, several experiments suggest indirectly that intracortical inhibitory mechanisms may also contribute to orientation selectivity. Whether cross-

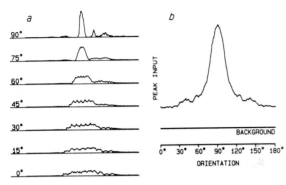

Fig. 10. a. Excitation from the LGN to the model simple cell of Fig. 9, evoked by stimuli of seven different orientations. Each curve was calculated in the same way as those in Fig. 8f and g. The stimulus orientation is indicated to the right of each curve. 0°, vertical; 90°, horizontal. b. The peak amplitude of the geniculate excitation as a function of stimulus orientation. The horizontal line (BACKGROUND) marks the sum of the spontaneous activity of the eighteen individual inputs.

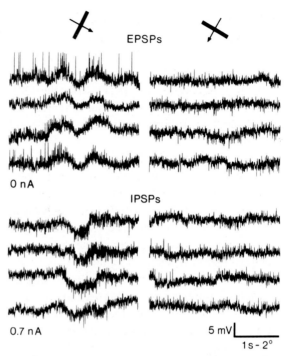

Fig. 12. A comparison of the preferred orientations of EPSPs and IPSPs evoked in a simple cell. Responses to a bar of optimal orientation for the EPSPs are shown to the left, EPSPs (recorded with 0 current injected through the recording electrode) above and IPSPs (recorded with 0.7 nA of depolarizing current injected through the recording electrode) below. To the right are responses to the bar swept at 90° to the optimal. Neither EPSPs nor IPSPs are evoked by such a stimulus.

oriented IPSPs are present in simple cells can be tested in the same way that the orientation selectivity of excitatory inputs was tested. To see IPSPs rather than EPSPs, the neuron is depolarized to near the equilibrium potential for EPSPs, as judged by the response to electrical stimulation of the LGN. Visually-evoked responses are then recorded, with the assumption that they, like the electrically-evoked records, will consist largely of IPSPs.

For the cell illustrated in Fig. 7, 0.7 nA of current was sufficient to completely suppress EPSPs evoked electrically from the LGN and to make visible instead a large IPSP (Fig. 8). This same depolarizing current also suppressed the EPSPs evoked by visual stimuli. Figure 11, which

was obtained using the same visual stimuli as those used in Fig. 7, shows that visually evoked depolarizations have disappeared. The hyperpolarizations evoked as the bar entered the OFF regions of the receptive field have been enhanced and broadened, however, indicating that they are in part the result of synaptic inhibition. The only IPSPs present, however, are those evoked by stimuli of the preferred orientation. Stimuli of the null orientation do not appear to evoke the IPSPs predicted by the cross-orientation inhibition models. Visually-evoked IPSPs and EPSPs have the same preferred orientation, rather than orthogonal orientations.

The orientation preference of EPSPs and IPSPs in a second simple cell is shown in Fig. 12.

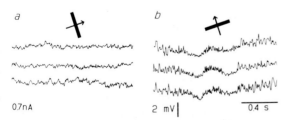

Fig. 11. Visually-evoked IPSPs recorded from the cell illustrated in Figs. 7 and 8. The same visual stimuli were used to obtain these records are was used in Fig. 7, but here the membrane was depolarized with 0.7 nA of injected current.

434

This cell's receptive field is made up of three subregions, a central OFF region flanked by two ON regions. An optimally-oriented bright bar swept across the receptive field evokes EPSPs from the ON regions, and IPSPs from the OFF regions (left-hand records). A null-oriented bar evokes neither EPSPs nor IPSPs (right-hand records).

While visual stimuli of the preferred orientation evoke both excitation and inhibition, these synaptic inputs do not directly antagonize one another. The EPSPs and IPSPs are separated in time and space within the receptive field so that the two inputs are never simultaneously active (Ferster, 1988). When Figs. 7 and 11 are compared, excitation and inhibition can be seen to alternate as the bar is swept across the receptive field. The same is true for the upper and lower records of Fig. 12. Whenever the bright bar entered an ON region or left an OFF region, it evoked EPSPs in the simple cell, which were interpreted as the activation of geniculate relay cells of the corresponding center type. Whenever the bar entered an OFF region or left an ON region, excitation was withdrawn, as indicated by the hyperpolarization in the EPSP-dominated records. But the IPSP-dominated records show hyperpolarization in the corresponding phases of the response; the withdrawal of excitation is accompanied by an increase in inhibition.

This is illustrated more clearly in Fig. 13, which contains the EPSPs and IPSPs evoked by flashing stimuli in the simple cell of Fig. 7. A bar was flashed within the ON region first with the cell hyperpolarized to show the EPSPs evoked by the stimulus. Depolarization occurs at light on, and hyperpolarization at light off, reflecting increases and decreases in excitation in these EPSP-dominated records. With the cell depolarized to reveal IPSPs, the only response to the stimulus is a hyperpolarization at light OFF, which in these records must represent an increase in inhibition. An analogous ON inhibition is present in the OFF region (not shown). The presence of this type of inhibition was first suggested by Hubel

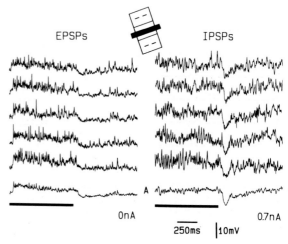

Fig. 13. Reciprocal OFF inhibition in the ON region of the simple cell illustrated in Fig. 7. Response to an optimally oriented bar flashed in the central ON region. The line beneath the traces indicates the duration of the flash. The bottom trace of each set (A) is an average of 10 individual records. The current injected through the electrode during the collection of each set of traces is indicated to the lower right. The bar evoked excitation at light on, and withdrawal of excitation at light off (a), accompanied by inhibition at light off (b).

and Wiesel (1962). Evidence for it in extracellular records has been presented by Palmer and Davis (1981) and Heggelund (1986).

The source of this inhibition is suggested by its properties. (1) The inhibitory interneurons must possess regions with pure ON or OFF responses. (2) The preferred orientation of the inhibitory interneurons must match the postsynaptic neuron. (3) The interneurons are likely to have little spontaneous activity, since visual stimuli evoke only increases in inhibition, no withdrawal of inhibition (for example at light-off in an OFF region). (4) The inhibitory interneurons are likely to receive direct excitation from the LGN, since the largest IPSPs evoked in simple cells by electrical stimulation are disynaptic. These properties best describe simple cells. Perhaps small spine-free stellate cells of layer 4 with simple receptive fields provide this push-pull inhibition to the subfields of their neighbors (Ferster, 1988). Neighboring simple cells have been described in which overlapping subregions of their receptive fields were of opposite response type (Palmer and Davis, 1981). Were one of the pair inhibitory to the other, it would produce IPSPs exactly like those seen in Figs. 11 and 13.

The function of this inhibition in building the receptive field of simple cells is unclear. One possible role, however, is to enhance disparity sensitivity. If a stimulus of appropriate non-zero disparity is presented to a binocular simple cell, its image will fall in the ON region of the receptive field of one eye and the OFF region of the receptive field in the other eye. At the onset of the stimulus, the ON inhibition from the OFF region will antagonize the ON excitation from the ON region, and prevent the neuron from responding. At zero disparity, when the stimulus falls within one ON region from each eye, the excitation it evokes from one region will reinforce the other.

### The arithmetic of EPSP-IPSP interactions

The activation of inhibitory synapses potentially could have two different means with which to decrease the activity of a postsynaptic neuron. Inhibitory synapses may either hyperpolarize the neuronal membrane, or they may directly shunt excitatory currents. Hyperpolarization occurs when the inhibitory channels open and negative current flows into the cell because of the electrochemical gradient on the ions to which the channels are permeable. This mechanism underlies all of the IPSPs visible in the records shown here. Shunting will occur if the conductance opened by the synapses is sufficient to reduce the input resistance of the soma or dendrites. By Ohm's law, such a reduction will reduce the depolarization that results from the injection of current by excitatory synapses (Blomfield, 1974; Fatt and Katz, 1953). Unlike hyperpolarization, however, shunting synapses could in theory decrease the excitability of a neuron without any visible change in membrane potential. If the reversal potential of an inhibitory synapse were near the resting membrane potential, that is, if the electrochemical gradient on the permeant ions were nearly

zero, then activating the synapse would not result in current flow or membrane hyperpolarization. By itself, the activation of the synapse would be undetectable in intracellular records, but the EPSPs generated distally to the site of the inhibition would reach the cell body with reduced amplitude because of the reduction in input resistance near the shunt.

Shunting has been proposed to provide neurons with a means of implementing AND-NOT logical operations between inhibitory and excitatory inputs. The nonlinear, multiplicative nature of shunting inhibition (all affected EPSPs are reduced in size by a constant proportion) could allow it to veto any incoming excitatory signal (Koch et al., 1983; Torre and Poggio, 1978). In addition, the veto mechanism could be performed selectively on a subset of excitatory inputs. Shunting synapses on a spine or a dendrite would antagonize any excitatory synapse located more distally in the dendritic tree, but would have little effect on synapses located nearer the soma or on other dendrites. These properties have been used to great advantage in models of cortical computation. Hyperpolarizing inhibition, in contrast, interacts with EPSPs in a linear fashion, the synaptic currents of the two inputs simply adding on the cell membrane.

Shunting inhibition has also been proposed as a possible mechanism for cross-orientation inhibition that might remain undetectable in intracellular records such as the ones shown in Fig. 11 (Koch and Poggio, 1985). Shunting inhibition would produce no changes in membrane potential detectable from a recording electrode in the soma, yet might substantially reduce the effectiveness of orientation-insensitive excitation arising from geniculate relay cells. Shunting inhibition located in the cell soma or proximal dendrites is ruled out by experiments like those in Fig. 11, however. Depolarizing the neuron by current injection should introduce a driving force on shunting ion channels so that activating them would produce a hyperpolarizing response. In addition, the increase in membrane conductance associated with the shunt would be detectable, yet it has not been observed (Douglas et al., 1988). What these experiments do not rule out, however, is the possibility that the shunting synapses might be located in regions of the dendrites that are electrically remote from the recording electrode. In that case, current reaching the synapses from the recording electrode would be greatly diminished, and only a fraction of the potentials generated at the synapses would reach the soma. While theoretical calculations of neuronal electrical properties suggest that dendrites are not electrically isolated from the soma (Koch et al., 1990), it is possible to test for the presence of remote shunting inhibition experimentally with a method that does not rely on current injection to shift the reversal potential or to reveal changes in input resistance.

We tested for the presence or absence of shunting inhibition by looking directly for their effect on EPSP amplitude (Ferster and Jagadeesh, 1991). A test EPSP was generated in a neuron of the cat visual cortex by electrical stimu-

lation of the LGN at a frequency of approximately 1 Hz. Simultaneously, visual stimuli were applied to the receptive field in order to activate inhibitory synapses. A bar of light was swept repeatedly across the receptive field at a slightly different frequency from that of the electrical stimulus. The asynchronous presentation of electrical and visual stimuli insured that each electrical stimulus occurred with the bar in a different position within the receptive field. If the bar evoked inhibition of the shunting type, the amplitude of the test EPSP would be decreased.

Before the electrical test stimulus was applied, visual stimuli alone were used to determine the receptive field structure. The intracellular records of Fig. 14 illustrate a simple cell whose receptive field was divided into four subregions, two ON regions and two OFF regions. A bar of the preferred orientation flashed in either ON region (Fig. 14a, 2 and 4) evoked depolarization at light on and hyperpolarization at light off. Flashing the bar in either OFF region (Fig. 14a, 1 and 3) evoked depolarization at light off and hyperpolar-

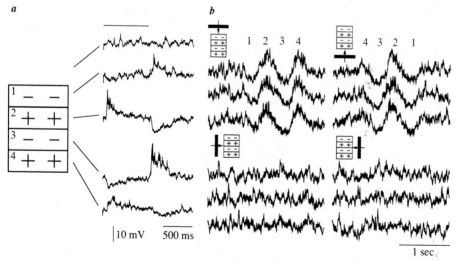

Fig. 14. a. A schematic diagram of the receptive field of a simple cell in area 17 of cat visual cortex. To the right of the diagram are shown intracellular responses of the cell to a stationary bright bar flashed in each of the four subregions (bottom four traces), together with the response to the bar flashed outside of the receptive field (top trace). The horizontal bar at the top of the traces indicate the time during which the stimulus bar was on. Each trace represents the average of the response to four separate presentations of the stimulus. b. The response of the cell to the bar being swept across the receptive field in four different directions, indicated by the inset above each set of traces. The responses to three consecutive stimulus presentations are shown for each direction of motion. Resting potential was −60 mV. These records and those of Figs. 15 and 16 were obtained with an in vivo modification of the whole-cell patch technique of Blanton et al. (Blanton et al., 1989).

ization at light on. When the bar was swept across the receptive field (Fig. 14b, top left traces), a series of depolarizations and hyperpolarizations occurred as the bar encountered each of the subfields, exactly analogous to the sequence of potentials visible in the records of Fig. 7. The four phases of the response to downward motion represent: (1) hyperpolarization as the bar enters OFF region 1; (2) depolarization as the bar enters ON region 2 and simultaneously leaves OFF region 1; (3) hyperpolarization as the bar enters OFF region 3 and leaves ON region 2; and (4) depolarization as the bar enters ON region 4 and leaves OFF region 3. This sequence is repeated in reverse order as the bar moves across the receptive field in the opposite direction (Fig. 14b, top right). (Although the receptive field consists of 4 distinct subfields, in extracellular records only 2 subfields would be visible. Visual stimuli in regions 1 and 4 evoked only small EPSPs which never triggered spikes. It is likely that regions 1 and 4 represent the surrounds of the geniculate

receptive fields whose centers underlie regions 2 and 3.) Sweeping the bar across the receptive field in the non-preferred orientation evokes only a small depolarization, which is barely visible in the individual traces (Fig. 14b, bottom).

Once the cell's receptive field structure was known, the LGN was stimulated electrically in order to evoke test EPSPs at the same time that the visual stimulus was moved through the receptive field. Examples of the responses of the simple cell to the electrical stimulus are shown in Fig. 15a. Both the early and late EPSP components of the response are mediated by monosynaptic connections: Component 1 is the monosynaptic input from geniculate relay cells, while component 2 is the monosynaptic input from antidromically-activated corticogeniculate cells in layer 6 (see above). That the test EPSP is generated by monosynaptic inputs is an important aspect of the method. A disynaptic test EPSP might vary in amplitude if the visual stimulus changed the excitability of the interneuron mediating the

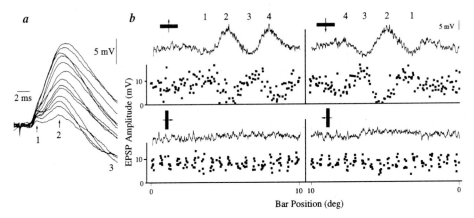

Fig. 15. a. Test EPSPs generated in the simple cell of Fig. 14 by electrical stimulation of the LGN. The three components of the response labelled 1–3 correspond to (1) a monosynaptic EPSP from the LGN, (2) a monosynaptic EPSP following antidromic activation of corticogeniculate neurons and their intracortical collaterals (Ferster and Lindström, 1985a,b) and (3) the beginning of a disynaptic IPSP, which lasted for 200 msec and reached an amplitude of 15 mV. Records were obtained while the visual stimulus was moving back and forth across the receptive field. The baselines of each trace have been matched, though during recording, the test-EPSPs were superimposed on the slow, visually-evoked fluctuations in membrane potential. b. Four graphs of test EPSP amplitude (measured at point 2 in a) against the position of the visual stimulus. The four different graphs correspond to four different directions of stimulus motion. Above each plot is shown the membrane potential changes evoked by the visual stimulus alone. The graph and the continuous curve are plotted in register: for a given bar position, the instantaneous membrane potential in the absence of electrical stimulation is located directly above the corresponding test EPSP amplitude. During the recording of all traces in the figure, the cell was held hyperpolarized with − 120 pA of current injected through the recording electrode. The amplitudes of both components of the test EPSP are similarly affected by bar position. Graphs of test EPSP amplitude vs. bar position based on measurements of EPSP amplitudes at point 1 part a of the figure are nearly identical to those shown.

input. These changes in excitability could be misinterpreted as shunting effects.

While the shape of the test EPSP varies little from trial to trial, the amplitudes of both EPSP components vary considerably. The graphs of Fig. 15b show that a large part of the variation is related to the position and orientation of the visual stimulus within the receptive field. In each graph, the amplitude of each test EPSP is plotted against the position of the bar at the time the electrical stimulus was delivered. Four separate graphs are shown for four different directions of bar motion. The continuous curve above is the response of the cell to the visual stimulus alone. These are averages of records similar to the ones shown in Fig. 14. Each graph is plotted in register with the intracellular record above it so that the membrane potential recorded in the absence of electrical stimulation is located directly above the test EPSP amplitude measured with the bar in the same position within the receptive field. All of the records in the figure were recorded with a small amount of negative current injected through the recording electrode. The current prevented the visual and electrical stimuli from triggering action potentials which would have confounded the amplitude measurements.

If the visual stimulus evoked shunting inhibition at any position or orientation within the receptive field, then the amplitude of the test EPSP would have been decreased significantly when the bar was in that position. A large decrease in amplitude, more than 80%, is visible when the bar passed through subregions 2 and 4 of the receptive field (Fig. 15b, top), but this decrease was almost certainly not caused by shunting inhibition. Regions 2 and 4 are the ON regions, ones in which a bright bar evokes maximal *excitation*. The decrease in test EPSP amplitude probably reflects simple saturation of the excitatory mechanism. As the cell becomes more and more depolarized towards the EPSP reversal potential, the driving force on EPSCs (excitatory postsynaptic currents) is greatly reduced. As a result, activating further excitatory synapses by

electrical stimulation results in a much smaller synaptic potential. In fact, the 80% reduction of EPSP size implies that the visually-evoked depolarization at the site of the excitatory synapses is 80% of the difference between the resting membrane potential and the EPSP reversal potential. Assuming a reversal potential near 0 mV, the visually-evoked depolarization may be as large as 40 mV, which is much larger than the 10 mV observed in the soma.

The visually-evoked depolarization might also affect EPSP amplitudes by opening voltage-sensitive channels in the cell membrane. These would reduce the cell's input resistance, and thereby reduce EPSP amplitude. No evidence for such a decrease in input resistance has been found, however (Douglas et al., 1988). A third possible mechanism for the decrease in test-EPSP amplitude is fatigue of the excitatory synapses by their visually-evoked activity. This is unlikely to be the cause of the decrease in EPSP amplitude, however. Geniculocortical synapses (which underlie component 1 of the test EPSP in Fig. 15a) are resistant to fatigue during repetitive electrical stimulation of the LGN at frequencies of greater than 100 Hz (not shown). The input from corticogeniculate neurons (component 2 of the test EPSP, Fig. 15a) is actually augmented by high-frequency stimulation.

The decrease in test-EPSP amplitude accompanying the visually-evoked depolarizations of regions 2 and 4 are matched by a slight increase in amplitude accompanying the visually-evoked hyperpolarizations of regions 1 and 3 (Fig. 15b, top). Here, the driving force on the synaptic currents of the excitatory synapses are increased by the hyperpolarization.

Finally, the bottom traces in Fig. 15b show the test-EPSP amplitudes recorded with the bar of the null orientation sweeping across the receptive field in a test for cross-oriented shunting inhibition. The lack of systematic variation of amplitude with bar position rules out the presence of such a shunt.

While the visual stimulus of the preferred ori-

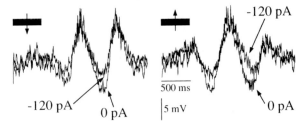

-120 pA

-120 pA    0 pA

500 ms

5 mV    0 pA

Fig. 16. Intracellular responses (of the same neuron as illustrated in Fig. 14) to the moving-bar stimulus. For each of two directions of motion, the two superimposed traces were recorded with and without a steady hyperpolarizing current (−120 pA) injected through the electrode. The injected current increased the resting potential significantly (approximately 10 mV), but the traces with and without current are superimposed in order to compare the amplitude of the stimulus-evoked changes in membrane potential. The hyperpolarizing components of the responses are smaller in the presence of hyperpolarizing current, indicating that these hyperpolarizations are in part generated by the activation of inhibitory synapses with a reversal potential below rest. Each trace is a smoothed average of four individual responses.

entation does not activate synaptic shunts of excitatory currents, it does evoke significant inhibition of the conventional hyperpolarizing type. As in the cell of Fig. 7, IPSPs contribute to the hyperpolarizations evoked when the bright bar enters an OFF region or leaves an ON region. This can be seen by comparing the response to visual stimulation with and without current injected through the recording electrode (Fig. 16). In this case, hyperpolarizing current was used to suppress the IPSPs (whereas in Fig. 11, depolarizing current was used to enhance them). The injection of current caused a decrease in size of the visually-evoked hyperpolarization by reducing the driving force on inhibitory postsynaptic currents (IPSCs). If these hyperpolarizations had been caused solely by a withdrawal of tonic excitation, rather than by hyperpolarizing inhibition, their amplitude would have been increased by the injected current, rather than decreased.

This experiment demonstrates directly that IPSPs evoked by the visual stimuli used here do not significantly shunt EPSPs anywhere within the dendritic tree. The synapses activated by the electrical stimulus, those of geniculate relay cells and

corticogeniculate neurons, are located throughout the dendritic trees of cortical cells, both near the soma and in the distal dendrites (Einstein et al., 1987; Freund et al., 1985; McGuire et al., 1984). Shunting inhibition anywhere within the dendritic tree would therefore have caused a decrease in the amplitude of the test EPSP. The absence of decreases (other than those attributable to visually-evoked depolarization) rules out the presence of a shunt. The primary mechanism by which cortical IPSPs reduce the excitability of cortical neurons appears to be by hyperpolarizing the membrane away from threshold. We have obtained results similar to those of Fig. 15 from a total of four simple cells (including the one illustrated in Figs. 14–16), each with resting potentials below −50 mV. In each, a decrease in test-EPSP amplitude of over 50% was observed during visual stimulation, but only during depolarizing phases of the visual response.

What the measurement of test-EPSP amplitudes does not rule out is the possibility that a shunt might occur between the soma and the axon hillock. The axon hillock of some neurons is encased in a synaptic cartridge that derives from cortical chandelier cells. These synapses could in theory shunt excitatory synaptic currents as they were conducted from the soma to the axon hillock where action potentials are initiated. In essence, these synapses could selectively raise the effective threshold of a neuron without producing a visible change in soma potential or input resistance.

## Conclusions

In some ways, the results described here are as noteworthy for what they show inhibition *not* to be doing, as much as for what they show what inhibition does contribute to cortical processing of visual input. While strong evidence from extracellular results and from models pointed to a significant contribution to orientation selectivity from cross-oriented inhibition, intracellular experiments reveal little trace of that contribution. So far, the role that intracellular experiments have unequivocally identified for inhibition in shaping the visual responses of cortical cells is in generating the mutual antagonism between subfields of simple cells.

Much remains to be done. Extracellular experiments have given very strong indications that inhibition is involved in end-stopping (Bolz and Gilbert, 1986) and direction selectivity (Emerson and Gerstein, 1977; Ganz and Felder, 1984). Though casual inspection of our intracellular records has so far not revealed strongly direction selective or length-dependent inhibition, rigorous experiments directed at understanding the origin of these receptive field properties may yet do so. Intracellular techniques are steadily improving. In vivo whole-cell patch recording, for example, provides stable and long-lasting penetrations of cortical cells more reliably than was previously possible with conventional sharp electrodes. The technique will make possible entirely new experiments, such as in vivo voltage clamp, intracellular studies with much more complex visual stimuli than are currently used, or intracellular application of pharmacological agents. Together these techniques have the potential to make intracellular studies of receptive field properties one of the most powerful methods of studying cortical integration.

## Acknowledgements

This work was supported by the National Eye Institute and the McKnight Endowment Fund for Neuroscience.

## References

Bishop, P.O., Coombs, J.S., et al. (1971) Interaction effects of visual contours on the discharge frequency of simple striate neurones. *J. Physiol. (London)*, 219: 659–687.

Bishop, P.O. and McLeod, J.G. (1954) Nature of potentials associated with synaptic transmission in lateral geniculate nucleus of cat. *J. Neurophysiol.*, 17: 387–414.

Blanton, M.G., Lo Turco, J.J., et al. (1989) Whole cell recording from neurons in slices of reptilian and mammalian cerebral cortex. *J. Neurosci. Methods*, 30: 203–210.

Blomfield, S. (1974) Arithmetical operations performed by nerve cells. *Brain Res.*, 69: 115–124.

Bolz, J. and Gilbert, C.D. (1986) Generation of end-inhibition in the visual cortex by interlaminar connections. *Nature*, 320: 362–365.

Connors, B.W., Malenka, B.W., et al. (1988) Two inhibitory postsynaptic potentials and GABA$_A$ and GABA$_B$ receptor-mediated responses in neocortex of rat and cat. *J. Physiol.*, 406: 443–468.

Daugman, J.G. (1980) Two-dimensional spectral analysis of cortical receptive field profiles. *Vision Res.*, 20: 847–856.

Davis, T.L. and Sterling, P. (1979) Microcircuitry of cat visual cortex: Classification of neurons in layer IV of area 17, and identification of patterns of lateral geniculate input. *J. Comp. Neurol.*, 188: 599–628.

Douglas, R.J., Martin, K.A.C., et al. (1988) Selective responses of visual cortical cells do not depend on shunting inhibition. *Nature*, 332: 642–644.

Dutar, P. and Nicoll, R.A. (1988) A physiological role for GABA$_B$ receptors in the central nervous system. *Nature*, 332: 156–158.

Einstein, G., Davis, T.L., et al. (1987) Pattern of lateral geniculate synapses on neuron somata in layer IV of the cat striate cortex. *J. Comp. Neurol.*, 260: 76–86.

Emerson, R.C. and Gerstein, G.L. (1977) Simple striate neurons in the cat. II. Mechanisms underlying directional assymetry and direction selectivity. *J. Neurophysiol.*, 40: 136–155.

Fatt, P. and Katz, B. (1953) The effect of inhibitory nerve impulses on a crustacean muscle fiber. *J. Physiol. (London)*, 121: 374–389.

Ferster, D. (1987) The origin of orientation selective EPSPs in simple cells of cat visual cortex. *J. Neurosci.*, 7: 1780–1791.

Ferster, D. (1988) Spatially opponent excitation and inhibition in simple cells of the cat visual cortex. *J. Neurosci.*, 8: 1172–1180.

Ferster, D. (1990a) X- and Y-mediated synaptic potentials in neurons of areas 17 and 18 of cat visual cortex. *Vis. Neurosci.*, 4: 115–133.

Ferster, D. (1990b) X- and Y-mediated current sources in area 17 and 18 of cat visual cortex. *Vis. Neurosci.*, 4: 135–145.

Ferster, D. (1990c) Binocular convergence of synaptic potentials in cat visual cortex. *Vis. Neurosci.*, 4: 625–629.

Ferster, D. and Jagadeesh, B. (1991) The synaptic arithmetic of EPSP-IPSP interactions in cat visual cortex. In preparation.

Ferster, D. and LeVay, S. (1978) The axonal arborization of lateral geniculate neurons in the striate cortex of the cat. *J. Comp. Neurol.*, 182: 923–944.

Ferster, D. and Lindström, S. (1983) An intracellular analysis of geniculocortical connectivity in area 17 of the cat. *J. Physiol. (London)*, 342: 181–215.

Ferster, D. and Lindström, S. (1985a) Augmenting responses evoked in area 17 of the cat by intracortical axons collaterals of cortico-geniculate cells. *J. Physiol. (London)*, 367: 217–232.

Ferster, D. and Lindström, S. (1985b) Synaptic excitation of neurones in area 17 of the cat by intracortical axon collaterals of cortico-geniculate cells. *J. Physiol. (London)*, 367: 233–252.

Freund, T.F., Martin, K.A.C., et al. (1985) Innervation of cat visual areas 17 and 18 by physiologically identified X- and Y-type thalamic afferents. I. Arborization patterns and quantitative distribution of postsynaptic elements. *J. Comp. Neurol.*, 242: 263–274.

Freund, T.F., Martin, K.A.C., et al. (1985) Innervation of cat visual areas 17 and 18 by physiologically identified X- and Y-type thalamic afferents. II. Identification of postsynaptic targets by GABA immunocytochemistry and Golgi impregnation. *J. Comp. Neurol.*, 242: 275–291.

Ganz, L. and Felder, R. (1984) Mechanism of direction selectivity in simple neurones of the cat's visual cortex analyzed with stationary flashed sequences. *J. Neurophysiol.*, 51: 294–324.

Gilbert, C.D. and Wiesel, T.N. (1979) Morphology and intracortical projections of functionally characterized neurons in the cat visual cortex. *Nature*, 280: 120–125.

Heggelund, P. (1986) Quantitative studies of enhancement and suppression zones in the receptive field of simple cells in cat striate cortex. *J. Physiol*, 373: 373.

Hornung, J.P. and Garey, L.J. (1981) The thalamic projection to cat visual cortex: Ultrastructure of neurons identified by Golgi impregnation or retrograde horseradish peroxidase transport. *Neuroscience*, 6: 1053–1068.

Hubel, D.H. and Wiesel, T.N. (1962) Receptive fields, binocular interaction and functional architecture in the cat's visual cortex. *J. Physiol. (London)*, 160: 106–154.

Humphrey, A.L., Sur, M., et al. (1985) Projection patterns of individual X- and Y-cell axons from the lateral geniculate nucleus to cortical area 17 in the cat. *J. Comp. Neurol.*, 233: 159–189.

Jones, J.P. and Palmer, L.A. (1987) The two-dimensional spatial structure of simple receptive fields in cat striate cortex. *J. Neurophysiol. (Bethesda)*, 58(6): 1187–1211.

Jones, J.P., Stepnoski, A., et al. (1987) The two-dimensional spectral structure of simple receptive fields in cat striate cortex. *J. Neurophysiol. (Bethesda)*, 58(6): 1212–1232.

Koch, C., Douglas, R., et al. (1990) Visibility of synaptically induced conductance changes: Theory and simulations of anatomically characterized cortical pyramidal cells. *J. Neuroscience*, 10: 1728–1744.

Koch, C. and Poggio, T. (1985) The synaptic veto mechanism: does it underlie direction and orientation selectivity in the visual cortex. *Models of the visual cortex*. New York: John Wiley, pp. 408–419.

Koch, C., Poggio, T., et al. (1983) Nonlinear interactions in a dendritic tree: Localization, timing, and role in information processing. *Proc. Natl. Acad. Sci. USA*, 80: 2799–2802.

LeVay, S. and Gilbert, C.D. (1976) Laminar patterns of geniculocortical projection in the cat. *Brain Res.*, 113: 1–19.

Lindström, S. and Wrobel, A. (1984) Separate inhibitory pathways to X and Y principal cells in the lateral geniculate nucleus of the cat. *Neurosci. Lett. Suppl.*, 18: 234S.

Martin, K.A.C. and Whitteridge, D. (1984) Form, function and intracortical projections of spiny neurones in the striate visual cortex of the cat. *J. Physiol. (London)*, 353: 463–504.

McGuire, B.A., Hornung, J.-P., et al. (1984) Patterns of synaptic input to layer 4 of the cat striate cortex. *J. Neurosci.*, 4: 3021–3033.

Morrone, M.C., Burr, D.C., et al. (1982) Functional implications of cross-orientation inhibition of cortical visual cells. I. Neurophysiological evidence. *Proc. R. Soc. London Ser. B*, 216: 335–354.

Newberry, N.R. and Nicoll, R.A. (1985) Comparison of the action of Baclofen with gamma-aminobutyric acid on rat hippocampal pyramidal cells *in vitro*. *J. Physiol.*, 360: 161–185.

Palmer, L.A. and Davis, T.L. (1981) Receptive-field structure in cat striate cortex. *J. Neurophysiol.*, 46: 260–276.

Ramoa, A.S., Shadlen, M., et al. (1986) A comparison of inhibition in orientation and spatial frequency selectivity of cat visual cortex. *Nature*, 321: 237–239.

Rose, D. (1979) Mechanisms underlying the receptive field properties of neurons in cat visual cortex. *Vision Res.*, 19: 533–601.

Sillito, A.M., Kemp, J.A., et al. (1980) A re-evaluation of the mechanisms underlying simple cell orientation selectivity. *Brain Res.*, 194: 517–520.

Singer, W., Tretter, F., et al. (1975) Organization of cat striate cortex: A correlation of receptive field properties with afferent and efferent connections. *J. Neurophysiol.*, 38: 1080–1098.

Soodak, R.E. (1986) Two-dimensional modeling of visual receptive fields using Gaussian subunits. *Proc. Natl. Acad. Sci. USA*, 83: 9259–9263.

Tanaka, K. (1983) Cross-correlation analysis of geniculostriate neuronal relationships in cats. *J. Neurophysiol.*, 49: 1303–1318.

Torre, V. and Poggio, T. (1978) A synaptic mechanism possibly underlying direction selectivity to motion. *Proc. R. Soc. London Ser. B*, 202: 409–416.

Tsumoto, T., Eckart, W., et al. (1979) Modification of orientation sensitivity of cat visual cortex neurons by removal of GABA-mediated inhibition. *Exp. Brain Res.*, 34: 351–363.

Vidyasagar, T.R. and Heide, W. (1984) Geniculate orientation biases seen with moving sine wave gratings: implications for a model of simple cell afferent connectivity. *Exp. Brain Res.*, 57: 196–200.

Wolf, W., Hicks, T.P., et al. (1986) The contribution of GABA-mediated inhibitory mechanisms to visual response properties of neurons in the kitten's striate cortex. *J. Neurosci.*, 6: 2779–2795.

R.R. Mize, R.E. Marc and A.M. Sillito (Eds.)
Progress in Brain Research, Vol. 90
© 1992 Elsevier Science Publishers B.V. All rights reserved

CHAPTER 21

# GABA-mediated inhibition in the neural networks of visual cortex

Neil J. Berman, Rodney J. Douglas and Kevan A.C. Martin

*MRC Anatomical Neuropharmacology Unit, Mansfield Road, Oxford OX1 3TH, England, UK*

## Introduction

The selective responses that are such a familiar feature of cortical neurons, have spurred many imaginative efforts to understand the machinery of neocortex. This program of research has, by any standards, been inordinately successful, particularly for the visual cortex (Hubel and Wiesel, 1977). Certainly more is known about the functional architecture of primary visual cortex, than for any other cortical area. In addition its extensive interconnections have been mapped (see reviews by Orban, 1984; Van Essen, 1985; Zeki and Shipp, 1988) and the component neurons have been studied in great anatomical detail (Lund, 1973; Szentágothai, 1973; Martin, 1984; Peters, 1987; Somogyi, 1989). Nevertheless, many issues remain unresolved.

Of all the components that make up the cortical machinery, the most difficult to place has been the GABA-mediated inhibitory system. That is not to say that inhibition is generally thought to be unimportant. On the contrary, inhibition has been used like leaven in bread for every model that requires selective responses from single neurons. In the visual cortex, for example, directionality is achieved by an inhibitory "veto" operation (Koch and Poggio, 1985), orientation selectivity by "cross-orientation" inhibition (Bishop et al., 1973), hypercomplexity or "end-stopping" by inhibitory end-zones (Hubel and Wiesel, 1965; Orban et al., 1979). The problem is that there is not

a coherent or consistent view of the role of inhibition in producing this selectivity. Indeed, there are now so many anomalous findings concerning cortical inhibition, that it seems inevitable that the biologists working in this area should find themselves suffering from a bad case of cognitive dissonance.

## Dissonant images of inhibition in visual cortex

In the visual cortex, dissonance has surfaced repeatedly, most notably about the issue of whether inhibition is involved in generating the property of orientation selectivity. Opposing positions have been succinctly and clearly stated. Sillito (1984) declared that "the inhibitory system is seen to be the architect of the orientation selectivity." Contrariwise, Ferster (1987) claimed "that orientation of cortical receptive fields is neither created nor sharpened by inhibition between neurons with different orientation preference." For the issues to be put so clearly, correctly implies that both have data to substantiate their own positions and explanations to account for the other's apparent misperceptions. Such dialectics are, of course, the stuff of science, but what they reveal in this instance, is not that the experimental designs are fatally flawed, nor that the results are incorrectly interpreted, nor that the critical experiments have yet to be carried out. Such fundamental disagreements about cortical inhibition occur, we believe,

444

because there has been a frank disconnection between the high-level explanations of the phenomena of selectivity, and considerations of the cellular mechanisms that are required to generate this selectivity.

In this chapter we set the issue of cortical inhibition in a different context, that of intra- and intercellular interactions. By doing so, we hoped to reconnect the phenomenology of the selective responses of single units to the rich database of structure and function of cortical neurons and microcircuits, thereby achieving some resolution of the incompatibilities in the experimental literature. At the outset it is worth re-stating three key sets of experimental observations, which are the prerequisites of our thesis. Firstly, cortical inhibition exists. It was found in the earliest single cell recordings from neocortex using intracellular (Phillips, 1959) and extracellular recording (Hubel and Wiesel, 1959). The pioneering pharmacological experiments of Sillito (1975) then established its importance in generating selective responses by demonstrating the deleterious effects of blocking GABA$_A$ receptors. Finally, the structural studies of neocortex, beginning with the Golgi studies of Ramón y Cajal (1911) and continuing with the contemporary technical wizardry of combining light and electron microscopy and immunocytochemistry (Jones, 1984; Somogyi and Freund, 1989; White, 1989), has revealed the rich diversity of the GABAergic components of the cortical circuits. Even taken individually, it is clear that from each of these key observations that there is something important to be understood about the nature and role of the inhibitory system in the neocortex.

## GABA-mediated synaptic inhibition: mechanisms

In the neocortex there is no structural evidence for the pre-synaptic inhibitory mechanisms that were described by Eccles (1964) in the spinal cord. Therefore, we assume that cortical inhibition acts primarily through postsynaptic mechanisms (but see Nelson, 1991). The action of the

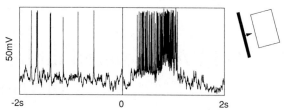

Fig. 1. Intracellular response of layer 3 pyramidal cell with a standard complex receptive field. Control period ($-2$ sec to 0 sec) is followed by 2 sec test period during which a dark bar appears and moves across the receptive field. (Douglas, Martin and Whitteridge, unpublished.)

inhibitory synapses is to produce an outward current that opposes the inward current produced by the excitatory synapses. In theoretical analyses of postsynaptic inhibition it has been convenient to divide the postynaptic effects into two types: hyperpolarizing inhibition and shunting inhibition. Both act by increasing the permeability or conductance of the membrane to ions whose reversal potentials are near (shunting), or more negative (hyperpolarizing) than the resting membrane potential. This distinction between shunting and hyperpolarizing inhibition is to some extent artificial, particularly in whole animal recordings where the concept of a "resting" membrane potential has to be considerably stretched to be an accurate description of the data (Fig. 1).

Hyperpolarizing inhibition drives an outward current across the membrane by inducing a small increase in conductance to potassium. The magnitude of the current produced depends on the voltage difference between the membrane potential (about $-50$ to $-70$ mV, at "rest") and the potassium reversal potential ($-90$ mV). Shunting inhibition also acts by producing an outward current. In this case the reversal potential of chloride ($-70$ mV) is closer to the "resting" membrane potential and so the outward current is driven by a relatively small potential difference. The magnitude of the outward current now depends largely on the size of the conductance increase for chloride.

During simultaneous activation of both excitatory and inhibitory synapses, the net inward current arriving at the axon hillock will determine whether the membrane reaches threshold. If the net current is sufficient to produce a suprathreshold depolarization, the magnitude of the excitatory current will determine the instantaneous rate at which the neuron will discharge. Theoretical analyses of cortical inhibition usually consider only the inhibitory effects on the sub-threshold membrane potential (Rall, 1964; Blomfield, 1974; Jack et al., 1975; Koch and Poggio, 1985). While it is mathematically convenient to consider only the subthreshold membrane potential, experimentally the effects of inhibition during natural visual stimulation have been assessed by measuring the changes in action potential discharge. The key is then to understand the effects of inhibition on the discharging neuron.

## Inhibitory control of cortical pyramidal neurons

We have approached this problem by a combination of computer simulation and experimental data. We developed a general program for simulating neuronal networks (CANON) that permits neurons to be specified as sets of interconnected compartments (Douglas and Martin, 1991a,b). The pyramidal cell, which is really the workhorse of the cortex, was the obvious focus for our analysis. The pyramidal cells used in the simulations were also chosen to straddle the limits of the morphological types seen in the visual cortex. From our catalogue of neurons, recorded intracellularly in vivo and injected with horseradish peroxidase, we selected two. One neuron was from layer 2, because these are the smallest pyra-

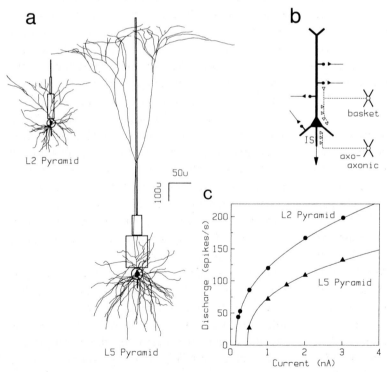

Fig. 2. Simplified compartmental models of cortical neurons. A. Reconstructed cortical pyramidal neurons (dendrites only) from layers 2 and 5. Idealized equivalent cylinder model cells used for simulations are superimposed. Scale bars: 100 $\mu$m, reconstructed neurons and vertical axis of model neurons; 50 $\mu$m, horizontal axis of model neurons only. B. Schematic of inhibitory inputs from basket and chandelier (axoaconic) cells to a typical pyramidal cell (filled shape). C. Current-discharge curves for the first interspike interval of the model cells shown in B. (See Douglas and Martin, 1990b.)

midal cells found in the cortex, the other neuron was from layer 5, which contains the largest pyramidal cells. The detailed structure of the dendritic arbour and soma was reconstructed in 3-D and then transformed into a simplified compartmental neuron (Fig. 2), which had the same input resistance and time constant as the original neuron recorded in vivo. The method for the simplification is described elsewhere (Douglas and Martin, 1990b; 1991a,b).

The pyramidal cells receive their inhibitory input from a number of sources (see Somogyi, 1989), but for our simulations we considered just two types of inhibitory neurons. One type, the chandelier, or axo-axonic cell, is a specialized GABAergic neuron that forms synapses exclusively on the axon initial segment of the pyramidal cell (Somogyi et al., 1982). Superficial layer pyramidal cells receive about 20–40 synapses from about 5 chandelier cells; deep layer pyramidal cells receive many fewer synapses (Freund et al. 1983; Fariñas and DeFelipe, 1990a,b). The axon initial-segment is a particularly sensitive site, since it is the region where the action potential is initiated, and thus the chandelier cell seems to offer a potent means of inhibiting the pyramidal cell output (for review, see Peters, 1984).

The other type we considered was the basket cell, which is the GABAergic cell most frequently encountered in both Golgi preparations (Ramón y Cajal, 1911) and in our intracellular recording from identified cells (Martin et al., 1983; see Martin, 1988). The basket cells form 85% of their synapses on the soma and dendrites of pramidal cells (Somogyi et al., 1983). Each pyramidal cell seems to receive a convergent input from 10 to 20 basket cells, each contributing about 5–10 synapses to each pyramid. These numbers are estimates based on small samples and there are certainly single instances where a single basket cell may provide many more synapses to an individual pyramidal cell (Kisvárday et al., 1987). However, they provide some limits for the parameters for the simulations.

Unitary synaptic conductances have not been measured for the synapses of identified chandelier or basket cells, so for the simulations we used a range of conductance values. For the soma and proximal dendrites the inhibitory conductances ranged between 0.1 and 1.0 $mS \cdot cm^{-2}$. For the axon initial segment they ranged between 1–10 $mS \cdot cm^{-2}$, because the initial segment has a higher density of GABAergic synapses. In the limiting case, each synapse produced a maximum conductance of about 0.3 nS, which is in excess of that suggested by recent patch-clamp studies (Kriegstein and LoTurco, 1990; Verdoorn et al., 1990). In the simulations, the average inhibitory conductance was held constant over the period of the excitatory current injection. This was done to approximate the sustained inhibition that would be required to prevent a response to non-optimal visual stimulation in vivo (Douglas et al., 1988).

The response of the model neurons to a step of excitatory current injected into the soma is shown in Fig. 3. These responses were essentially indistinguishable from those of pyramidal cells recorded in vivo or in vitro. In this study we were only concerned with the peak frequency of the action potential discharge, before the conductances associated with spike adaptation took effect and slowed the discharge rate (Berman et al., 1989a; Douglas and Martin, 1991b). If the first interspike interval was plotted as a function of excitatory current, then the data points were well-fit with a power function (Fig. 2C). The difference between the superficial and the deep layer pyramid is explained by the decreased current load offered by the smaller dendritic arbour of the layer 2 pyramidal cell.

It seems obvious that an excitatory current just sufficient to produce a suprathreshold depolarization of the membrane could be offset by an inhibitory current, which would then keep the membrane potential below threshold and prevent action potentials from being produced. A large excitatory current, however, would overcome the inhibition and produce an action potential discharge. But the frequency of discharge would be reduced in the face of inhibition, because part of the excitatory current would be used to offset the inhibitory current. Inhibition would seem to have two effects. One is to raise the current threshold for action potential discharge. The second is to reduce the peak discharge rate. Both effects have been predicted in a formal model using idealized neurons (Blomfield, 1974) and apparently confirmed experimentally (Rose, 1977; Burr et al., 1981).

Our simulations confirmed that the principal effect of both types of inhibition, hyperpolarizing and shunting, was to increase the current threshold before action potentials were produced. Once threshold was reached, however, the increase in the frequency of firing for a given increase in excitatory current was greater for the inhibited

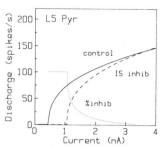

Fig. 4. Simulated effect of axoaxonic cell inhibition on current-discharge relationship of model layer 5 pyramidal neuron (see Fig. 2.). Fitted power curves of current-discharge shown before (continuous line, control) and after (dashed line) initial segment inhibition (5 mS·cm$^{-2}$; $E_{rev}$ −80 mV). Difference between the control and inhibited expressed as percent inhibition (dotted line). (See Douglas and Martin, 1990b.)

than for the non-inhibited case (Fig. 4). This effect was related to the magnitude of the conductance change, and was more marked for shunting than for hyperpolarizing inhibition. For large excitatory currents there was little difference in the discharge rates for the inhibited and non-inhibited case. If the effect of inhibition is expressed as the percentage of the difference between firing rate of the control and the inhibited case ("% inhib" curve in Fig. 4), then it is immediately evident that the effectiveness of the inhibition decreases with increasing excitatory current. Experimentally, sometimes the peak firing rate during inhibition was higher than control, sometimes a little lower, as illustrated in Figs. 5 and 7.

The pattern was not dependent on the site of the inhibition. The same result was obtained regardless of whether the inhibition was applied by chandelier cells (to the axon initial segment), or basket cells (to the soma), or both together. On a synapse for synapse basis, chandelier inhibition was more efficient than the inhibition applied to the soma by basket cells, simply because the density of inhibitory synapses was so much higher on the initial segment than on the soma (Fariñas and DeFelipe, 1990a,b). The lack of obvious functional differences between the chandelier and the basket cells in the simulation, despite the differences in their postsynaptic targeting, raises the

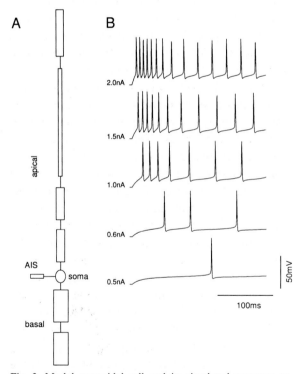

Fig. 3. Model pyramidal cell and its simulated response to excitatory current steps. A. Compartmental model of HRP-filled layer 5 neuron shown in Fig. 13A. Each compartment is allocated appropriate profiles of passive and active conductances based on biophysical data from the recorded cell itself and the literature. B. Response of model cell to simulated depolarizing current step injection. (Details in Douglas and Martin, 1991a,b.)

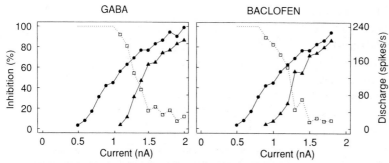

Fig. 5. Inhibition of discharge in a layer 2/3 neuron in rat visual cortex in vitro. Current-discharge curves (right ordinate) for the 1st interspike interval were obtained from current step injections before (closed circles) and during (closed triangles) iontophoretic applications of GABA (19 nA, left graph) and baclofen (20 nA, right graph) to the same neuron. Both GABA and baclofen increased the conductance of the cell by 21% (5 nS) and 74% (18 nS), respectively. The effectiveness of the inhibition is expressed as percentage inhibition (open squares, left ordinate). (Berman, N.J., Douglas, R.J. and Martin, K.A.C., unpublished.)

possibility that the synapses on the initial segment do not act by the conventional mechanisms we modelled.

The simulations showed that there was little difference between inhibition applied by hyperpolarizing or shunting mechanisms. Both increased the current threshold and both had little effect on the instantaneous frequency of firing for large excitatory currents, if only the first action potentials were considered. This result was to us unexpected, but in retrospect the explanation was blindingly simple. The maximum sodium and potassium spike conductances are about 10 times larger than the synaptic and adaptation conductances. Thus, while inhibition tends to prevent the activation of the action-potential current, it does not have much effect on the trajectory of the action potential once it has been initiated, because this phase is dominated by the spike conductances. During the interspike interval the membrane is once more strongly influenced by the synaptic and adaptive conductances. When the discharge rate increases in response to stronger excitatory currents, the spike conductances (particularly the delayed rectifying potassium conductance) do not relax completely. Thus, for strong excitatory currents, the spike conductances dominate at all phases, including the interspike interval, and drive the current-discharge relation into saturation. The theoretical analysis

by Blomfield (1974) did not take into account the active action potential conductances and thus he did not predict the reduced effectiveness of inhibition for strong excitatory currents. In the light of our analysis, the apparent experimental support (Rose, 1977; Burr et al., 1981) for the Blomfield theory will need to be reinterpreted.

Our simulation showed that if sufficient excitatory current can be delivered to the axon hillock, the neuron will always be able to fire at near peak discharge rates. The "sufficient current" depends on the input resistance and the membrane time-constant of the neuron. The activity of the GABA synapses reduces the membrane time-constant by increasing the membrane conductance. The shorter time-constant permits the membrane to recharge more rapidly after each action potential, so the neuron fires at a higher rate for a given current. This explains the increased slope of the current-discharge curve once the excitatory current is suprathreshold. Theoretically, the peak discharge rate could be marginally higher in the presence of GABA than in the non-inhibited case, but at high input currents the spike discharge saturates.

If the chandelier and basket cells were required to inhibit the neuron completely via the mechanisms we have modelled, they could approximate complete blockade only by forcing the threshold to the upper end of the operational range of excitatory current (approx. 1.5–2.0 nA). The conductance required to produce such an enormous increase in threshold would have to be of the same size as the spike conductances. Even so, if the excitatory current did exceed threshold during the period of inhibition, there would be a catastrophic failure of inhibition: the neuron would respond immediately at a high discharge rate. Most models of cortical selectivity unsuspectingly run the gauntlet between complete suppression of maximal excitation and a catastrophic break-through discharge. In these models, the absence of response to a stimulus arises through inhibition of a strong excitatory discharge. Our theoretical work shows that strong excitatory transients are very difficult to suppress, unless the magnitude of the inhibition is very large indeed. We have tested our hypothesis experimentally, and the results will be discussed below.

## GABA-mediated post-synaptic inhibition: in the dish

The simulations emphasised that the difficulty of GABA-mediated postsynaptic inhibition to contain strong excitation was not dependent on the location of the inhibitory synapses. This allowed us to test our theory by iontophoresing GABA directly onto the postsynaptic membrane of cortical neurons to assess its effect on the current-discharge relationship. The experiments were performed on slices of rat visual cortex, maintained in vitro (Berman, N.J., Douglas, R.J. and Martin, K.A.C., unpublished). Neurons in various layers were impaled and excited by injections of current through the recording pipette. Most of the neurons responded to a step of constant current by discharging initially at a high rate and then rapidly adapting. This pattern is typical of pyramidal neurons (Connors et al., 1982; McCormick, 1990). When GABA was then iontophoresed onto the neurons, the input conductance of the neuron increased and the membrane potential showed a complex sequence of hyperpolarization and depolarization before settling to a constant value. The

change in the current-discharge curve was as our theory predicted (Fig. 5). The current threshold was raised, but once the threshold was crossed, the neurons rapidly reached near-control rates of firing. This effect is reflected in the rapid decrease of the percent inhibition curve. Very similar results were obtained if the $GABA_B$ receptor agonist, baclofen, was iontophoresed onto the same neurons (Fig. 5).

Our results using baclofen agree well with a similar study by Connors et al. (1988). They also found that iontophoresis of baclofen increased the current threshold, steepened the initial slope of the current-discharge curve, but had little effect on the discharge rates produced by large currents. The increased threshold is explained by the additional outward currents, which result from activation of the $GABA_B$ conductances, and which offset the inward excitatory currents. The steepened slope of the current-discharge curve is due to the reduction in the membrane time-constant induced by the $GABA_B$ agonist.

Our results using GABA, which of course acts on both the $GABA_A$ and the $GABA_B$ receptors, appear to contradict those of Connors et al. (1988), who were unable to elicit two sequential spikes during GABA iontophoresis. The difference between their results and ours is simply that we carefully titrated the GABA iontophoresis so that the increase in the current threshold and input conductance remained within physiological ranges. With larger iontophoretic currents it was possible to prevent the membrane from reaching threshold with the maximum excitatory currents used here (3 nA). Similar results have been observed in extracellular recordings that have used iontophoretically-applied GABA to inhibit visual responses (Rose, 1977; Hess and Murata, 1974). However, the membrane conductance was not measured in those studies. In our in vitro study, blocking discharge was only achieved by applying amounts of GABA that drove the membrane conductance to levels far in excess of anything seen during the peak of an electrically-evoked IPSP, or during visually-evoked inhibition (Ber-

450

man et al., 1989b, 1991). The fact that conductance changes outside the normal physiological range can be obtained by iontophoresis, does raise the further important issue of what receptors are actually being activated during the extracellular GABA application.

With the development of specific antibodies to subunits of the GABA receptor, it has now become possible to map out the distribution of the GABA receptor at the subcellular level. This has been done for the cortical pyramidal cells using antibodies directed against the alpha-subunit of the benzodiazepine/$GABA_A$/chloride channel complex (Somogyi, 1989). The results were clear-cut, but rather disturbing for physiologists, because they showed that there were a large number of extrasynaptic sites that were immunoreactive. If the immunoreactivity does indeed indicate the sites of active receptors, the observation raises the possibility that many of the receptors activated during iontophoretic application of GABA are not those involved in normal synaptic transmission (but see Somogyi, 1989). In fact it seems conceivable that the receptors lying beneath the synaptic boutons may be relatively protected from the GABA delivered by extracellular application. Thus, the results of iontophoretic experiments, including our own, should be interpreted with a degree of caution. They may not give much insight into the mechanisms that operate during normal function.

In view of the ambiguity in the interpretation of these results, we took the analysis one step further and studied the effects of synaptically-applied neurotransmitter. We stimulated the white matter underlying the cortex to produce IPSPs in the recorded neurons. We could then show that excitatory currents delivered through the recording pipette could break through a synaptically-evoked IPSP to produce a discharge (Fig. 6). Using this protocol we were not able to construct a current-discharge curve because the inhibition was not in steady state, but varied both in the magnitude of the conductance and in the membrane potential over the duration of the IPSP.

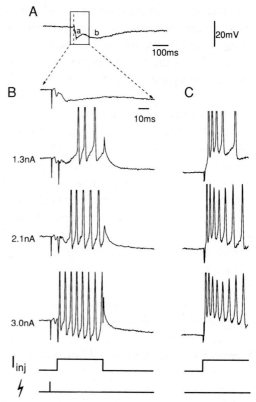

Fig. 6. Breakthrough discharge during synaptically evoked IPSP. A. Typical response of layer 5 neuron in rat visual cortex in vitro to electrical stimulation of white matter (vertical dashed line). Short duration EPSPs are followed by short $GABA_A$ (a) and long $GABA_B$ (b) IPSPs. B. Region dominated by $GABA_A$ IPSP in A shown on expanded timebase in first trace. Subsequent traces show the response to injection of current steps ($I_{inj}$) timed to coincide with the $GABA_A$ IPSP (8–50 msec) following white matter stimulation (bolt). C. Control responses to identical current injections without white matter stimulation. (Berman, N.J., Douglas, R.J. and Martin, K.A.C., unpublished.)

Nevertheless, in the face of strong transient excitation, the inhibitory synaptic mechanisms failed to prevent the excitatory current from reaching threshold and producing action potentials. This observation clearly raises problems for any model that requires inhibition to quench strong excitation.

We should emphasize that these experiments, like most laboratory models, are concerned with the limits of the behaviour of the system, not the normal dynamics. Although we have kept the discharge rates within physiological ranges, it is clear that simply looking at the first interspike interval of a current-discharge curve gives only one part of the picture. The same neurons in vivo are required to respond to a stimulus for durations of hundreds of milliseconds, even seconds. While inhibitory control of the transient excitatory response is clearly necessary, inhibition is also required to act on sustained discharges. We have thus examined in some detail the action of GABA on neurons in the adapted state.

Adaptation of discharge is achieved by turning on intrinsic potassium conductances, which produce outward currents (Connors et al., 1982; Rudy, 1988; Schwindt et al., 1988a,b; Berman et al., 1989a; Douglas and Martin, 1990a; McCormick, 1990). These intrinsic adaptive currents act in concert with the synaptically-induced inhibitory currents to oppose the excitatory inward currents, which themselves arise both from intrinsic membrane currents and synaptic currents. In the adapted phase of the current-discharge curve, the response is dominated by the intrinsic adaptive potassium conductances (Schwindt et al.,

1988a,b; McCormick, 1990). Under these conditions the effect of GABA is simply to shunt some excitatory current. This will displace the adapted current-discharge curve to the right on the current axis. The magnitude of this displacement will depend on the relative state of adaptation and the magnitude of GABA-mediated conductances. We have found in vitro that the iontopheretic GABA-mediated inhibition is still unable to prevent strong excitatory currents from reaching threshold and producing a discharge, despite the assistance of the adaptive conductances (Fig. 7). This is a remarkable finding that forces us to re-examine the whole basis of response selectivity meditated by GABA in the visual cortex.

## Can GABAergic neurons inhibit visual responses?

Generations of physiologists have recorded the extracellular responses of single neurons in the visual cortex. These recordings have indicated that the firing frequency of cortical neurons in response to optimal stimuli can be in excess of

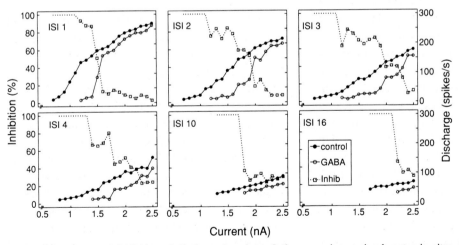

Fig. 7. Adaptation and inhibition of discharge in a layer 2/3 neuron in rat visual cortex in vitro. Current-discharge curves and percent inhibition plotted as for Fig. 5. Each graph shows the current-discharge curve before (closed circles) and during GABA application (open circles), and net inhibitory effect (open circles) for the interspike interval (ISI) indicated. GABA was iontophoresed in the vicinity of the soma. Full adaptation is reached by ISI 10. Control current threshold was 0.6 nA (note abscissa begins at 0.5 nA). Data was obtained after the GABA-induced conductance increase (38%, 9 nS) had stabilized (Scharfman and Sarvey, 1987). (Berman, N.J., Douglas, R.J. and Martin, K.A.C., unpublished.)

100 spikes/sec (Orban, 1984). Comparison of these responses with the current-discharge curves from similar neurons in vitro, gives some estimate of the magnitude of the excitatory current involved. Assuming the in vitro data is directly applicable to the in vivo situation, it seems unavoidable that at least 1–2 nA of excitatory current would be required to produce a reasonable discharge rate if the neuron was in the adapted state. Many of the proposed models for cortical selectivity require the inhibitory mechanisms to oppose this amount of excitatory current. For example, there are a number of models for selectivity of simple cells in layer 4 of visual cortex (Heggelund, 1981a; Wiesel and Gilbert, 1983) that use the same basic principles to achieve their effect: excitation is provided by thalamic afferents and inhibition via inhibitory interneurons, which themselves are excited by thalamic afferents or intracortical excitatory pathways.

The most transparent realization of these principles is Heggelund's circuit for the simple cell, illustrated in Fig. 8. We have pointed out previously that this circuit bears close resemblances to the circuit suggested by Barlow and Levick (1965) to account for directional selectivity in rabbit retinal ganglion cells, and later transplanted to the visual cortex by Barlow (1981). Here, as in most models of cortical selectivity, inhibition operates as negative excitation. That is, the purpose of the inhibition is to cancel out inappropriate excitatory responses. Using this inhibition, the concentric centre-surround fields of the thalamic afferents can thus be chiselled, filed, and smoothed into receptive fields of any desired size, shape, or texture (see Martin, 1988).

For the Barlow-Levick model, the spatial offset of the sets of excitatory afferents to the inhibitory neuron and the delay inserted by the additional synapses in the inhibitory circuit ensures that inhibition arrives after the direct excitation in the optimal direction of motion. In the non-preferred direction, excitation and inhibition arrive simultaneously and cancel. There is convincing evidence from a number of single unit

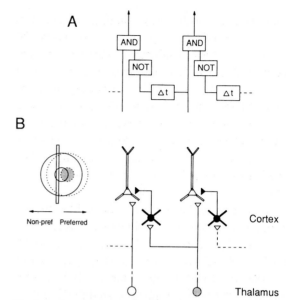

Fig. 8. Barlow and Levick (1965) model of direction selectivity. A. Two non-directional receptors (e.g., thalamic relay cells) are connected to a logical AND-NOT gate, one via a delay, $\Delta t$. B. Barlow and Levick (1965) model used to explain how the direction selectivity of cortical cells is derived from the non-directional thalamic input. The spatially displaced, circular symmetric receptive fields of thalamic neurons are shown on the left (shaded cell responds to shaded field). Pyramidal neurons receive direct excitation from thalamic neurons, and a synaptically delayed input from inhibitory cells (filled) in cortex.

studies that such a sequence of excitation and inhibition occurs (Bishop et al., 1971; Emerson and Gerstein, 1977; Palmer and Davis, 1981; Bullier et al., 1982; Ganz and Felder, 1984). Strong support for the circuit also arises from pharmacological studies in which directionality is lost when the action of inhibitory interneurons are impaired by blocking the $GABA_A$ receptors using bicuculline (Sillito, 1975). Further support arrives in the form of intracellular recordings, in which a sequence of depolarization followed by hyperpolarization was elicited when the stimulus moved in the optimal direction (Douglas et al., 1991).

Missing from these analyses of the directional response is a quantitative estimate of the relative magnitude of excitation and inhibition. Implicit in the Barlow-Levick model is that the inhibition is strong enough to cancel the excitation in the non-preferred direction, but this calculation has not been made from experimental data. However, the separation of excitation and inhibition in simple receptive fields permits a relatively straightforward calculation to be made of the relative magnitudes of inhibition and excitation. This estimate can even be made from extracellular recordings in which the depth of the inhibition can be judged by the degree to which it can suppress the spontaneous discharge of the neuron. The estimate can also be made using intracellular recordings where the actual degree of hyperpolarization of the membrane can be assessed. Both these measures are illustrated for the same simple cell (Fig. 9). The neuron was located in layer 4 and was shown by electrical stimulation to be excited monosynaptically by thalamic afferents. In this example (Fig. 9A) it is clear that the inhibition following the excitation for the optimal direction of motion was not sufficiently strong to reduce the spontaneous activity to zero. The excitatory response was at least twice the baseline spontaneous activity, i.e., excitation in this neuron pro-

duced more action potentials than the inhibition suppressed.

This difference in the magnitude of excitation vs inhibition is also evident in the intracellular records (Fig. 9B). The magnitude of the hyperpolarization, which results in inhibition of the action potential discharge, is small. The amount of outward current required to produce a 5 mV hyperpolarization is about 0.2 nA for a neuron with an input resistance of 25 M$\Omega$. The excitatory current required to drive the neuron to threshold is at least this value. Thus additional excitatory current is required to produce the frequency of action potential discharge seen here. It seems that for this simple cell at least, the directional response cannot be explained by the cancelling of inhibition and excitation: the apparent magnitude of the inhibition is insufficient. This simple observation and calculation, which could have been made at any time over the past 30 years, clearly raises a host of interrelated questions concerning the nature and mechanisms of action of GABA in generating response selectivity.

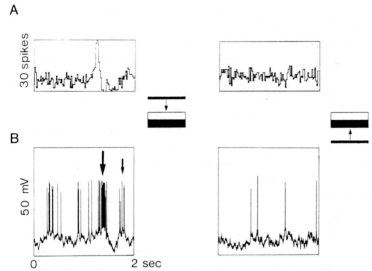

Fig. 9. Response of directional simple cell to a moving bar. Layer 4 neuron monosynaptically activated from LGN. A. Extracellular response to the moving bar in the preferred (left) and non-preferred direction (right). B. Intracellular record of membrane potential changes underlying the extracellular response in A. In the preferred direction the strong ON response (large arrow) is followed by a hyperpolarization and then a smaller excitatory response (small arrow). (From Douglas et al., 1991.)

## The story inside

The case for the simple cell described above is clear enough from the extracellular records. The intracellular recording serves only to confirm the conclusion that the inhibition does not seem strong enough to explain the direction selectivity. But, one swallow does not make a summer. In other neurons, for example, the spontaneous activity recorded by the extracellular electrode is reduced to zero by the inhibition. In such cases the magnitude of the inhibition can only be guessed at (Palmer and Davis, 1981). Only intracellular recording can resolve the issue. We have recorded intracellularly from neurons in the visual cortex, stimulating them with conventional visual stimuli. The general pattern of inhibition as it relates to the membrane potential can be summarized quite briefly. The magnitude of the hyperpolarizations was greatest when the neuron was stimulated with the optimal stimulus. Stimuli that are not optimally oriented, or which move in non-optimal directions, do not elicit strong hyperpolarizations. The intracellular records from the simple cell illustrated in Fig. 9 are then typical.

Hubel and Wiesel (1962) envisaged orientation selectivity as being set up once and for all in layer 4 and then relayed by excitatory connections to other layers. The spectre of their schema has haunted considerations of inhibition in the visual cortex. If the selectivity of the neurons has been generated at a prior stage of processing, then what appears to be inhibition would not be postsynaptic inhibition at all, but removal of excitation. Indeed, all the data presented above could potentially be explained in terms of removal of excitation. A variant of this has been provided by Nelson (1991), who has proposed, on the basis of extracellular recordings, that the inhibition present in the visual cortex acts by a presynaptic mechanism directed only at the thalamocortical synapse in layer 4. In other words, there is no postsynaptic inhibition, only a mechanism that removes the initial thalamocortical excitation. Against this, there are several lines of evidence

that point to the existence and effectiveness of postsynaptic inhibitory mechanisms. One line is the accumulation of structural and physiological evidence, which shows that every neuron in the cortex receives a rich GABAergic input (see Somogyi, 1989). Add to this the extensive studies of the physiology of the GABAergic neurons, which have shown that they have quite normal receptive fields (Gilbert and Wiesel, 1979; Martin et al., 1983; Martin, 1988). In sum, there is no reason to suppose that the GABA neurons are not activated by the conventional stimuli that are used. On these grounds alone, it seems likely that postsynaptic inhibition would be evident under most stimulus conditions.

The presence of postsynaptic inhibition can be demonstrated using conventional biophysical techniques (see Ferster, 1986). The strategy is to current clamp the membrane potential at different values and show that the amplitude of the "inhibitory" potential changes in the direction expected for a postsynaptic mechanism. This is shown for a layer 5 pyramidal neuron (Fig. 10). A hyperpolarizing potential was evoked by flashing a dark bar on its "ON" subfield. If the "hyperpolarization" is due to a reduction in excitatory depolarization then the amplitude of the hyperpolarization should hardly be affected by a sustained polarizing current. When depolarizing current was injected into the neuron, we found that the amplitude of the inhibitory hyperpolarization increased in magnitude. This indicates that the inhibition is not presynaptic. The depolarization increases the difference between the membrane potential and the reversal potential of the inhibitory synapses, so providing a larger driving potential for the inhibitory current.

The central difficulty is that inhibition measured by these biophysical techniques does not appear to be powerful. Yet strong inhibition is required, it seems, if strong excitatory responses are to be quenched. However, there remain several escape routes for those wedded to the necessity of omnipotent inhibition. One is the possibility that the hyperpolarization does not accurately

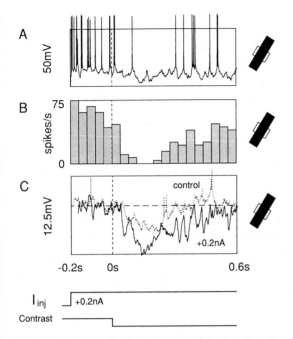

A    50mV

B    75
     spikes/s
     0

C    12.5mV
     control
     +0.2nA

-0.2s    0s              0.6s

I_inj ⌐ +0.2nA

Contrast

Fig. 10. Response of a layer 5 pyramidal cell with a simple receptive field (S1) to flashed bar. Excitatory current was injected to raise firing rate ($I_{inj}$, $t = -0.2$ sec, $+0.2$ nA), while a dark bar appeared (Contrast, $t = 0$ sec) which remained for the test duration. A. Intracellular response to the current step and flash onset (vertical dashed line). B. Histogram showing effect on spike rate averaged over 7 trials. Flash initially suppressed firing (latency 40 msec), but the effect diminished from 250 msec onwards. C. Average membrane polarizations, (7 trials) associated with flash-induced inhibition of firing, with (solid line) and without (dotted line) conditioning current step ($I_{inj}$). (From Berman et al., 1991.)

reflect the magnitude of the inhibition. If inhibition acts by shunting the excitatory current it would not induce much change in membrane potential. Shunting inhibition would at least account for directional and orientation selectivity in cases where the magnitude of the hyperpolarization appears too small to account for the elimination or reduction of response seen with non-optimal stimuli. Experimentally, the signature of shunting inhibition is a large increase in the input conductance of the neuron. For shunting inhibition to be effective against visually-driven excitation, it must be sustained for the duration of flow of the excitatory current. We could examine this in vivo using the standard technique of injecting a

series of constant-current pulses to measure the conductance, while stimulating the neuron visually. If the inhibition was associated with large increases in conductance, then the amplitude of the voltage deflections produced by the constant current pulses should fall dramatically during inhibition.

We tested a range of neurons using this method (Douglas et al., 1988). The results were clear-cut. Large sustained conductance changes were not found, although a wide range of conditions were tested. Regardless of the contrast of the stimulus, the receptive field of the neuron (simple or complex), the receptive field property being examined (subfield antagonism of simple cells, orientation, or directionality), or whether the neuron was driven directly or indirectly by thalamic afferents, the input conductance of the neuron did not increase more than about 10–40% of the initial conductance. This was insufficiently large to account for the inhibition of the excitatory response.

To illustrate this point we give two examples: one using a stationary flashed stimulus, the other using a moving stimulus. We used a stationary stimulus to activate the inhibitory mechanisms that underlie the subfield antagonism of simple cells originally reported by Hubel and Wiesel (1959, 1962). A dark bar was placed over the "ON" field of a layer 5 neuron. With the onset of the stimulus, the membrane hyperpolarized and remained hyperpolarized for the entire duration of the stimulus (Fig. 11). Constant current pulses were then injected into the neuron through the recording pipette during a control and test period. The derived input conductance was plotted as a percent of the conductance of the neuron measured during the control period. The onset of the stimulus induced a clear increase in the conductance of the neuron, which endured for the duration of the stimulus. Thus the inhibition and hyperpolarization was associated with an increase in input conductance of about 20%.

We could further demonstrate that the degree of hyperpolarization seen with visual stimulation does not reflect the limit of postsynaptic inhibition available to the neuron. Electrical stimulation is the most effective means we know of for inducing an IPSP, presumably because the pulse stimulus provides a volley of excitation to the cortex that is not matched even by the flashed stimulus. During electrical stimulation a large fraction of the cortical neurons are activated simultaneously and summate their effect. Comparison of the visual and the electrical response for the same neuron (Fig. 11) indicates that the magnitude of the hyperpolarization elicited by the electrical pulse is greater than that of the flash stimulus. The single pulse activation of the inhibitory synapses endures for several hundred msec. This is not due to repetitive excitation of the inhibitory population, since every neuron we have tested in this way shows the same pattern of a brief EPSP followed by an extended IPSP. Thus the whole visual cortex becomes silent during the period of an electrically-evoked IPSP.

The second example is that of a simple cell from layer 6, which we stimulated with a moving bar (Douglas et al., 1988). This neuron showed a sequence of excitation followed by inhibition in the preferred direction of motion (Fig. 12). In the reverse direction, inhibition was also evoked, but now superimposed on the excitatory response, as might be predicted from the Barlow and Levick (1965) model. Constant current pulses were injected to measure the conductance. The start of the regular pulse train was staggered from trial to trial. This reduced the sensitivity of the method, because we could not average several trials, but ensured that the entire period of recording was sampled. We estimated that conductance changes smaller than 15% of control would not be detected by our method.

These measurements showed that in neither the preferred direction, nor the reverse direction, was there any evidence of a marked increase in conductance, except during the period of maxi-

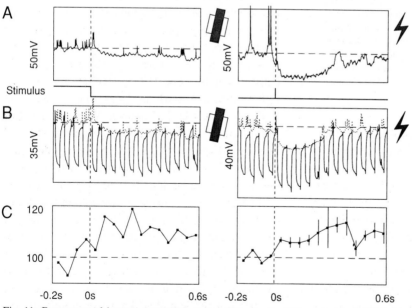

Fig. 11. Responses of layer 6 pyramidal neuron with simple (S1) receptive field to dark bar flash (left column) and electrical stimulation (bolt) of afferents from OR2 (right column). A. Intracellular membrane potential responses to flash (6 trials) and OR2 stimulation (single sweep). B. Averaged responses with hyperpolarizing constant current pulses (solid lines) to flash (6 trials) and OR2 (5 trials) stimulation. Dotted trace shows average responses without current pulses, for comparison. C. Mean percentage change in input conductance (normalized against control mean) derived from the average responses above for flash ($n = 7$) and OR2 response ($\pm$ S.E.M., $n = 5$). (From Berman et al., 1991.)

mal excitation. The regions of distinct hyperpolarization were not associated with increase in the conductance of more than 20%. The results of the moving stimulus are compatible with those of the flashed stimulus. The flashed stimulus might be expected to produce a larger change in conductance because there is a more coherent volley of excitation arriving at the cortex, and because the response evoked is more "pure". The moving bar inevitably evokes both excitation and inhibition through its leading and trailing edges.

The evidence that visually-evoked inhibition is not associated with large changes in membrane potential or input conductance, added to the case against selectivity being produced by strong inhibition. We remained concerned that we were underestimating the magnitude of the inhibition. Perhaps the intracellular recording pipette lo-

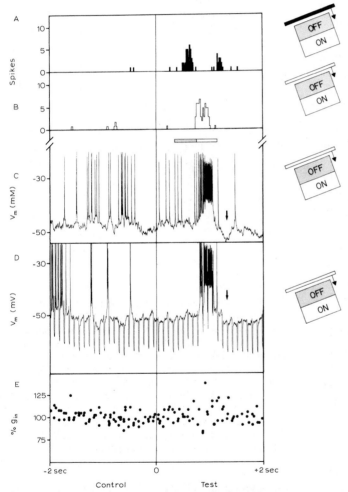

Fig. 12. Responses of layer 6 pyramidal neuron with S2 receptive field to moving bars. Neuron received monosynaptic activation from LGN. Same protocol as Fig. 1. A and B. Extracellularly recorded action potential discharge evoked by light and dark bars in most preferred direction and orientation. C. Intracellular recording of membrane potential response underlying extracellular response in B. Rapid discharge is followed by a hyperpolarization (arrow). D. Membrane potential response to visual stimulus with injection of current pulses ($-0.1$ nA, 30 ms, 10 Hz). E. Input conductances (normalised against control mean) derived from 3 trials similar to D. There is no large and sustained change in the conductance of the neuron anywhere in the response. (Bar width, 0.3°; length, 13.1°; velocity, 3.3°/sec). (See Douglas et al., 1988; Berman et al., 1991.)

458

cated in the soma was unable to detect conductance changes occurring out on the dendrites. We needed to secure quantitative estimates of two central issues: firstly, how visible are inhibitory conductances and, secondly, how large do they need to be to sink the excitatory currents? The quickest way of answering these questions seemed to be to do the calculations.

## Visibility of synaptic conductances

We derived theoretical expressions for the change in input conductance produced by synapses, which could be positioned at any location on a passive dendritic tree (Koch et al., 1990). For the case of an idealized neuron with an infinite dendritic cylinder, the analysis demonstrated that the change in conductance produced by a single synapse decays exponentially with the distance of the synapse from the recording site. As we might expect, the visibility of a conductance change was highly dependent on the relative location of the active synapses and the recording pipette. The visibility of the conductance change decayed more rapidly with distance in neurons with long thin dendrites (e.g., beta-type retinal ganglion cells) than in those with shorter thicker dendrites (e.g., pyramidal neurons). Fortunately, the visibility did not depend on the synaptic reversal potential, so that conductance changes that were hyperpolarizing, depolarizing or shunting, were all equally visible. The changes in the somatic input conductance produced by multiple synaptic activation were always less than the sum of the conductance changes produced by individual synapses acting on their own. This was a case of more giving less due to the non-linear interactions between the multiple conductance inputs. Finally, we found that the absolute change in the somatic input conductance was independent of the leak produced by damage to the somatic membrane by the recording pipette.

We then used our anatomical data to simulate the effects of activating basket cell synapses made at known locations on the dendritic trees of ac-

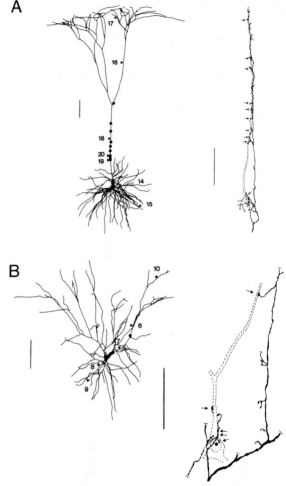

Fig. 13. Location of inhibitory inputs on pyramidal cells used in simulations of conductance visibility. A. Computer plot of a reconstructed layer 5 pyramidal cell (left) showing siting of inhibitory inputs (filled circles) and excitatory inputs on spines (numbers 15–20). Locations of inhibitory sites were based on the synaptic contacts (arrows, right) formed by an HRP-filled GABAergic basket cell axon on a layer 5 pyramidal cell. B. Reconstruction of an HRP-filled layer 2 pyramidal cell (left) and siting of inhibitory (circles) and excitatory (numbers 6–10) inputs. Inhibitory site location based on identified basket cell input to a similar cell (right, arrows) in layer 2/3. Scale bars: 100 μm in A; 50 μm in B. (See Koch et al., 1990.)

tual pyramidal cells (Fig. 13). We selected examples of the largest (from layer 5) and smallest (from layer 2) pyramidal cells from our catalogue of physiologically-characterized and morphologically-identified neurons. For these simulations we did not reduce the detailed 3-dimensional reconstruction of the dendritic tree to the simplified compartmental model (see Fig. 2). The specific locations of basket cell synapses made on such pyramidal cells were obtained from our catalogue of neurons (Somogyi et al., 1983; Kisvárday et al., 1987). The basket cell synapses were assumed to act by either $GABA_A$ (chloride-mediated, shunting) or both $GABA_A$ and $GABA_B$ (potassium-mediated, hyperpolarizing) synapses.

Various combinations of excitatory and inhibitory interactions were simulated. In all the various conditions, the inhibitory synapses had to increase the input conductance of the neuron by at least 100% to reduce the excitatory current by 50%. To achieve complete inhibition of moderate excitation required very much larger increases in conductance: up to 1600% in one example. In most cases, over 80% of the total inhibitory conductance would be visible to a recording pipette located in the soma. This is perhaps not surprising, given that the basket cell synapses are located on the proximal dendrites and soma. Of the reduction in visibility that occurs, most is due to proximal $GABA_A$ conductances shunting the inhibitory synapses that are located more distally on the dendritic tree.

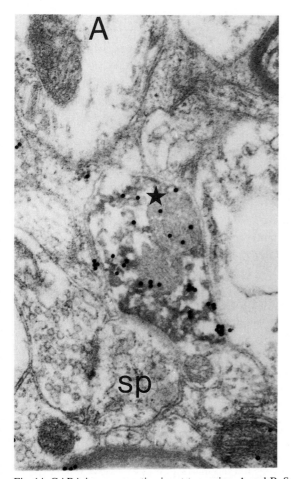
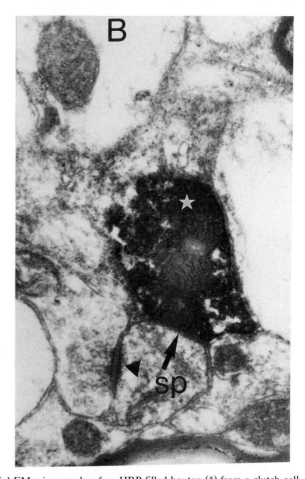

Fig. 14. GABA-immunoreactive input to a spine. A and B. Serial EM micrographs of an HRP-filled bouton (*) from a clutch cell that formed a type 2 synapse (inhibitory) on a spine (sp). The same spine also receives a type 1 synapse (presumably excitatory) from another bouton. The HRP-filled bouton (*) was shown to be GABA-positive in the adjacent section in A, by GABA-immunoreactive labelling. Scale bar: 0.5 $\mu$m. (modified from Somogyi and Soltész, 1986.)

460

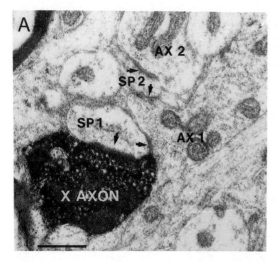

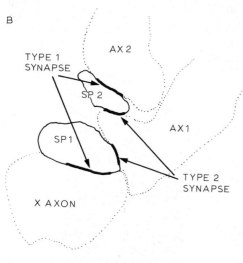

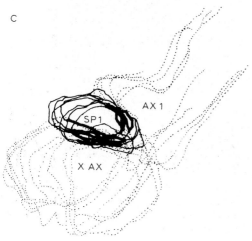

## Synaptic "veto" on dendritic spines

One further issue needs consideration, and that is whether significant inhibition occurs at the level of the spine. The notion of an inhibitory veto operating on the dendritic spines has been mooted repeatedly (Diamond et al., 1970; Jack et al., 1975; Torre and Poggio, 1978; Koch and Poggio, 1985). Spines are the site of most of the excitatory input to cortical spiny neurons (Garey and Powell, 1971; Szentágothai, 1973), and thus a shunting inhibitory synapse located on a particular spine would provide a means of selectively inhibiting the excitatory input to that spine. Spines are distanced electrotonically from the soma by the intervening impedance properties of the dendritic shaft, and the spine neck, which is thought to have a high axial resistance. Thus, the conductance changes wrought by the action of synapses on the spine head would be masked from our recording pipette, whose tip is generally impaled in the soma or proximal dendrites.

It is impossible to test the hypothesis that a selective inhibitory veto acts at the level of a spine using contemporary electrophysiological techniques. However, we could do the next-best thing, which was to see whether the necessary circuitry exists (Dehay et al., 1991). There is clear evidence that spines do receive synapses from GABAergic boutons (see Fig. 14) (e.g., Somogyi and Soltész, 1986). We also know the source of many of these GABAergic synapses: the large and small (clutch) basket cells both provide be-

Fig. 15. Dual input to a thalamorecipient dendritic spine. A. EM micrograph showing a spine head (sp1) receiving asymmetric (type 1) input from an identified HRP-filled thalamic X-axon, and symmetric (type 2) from an unidentified axon (AX 1). B. Computer plot of profiles show in A. A nearby spine head (SP 2) also receives both type 1 and type 2 input. C. Wire frame montage of several sections through the structures contacting spine 1 in A, showing the extent of the dual inputs. Scale bar 0.5 mm. (See Dehay et al., 1991.)

tween 20–40% of their output to spines (Somogyi et al, 1983; Kisvárday et al., 1986; Somogyi and Soltész, 1986). The double bouquet cell also provides input to spines (Somogyi and Cowey, 1981). Only about 7% of spines receive a synapse from a GABAergic bouton in addition to the excitatory synapse (Beaulieu and Colonnier, 1985; Dehay et al., 1991). In layer 4 it seems most likely that the excitatory input needs to inhibited at the earliest stage possible. This means that the excitation provided by the thalamic afferents themselves has to be inhibited, because it is out of their non-oriented, non-directional receptive fields that the selective cortical fields are built. It seems possible that the inhibitory synapses were targeting the spines that received an excitatory synapse from a thalamocortical bouton. We examined this possibility using a combined physiological and anatomical method (Dehay et al., 1991).

We recorded from single axons as they coursed through the optic radiations, and identified them physiologically as arising from either X- or Y-type relay cells in the lateral geniculate nucleus of the thalamus. The axons were then injected intra-axonally with horseradish peroxidase, which fills the entire axonal arbour. Using the electron microscope we were then able to identify spines that received excitatory synapses from the horseradish peroxidase labelled boutons (Fig. 15A). Most spines received only a single synaptic input. Occasionally the spine received a second synapse, whose morphology identified it as originating from a smooth GABAergic interneuron (Fig. 15). When the results were totted-up from a total of 76 boutons examined from 4 axons, we found that less than 7% of the spines that made synapses with thalamic afferent boutons received a second synapse (Dehay et al., 1991). For the vast majority of thalamocortical synapses on spines, the excitatory current they provide flows unscathed by shunting inhibition to the parent dendritic shaft. Even for spines that receive a GABAergic synaptic input, there is some doubt as to the selectivity of the inhibition. In some instances we were able to trace the axon making the synapse on the spine

and show that it made an additional synapse on the parent dendritic shaft. These observations provide a clear and quantitative answer to the issue of whether a synaptic veto mechanism was located at the level of the dendritic spine and could be used to gate effectively the primary source of excitation to visual cortex. We cannot explain away our experimental failure to find large inhibitory conductances by supposing they are located on electrotonically distant spine heads. Nelson (1991) has suggested that the thalamocortical synapse may be subject to presynaptic inhibition. This convenient explanation of our physiological result is ruled out by our morphological observation that none of the thalamic afferent boutons received a synaptic input, as would be required for presynaptic inhibition.

We seem to have returned to the place where we first began: faced with the problem of understanding what GABAergic inhibition is doing in the cortex. However, we are wiser for the exercise we have summarised above. Through experiment and simulation we have been able to define some of the limits of the behaviour when excitatory and inhibitory synapses interact. Our failure to find significant increases in conductance during non-optimal stimulation cannot be explained by an inherent inability of our technique to detect such conductance changes if they are occurring: it would be impossible, even for physiologists of limited competence, to miss conductance changes of the magnitude required (Koch et al., 1990). The anatomical investigation confirmed that there is no special synaptic organization that might prevent inhibition being visible to normal recording methods. Taken together, the theory and experiment imply that synaptically-mediated inhibition cannot play the dominant role that has traditionally been assigned to it. Instead, the excitatory gain of the cortex appears to be controlled by a relatively weak inhibition. To make further progress on this problem we scrambled out of the thickets of synaptic interactions and headed for higher ground. What we needed was a wider view of the operation of local circuits in the cortex.

## Solutions through cortical microcircuits

From time to time, neurophysiologists and neuroanatomists have suggested that the circuitry of the neocortex is highly conserved, with the same basic "bauplan" being used in all cortical areas (Szentágothai, 1975; Creutzfeldt, 1977; Powell, 1981). Amongst physiologists, Hubel and Wiesel (1977) found evidence for repeated functional units in the primary visual cortex, which they named "hypercolumns". They introduced the notion of the functional uniformity of striate cortex and suggested that the reason for this might be that cortical area 17 consists of a series of stereotyped machines, repeated over and over (Hubel and Wiesel, 1974). Their idea that area 17 has a crystal-like structure has not been explored in depth by physiologists or neuroanatomists, and certainly no-one has gone much beyond speculating that the concept might be extended to include the entire neocortex.

Neuroanatomists, to be sure, have provided a great deal of information about the types of neurons that are found in neocortex, and their relative numbers (Lorente de Nó, 1949; Scholl, 1956; Rockel et al., 1980; Jones, 1984; Gabbott and Somogyi, 1986; Peters, 1987). It has largely been left to physiologists to assemble these components into functional circuits. But, their circuits have been configured for particular functions. For example, the layer 6 pyramidal neurons send a local collateral projection to the middle layers of the cortex. Wiesel and Gilbert (1983) and Bolz and Gilbert (1986) used this anatomical information to show how the specific property of end-inhibition might be achieved by this circuit. However effective their explanation is for the visual cortex, and it is controversial (Murphy and Sillito, 1987; see Martin, 1988, Somogyi, 1989), it sheds no light on what the equivalent projection might be doing in all the other cortical areas.

The natural question arises as to why we should not be content with explaining the role of a stereotyped connection in terms of a specific function. It is self-evidently difficult enough to tease out a single function for any of the intracortical circuits even in well-worked areas like the visual cortex. Our saga with GABA-mediated inhibition showed that we might be in danger of becoming too focused on GABA-mediated inhibition alone. Unless we deliberately took a wider look, with GABA-mediated inhibition forming a part rather than the whole of the picture, we might miss out on understanding basic principles of cortical operation. Hence our present endeavour to find a more general solution to the problem of cortical function, rather than simply to explain the orientation or direction selectivity of neurons in the visual cortex. The task we set ourselves was to develop a "canonical" microcircuit for neocortex (Douglas et al., 1989; Douglas and Martin, 1991a,b). "Canonical" is meant in the mathematical sense of simplest, or clearest form of microcircuit. The general properties that emerge from the abstract circuit we have developed, have provided novel insights into the possible mechanisms underlying the response selectivity of neurons in the visual cortex and the role of GABA-mediated inhibition in particular.

Ten years ago it was not possible to envisage such a project. There were still too many unknowns. Now the situation is very different. A compendium of new techniques has produced a veritable flood of information about the nuts and bolts of neocortex. In particular, methods that enabled the anatomical identification of neurons that had been studied physiologically meant that, for the first time ever, a direct bridge could be built between the microstructural studies and the physiological studies of single neurons. Another major tool is the computer, whose value we have demonstrated here for the analysis of interneuronal interactions. In the development of the canonical microcircuit the computer simulations were especially invaluable for exploring facets of the function of the circuitry that could not be studied experimentally.

The starting point for the microcircuit was the biology. The first step was to decide on the components to be included in our preliminary sketch of the cortical circuits. For this, we could draw on an extensive database of neurons whose receptive fields were mapped, whose afferent connections were studied using electrical stimulation, and whose morphology was identified by intracellular filling with horseradish peroxidase (Martin and Whitteridge, 1984). The major additional advantage of filling the neuron with horseradish peroxidase is that the intracortical collaterals of the axon can be completely labelled. This is not true with any other method, including the invaluable Golgi-staining technique. Thus the three-dimensional reconstructions of the dendritic arbours allowed us to derive the "simplified" neurons that were used here and in the theoretical analysis of inhibition described above. The detailed reconstructions of the axonal arbours of these neurons allowed us to produce an accurate picture of the stereotyped interlaminar connections of the various types of neurons in the different

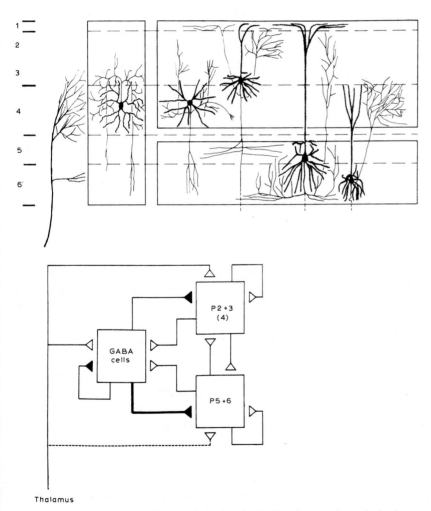

Fig. 16. Cortical circuitry and the canonical microcircuit. Top diagram shows the basic neuronal types in cortex, their typical axonal arborizations and the laminar boundaries. The cell types grouped in the 3 boxes are represented below in their respective positions in the canonical circuit. Superficial (P2 + 3(4)) and deep (P5 + 6) pyramidal cells are interconnected with a single pool of GABA cells. Heavy solid line indicates stronger inhibitory input, and dashed line indicates weaker thalamic input, to deep cells. (See Douglas et al., 1989; Douglas and Martin, 1991a,b.)

cortical layers (Martin and Whitteridge, 1984). These connections, and their reduction to the canonical form, are shown in Fig. 16. We are obviously aware that there are many varieties of smooth, GABAergic neurons, but in the light of our theoretical analysis of axoaxonic and basket cell inhibition, we are as yet unable to offer any compelling argument for differentiating them into functional subgroups. To avoid unnecessary overcomplication we have used a basket cell that makes connections to superficial and deep cortical layers as the generic functional representative of the population of GABAergic neurons.

Ultrastructural studies of the synaptic connections made by identified neurons provide the statistics of the basic connections between the different components of the neocortex (see Martin, 1984, 1988). These studies show that spiny cells receive about 85% of the synapses made by any cell type in the cortex. Since 70% of the cortical neurons are pyramidal, this means that pyramidal neurons are the focus of connectivity. Even in layer 4, the main thalamorecipient zone, we found a surprising number of "star" pyramidal neurons (Martin and Whitteridge, 1984). The spiny stellate neurons, which are found only in layer 4, probably form less than 10% of neurons even in the granular cortical areas, such as visual cortex. Their percentage falls even lower in the agranular areas such as somatomotor cortex, where layer 4 is virtually absent and layer 3 becomes the main thalamorecipient zone (see Jones, 1984). The traditional view of layer 4, and the spiny stellate cells in particular, as unique recipients of thalamic input is quite incorrect. Both physiological studies (Hoffman and Stone, 1971; Bullier and Henry, 1979; Ferster and Lindström, 1983; Martin and Whitteridge, 1984) as well as detailed anatomical studies (Freund et al., 1985a,b; see White, 1989) show that neurons in every lamina receive direct thalamocortical input.

Our electrophysiological studies (Martin and Whitteridge, 1984; Douglas et al., 1989) provided estimates of the conduction times and synaptic delays, which were incorporated into the simula-tions. What we have not yet been able to establish is how the weighting of the thalamic input varies for the different target neurons. Layer 5 pyramidal cells, whose apical dendrite pass unbranched through layer 4, probably receive fewer thalamocortical synapses than neurons that have a large fraction of their dendritic arbour in layer 4 (see White, 1989). It should be noted that even in layer 4 of visual cortex, the thalamic afferents contribute only 5–30% of the synapses (Garey and Powell, 1971; LeVay and Gilbert, 1976). The majority of excitatory synapses, even in layer 4, come mainly from the intracortical collaterals of spiny cells.

In the absence of sufficient information concerning the distribution and conductances of the NMDA receptor in the visual cortex, we assumed only an AMPA-like receptor for the excitatory synapses. In our simulations the thalamocortical afferents provided 10–20% of the total excitatory conductance of spiny cells of the superficial layers (including layer 4), and 1–10% for the deep layer pyramids. As for the superficial layer spiny cells, the thalamocortical afferents supplied 10–20% of their total excitatory conductance. The remainder of the excitatory conductance comes from the intracortical collaterals of the spiny neurons. We arranged that spiny cells in layer 2 + 3 + 4 received half their intracortical excitation from spiny neurons in layer 2 + 3 and half from neurons in layer 5 + 6. A similar arrangement applied to the pyramids of layers 5 + 6. We did not assume that all neurons receive the same pattern of inputs. If we open up the boxes (Fig. 17) we find various patterns of connectivity of the components, e.g., some receive direct thalamocortical input, some none. For the purposes of the simulation it was convenient to consider the activity of the "average" neuron, which had the "average" connectivity. In the comparisons given below we compare the response of individual neurons recorded in vivo, and the average simulated response of the superficial or deep layer pyramidal cell populations.

All the pyramidal neurons appear to have both

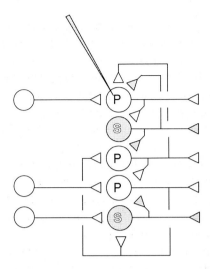

Thalamus          Cortex

Fig. 17. Principles of connectivity between the different neurons in the microcircuit. Excitatory (open triangles) input from thalamus innervates some of the pyramidal cells (P) and smooth cells (S) in cortex. They in turn are interconnected with excitatory (open triangles) and inhibitory (shaded triangles) synapses. The performance of the circuit is monitored by "recording" the averaged response of one group of neurons.

GABA$_A$ and GABA$_B$ receptors (Connors et al., 1988; Douglas et al., 1989), and these were incorporated into the canonical microcircuit. In terms of the function of the GABA conductances, the microcircuit we constructed required one important assumption for which we have only a physiological justification. When we recorded from identified pyramidal neurons in the superficial and deep layers we found what so many before us had found, the standard receptive field types described originally by Hubel and Wiesel (1962). However, there was one clear and robust difference between superficial and deep layer pyramidal neurons that was independent of receptive field type (Douglas et al., 1989; Douglas and Martin, 1991a,b). When the cortex is activated by a brief electrical pulse stimulus to the white matter, an action potential is generated simultaneously in a large number of thalamocortical afferents. The arrival of this synchronous volley of action potentials in the cortical grey matter evokes in every neuron the well-described sequence of

an EPSP followed by an IPSP (Fig. 18A). The difference we found was that in the deep layer pyramidal cells, the latency from stimulus onset to maximum hyperpolarization was consistently much shorter than for the superficial layer cells (Fig. 18B). It appeared functionally as if the GABA$_A$-mediated inhibition was stronger for pyramidal cells in the deep layers. This aspect was incorporated in our simulation by making the GABA$_A$ inhibition twice as strong for the deep layer compared to the superficial layer pyramidal neurons. A structural explanation for this difference has yet to be found.

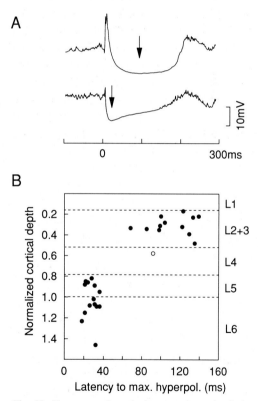

Fig. 18. Response of cortical neurons to stimulation of the optic radiation. A. Averaged intracellular response of typical superficial (top trace, layer 2/3) and deep (bottom trace, layer 5/6) neurons. Arrows indicate the position of maximum hyperpolarization. B. Relationship between cortical depth (layer on right) and latency to maximum hyperpolarization for 26 identified pyramidal (filled circles) and one spiny stellate cell (open circle). (See Douglas and Martin, 1989, 1991a,b.)

## Validation of the canonical microcircuit

The simplest way of comparing the performance of the microcircuit to that of the visual cortex was to simulate the electrical pulse stimulus applied to the thalamic afferents. This avoided all the complications and computational overload of simulating a visual stimulus. The pulse stimulus could also be used in combination with the pharmacological tools that now exist for manipulating the GABA receptors. By blocking or activating components of the GABA receptors in actual cortical neurons in vivo, and stimulating the afferents with an electrical pulse, we could see whether the canonical microcircuit would predict similar behaviour. In the event the microcircuit predicted the in vivo results with remarkable accuracy. For example, iontophoresing the $GABA_A$ antagonist $N$-m-bicuculline onto the neuron appeared to eliminate the early portion of the IPSP, allowing more excitation to predominate (Fig. 19A). In the deep layer pyramidal cell population, this had the effect of producing a response that resembled that of the superficial layer pyramidal cells. The

latter part of the IPSP appeared to be insensitive to bicuculline application, even after 5–10 min of iontophoresis. The rapidly developing and short-duration component of the IPSP is probably due to the bicuculline-sensitive $GABA_A$ receptors, while the slower-developing and longer-lasting component is probably due to the bicuculline-insensitive $GABA_B$ receptors, as has been found in vitro (Connors et al., 1988). Clearly, in our in vivo recording, both the $GABA_A$ and the $GABA_B$ responses are hyperpolarizing. In in vitro recording the reversal potential of the $GABA_A$ synapse is nearer the resting membrane potential.

In our experiments, the tip of the multibarrel pipette containing the drugs was only 20–30 $\mu$m from the tip of the intracellular pipette. The localized effect of $N$-m-bicuculline iontophoresis was simulated by modifying the effect of the $GABA_A$ conductances in a subset of pyramidal and smooth neurons in the appropriate layers. In this subset the $GABA_A$ component of the inhibitory conductance was reduced to 20% of its original value. The simulations show that the modelled responses reflect quite accurately the

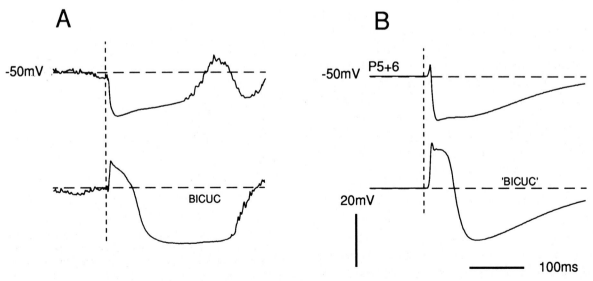

Fig. 19. Comparison of neuron and canonical model response to afferent stimulation and the effect of bicuculline. A. Normal response of a deep layer neuron (top trace) to afferent stimulation (vertical dashed line in all figures) and during iontophoresis of bicuculline (BICUC, bottom trace). B. Response of a deep neuron in the model representing the average response to afferent stimulation (top). Simulation of blockade of $GABA_A$ "receptors" ("BICUC") (bottom). (See Douglas and Martin, 1991a)

response obtained in the actual neurons (Fig. 19B). The effect of GABA, or GABA in combination with *N*-m-bicuculline was also examined (Fig. 20). In the in vivo recordings, application of GABA produced a hyperpolarization of the membrane. The absolute size of the IPSPs decreased, presumably because the resting potential had moved closer to the GABA reversal potential (Fig. 20A). When *N*-m-bicuculline was added to the GABA iontophoresis, the membrane hyperpolarized further and the amplitude and duration of the EPSP increased. We interpret the latter as the release from $GABA_A$ inhibition, and the former as evidence for different reversal potentials of the $GABA_A$ and the $GABA_B$ receptor (Connors et al., 1988; Douglas and Martin, 1990a). The $GABA_B$ response is thought to be mediated

by potassium, which has a reversal potential of about $-90$ mV, whereas the $GABA_A$ response is thought to be mediated by chloride, which has a membrane reversal potential of about $-70$ mV (for review, see Douglas and Martin, 1990a). Thus, when the chloride-mediated response is blocked by bicuculline, the membrane moves towards the still-active $GABA_B$ reversal potential. The responses to GABA in the microcircuit were simulated by activating 50% of the $GABA_A$ and the $GABA_B$ conductances (Fig 20B). *N*-m-Bicuculline effects were modelled as described above. The simulated responses provided as remarkable agreement with the experimental data.

A final test was to use baclofen to activate the $GABA_B$ receptors (Fig. 21). When baclofen was iontophoresed onto neurons, the membrane hy-

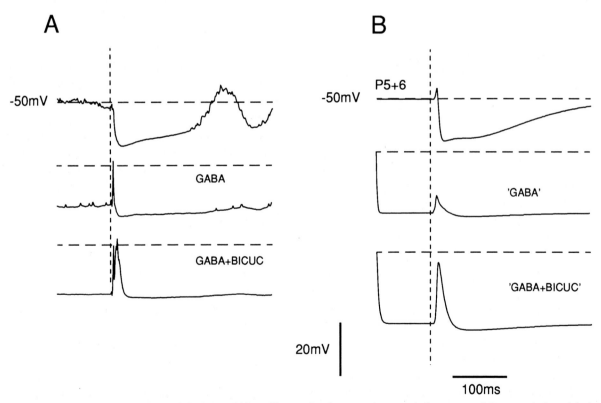

Fig. 20. Comparison of the effects of GABA and bicuculline application on a deep cortical neuron and the canonical model. A. Normal response of deep layer neuron (top), response during GABA iontophoresis (middle) and with additional iontophoresis of bicuculline (bottom). B. Response of a deep layer neuron in the canonical model (top). Simulation of GABA application (middle) and additional bicuculline application (bottom). (See Douglas and Martin, 1991a.)

468

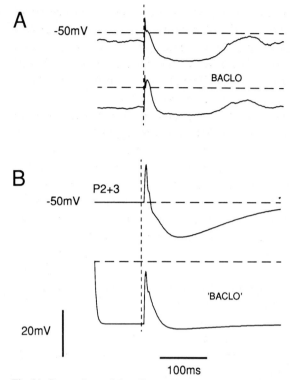

A
-50mV

BACLO

B

P2+3
-50mV

'BACLO'

20mV

100ms

Fig. 21. Comparison of the effects of baclofen application on a cortical neuron and the canonical model. A. Typical response of layer 2 neuron to afferent stimulation (top) and during iontophoresis of baclofen (bottom). B. Response of a superficial neuron in the canonical model (top) and response during simulation of baclofen application (bottom). (see Douglas and Martin, 1991a.)

perpolarized and the late component of the IPSP flattened. This effect was simulated by activating 50% of the $GABA_B$ conductances in the test neurons of the microcircuit. The response of the model neuron differed from the actual neurons only in that activation of the $GABA_B$ receptors appeared to be more effective in the simulation. In other respects the response of the microcircuit to the simulated action of baclofen agreed well with that of the experimental data.

These results show, inter alia, that the dynamics of the $GABA_B$ inhibition are quite different from that of $GABA_A$. The $GABA_B$, acting as it does through a second messenger system, has a response that is governed by time-constants that are an order of magnitude greater than those of

the $GABA_A$ response. Consequently, the $GABA_B$ mechanism behaves like a leaky integrator. With continued inhibitory stimulation, the inhibitory effect accumulates, gradually hyperpolarizing the membrane over hundreds of milliseconds, so increasing the current threshold for action potential generation. In this context, $GABA_B$ inhibition can be viewed as an adaptive process that acts via an inhibitory interneuron. The adaptive modification of the threshold depends both on the activity of the neuron being inhibited, and on the averaged activity within the population of neurons in which it is embedded. This latter aspect means that the response of a particular neuron can be referenced against the average activity of the population. The $GABA_B$ system might therefore be involved in adaptive processes, such as contrast gain control (Ohzawa et al., 1986). Indeed, the work of DeBruyn and Bonds (1986) suggests that the $GABA_A$ receptors are not involved in contrast gain control. The selective responses of neurons are generally thought to be exclusively mediated by the $GABA_A$ system (Baumfalk and Albus, 1987, 1988), but in the canonical microcircuit the $GABA_B$ system is inextricably involved in the structuring of receptive fields. This may explain why blocking $GABA_A$ does not always eliminate the selectivity of the neuron for the orientation or direction of the stimulus (e.g., Sillito, 1977; Nelson, 1991).

**Canonical criticisms**

The similarity of the model responses to the experimental data gave further confidence in the values of the parameters we had used for the model. Sceptics might put forward the proposition that with so many parameters to tweak it would be inept indeed not to have achieved such a close correspondence between experiment and theory. It is the nature of complex systems that they are under-determined by data. We have attempted to constrain as many parameters as possible by reference to biological data. Another line of criticism would say that the microcircuit is obviously too simple, it lacks NMDA receptors, it does not differentiate between the different GABAergic neurons, it takes no account of the corticothalamic projection, or any of the many other projections to cortex that are known to exist. Of these deficiencies we are well aware, since these aspects were deliberately not included. Nevertheless, it is difficult for us to see the microcircuit as an oversimplification. Instead we view it as an example of our "minimalist" approach, a necessary use of Occam's razor to shave the number of variables to a minimum.

Our "minimalist" approach is an alternative to the "rococo" approach used by others to explain the selectivity of cortical neurons. Adherents of the rococo approach include everything (kitchen sink excepted) in their models (e.g., Wehmeier et al., 1989; Wörgötter and Koch, 1991). In contrast, we are not offering a comprehensive description of the cortical microcircuits. Rather, the canonical microcircuit is the minimum set of necessary connections from which more complex patterns of interconnections can be elaborated. In deriving the microcircuit we have made the fewest possible assumptions about the circuitry and the synaptic functions, while keeping our hypothetical circuit closely matched to the quality of the actual anatomical and physiological data from which it was derived.

In support of our approach there are several further points worth considering. One is that over 100 years of study of the cortical machinery has not produced a consensus as to what the cortical microcircuits are, or even how many of them there are. We offer a microcircuit that seems to represent the average connectivity and physiology of a patch of cortex. We do not claim that the connectivity of cortex is homogeneous. Indeed our own results from reconstructed neurons (see Martin and Whitteridge, 1984; Martin, 1988) show that it is not. The claim is simply that over the temporal scale of the electrical pulse response, the cortex behaves as if it had a rather simple connectivity. We anticipate that such canonical microcircuits are elaborated to perform many dif-

ferent functions in the different cortical areas. Our view contrasts with the view of neocortex as a collection of ad hoc specialist circuits, with different circuit designs for the different cortical areas, each surviving by evolutionary opportunism and designed to perform a special function like form or motion analysis. By suggesting the form of a canonical microcircuit we have at least provided a clear target by which alternatives can be judged, so that through this process we may arrive at some consensus as to what the form of the cortical microcircuits actually are.

### Demonstration of the competence of the microcircuit

In describing the testing of the canonical microcircuit we concentrated on the effects the GABA agonists and antagonists had on the IPSP. Indeed, the pulse response is so dominated by the substantial and long-lasting hyperpolarizing IPSP, that it is not difficult to miss the brief and relatively small EPSP that precedes the IPSP. However, in many ways, it is the excitatory response that is most critical. The most notable facet of the circuit is that the thalamic neurons only provide a small (10–20%) component of the cortical excitation (Douglas et al., 1989; Douglas and Martin, 1991a,b). The major drive to cortical neurons is from other cortical neurons. What we need most to understand is how this excitation is controlled by the GABA-mediated inhibition.

We have approached this problem in several ways, using both experimental and theoretical approaches. The clearest understanding is perhaps provided by returning to the example of direction selectivity. In our consideration of the conventional models for directionality, we provided evidence from both experiments and theory that these models could not account for the response seen. In particular, the magnitude of the inhibition was not large enough to quench the strong excitatory response evoked by stimuli moving in the optimal direction. This problem is pointed up by a glance at the schematic circuit

(Fig. 16), which shows that positive, excitatory feedback is everywhere in evidence. But, it is the rich interconnections between the excitatory populations that are at the heart of our solution to the problems of deriving the selective responses of cortical neurons.

The paradoxical absence of strong inhibition in our in vivo data may be explained if we reconsider the traditional role of the thalamic afferent excitation. In all other models, the thalamic afferents provide the major drive to simple cells, and perhaps some complex cells as well (Hubel and Wiesel, 1962; Heggelund, 1981b). In the canonical microcircuit, the thalamic afferents serve only to provide a primary source signal that is strongly amplified by the recurrent collaterals of the pyramidal cells. This provides the key to reconciling the apparently weak inhibition with the control of strong excitation. The simple explanation that emerges is that if the relatively weak excitatory input from the thalamic afferents is inhibited, then the pathways available for cortical re-excitation will not be engaged, or only weakly so. Rapid activation of inhibitory neurons by the thalamic afferents can shape the cortical response by controlling access to the cortical amplifier. If no inhibition is present, the weak geniculate excitation will be amplified by the local excitatory circuitry, which will eventually produce the strong excitation associated with optimal stimulation. The prime advantage of this process is that the inhibition need only control a small component of the excitation, not the full-blown response.

**Selectivity explained**

To demonstrate how stimulus-selectivity might be generated by this mechanism, we have taken the example of a direction-selective neuron that is monosynaptically excited by the non-directional thalamic neurons (Douglas and Martin, 1991a,b). This is the most difficult example to account for in terms of conventional models, since the thalamic excitation is identical for both directions of motion, only the timing of the inputs is different.

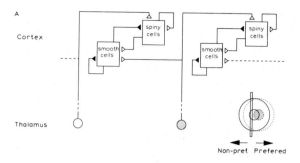

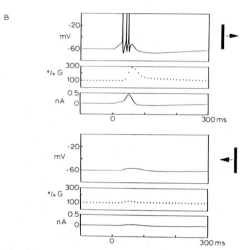

Fig. 22. Simulation of directionality with the canonical microcircuit. A. Two identical modules of the canonical microcircuit are linked to simulate directionality. For simplicity, only neurons in layer 4 were simulated. The two modules received thalamic input from "cells" with displaced receptive fields (shaded and unshaded field). B. Directional responses of the model. Top three windows: Response of an average "neuron" to preferred direction; membrane potential (top), input conductance changes (middle) and total current arriving at the soma (bottom). Bottom three windows: Response of an average "neuron" to non-preferred direction. Membrane potential (top), associated conductance increase (middle), and total current (bottom) arriving at the soma. (See Douglas and Martin, 1991a.)

To simulate this we have linked together two modules, each containing the identical canonical microcircuit (Fig. 22A). To simplify the calculations we considered only the neurons within layer 4, but the same principles apply to the whole microcircuit. To achieve the bias necessary for direction-selectivity we arranged that the smooth inhibitory neurons were excited by thalamic afferents whose receptive fields were slightly displaced from those of the afferents supplying the spiny neurons in the same module. Obviously, this is not the only manner in which a bias could be built into the circuit, but it is simple and consistent with the non-uniform distribution of the synaptic boutons of single thalamic afferent arbours (Gilbert and Wiesel, 1983; Freund et al., 1985a; Humphrey et al., 1985).

It is evident from the circuit that when the stimulus is moved in the preferred direction, the spiny neurons will be excited slightly ahead of the smooth neurons in the same module. Inhibition is then too late to prevent intracortical re-excitation, resulting in a strong response. In the non-preferred direction the smooth neurons will be excited slightly in advance of the spiny neurons they inhibit. Now the smooth neurons are able to inhibit the primary excitation provided by the thalamus, and so prevent the cortical amplification circuits from being engaged. The simplified neurons used for the simulations had biophysical properties that were, in the required respects, indistinguishable from the actual reconstructed neurons from which they were derived. We were therefore able to make precise measurements of the magnitude of the various currents and conductances during the different stimulus conditions. The net synaptic currents that arrive at the axon hillock, and the normalized conductance changes associated with these currents are shown in Fig. 22B. In the preferred direction of motion the net synaptic current is initially inward and leads to a depolarization and action potential discharge. After the discharge, the net current is outward and leads to a post-discharge hyperpolarization similar to that seen in actual neurons (Berman et al., 1991; Douglas and Martin, 1991a). This outward current is due to the extended time-course of the $GABA_B$ response. The high conductance changes associated with the response are mainly due to the excitatory currents. In actual neurons some of the conductance change at the spine head would be masked from the soma recording site by the impedance of the spine neck and dendritic shaft. In the non-pre-

ferred direction the net synaptic current is small and produces a depolarization of 4 mV. The conductance change is mainly due to the activity of the inhibitory synapses. In this case it is an increase of about 20% above control, which is near the lower limit of what we were able to measure experimentally in vivo. Thus the model provides a resolution to the paradox of the absence of strong inhibition.

The concept we have introduced here, of inhibition acting against a small primary excitation, not the full-blown secondary excitation, provides elucidation of a number of morphological observations we have made during our studies of the cortical microcircuitry. From the design of the canonical microcircuit it follows that the spiny cells operate in tandem with the smooth cells in the same module. Thus the smooth cells will produce the strongest recurrent inhibition when the spiny cells they inhibit are driven optimally. Conversely, non-optimal stimulation, which provides weak re-excitation, will drive the smooth cells weakly. This means that the smooth cells and the spiny cells they inhibit can co-exist in the same cortical column and have the same stimulus selectivity. This explains the physiological observation of simple cell responses, where the strongest inhibition is seen with the optimal stimuli (Bishop et al., 1973; Ferster, 1986; Douglas et al., 1991). Most models predict that a lack of response is due to strong inhibition (e.g., Sillito, 1984), while a strong response is taken to mean that inhibition is absent (e.g., Ferster, 1987). Because the canonical microcircuit functions in the opposite manner, it alone can explain the otherwise puzzling observation that smooth neurons provide their strongest innervation to their own cortical columns (Freund et al., 1983; Kisvárday et al., 1985a,b).

The necessity for the primary excitation to be inhibited effectively during non-optimal stimulation, also provides an explanation for the innervation of smooth neurons by thalamic afferents. In our study of X and Y-type afferents, we found that the only neurons that received direct synaptic input onto their somata were the GABAergic neurons (Freund et al., 1985b). We also noted that the collateral branches of the afferents that formed these somatic synapses were myelinated up to the bouton. The morphological picture suggested that thalamic excitation of the smooth neurons has to be very secure and rapid, hence excitation is delivered by myelinated axons as close to the axon hillock as possible, by-passing the cable properties of the dendrites. From the example of directionality given here, it is clear that inhibition cannot be delayed or else the intracortical circuits will engage and amplify the small thalamic signal.

## Canonical benefits

The canonical microcircuit provides a secure and definable place for the GABA-mediated inhibitory system. Indeed, from the perspective of the canonical microcircuit, inhibition and excitation are as inseparable as white on rice. Structurally, inhibitory and excitatory neurons are richly interconnected. Functionally they operate in tandem. Changes in the bias or strength of one has immediate and profound consequences for the other. Thus, when viewed from the perspective of the canonical microcircuit, debates about whether the inhibitory system is involved in a particular response property of neurons in visual cortex, fade into history.

The insights we have gained into the GABAergic inhibitory system have come by looking at the system from both a structural and a functional viewpoint. In clarifying our intuitions, the importance of formal modelling cannot be over-emphasized. The theoretical work has provided a landscape in which the experimental results appear in sharp relief. In this landscape many of the current conceptual confusions about cortical processing appear to be due to a fixation on the single neuron. It is now clear to us that to think only in terms of single neurons is doomed to frustration. It is its context in the local circuits that determine the behaviour of the single neuron. Herein lies

perhaps the canonical microcircuit's greatest strength, for if nothing else it draws attention to the properties of circuits, not single units.

The microcircuit provides the means of linking many different pieces of experimental data and offers novel explanations of operations at subcellular, cellular and microcircuit levels. The principles of operation of the canonical microcircuit, demonstrated here for direction selectivity, can be directly applied to other cases of selectivity, such as orientation, end-inhibition, and depth tuning. In the context of the microcircuit many of the apparently contradictory experimental results concerning GABA inhibition have been reconciled. The canonical microcircuit also offers a route through to important, but little explored areas, like adaptive gain control, recurrent pathways, and analogue parallel processing. It may also serve as a basis for understanding the microcircuits in areas where pathways other than the thalamic afferents provide the "seed" excitation. It thus provides strong direction for the coherent development of unifying theories and experimental work across a broad front.

## Acknowledgments

Professor D Whitteridge, F.R.S. continued to educate, examine and entertain us. Conversations with Christof "Rococo" Koch were inspirational. John Anderson and Charmaine Nelson were liberal with their considerable skills. We thank the Wellcome Trust and the Royal Society for additional support to KACM. NJB was the Blaschko Scholar and the Herbert von Karajan Neuroscience Trust Scholar for part of the period of this research. RJD received support from the Human Frontier Science (T. Tsumoto, P.I.) and the Mellon Foundation. KACM is the Henry Head Research Fellow of the Royal Society.

## References

Barlow, H.B. (1981) Critical limiting factors in the design of the eye and visual cortex. The Ferrier Lecture. *Proc. R. Soc. (London) B*, 212: 1–34.

Barlow, H.B. and Levick, W.R. (1965) The mechanism of directionally selective units in the rabbit's retina. *J. Physiol.*, 178: 477–504.

Baumfalk, U. and Albus, K. (1987) Baclofen inhibits the spontaneous and visually evoked responses of neurons in the striate cortex of the cat. *Neurosci. Lett.*, 75: 187–192.

Baumfalk, U. and Albus, K. (1988) Phaclofen antagonizes baclofen-induced suppression of visually evoked responses in the cat's striate cortex. *Brain Res.*, 463: 398–402.

Beaulieu, C. and Colonnier, M. (1985) A laminar analysis of the number of round-asymmetrical and flat-symmetrical synapses on spines, dendritic trunks, and cell bodies in area 17 of the cat. *J. Comp. Neurol.*, 231: 180–189.

Berman, N.J., Bush, P.C. and Douglas, R.J. (1989a) Adaptation and bursting may be controlled by a single fast potassium current. *Q.J. Exp. Physiol.*, 74: 223–226.

Berman, N.J., Douglas, R.J. and Martin, K.A.C. (1989b) The conductances associated with inhibitory postsynaptic potentials are larger in visual cortical neurons in vitro than in similar neurons in intact, anaesthetized rats. *J. Physiol.*, 418: 107P.

Berman, N.J., Douglas, R.J., Martin, K.A.C. and Whitteridge, D. (1991) Mechanisms of inhibition in cat visual cortex. *J. Physiol.*, 440: 697–722.

Bishop, P.O., Coombs, J.S. and Henry, G.H. (1971). Responses to visual contours: Spatio-temporal aspects of excitation in the receptive fields of simple striate neurons. *J. Physiol.*, 219: 625–657.

Bishop, P.O., Coombs, J.S. and Henry, G.H. (1973) Receptive fields of simple cells in the cat striate cortex. *J. Physiol.*, 231: 31–60

Blomfield, S. (1974) Arithmetical operations performed by nerve cells. *Brain Res.*, 69: 115–124.

Bolz, J. and Gilbert, C.D. (1986) Generation of end-inhibition in the visual cortex via interlaminar connections. *Nature*, 320: 362–365.

Bullier, J. and Henry, G.H. (1979) Ordinal position of neurons in cat striate cortex. *J. Neurophysiol.*, 42: 1251–1263.

Bullier, J. Mustari, M.J. and Henry, G.H. (1982) Receptive-field transformations between LGN neurons and S-cells of cat striate cortex. *J. Neurophysiol.*, 47: 417–438.

Burr, D., Morrone, M.C. and Maffei, L. (1981) Intracortical inhibition prevents simple cells from responding to visual patterns. *Exp. Brain Res.*, 43: 455–458.

Colonnier, M. (1964) The tangential organization of the cortex. *J. Anat.*, 98: 327–344.

Connors, B.W. Gutnick, M.J. and Prince, D.A. (1982) Electrophysiological properties of neocortical neurons in vitro. *J. Neurophysiol.*, 48: 1302–1320.

Connors, B.W., Malenka, R.C. and Da Silva, L.R. (1988) Two inhibitory postsynaptic potentials, and $GABA_A$ and $GABA_B$ receptor-mediated responses in neocortex of rat and cat. *J. Physiol.*, 406: 443–468.

Creutzfeldt, O.D. (1977) Generality of the functional structure of the neocortex. *Naturwissenschaften*, 64: 507–517.

DeBruyn, E.J. and Bonds, A.B. (1986) Contrast adaptation in cat visual cortex is not mediated by GABA. *Brain Res.*, 383: 339–342.

Dehay, C., Douglas, R.J., Martin, K.A.C. and Nelson, C. (1991) Excitation by geniculocortical synapses is not "vetoed" at the level of dendritic spines in cat visual cortex. *J. Physiol.*, 440: 723–734.

Diamond, J., Gray, E.G. and Yasargil G.M. (1970) The function of the dendritic spine: an hypothesis. In: P. Anderson and J.K.S Jansen (Eds.), *Excitatory Synaptic Mechanisms*, Oslo: Universitets Forlaget, pp. 213–222.

Douglas, R.J. and Martin, K.A.C. (1990a) Neocortex. In: G. Shepherd, (Ed.), *Synaptic Organisation of the Brain*, New York: Oxford University Press, pp. 220–248.

Douglas, R.J. and Martin, K.A.C. (1990b) Control of neuronal output by inhibition at the axon initial segment. *Neural Computation*, 2: 283–292.

Douglas, R.J. and Martin, K.A.C. (1991a) A functional microcircuit for the visual cortex. *J. Physiol.*, 440: 735–769.

Douglas, R.J. and Martin, K.A.C. (1991b) Exploring cortical microcircuits: A combined anatomical, physiological and computational approach. In: T. McKenna, J. Davis and S. Zornetzer (Eds.), *Single Neurone Computation*, Boston: Academic Press, in press.

Douglas, R.J., Martin, K.A.C. and Whitteridge, D. (1991) An intracellular analysis of the visual responses of neurons in cat visual cortex. *J. Physiol.*, 440: 659–696.

Douglas, R.J., K.A.C. Martin, and Whitteridge, D. (1988) Selective responses of visual cortical cells do not depend on shunting inhibition. *Nature*, 332: 642–644.

Douglas, R.J., Martin, K.A.C. and Whitteridge, D. (1989) A canonical microcircuit for neocortex. *Neural Computation*, 1: 479–487.

Eccles, J.C. (1964) The Physiology of Synapses. Berlin: Springer.

Emerson, R.C. and Gerstein, G.L. (1977) Simple striate neurons in the cat. I. Comparison of responses to moving and stationary stimuli. *J. Neurophysiol.*, 40: 766–783.

Fariñas, I. and DeFelipe, J. (1990a) Patterns of synaptic input on corticocortical and corticothalamic cells in the visual cortex. I. The cell body. *J. Comp. Neurol.*, 304: 53–69.

Fariñas, I. and DeFelipe, J. (1990b) Patterns of synaptic input on corticocortical and corticothalamic cells in the visual cortex. II. The axon initial segment. *J. Comp. Neurol.*, 304: 70–77.

Ferster, D. (1986) Orientation selectivity of synaptic potentials in neurons of cat primary visual cortex. *J. Neurosci.*, 6: 1284–1301.

Ferster, D. (1987) Origin of orientation-selective EPSPs in simple cells of cat visual cortex. *J. Neurosci.*, 7: 1780–1791.

Ferster, D. and Lindström, S. (1983) An intracellular analysis of geniculo-cortical connectivity in area 17 of the cat. *J. Physiol.*, 342: 181–215.

Freund, T.F., Martin, K.A.C., Smith, A.D., and Somogyi, P. (1983) Glutamate decarboxylase-immunoreactive terminals of Golgi-impregnated axo-axonic cells and of presumed basket cells in synaptic contact with pyramidal neurons of the cat's visual cortex. *J. Comp. Neurol.*, 221: 263–278.

Freund, T.F., Martin, K.A.C. and Whitteridge, D. (1985a) Innervation of cat visual areas 17 and 18 by physiologically identified X and Y-type thalamic afferents. I. Arborisation patterns and quantitative distribution of postsynaptic elements. *J. Comp. Neurol.*, 242: 263–274.

Freund, T.F., Martin, K.A.C., Somogyi, P. and Whitteridge, D. (1985b) Innervation of cat visual areas 17 and 18 by physiologically identified X and Y-type thalamic afferents. II. Identification of postsynaptic targets by GABA immunocytochemistry and Golgi impregnation. *J. Comp. Neurol.*, 242: 275–291.

Gabbott, P.L.A. and Somogyi, P. (1986) Quantitative distribution of GABA-immunoreactive neurons in the visual cortex (area 17) of the cat. *Exp. Brain. Res.*, 61: 323–331.

Ganz, L. and Felder, R. (1984) Mechanisms of directional selectivity in simple neurons of the cat's visual cortex analyzed with stationary flash sequences. *J. Neurophysiol.*, 51: 294–324.

Garey, L.J. and Powell, T.P.S. (1971) An experimental study of the termination of the lateral geniculo-cortical pathway in the cat and monkey. *Proc. R. Soc. London B*, 179: 41–63.

Gilbert, C.D. and Wiesel, T.N. (1979) Morphology and intracortical projections of functionally characterised neurons in the cat visual cortex. *Nature,* 280: 120–125.

Gilbert, C.D. and Wiesel, T.N. (1983) Clustered intrinsic connections in cat visual cortex. *J. Neurosci.,* 3: 1116–1133.

Heggelund, P. (1981a) Receptive field organization of simple cells in cat striate cortex. *Exp. Brain Res.,* 42: 89–98.

Heggelund, P. (1981b) Receptive field organization of complex cells in cat striate cortex. *Exp. Brain Res.,* 42: 99–107.

Hess, R. and Murata, K. (1974) Effects of glutamate and GABA on specific response properties of neurons in the visual cortex. *Exp. Brain. Res.,* 21: 285–298.

Hoffman, K.-P. and Stone, J. (1971) Conduction velocity of afferents to cat visual cortex: A correlation with cortical receptive field properties. *Brain Res.,* 32: 460–466.

Hubel, D.H. and Wiesel, T.N. (1959) Receptive fields of single neurons in the cat's striate cortex. *J. Physiol.,* 148: 574–591.

Hubel, D.H. and Wiesel, T.N. (1962) Receptive fields, binocular interaction and functional architecture in the cat's visual cortex. *J. Physiol.,* 160: 106–154.

Hubel, D.H. and Wiesel, T.N. (1974) Sequence regularity and geometry of orientation columns in the monkey striate cortex. *J. Comp. Neurol.,* 158: 267–294.

Hubel, D.H. and Wiesel, T.N. (1977) Ferrier Lecture: Functional architecture of macaque monkey visual cortex. *Proc. R. Soc. (London) B*, 198: 1–59.

Hubel, D.H. and Wiesel, T.N. (1965) Receptive fields and functional architecture in two non-striate visual areas (18 and 19) of the cat. *J. Neurophysiol.,* 28: 229–289.

Humphrey, A.L., Sur, M., Ulrich, D.J. and Sherman, S.M. (1985) Projection patterns of individual X- and Y-cell axons from the lateral geniculate nucleus to cortical area 17 in the cat. *J. Comp. Neurol.,* 233: 159–189.

Jack, J.J.B., Noble, D. and Tsien, R.W. (1975) *Electric Current Flow in Excitable Cells*, Oxford: Oxford University Press.

Jones, E.G. (1984) Identification and classification of intrinsic circuit elements in the neocortex. In: G.M. Edelman, W.E. Gall, and W.M. Cowan, (Eds.), *Dynamic Aspects of Neocortical Function*, New York: John Wiley, pp. 7–40.

Kisvárday, Z.F., Martin, K.A.C., Whitteridge, D. and Somogyi, P. (1985a) The physiology, morphology and synaptology of basket cells in cat's visual cortex. *J. Comp. Neurol.,* 241: 111–137.

Kisvárday, Z.F., Martin, K.A.C., Whitteridge, D. and Somogyi, P. (1985b) Synaptic connections of intracellularly filled clutch cells: a type of small basket cell in the visual cortex of the cat. *J. Comp. Neurol.,* 241: 111–137.

Kisvárday, Z.F., Martin, K.A.C., Freund, T.F., Maglocsky, Z.S., Whitteridge, D. and Somogyi, P. (1986) Synaptic targets of HRP-filled layer III pyramidal cells in the cat striate cortex. *Exp. Brain Res.,* 64: 541–552.

Kisvárday, Z.F., Martin, K.A.C., Friedlander, M.J. and Somogyi, P. (1987) Evidence for interlaminar inhibitory circuits in striate cortex of cat. *J. Comp. Neurol.,* 260: 1–19.

Koch, C. and Poggio, T. (1985) The synaptic veto mechanism: does it underlie direction and orientation selectivity in the visual cortex? In: D. Rose and V.G. Dobson (Eds.), *Models of the Visual Cortex*, Chichester, New York: John Wiley, 408 pp.

Koch, C., Douglas, R.J. and Wehmeier, U. (1990) Visibility of synaptically induced conductance changes: Theory and simulations of anatomically characterized cortical pyramidal cells. *J. Neurosci.,* 10: 1728–1744.

Kriegstein, A.R. and LoTurco, J.J. (1990) GABAergic synaptic currents in slices of neocortex analyzed with whole-cell and cell-detached patch-clamp techniques. *Soc. Neurosci. Abstr.,* 16(1): 57

Le Vay, S. and Gilbert, C.D. (1976) Laminar patterns of geniculocortical projection in the cat. *Brain Res.,* 113: 1–19.

Lorente de No (1949) Cerebral cortex. Architecture, intracortical connections, motor projections. In: J.F. Fulton (Ed.), *Physiology of the Nervous System.* 3rd Edn. New York: Oxford University Press, pp. 288–312.

Lund, J.S. (1973) Organization of neurons in the visual cortex, area 17 of the monkey (*Macaca mulatta*). *J. Comp. Neurol.,* 147: 455–495.

Martin, K.A.C. (1984) Neuronal circuits in cat striate cortex. In: E.G. Jones and A. Peters (Eds.), *Cerebral Cortex, Vol. 2, Functional Properties of Cortical Cells*, New York: Plenum Press, pp. 241–284.

Martin, K.A.C. (1988) From enzymes to visual perception. A bridge too far? *Trends Neurosci.,* 11: 380–387.

Martin, Ķ.A.C. and Whitteridge, D. (1984) Form, function and intracortical projections of spiny neurons in the striate visual cortex of the cat. *J. Physiol.,* 353: 463–504.

Martin, K.A.C., Somogyi, P. and Whitteridge, D. (1983) Physiological and morphological properties of identified basket cells in the cat's visual cortex. *Exp. Brain Res.,* 50: 193–200.

McCormick, D.A. (1990) Membrane properties and neurotransmitter actions. In: G. Shepherd (Ed.), *Synaptic Organization of the Brain*, 3rd Edn. New York: Oxford University Press, pp. 220–243.

Murphy, P.C. and Sillito, A.M. (1987) Corticofugal feedback influences the generation of length tuning in the visual pathway. *Nature*, 329: 727–729.

Nelson, S.B. (1991) Temporal interactions in the cat visual system. III. Pharmacological studies of cortical suppression suggest a presynaptic mechanism. *J. Neurosci.*, 11: 369–380.

Ohzawa, I., Sclar, G. and Freeman, R.D. (1985) Contrast gain control in the cat's visual system. *J. Neurophysiol.*, 54: 651–667.

Orban, G.A., Kato, H. and Bishop, P.O. (1979) End-zone regions in receptive fields of hypercomplex and other striate neurons in the cat. *J. Neurophysiol.*, 42: 818–832.

Orban, G.A. (1984) *Neuronal Operations in the Visual Cortex*, Berlin, Heidelberg: Springer Verlag.

Palmer, L.A. and Davis, T.L. (1981) Comparison of responses to moving and stationary stimuli in cat striate cortex. *J. Neurophysiol.*, 46: 277–295.

Peters, A. (1984) Chandelier cells. In *Cerebral Cortex, Vol. 1, Cellular components of Cerebral Cortex*, New York: Plenum Press, pp. 361–380.

Peters, A. (1987) Numbers of neurons and synapses in primary visual cortex. In: E.G. Jones and A. Peters (Eds.), *Cerebral Cortex, Vol 6, Further Aspects of Cortical Function including Hippocampus*, New York: Plenum Press, pp. 267–294.

Phillips, C.G. (1959). Intracellular records from Betz cells in the cat. *Q.J. Exp. Physiol.*, 44: 1–25.

Powell, T.P.S. (1981) Certain aspects of the intrinsic organisation of the cerebral cortex. In: O. Pompeiano and A. Marsan (Eds.), *Brain Mechanisms and Perceptual Awareness*, New York: Raven Press, pp. 1–19.

Rall, W. (1964) Theoretical significance of dendritic trees for neuronal input-output relations. In: R.F. Reiss (Ed.), *Neural Theory and Modelling*, Stanford: Stanford University Press, pp. 73–97.

Ramón y Cajal, S. (1911) *Histologie du Systeme Nerveux de l'Homme et des Vertebres II*, trans. Alouzay, L. Paris: Maloine.

Rockell, A.J., Hiorns, R.W. and Powell, T.P.S. (1980) The basic uniformity in structure of the neocortex. *Brain*, 103: 221–223.

Rose, D. (1977). On the arithmetical operation performed by inhibitory synapses onto the neuronal soma. *Exp. Brain Res.*, 28: 221–223.

Rudy, B. (1988) Diversity and ubiquity of K$^+$ channels. *Neuroscience*, 25: 729–749.

Scharfman, H.E. and Sarvey, J.M. (1987) Responses to GABA recorded from identified rat visual cortical neurons. *Neuroscience*, 23: 407–422.

Scholl, D.A. (1956) *The Organisation of the Cerebral Cortex*, London: Methuen, pp. 102.

Schwindt, P.C. Spain, W.J., Foehring, R.C., Stafstrom, C.E., Chubb, M.C. and Crill, W.E. (1988a) Multiple potassium conductances and their functions in neurons from cat sensorimotor cortex in vitro. *J. Neurophysiol.*, 59: 424–449.

Schwindt, P.C. Spain, W.J., Foehring, R.C., Chubb, M.C. and Crill, W.E. (1988b) Slow conductances in neurons from cat sensorimotor cortex in vitro and their role in slow excitability changes. *J. Neurophysiol.*, 59: 450–467.

Sillito, A.M. (1975) The contribution of inhibitory mechanisms to the receptive field properties of neurons in the striate cortex of the cat. *J. Physiol.*, 250: 305–329.

Sillito, A.M. (1977) Inhibitory processes underlying direction specificity of simple, complex and hypercomplex cells in the cat's striate cortex. *J. Physiol.*, 271: 299–720.

Sillito, A.M. (1984) Functional considerations of the operation of GABAergic inhibitory processes in the visual cortex. In: E.G. Jones and A. Peters (Eds.), *Cerebral Cortex, Vol. 2, Functional properties of cortical cells*, New York: Plenum Press, pp. 91–117.

Somogyi, P. (1989) Synaptic organization of GABAergic neurons and GABA$_A$ receptors in the lateral geniculate nucleus and visual cortex. In: D.K.-T. Lam and C.D. Gilbert (Eds.), *Neural mechanisms of visual perception*, Houston, Texas: Portfolio Pub. Co., pp. 35–62.

Somogyi, P. and Cowey, A. (1981) Combined Golgi and electron microscopes study on the synapses formed by double bouquet cells in the visual cortex of the cat and monkey. *J. Comp. Neurol.*, 195: 547–566.

Somogyi, P. and Freund, T.F. (1989) Immunocytochemistry and synaptic relationships of physiologically characterized HRP-filled neurons. In: L. Heimer and L. Zaborszky (Eds.), *Neuroanatomical Tract-Tracing Methods, 2* New York: Plenum, pp. 239–264.

Somogyi, P. and Soltész, I. (1986) Immunogold demonstration of GABA in synaptic terminals of intracellularly recorded, horseradish peroxidase-filled basket cells and clutch cells in the cat's visual cortex. *Neuroscience*, 19: 1051–1065.

Somogyi, P., Freund, T.F., and Cowey, A. (1982) The axoaxonic interneuron in the cerebral cortex of the rat, cat and monkey. *Neuroscience*, 7: 2577–2608.

Somogyi, P., Kisvárday, Z.F., Martin, K.A.C., and Whitteridge, D. (1983) Synaptic connections of morphologically identified and physiologically characterised large basket cells in the striate cortex of cat. *Neuroscience*, 10: 261–294.

Szentágothai, J. (1973) Synaptology of visual cortex. In: R. Jung (Ed.), *Handbook of Sensory Physiology, Vol. VII / 3, Central Visual Information*, Berlin: Springer-Verlag, pp. 269–324.

Szentágothai, J. (1975) The "module-concept" in cerebral cortex architecture. *Brain Res.*, 95: 475–496.

Torre, V. and Poggio, T. (1978) A synaptic mechanism possibly underlying directional selectivity to motion. *Proc. R. Soc. (London) B*, 202: 409–416.

Van Essen, D. (1985) Functional organisation of the primate visual cortex. In: A. Peters and E.G. Jones (Eds.), *Cerebral Cortex, Vol. 3, Visual Cortex*, New York: Plenum Press, pp. 259–329.

Verdoorn, T.A., Kass, R.S., Seeburg, P.H. and Sakmann, B. (1990) Single channel properties of heterooligomeric rat GABA$_A$ receptors expressed using different alpha subunit variants. *Soc. Neurosci. Abstr.*, 16(1): 379.

Wehmeier, U., Dong, D., Koch, C. and Van Essen, D. (1989)

Modeling the Mammalian Visual System. In: C. Koch and I. Segev (Eds.), *Methods in Neural Modeling*, Cambridge, MA: MIT Press, pp. 335–359.

White, E.L. (1989) *Cortical Circuits: Synaptic Organization of the Cerebral Cortex. Structure, Function and Theory*, Boston: Birkhauser.

Wiesel, T.N. and Gilbert, C. (1983) The Sharpley-Schafer Lecture. Morphological basis of visual cortical function. *Q.J. Exp. Physiol.*, 68: 525–543.

Wörgötter, F. and Koch, C. (1991) A detailed model of the primary visual pathway in the cat: comparison of afferent excitatory and intracortical inhibitory connection schemes for orientation selectivity. *J.Neurosci.*, 11: 1959–1979.

Zeki, S. and Shipp, S. (1988) The functional logic of cortical connections. *Nature*, 335: 311–317.

R.R. Mize, R.E. Marc and A.M. Sillito (Eds.)
Progress in Brain Research, Vol. 90
© 1992 Elsevier Science Publishers B.V. All rights reserved

CHAPTER 22

# Organization and plasticity of GABA neurons and receptors in monkey visual cortex

Stewart Hendry and Renee K. Carder

*Department of Anatomy and Neurobiology, University of California, Irvine, CA 92717, USA*

## Introduction

GABA interneurons, the principal mediators of intracortical inhibition, are a heterogeneous group that displays marked diversity in morphological and chemical characteristics. Within the primary visual area (area 17 or V1) of the monkey cerebral cortex, a much larger density of GABA immunoreactive neurons is present than in other cortical areas (Hendry et al., 1987). However, because of the greatly increased density of all neurons in this area (Rockel et al., 1980), the proportion of GABA cells is lower than in other areas of monkey cortex and approaches 20% of the total population (Hendry et al., 1987). These neurons appear to be responsible for establishing and reinforcing many of the physiological properties, such as orientation, direction specificity and end inhibition, that are characteristic of the cerebral cortex (Sillito, 1984). In what follows, several aspects of the organization and plasticity of GABA neurons are accented. These include the division of the GABA population in monkey area 17 into morphological and chemical subpopulations, the normal distribution of GABA neurons in specific layers and compartments, and the ability of the GABA neurons in the adult cortex to change chemical properties following loss of input from one eye. The findings that GABAergic properties change with monocular deprivation are correlated with data that suggest certain morphological classes are preferentially affected by deprivation and that the deprivation may lead to changes in physiological properties of the cortical cells.

## Morphological features of GABA neurons

GABA neurons are non-pyramidal cells with smooth or beaded dendritic processes (Houser et al., 1984) and thus belong to the general group of aspiny or sparsely spiny neurons (Fig. 1), characterized by the presence of both symmetric and asymmetric synapses on their somata and by the exclusively symmetric synapses they form with postsynaptic structures. Based primarily on axonal ramifications, and terminations, four classes of GABA neurons have been identified in monkey visual cortex:

### (1) Double bouquet cells

The axons of double bouquet cells branch into several vertically oriented collaterals close to their cell bodies and span layers II–VI in relatively narrow, vertically oriented cylinders (Somogyi and Cowey, 1981; Somogyi et al., 1981, 1984; Werner et al., 1989). This class of cell has been identified as GABAergic in other areas of the monkey cerebral cortex, where the morphology of neurons immunostained for peptides and proteins that coexist with GABA (see below) leave no doubt that they are double bouquet cells (deLima and Morrison, 1989; DeFelipe et al., 1990). Small

478

intracortical injections of $^3$H-GABA into monkey area 17 have revealed a vertical organization of GABA-accumulating intrinsic neurons which is presumably based upon the retrograde labeling of double bouquet cells (Somogyi et al., 1981, 1984).

## (2) Clutch cells

The clutch cell is characterized by its profusely branched and crowded varicose axon which is densely packed with large bulbous boutons (Kisvarday et al., 1986). The dendritic shafts and

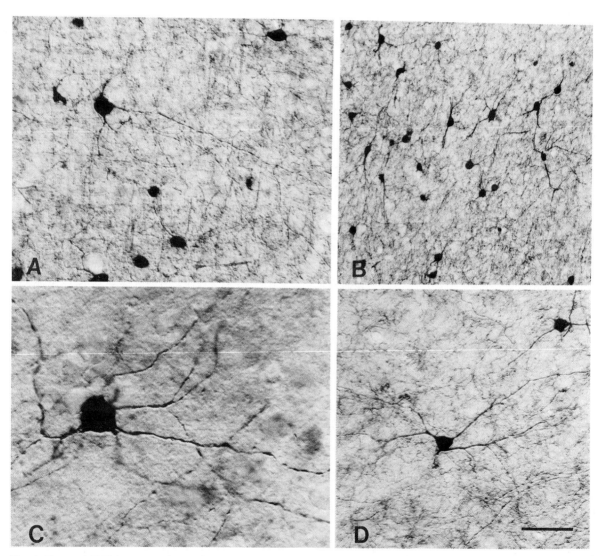

Fig. 1. Types of GABA neurons in monkey area 17. A,C. GABA neurons immunostained with an antibody to the protein, parvalbumin. Large numbers of these cells are present in deep part of layer III, layers IVA and IVC and layer VI. The sizes of the somata vary from small (approximately 8 $\mu$m in diamter) to large (greater than 15 $\mu$m in diameter). Large multipolar neurons with long dendrites (C) are most common in layers IV and VI. The large size of the somata, the multipolar dendritic morphology and the axonal terminations onto the somata of pyramidal neurons indicates that many of the parvalbumin-immunoreactive neurons are large basket cells. The smaller cells may include chandelier neurons. B,D. GABA neurons immunostained with an antibody to the protein, calbindin. Numerous small somata with thin dendrites are present in layers II and III (B). These may include the class of double bouquet cells. Larger somata with more elongated dendrites are present in layers V and VI. Bar: 40 $\mu$m in A,D; 65 $\mu$m in B; 20 $\mu$m in C.

spines of spiny stellate cells appear to be its major postsynaptic target. This cell type has been positively identified as GABAergic in both monkey and cat area 17 (Kisvarday et al., 1986; Somogyi and Soltesz, 1986).

### (3) Basket cells

These multipolar neurons (Marin-Padilla 1969; Jones, 1975) have axon arbors that form terminal nests around the somata and primary dendrites of pyramidal neurons. The basket cell axons form symmetric synapses principally on pyramidal somata, spines and apical and basal dendrites of pyramidal cells, but may also contact somata and dendrites of non-pyramidal cells (Somogyi et al., 1983). Although most extensively studied in other areas of the monkey cortex, basket cells have been described in monkey area 17 (Lund., 1987; Lund et al., 1988) and neurons of similar morphology have been identified as GABA immunoreactive (Fitzpatrick et al., 1987).

### (4) Chandelier cells

The axonal arborizations of chandelier cells terminate in a series of vertically oriented boutons that resemble candlesticks. Chandelier cells form symmetric synapses exclusively with axon initial segments of pyramidal neurons primarily located in layers II and III (Peters et al., 1982; Somogyi et al., 1982; Freund et al., 1983; Werner et al., 1989). In other cortical areas chandelier cells have been conclusively identified as GABAergic (Somogyi et al., 1981; DeFelipe et al., 1985).

### Chemically characterized subpopulations

GABA neurons of the cerebral cortex can be subdivided based on the presence within them of neuropeptides and intracellular proteins and by the presence of specific cell-surface proteoglycans along the external surfaces of their plasma membranes (Fig. 2). The great majority of neurons in the monkey cerebral cortex immunoreactive for neuropeptide Y (NPY), somatostatin (soma-

totropin release inhibiting factor or SRIF), cholecystokinin octapeptide (CCK), substance P (SP) and a related tachykinin, substance K (SK) are subpopulations of GABA cells (Hendry et al., 1984b, 1988; Jones and Hendry, 1986; Jones et al., 1988). The total population of cortical GABAergic neurons immunoreactive for one or more of these peptides is an estimated 40% (10% for non-tachykinins and 30% for tachykinins; Jones and Hendry, 1986; Jones et al., 1988). Two well-recognized morphological classes of GABA neurons are immunoreactive for none of the peptides listed above: the relatively small size of the neurons immunostained for CCK, SRIF, NPY or the tachykinins, and the absence of peptide immunostained terminals surrounding the somata of pyramidal cells or contacting the initial segments of pyramidal cell axons suggests that none of the known neuropeptides are expressed by large GABAergic basket cells or by chandelier cells (Hendry et al., 1983, 1984; DeLima and Morrison, 1989). Recent findings indicate that chandelier cells of the monkey prefrontal cortex are immunoreactive for the peptide, corticotropin releasing factor (CRF; Lewis and Lund, 1990). Whether chandelier cells of area 17 are also CRF-positive is unknown.

Two $Ca^{2+}$ binding proteins, calbindin (28 kDa vitamin D-dependent $Ca^{2+}$ binding protein) and parvalbumin have been localized in two, largely separate populations of GABA neurons in the neocortex of Old World monkeys (Fig. 2C–F; Hendry et al., 1989). Parvalbumin-containing cells have somata that range in size from greater than 15 $\mu$m to less than 10 $\mu$m, the largest of which has all of the features of classical basket cells (Fig. 1C; Marin-Padilla, 1969; Jones, 1975; DeFelipe et al., 1986): (1) they are concentrated in layers III and V; (2) their soma exceed 15 $\mu$m in diameter; (3) they are multipolar and give rise to very extensive ascending and descending processes; (4) the terminal sites of the large basket cells, the somata and proximal dendrites of pyramidal neurons, are surrounded by parvalbumin immunoreactive multiterminal endings. The pres-

480

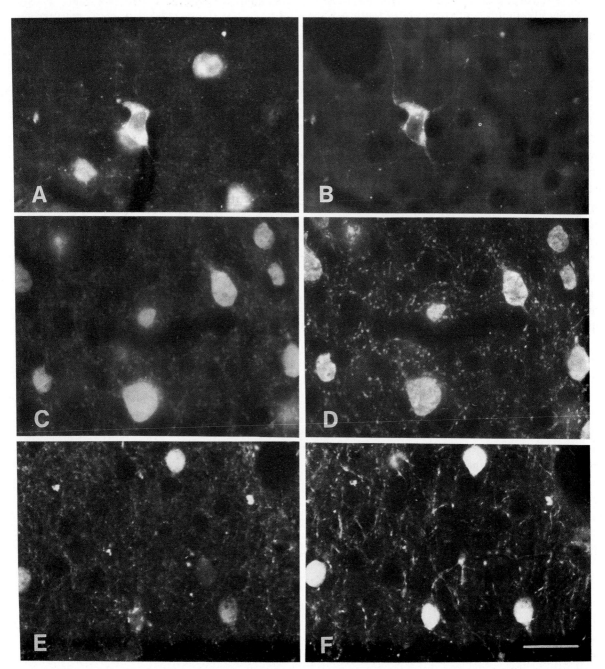

Fig. 2. Coexistence of proteins and peptides in GABA neurons of monkey area 17. A,B. GABA (A) and NPY (B) immunoreactivity detected with a simultaneous localization method. Of the several GABA immunoreactive neurons seen in layer II, one is also NPY immunoreactive. C,D. GABA (C) and parvalbumin (D) immunostaining in layer IVC of monkey area 17. All of the GABA immunoreactive neurons in this field and the great majority throughout layer IVC are also parvalbumin immunoreactive. E,F. GABA (E) and calbindin (F) immunostaining in layer II. Many of the GABA somata in periodic patches of layer III are calbindin immunoreactive. Bar: 20 $\mu$m.

ence of parvalbumin immunoreactivity in axon terminations that synapse onto pyramidal cell axon initial segments has also been used to identify a second population of parvalbumin neurons as chandelier cells (DeFelipe et al., 1989). By contrast, calbindin-immunoreactive somata that are small, present in layers II and V, and give rise to radial bundles of axons are interpreted to be double bouquet cells (DeFelipe et al., 1990).

Cell-surface proteoglycans, which can be visualized with specific antibodies or lectins, have also been used to identify subpopulations of GABA neurons in the cerebral cortex (for review, see Naegle and Barnstable, 1989). By its recognition of a complex proteoglycan, the monoclonal antibody, Cat-301, stains a heterogeneous population of neurons in the monkey area 17 (Hendry et al., 1986; DeYoe et al., 1990). While a small number of Cat-301 neurons have the characteristic features of pyramidal neurons, a prominent class is immunoreactive for GABA and comprises approximately half the GABA population (Hendry et al., 1988a). The majority of the GABA/Cat-301 neurons display no peptide immunoreactivity. A similar pattern of GABA cell labeling is seen with the lectin, *Vicia villosa* (VVA; Mulligan et al., 1989). Seventy-eight percent of the VVA labeled cells display GABA immunoreactivity and 30% of the GABA immunoreactive neurons are also labeled for VVA. Although the distribution of VVA positive cells overlaps with that of the neuropeptides, preliminary results indicate that neither SP nor NPY are present within VVA stained neurons (Mulligan et al., 1989). Based on the size and morphology of labeled neurons it appears that Cat-301 and VVA label more than one subpopulation of GABA cells, with the larger VVA- and Cat-301-positive cells possessing features that are reminiscent of the large basket cell (Marin-Padilla, 1969; Jones, 1975; DeFelipe et al., 1986).

These findings demonstrate that the large population of GABA neurons in monkey area 17 is composed of distinct subpopulations, each containing specific intracellular or cell-surface pro-

teins and peptides. In some cases, the chemical characteristics serve as signatures for specific morphological classes of GABA cells. In the following section, the distribution of these chemical subpopulations of GABA cells within specific layers and compartments in area 17 is discussed.

## Laminar distribution of GABA neurons

GABA neurons are present through the thickness of monkey area 17 but they and the $GABA_A$ receptors are unevenly distributed across layers (Fig. 3). At least half of the GABA neurons in area 17 are present in the supragranular layers, and 35% are within layer IV, particularly layers IVA and IVC (Fitzpatrick et al., 1987; Hendry et al., 1987), which receive the densest innervation from axons of the LGN. Of the three major subdivisions of layer IV, the most superficial (layer IVA) contains the highest percentage of GABA neurons (35%), while in the remaining two layers (layers IVB and IVC) the GABA cells comprise 15–20% of the total neuronal population (Hendrickson et al., 1981; Fitzpatrick et al., 1987; Hendry et al., 1987). Layer IVC can be further subdivided into $IVC\alpha$ and $IVC\beta$, and while $IVC\alpha$ contains a class of large GABAergic neurons, $IVC\beta$ has an increased density of GABAergic neurons (Fitzpatrick et al., 1987). Hybridization with a cRNA probe for the GABA synthesizing enzyme, glutamate decarboxylase (GAD) reveals a similar laminar organization of neurons expressing the GAD gene although their distribution within $IVC\alpha$ and $IVC\beta$ further divides those layers into sublaminae (Benson et al., 1991).

In addition to the GABA somata, GABA axon terminals and $GABA_A$ receptors are also very dense in the layers most heavily innervated by axons from the LGN (i.e., layers IVA and IVC; Fig. 3). This preferential distribution of terminals is so prominent, in part due to the presence of a specific populations of larger GABAergic axon terminals in layers IVA and IVC (Fitzpatrick et al., 1987). Both autoradiographic and immunocytochemical methods indicate that the distribution

482

of GABA$_A$ receptors matches that of GABA neurons and terminals, with high densities in layers IVA and IVC$\beta$, as well as in layers II–III and VI (Shaw and Cynader, 1986; Rakic et al., 1988; Hendry et al., 1990).

The data on the localization of the entire population of GABA somata, terminals and receptors indicate a preferential distribution within layers that are directly innervated by axons from the LGN. Within the total GABA population, each of the subpopulations characterized by the coexistence of a particular peptide, protein or cell-surface carbohydrate has a unique distribution, but all can be included into one of two broad groups: neurons primarily in the geniculo-cortical-recipient zones, and neurons in the regions outside of these recipient zones. Included in the former are GABA neurons immunoreac-

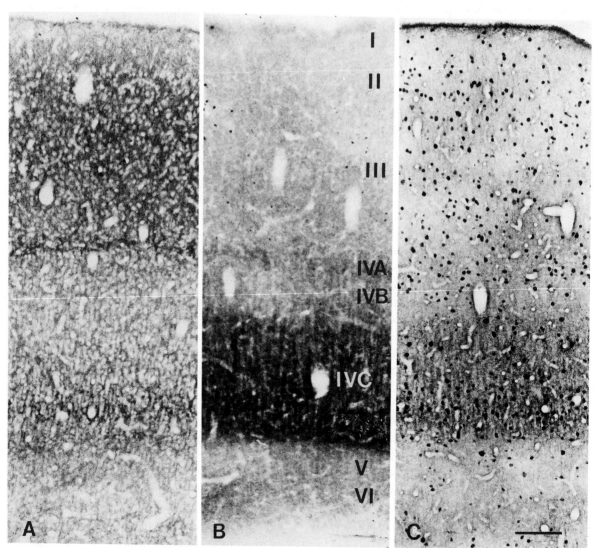

Fig. 3. Laminar distribution of GABA systems in monkey area 17. A. Immunoreactivity for the $\beta_2/\beta_3$ subunit of the GABA$_A$ receptor. By comparison with the pattern of CO histochemical staining (B), the densest receptor immunostaining is found in layers II–III, IVA and the bottom half of layer IVC (IVC$\beta$). B. Histochemical staining for CO allows for accurate assignment of laminar borders in area 17. C. GABA immunostaining is made up of numerous somata and puncta (axon terminals). Both are extremely dense in layer IVC$\beta$, as well as layer IVA and layers II–III. Bar: 150 $\mu$m.

tive for tachykinins (Hendry et al., 1988b) or parvalbumin (Omidi et al., 1988) or labeled with VVA (Mulligan et al., 1988). These are preferentially located within laminae receiving geniculocortical inputs. By contrast, subpopulations of GABA neurons immunoreactive for CCK, SRIF and NPY (Hendry et al., 1984a,b) or calbindin (Omidi et al., 1988) are concentrated in layers that are not directly innervated by geniculocortical axons.

Within two levels in area 17, geniculocortical axons terminate unevenly: they occupy a regular series of patches in layers II–III and the walls of an irregular honeycomb in IVA (Hendrickson et al., 1978; Hendrickson, 1982; Itaya et al., 1984). This distribution of LGN axons is reflected in the histochemical staining pattern for the enzyme, cytochrome-$c$ oxidase (CO; Fitzpatrick et al., 1983; Livingstone and Hubel, 1984). The periodic patches of high CO activity and LGN terminations in layers II and III line up in rows at the centers of ocular dominance columns and are surrounded by regions that are less intensely stained for CO and do not receive LGN terminations (Fig. 4; Horton and Hubel, 1981; Humphrey and Hendrickson, 1983; Wong-Riley and Carroll, 1984; Horton, 1984). Within the CO patches are chemically specific subpopulations of neurons. The GABA neurons are, themselves, inhomogeneously distributed but the highly irregular variation in GABA cell density exhibits no correlation with the presence of CO-stained patches (Fig. 4A–B; Fitzpatrick et al., 1987; Hendry et al., 1987). However, distinct subpopulations of GABA neurons that display parvalbumin (Fig. 10; Omidi et al., 1988) and Cat-301 immunostaining (Fig. 4E–F; Hendry et al., 1988a) are concentrated within the CO patches. The patches of GABA/Cat-301 neurons are smaller than their CO stained counterparts and occupy the most darkly stained cores of the CO patches. Evidence that neurons within the cores differ physiologically from the surrounding shell of CO patches (Livingstone and Hubel, 1984), suggests that the Cat-301 cells are a subpopulation of GABA neu-

rons that are functionally distinct as well as chemically distinct. An additonal subpopulation of GABA neurons, which displays tachykinin-like immunoreactivity, is also more intense within the CO-stained patches (Hendry et al., 1988b). However, this pattern is due to a greater density of immunostained punctate profiles rather than a preferential distribution of the tachykinin-positive somata, themselves. Finally, and perhaps most significantly for the functional organization of area 17, GABAergic terminals (Fig. 4A–B; Hendrickson et al., 1981; Fitzpatrick et al., 1987) and the $\beta_2/\beta_3$ subunit of the GABA$_A$ receptor (Fig. 4C–D; Hendry et al., 1990) are localized preferentially within the CO patches of layers II and III.

Other chemically specific subpopulations of GABA neurons selectively occupy the regions surrounding the CO patches. In both New World (Celio et al., 1986) and Old World monkeys (Omidi et al., 1988) calbindin-immunostained GABA neurons are concentrated in regions outside the patches (Fig. 11). In addition, GABA/NPY-positive somata are much more common outside the regions of the CO-stained patches than inside the patches (Kuljis and Rakic, 1989). These data indicate that, although the total GABA neuronal population is distributed without any consistent relationship to the CO patches (Fitzpatrick et al., 1987; Hendry et al., 1987), separate and distinct subpopulations of GABA neurons occupy either the regions of the patches or the regions around them.

In layer IVA, geniculocortical terminations are distributed in a honeycomb pattern which closely matches the pattern seen with CO staining (Hendrickson et al., 1978; Hendrickson, 1982; Blasdel and Lund, 1982; Itaya et al., 1984). Although GABA somata are homogeneously distributed in this layer, the GABA terminals occupy the walls of a honeycomb that coincides precisely with the pattern of intense CO staining (Fitzpatrick et al., 1987). In addition, the distribution of the $\beta_2/\beta_3$ subunit of the GABA$_A$ receptor in layer IVA is characterized by a lattice

484

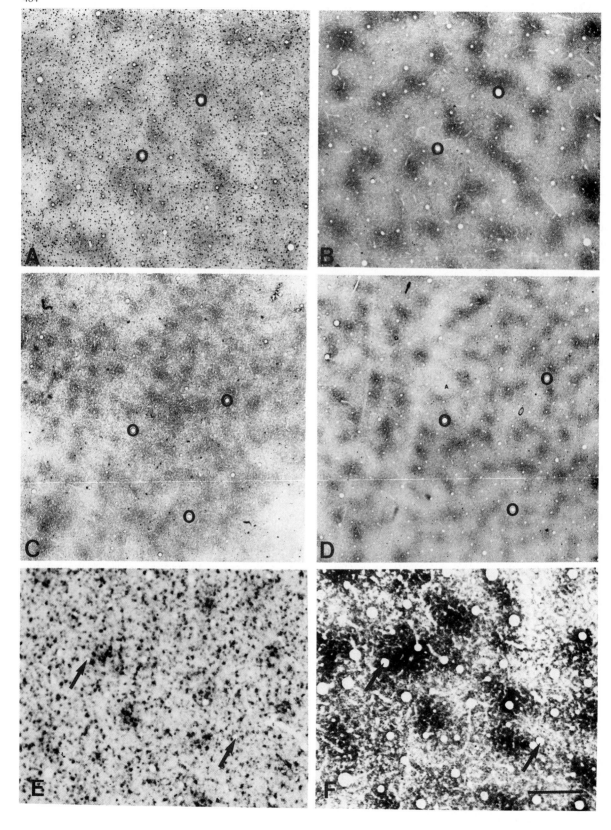

consisting of many long strands of puncta stacked on top of one another. This lattice of intense receptor immunostaining also corresponds precisely to the honeycomb of CO staining (Hendry et al., 1990). Thus, the distribution of geniculo-cortical afferents, CO staining and GABA terminal and receptor distribution reveals IVA to be a composite lamina, made up of an irregular, intensely active lattice of thalamic and intrinsic GABAergic interactions and interspersed regions that more closely resemble the neuropil of the underlying layer IVB.

These findings on the morphological and chemical subivisions of GABA neurons and their distribution within specific layers and compartments within monkey area 17 demonstrate that when the entire GABA population is considered, a preferential but not exclusive distribution of cells within geniculocortical recipient zones exists. Furthermore, subpopulations of GABA neurons are present in area 17, some present within compartments (e.g., the CO patches of layers II–III and the lattices of layer IVA) that receive LGN inputs and others present within regions (the inter-patch regions in layers II–III) that do not. It is also very clear that in the normal monkey, the distribution of GABA neurons and subpopulations of GABA neurons may vary *within* ocular dominance columns (CO patch vs. interpatch) but the distribution does not vary *across* ocular dominance columns. That is, the systems of right- and left-eye dominance columns contain the same densities and distributions of GABA neurons and GABA subpopulations (see below). In the following sections, data will be presented

and discussed which indicates this homogeneous distribution is definitely not the case for monkeys deprived of visual input from one eye in adulthood. Under those circumstances, dramatic changes in the total GABA population and in specific subpopulations occur across ocular dominance columns and within select compartments of the columns.

**Visual cortical plasticity**

A growing body of data indicates that in both the peripheral and central nervous systems changes related to the levels of synaptic input produce changes in the molecular features of specific neuronal populations (LaGamma et al., 1985; White et al., 1987; Morris et al., 1988; Warren et al., 1989; Welker et al., 1989; Neve and Bear, 1989; Feldblum et al., 1990). For example, the changes produced by denervation of different groups of neurons include increased or reduced levels of neurotransmitters, neuropeptides, related enzymes, receptors and second messenger molecules (Baker et al., 1983; Black et al., 1984; Kosaka et al., 1987). The functional significance of these changes can be appreciated from both classical and recent studies of denervation supersensitivity, in which loss of an afferent produces a pronounced increase in neuronal response to the afferent's neurotransmitter (Lomo and Rosenthal, 1972; Frank et al., 1975). Within some systems, the plastic response to changes in inputs is restricted to specific neuronal populations, possibly to specific neuronal classes. Of particular interest is whether such changes detected in sim-

Fig. 4. Patterns of immunoreactivity in the periodic patches of CO staining in layers II–III of monkey area 17. A,B. Comparison of GABA (A) and CO (B) staining in adjacent tangential sections through layers II and III. Although patches of GABA immunostaining are present (A) and these coincide with the patches of CO staining (B), the GABA patches appear diffuse because they represent terminal immunostaining. The density of GABA somata is no greater inside the patches than outside. C,D. Comparison of GABA$_A$ receptor immunostaining (C) and CO staining (D) in layers II–III. In approximately 80% of the CO patches, a heightened immunostaining of receptors is evident. E,F. Comparison of Cat-301 and CO staining. Clusters of Cat-301 immunostained GABA neurons are present in layers II–III (E) and in layers IVB and VI. These clusters coincide with the core regions of the CO patches in layers II–III (F). The profiles of the same blood vessels in the pairs of sections are indicated by circles in A–D and by arrows in E,F.

pler systems also occur in the most complex neuronal system, the cerebral cortex. Are the chemical traits of cortical neurons changeable and are those changes restricted to certain neuronal subpopulations?

For a brief period during the development of the monkey cerebral cortex, manipulations of one eye alter the physiology and connectivity of the primary visual area (Hubel et al., 1977; LeVay et al., 1980). The most dramatic of the changes is the expansion of regions or "columns" dominated by the normal eye and the shrinkage of columns dominated by the deprived eye. Such changes in column size are apparent with two types of method: (1) physiological methods that examine the receptive fields of cortical neurons, in which case the territories of cortical neurons excited by the normal eye are found to be abnormally large while those excited by the deprived eye are small and contain neurons that are difficult to activate; (2) anatomical methods that examine the indirect inputs from the two retinae (deprived and normal) through the relay in the LGN, in which case retinogeniculocortical axons of the normal eye occupy much wider regions in area 17 than similar axons of the deprived eye. Current understanding of this and related aspects of developmental plasticity indicates the physiological expansion occurs because of the sprouting of geniculocortical afferents driven by the normal eye. The various anatomical and physiological components of developmental plasticity end in the first 4–12 months of postnatal life.

The ability of the cerebral cortex to change does not end in childhood. In the monkey first somatic sensory cortex significant functional reorganization has been reported to occur following partial deafferentation of the digits or other manipulations of the sensory periphery in the adult monkey (Kaas et al., 1983; Wall et al., 1986; Clark et al., 1988). Many of the changes of the somatic sensory cortex in this and other species take place too quickly (a matter of hours) to be accounted for by the sprouting of central axons. These findings are in keeping with the idea that areas of the neocortex, unlike the hippocampus (Lynch et al., 1972), are incapable of anatomical reorganization past a certain early age but the findings indicate that functional plasticity persists into adulthood.

How is functional plasticity possible in a hardwired system? One obvious possibility is through changes in neuronal chemistry, particularly in the neurotransmitter and receptor properties of cortical neurons. Such changes would be particularly provocative if they occurred in the GABA system of the cerebral cortex, for as outlined above, GABA transmission is reported to be vital for the construction of various visual cortical receptive field properties, and anatomically, the greatest concentrations of GABA neurons in monkey area 17 are in the geniculocortical recipient layers. Studies over the past four years have shown that in area 17 of monkeys, reductions in neuronal activity selectively reduce levels of immunoreactivity for several substances, including GABA and related proteins and peptides, increase levels of other proteins and leave a great many unaffected. Conversely, increased neuronal activity produces increased immunoreactivity for certain proteins and peptides. The responses exhibited by individual neurons appear to be selective for specific subpopulations of GABA neurons and may be related to their synaptic organization. Some, but not all, of the effects on protein levels are exerted at the level of gene transcription.

## Activity-dependent regulation in GABA neurons

When the neuronal activity in one retina is eliminated, either by enucleation of the eye or injection of the voltage-gated sodium channel blocker, tetrodotoxin (TTX), into the vitreous body of the eye, the metabolic activity in area 17 of adult monkeys is rapidly affected. Within four or five days, the histochemical staining for CO is markedly reduced in columns dominated by the manipulated eye (Wong-Riley and Carroll, 1984; Trusk et al., 1990). In tangential sections through the major thalamic-recipient layer, IVC, the reduced staining in the removed/injected-eye columns and the normal, dark staining of the intact-eye columns appear as series of elongated light and dark stripes, each approximately 0.5 mm wide (Fig. 5B,D,F). When adjacent sections of the same adult monkeys are immunocytochemically stained for the amino acid neurotransmitter, GABA, identical patterns of alternating light and dark stripes are apparent (Fig. 5A,E; Hendry and Jones, 1986, 1988a). These CO and GABA patterns contrast with the homogeneous staining for both in layer IVC of normal adult monkeys. Comparisons of the CO and GABA staining in layer IVC of deprived monkeys reveals that the lightly stained CO stripes correspond to the lightly stained GABA stripes. That is, the GABA immunostaining is reduced in the injected/removed-eye columns of adult monkeys (Figs. 5 and 6; Hendry and Jones, 1986, 1988a). The qualitative impression of reduced immunostaining is seen as a reduction in the numerical density of immunocytochemically stained somata and puncta (terminals) to approximately half the density seen in layer IVC of a normal monkey and in the normal-eye stripes in layer IVC of a monocularly deprived monkey. Similar reductions in the number of GABA immunostained neurons are apparent in stripes through layer IVA. In layers II and III the reductions in GABA-immunoreactive neurons in the deprived-eye columns are evident in the regions of the CO patches and in the regions between the patches (Fig. 6; Hendry and Jones, 1988a).

That the reduction in GABA immunoreactivity of the adult monkey visual cortex is dependent on neuronal activity can be inferred from several observations.

(1) The cortical reduction following retinal manipulations occurs across at least one synapse, which takes place in the LGN, and is not a result of direct deafferentation. In the LGN, itself, the metabolic activity and CO staining of neurons that receive inputs from a deprived eye are quickly reduced but the GABA immunostaining remains normal 3 weeks *after* the cortical immunostaining has been reduced (Hendry, 1991).

(2) Reduction in cortical immunostaining occurs with injections of TTX, which silences retinal ganglion cells but does not grossly affect their axonal transport (Hendry and Jones, 1988a).

(3) Reduced immunostaining occurs, at least in juvenile animals, when the levels of light reaching the retina are reduced but not eliminated by lid suturing (Fig. 5A–B). In that case, several weeks and not simply four or five days of deprivation (as in the case of enucleation or TTX injections) are necessary to reduce the levels of GABA immunostaining (Hendry and Jones, 1986, 1988a).

(4) The reduced number of GABA immunoreactive neurons is seen without a loss in the total number of neurons in layer IVC, indicating that the GABA neurons do not die as a result of the eye manipulations (Hendry and Jones, 1986, 1988a).

(5) Perhaps most significantly, the GABA immunostaining of layer IVC can be returned to normal if TTX-injected monkeys are allowed relatively long periods of renewed binocular vision (Fig. 7). Those experiments involved the taking of biopsies from area 17 of monkeys injected with TTX, after which the monkeys were allowed to recover without further injections for several weeks and then sacrificed. The biopsies showed stripes of reduced CO and GABA staining but blocks of area 17 stained following the return to binocular vision were qualitatively and quantitatively normal (Hendry and Jones, 1988a).

(6) Reductions in GABA immunoreactivity can be detected quantitatively in and around the CO-rich patches in layers II and III that overlie the centers of the deprived-eye columns (Fig. 6; Hendry and Jones, 1988a). Only in the CO patches that overlie the centers of the intact-eye columns, where neurons are driven exclusively by the intact

488

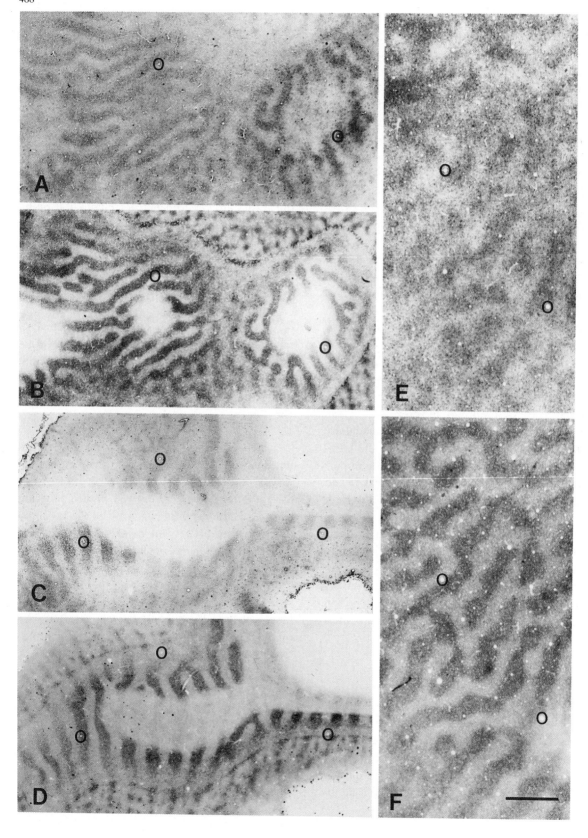

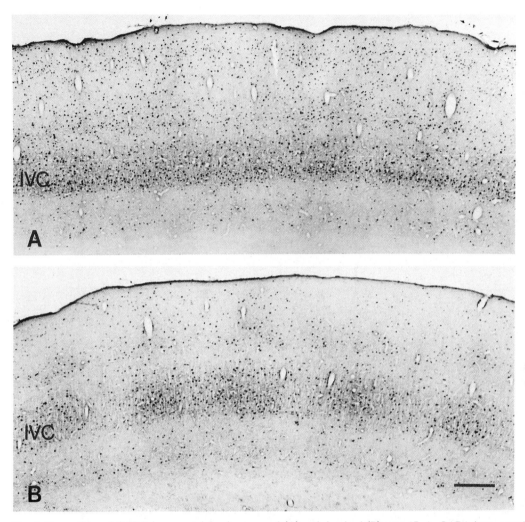

Fig. 6. Comparison of GABA immunostaining in a normal (A) and deprived (B) area 17. A. GABA immunostained somata and terminals in a normal adult monkey are very dense and virtually uniform within layer IVC. Numerous immunostained somata are also present in layers II–III.B. In an adult monkey in which activity in one retina has been eliminated, the distribution of GABA somata and terminals in layers IVA and IVC consists of alternating light and dark regions, corresponding with deprived- and normal-eye columns. In addition, the immunostaining of layers II and III is also noticeably reduced. Bar: 250 $\mu$m.

Fig. 5. Reduction in GABA and GAD immunostaining in ocular dominance stripes through layer IVC of area 17. A,B. Pair of adjacent tangential sections principally through layer IVC of a monocularly deprived young adult macaque monkey. GABA immunostaining (A) and CO staining (B) both consist of darkly and lightly stained stripes. By lining up the same blood vessel profiles in the two sections (circles) one can determine that the darkly stained GABA and CO stripes coincide and the lightly stained GABA and CO stripes coincide. C,D. Tangential sections through layer IVC of an adult macaque monkey that received monocular injections of TTX. Comparison of the positions of the same blood vessels (circles) reveals that the dark and light stripes immunostained for GAD (C) coincide with dark and light stripes histochemically stained for CO (D). E,F. GABA immunostaining (E) and CO staining (F) of layer IVC in area 17 of a Cebus monkey that received monocular injections of TTX. The irregular stripes of dark and light GABA immunostaining correspond to similar stripes of CO staining, demonstrating that in New World monkeys with ocular dominance columns, loss of input from one eye reduces the GABA immunostaining in the corresponding ocular dominance columns. Bar: 1.8 mm in A,B; 1.4 mm in C,D; 1 mm in E,F.

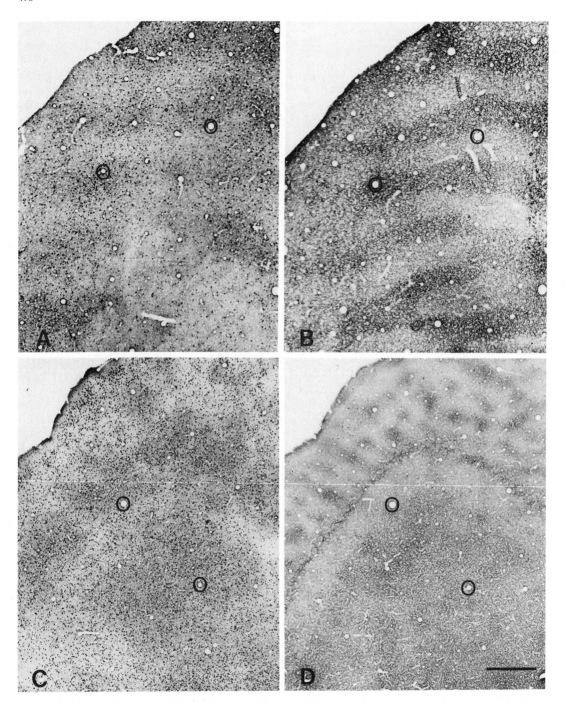

Fig. 7. Restoration of normal GABA immunostaining in area 17. A,B. GABA (A) and CO (B) staining of area 17 from a block taken as a surgical biopsy from a monkey that had received an injection of TTX into one eye. Both A and B include layer IVC and contain alternating stripes of greater and lesser staining. Comparison of the same blood vessel profiles in these two adjacent sections (circles) shows the lightly stained CO stripes (i.e., injected-eye columns) contain a reduced number of GABA somata and terminals. C,D. GABA (C) and CO staining (D) of area 17 from the same monkey as in A,B following several weeks in which the TTX injections were stopped, thus restoring binocular vision to the monkey. Stripes are seen in neither preparation and quantitative measures show that the numerical density and proportion of GABA neurons in layer IVC is returned to normal. The lighter staining in the lower left corner in C is due to the protrusion of layer V into the plane of the section. Bar: 0.6 mm in A; 1.5 mm in B.

eye (Livingstone and Hubel, 1984), is the GABA population normal. Thus, wherever the effects of monocular deprivation would effect neuronal activity, changes in GABA immunoreactivity are apparent.

(7) Reduced GABA immunostaining is seen in deprived-eye columns in layer IVC of Cebus monkeys (Carder et al., 1990), a species of New World monkeys whose primary visual cortex possesses ocular dominance columns (Hess and Edwards, 1987). However, in cat visual cortex, where ocular dominance columns also exist (Hubel and Wiesel, 1963; Shatz et al., 1977) but where individual neurons of layer IV display greater binocular properties than cells in layers IVA and IVC of monkey visual cortex (Shatz and Stryker, 1978), deprivation-induced changes in GABA and GAD expression do not occur (Bear et al.,1985; Benson et al., 1989). Thus, in species whose visual cortical neurons are dependent on one eye for the bulk of their visual input, changes in transmitter expression are apparent, but in at least one species whose neurons are driven by both eyes, the level of neuronal activity may be sufficient to maintain normal transmitter expression.

These findings have led to the conclusion that the loss of half the GABA immunostained neurons in layer IVC of deprived-eye columns represents an activity-dependent reduction in the concentration of GABA in individual cells, to the point that they can no longer be stained by immunocytochemical methods (Hendry and Jones, 1986; 1988a). Recent findings indicate, however, that the simple loss of activity is not sufficient to reduce GABA immunoreactive levels. When visually driven neuronal activity reaching area 17 from both eyes is eliminated by lesioning the LGN, the GABA immunostaining of the cortex is qualitatively and quantitatively normal: there is no sign of reduced immunostaining and the numerical density and proportion of GABA immunoreactive neurons remains normal in the deafferented visual cortex. Furthermore, the GABA immunostaining in the monocular segment of area 17, driven by a TTX-injected eye, is unaffected by the deprivation and is qualitatively and quantitatively identical to the immunostaining of normal-eye columns (unpublished observations). These data suggest that a competition between ocular dominance columns may be necessary for the chemical make-up of visual cortical neurons to be changed.

## Changes in GABA-related substances

Levels of neuronal GABA could be reduced by several mechanisms, including changes in synthesis, degradation, reuptake or intracellular processing. While not excluding the others, observations on the immunostaining for GAD suggest that reduction in the synthesis of GABA plays a major role in the plasticity of deprived-eye columns. The GAD immunoreactivity shows a 50% reduction in the numerical density of GAD-positive somata in layer IVC of deprived-eye columns (Fig. 5C–D; Hendry and Jones, 1986, 1988a; see also Hendrickson, 1982). Dramatic reductions in the density of immunostained puncta were also observed. From these results, it appears that the most likely cause for the apparent reduction in neuronal GABA levels is a reduction in GAD in half of the deprived neurons. As seen with GABA immunostaining, the reductions in GAD immunoreactivity occur most dramatically in neurons of layers IVC and IVA, where the bulk of geniculocortical axons terminate in area 17.

GABA is a powerful inhibitory neurotransmitter in the cerebral cortex which exerts many of its postsynaptic effects through the $GABA_A$ receptor subtype (Krnjevic, 1984; Sillito, 1984). This subtype possesses binding sites for GABA, benzodiazepines and barbiturates and contains a chloride channel that is opened when GABA occupies the receptor (Olsen and Tobin, 1990). Clearly, the functional consequence of reductions in the levels of GABA contained and released by

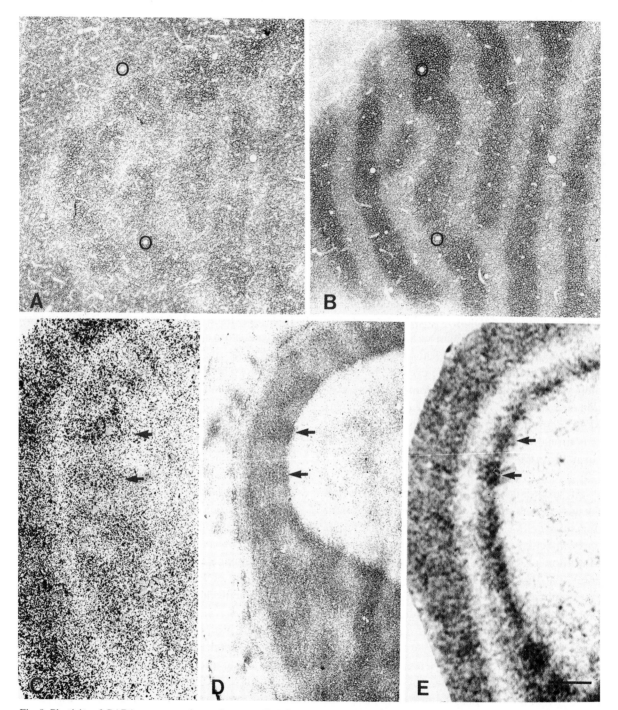

Fig. 8. Plasticity of GABA$_A$ receptors in monkey area 17. A,B. Adjacent sections through layer IVC of a monkey that had received TTX injections into one eye. The immunostaining for the $\beta_2/\beta_3$ subunit of the GABA$_A$ receptor in layer IVC is broken up into elongated darkly and lightly stained stripes (A) which, by comparing the positions of the same blood vessel profiles (circles) in the adjacent CO stained section (B) correspond to normal-eye and injected-eye columns, respectively. A similar down-regulation of receptors is also seen when the binding of [$^3$H]flunitrazepam (C) and [$^3$H]muscimol (E) is compared with the CO staining (D) in adjacent sections. Arrows indicate the positions of the same intensely radioactive, normal-eye columns, determined by comparing blood vessel profiles in the three sections. Bar: 0.6 mm in A,B; 1.0 mm in C–E.

deprived cortical neurons would depend on the response of the GABA$_A$ receptors. If, as seen for the vast majority of neurotransmitter receptors, the number or affinity of the receptors is increased when neurotransmitter levels are reduced (e.g., denervation supersensitivity; Kuffler, 1943; Brown, 1969) then the effects of reduced GABA levels might be offset by increased receptor levels or sensitivity. Such an increase in GABA$_A$ receptors has been reported for the deprived kitten visual cortex (Shaw and Cynader, 1988). If, on the other hand, the receptor levels are reduced in parallel with GABA levels then the reduction in GABA transmission would most likely be magnified. The latter appears to be the case. Immunocytochemical experiments with a monoclonal antibody to the $\beta_2/\beta_3$ subunit of the GABA$_A$ receptor (deBlas et al., 1988) show that enucleation and TTX injections reduce the levels of receptor immunoreactivity in layers IVA and IVC of the deprived-eye columns (Fig. 8A,B; Hendry et al., 1990). Radioligand binding experiments confirm a change in the receptors and demonstrate that a 25% reduction in the binding of both a GABA agonist, muscimol, and the benzodiazepine, flunitrazepam (Fig. 8C–E). Preliminary Scatchard analysis suggests that this reduction in binding occurs through reduced numbers of receptors and not in the affinity of the receptors. The immunocytochemical and ligand-binding studies indicate, then, that GABA-binding and benzodiazepine-binding subunits of the GABA$_A$ receptor in the visual cortex are reduced by loss of input from one eye. The reduced receptor levels are found in the same geniculocortical recipient layers, IVC and IVA, as those displaying reduced GABA and GAD levels (Fig. 8A,B). Together, reductions in presynaptic GABA levels and postsynaptic receptor levels might greatly reduce the levels of inhibition in deprived-eye columns.

As outlined above, a variety of neuropeptides and proteins are present in subpopulations of GABA neurons. Two of these coexisting substances, the tachykinin neuropeptide family and the calcium binding protein, paravalbumin, are present within GABA neurons of the geniculocortical recipient layer IVC: tachykinins are present in approximately half of the GABA neurons in this layer (Hendry et al., 1988b) and parvalbumin in virtually all of them (Omidi et al., 1988). Both display dramatic reductions in immunoreactive levels following TTX injections into one eye (Hendry et al., 1988b; Omidi et al., 1988). Very little tachykinin immunoreactivity remains in deprived-eye columns, as more than four out of five neurons lose their immunostaining within five days of retinal silence (Fig. 9). Parvalbumin very closely follows GABA, with reductions in the numerical density of immunostained neurons by one-half (Fig. 10C,D). These data demonstrate that molecules tied to the GABA system of the primary visual cortex remain plastic in adulthood and show rapid reductions in immunoreactive levels following loss of input from one eye.

The reduced immunoreactivity following monocular deprivation does not arise from a general reduction in protein synthesis by cortical neurons. Instead, the effects of monocular deprivation in the adult monkey visual cortex are selective, producing increased levels in certain proteins and no changes in a large number of substances. Thus, in layer IVC$\beta$ of adult monkey visual cortex, the immunoreactivity for the alpha subunit of type II calmodulin-dependent protein kinase (type II CaM kinase) is greater within neurons of deprived-eye columns than in cells of neighboring normal-eye columns and in cells of normal area 17 (Hendry and Kennedy, 1986). This increased kinase immunostaining of cortical neurons is paralleled by an increase in histochemical staining for cortical fibers that contain acetylcholinesterase (AChE), which was the first of the neurotransmitter-related proteins in adult primate area 17 found to be regulated by neuronal activity (Graybiel and Ragsdale, 1982; Horton, 1984). Many other proteins and peptides, including synapsin I (Hendry and Kennedy, 1986), neuron specific enolase, non-phosphorylated neurofilament proteins, neuropeptide Y and somatostatin show no changes in immunoreactivity with

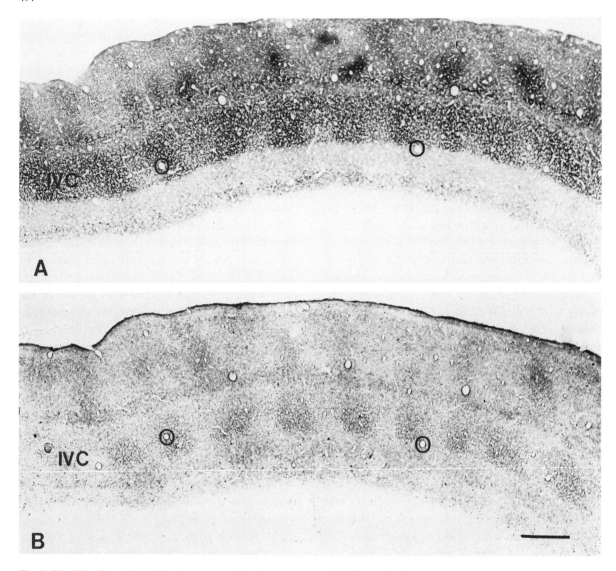

Fig. 9. Plasticity of tachykinin-like immunoreactivity in monkey area 17. CO staining (A) and tachykinin immunostaining (B) in a TTX-injected monkey. Both the CO staining and tachykinin immunostaining in layer IVC are made up of dark and light bands. Comparison of the positions of the same blood vessels (circles) in the two sections indicates that the light tachykinin immunostaining, which represents an 80% loss of immunoreactivity in somata and terminals, coincide with injected-eye columns. Normal immunostaining is found in the intact-eye columns. Bar: 1.0 mm.

monocular deprivation (unpublished observations).

## Up-regulation of neuronal proteins

The increased immunostaining for the alpha subunit of type II CaM kinase results from a greater staining of individual neurons rather than the staining of more neurons (Hendry and Kennedy, 1986). Whether the increased levels of AChE staining represent greater levels or activity of the enzyme in "old" fibers or the presence of the enzyme in "new" fibers is not known. However, recent studies suggest that increased neuronal activity does lead to the immunostaining of novel populations of cells in monkey area 17. These

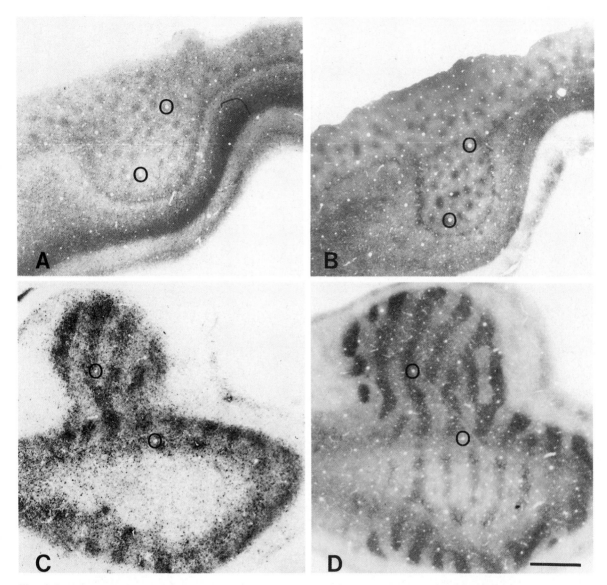

Fig. 10. Parvalbumin immunoreactivity in monkey area 17. A,B. Distribution of parvalbumin immunoreactive elements (A) and CO staining (B) in closely neighboring tangential sections through area 17 of a normal monkey. The sections, cut tangentially through layers II and III, reveal patchy immunostaining and CO staining. Comparison of the positions of the same blood vessel profiles (circles) demonstrates that the patches of parvalbumin immunoreactivity coincide with the patches of intense CO staining. In addition, parvalbumin neurons are very dense in layers IVA and IVC. C,D. Parvalbumin (C) and CO (D) staining in layer IVC of a monkey that received TTX injections into one eye. In both of the adjacent sections, stripes of intense and light staining are present. Comparison of the same blood vessel profiles (circles) demonstrates that the light immunostaining, which represents a reduction in the immunoreactivity of somata and terminals, coincides with the light CO staining (i.e., injected-eye columns). Bar: 2.5 mm in A,B; 1.5 mm in C,D.

studies have focussed on the periodic CO patches in layers II and III of area 17. As outlined, above, the CO-stained patches normally form rows that overlie the centers of ocular dominance columns for each eye. With prolonged silencing of one eye by repeated TTX injections or with chronic blur-

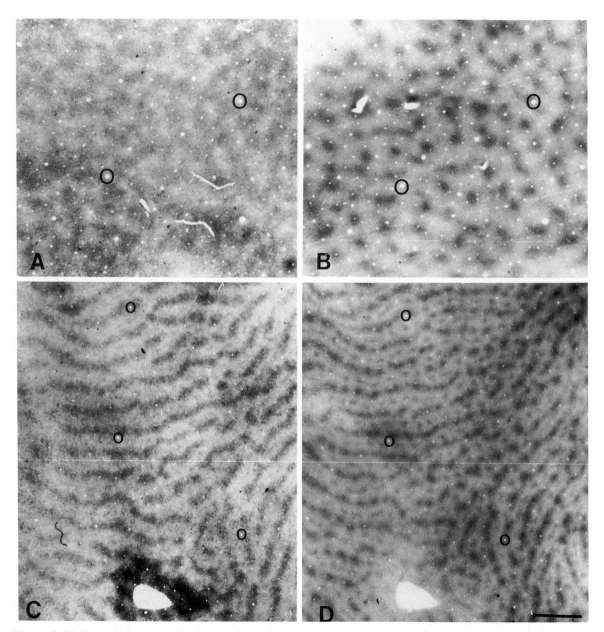

Fig. 11. Calbindin immunoreactivity in monkey area 17. A,B. Calbindin immunostaining (A) and CO staining (B) in a tangential section through layers II and III of a normal monkey. The distribution of immunoreactive somata and terminals is inhomogeneous in the superficial layers and consists of a matrix of intensely immunostained elements surrounding lightly stained core regions. Comparison of the positions of the same blood vessel profiles in the adjacent sections (circles) shows that the intense immunostaining is in the regions lightly stained for CO. The lightly immunostained cores thus correspond to the regions of the CO patches. C,D. In layers II–III of a monkey that had received injections of TTX into one eye, both the calbindin immunostaining (C) and the CO staining (D) is abnormal. In the CO stained section, every other row of patches forms a more continuous line than normal while the patches in the alternating rows are shrunken. Correlation of these sections with those through layer IVC reveals that the elongated rows lie at the centers of intact-eye columns and the rows of shrunken patches to lie at the centers of injected-eye columns. Comparison of the positions of the same blood vessel profiles (circles) in the CO and calbindin sections shows that the calbinin immunostained neurons and terminals occupy not only the inter-patch regions but also the patches of the intact-eye columns. Bar: 1.5 mm in A,B; 2.4 mm in C,D.

ring of one eye by removal of the crystalline lens, the blobs in every other row shrink while those in the alternating rows expand to fill in the gaps between them (Fig. 11; Trusk et al., 1989; Hendry et al., 1988b). Those blobs which expand overlie the centers of *normal-eye* columns. For at least the tachykinin neuropeptide family, the increased CO staining, which is indicative of increased metabolic activity, leads to immunocytochemically detectable levels in an abnormally large population of cortical neurons in and between the CO patches. These findings indicate that the tachykinin immunostaining is present in novel groups of neurons.

The increased staining of one protein, calbindin, is dramatic for the speed and precision with which it occurs. Calbindin is, in normal monkeys, present within neurons that surround the blobs (Fig. 11A,B; Celio et al., 1986; Omidi et al., 1988). However, within a matter of days following injection of TTX into one eye, the calbindin immunostaining in the rows overlying the normal-eye columns is present both in the blobs and around them (Fig. 11C,D). The novel population of calbindin neurons in the blobs closely resembles the normal population that surrounds the blobs: the cells are small, superficially-placed non-pyramidal neurons in which immunoreactivity for GABA coexists but immunoreactivity for parvalbumin is excluded. Thus, in their laminar position, morphology and chemical properties the normal and novel calbindin populations are indistinguishable, yet only one contains immunocytochemically detectable levels of the protein under normal visual conditions. One possible explanation for these findings is that the ability to synthesize calbindin is restricted to certain classes of cortical neurons; changes in neuronal activity can lead members of those classes to express or increase that synthetic capability but cannot lead members of other classes to do so.

The changes in the normal-eye columns of monocularly deprived monkeys are consistent with the observations that functionally, the inputs from the two eyes continue to compete in the cortex of adult animals. The source of the interocular interactions in area 17 is most likely the intracortical connections between neighboring columns. For the neurons of layer IVC, where the most robust changes in neuronal immunostaining occur, dendrites remain largely confined to the ocular dominance column in which their cell body is situated, but axons of these neurons and probably of neurons in other layers that innervate layer IVC cross column boundaries (Katz et al., 1989). One might predict that the intercolumnar projections and their terminations onto GABA neurons are a critical component of the regulation of immunoreactive levels in area 17. However, findings of synaptic inputs to GABA cells of layer IVC$\beta$ have implicated the geniculocortical inputs in determining which GABA cells cease to stain and which continue to stain (Hendry and Jones, 1988b). That study indicated that the subpopulation of GABA neurons which is sensitive to monocular deprivation in adults and loses its GABA immunoreactivity receives relatively few synaptic contacts on somata and proximal dendrites but that a relatively large proportion of these synapses arise from the LGN. By contrast, the neurons that continue to display GABA immunoreactivity are relatively densely innervated but receive a small proportion of their synaptic inputs from geniculocortical axons.

It is not clear if the two populations of GABA cells, those sensitive to visual deprivation and those relatively resistant to change, correspond to the different morphological classes described previously. The most closely studied class of GABA neuron in monkey area 17, the clutch cell, is reported to be lightly innervated (Kisvarday et al., 1986) and may be part of the GABA population that is sensitive to deprivation. The large basket cell is, in other areas of the monkey cerebral cortex, generally described as densely innervated (Jones and Hendry, 1984) and might on that basis be considered resistant to deprivation. However, analysis of the somal diameters of GABA in normal- and deprived-eye columns indicates that large and small neurons are equally affected by visual deprivation: in layer IVC of the deprived-eye columns, approximately half the GABA neurons over 15 $\mu$m in diameter and approximately half under 15 $\mu$m in diameter are no longer immunoreactive following loss of input from one eye (Hendry and Jones, 1988b). These data suggest that the effects of deprivation may target some classes preferentially but are probably felt by members in each of the GABA cell classes of layer IVC.

## Cellular mechanisms of neurochemical plasticity in area 17

Changes in neurotransmitter and neuropeptide immunoreactivity within the central nervous system are commonly correlated with changes in the levels of the mRNAs encoding for the particular neurotransmitter enzyme or neuropeptide (White et al., 1987; Morris et al., 1988). In area 17 of adult monkeys, the deprivation-induced changes in type II CaM kinase apparently occur through changes in mRNA levels while the changes in GAD do not. In situ hybridization histochemistry reveals dramatic increases in the levels mRNAs encoding the alpha subunit of type II CaM kinase in layer IVC of area 17 (Benson et al., 1991; Jones et al., 1991). The increased hybridization signal is found in deprived-eye columns, where increased immunoreactivity for the alpha subunit also occurs (Hendry and Kennedy, 1986); levels of mRNAs in the normal-eye columns remain unchanged (Benson et al., 1991). By contrast with these findings, in situ hybridization histochemistry reveals no changes in the levels of GAD message in area 17, either in the deprived-eye columns or the normal-eye columns of monocularly deprived monkeys (Benson et al., 1991; Jones et al., 1991). Instead, the levels of mRNA encoding for GAD appear normal throughout layers IVA and IVC. These data suggest that while the regulation of the alpha subunit of type II CaM kinase occurs at the level of gene transcription, the regulation of GAD is most likely a post-transcriptional and possibly a post-translational event.

## Functional consequences

It is generally accepted that past a certain stage in development, the primary visual area of the monkey cerebral cortex is incapable of plasticity. Certainly, there is no evidence that area 17 of the adult monkey is capable of morphological plasticity, but two lines of evidence suggest that this area displays functional plasticity. With one line of research, the effects of adult enucleation of the fixating eye in an amblyopic monkey indicates that the deprived eye is actively suppressed by the fixating eye. With removal of the fixating eye in adulthood, the psychophysically measured contrast and spectral sensitivities of a strabismic eye improve dramatically (Harweth et al., 1986). With the second line of evidence, brief reports of electrophysiologically recorded changes in area 17 of monkeys enucleated as adults indicate that the properties of single neurons may remain plastic throughout life. Thus, LeVay and co-workers (1980) report that removal of one eye in an adult monkey results not in alternating half-millimeter wide silent and visually-responsive zones but in long regions of cells driven by the remaining eye, interrupted by very narrow silent zones. These findings suggest that the amount of cortex responsive to the intact eye has expanded, even though no evidence of sprouting by geniculocortical axons was seen in a second adult enucleated monkey (LeVay et al., 1980). Both lines of research could be interpreted to suggest that basic functional properties of cortical neurons, including the responsiveness to retinal inputs, are defined by inhibitory, presumably GABAergic mechanisms. The studies outlined in this section suggest that removal of inputs from one retina, even in adulthood, reduces the level of GABA-mediated effects (by reducing both GABA and GABA receptors) in columns dominated by that retina. It may be the reduction in these GABAergic properties that allows inputs from the remaining eye to be released from a tonic inhibition, thus producing changes in the functional properties of visual cortical neurons.

## Summary

The GABA neurons of monkey area 17 are a morphologically and chemically heterogeneous population of interneurons that are normally distributed most densely within the geniculocortical recipient zones of the visual cortex. In adult monkeys deprived of visual input from one eye, the levels of immunoreactivity for GABA and GAD within neurons of these geniculocortical zones is reduced. Similar changes are seen in the levels of proteins that make up the $GABA_A$ receptor sub-type. The effects of monocular deprivation on other substances suggest that specific types of GABA neurons, such as those in which the tachykinin neuropeptide family and parvalbumin coexist with GABA, are greatly influenced by changes in visual input. That some proteins remain normal within deprived-eye neurons and that other proteins are increased indicates the changes in the GABA cells of the cortex are not the result of a general reduction in protein synthesis. Comparisons of what is known about the morphological and synaptic features of GABA cells in area 17 and the characteristics of cells affected by monocular deprivation suggests that certain classes, such as the clutch cell, may be preferential targets of deprivation. Such a selective loss of certain GABA neurons would have broad implications for the possible physiological plasticity of cortical cells, for if ongoing studies determine that specific receptive field properties are affected by monocular deprivation in adults, the correlation of functional properties and classes of GABA cells would be possible.

## References

Baker, H., Kawano, T., Margolis, F.L. and Joh, T.H. (1983) Transneuronal regulation of tyrosine hydroxylase expression in olfactory bulb of mouse and rat. *J. Neurosci.*, 3: 69–78.

Bear, M.F., Schmechel, D.E. and Ebner, F.F. (1985) Glutamic acid decarboxylase in the striate cortex of normal and monocularly deprived kittens. *J. Neurosci.*, 5: 1262–1275.

Benson, D.L., Isackson, P.J., Hendry, S.H.C. and Jones, E.G. (1989) Expression of glutamic acid decarboxylase mRNA in normal and monocularly deprived cat visual cortex. *Mol. Brain Res.*, 5: 279–287.

Benson, D.L., Isackson, P.J., Gall, C.M. and Jones, E.G. (1991) Differential effects of monocular deprivation on glutamic acid decarboxylase and type II calcium-calmodulin-dependent protein kinase gene expression in the adult monkey visual cortex. *J. Neurosci.*, 11: 31–47.

Black, I.B., Adler, J.E., Dreyfus, C.F., Jonakait, G.M., Katz, D.M., LaGamma, E.F. and Markey, K.M. (1984) Neurotransmitter plasticity at the molecular level. *Science*, 225: 1266–1270.

Blasdel, G.G. and Lund, J.S. (1982) Termination of afferent axons in macaque striate cortex. *J. Neurosci.*, 3: 1389–1413.

Brown, D.A. (1969) Responses of normal and denervated cat superior cervical ganglia to some stimulant compounds. *J. Physiol. (London)*, 201: 225–236.

Carder, R.K., Hendry, S.H.C. and Jones, E.G. (1990) Neurotransmitter regulation in ocular dominance columns of new world monkeys. *Soc. Neurosci. Abstr.*, 14: 707.

Celio, M.R., Scharer, L., Morrison, J.H., Norman, A.W. and Bloom, F.E. (1986) Calbindin immunoreactivity alternates with cytochrome c-oxidase-rich zones in some layers of the primate visual cortex. *Nature*, 323: 715–717.

Clark, S.A., Allard, T., Jenkins, W.M. and Merzenich, M.M. (1988) Receptive fields in the body-surface map in adult cortex defined by temporally correlated inputs. *Nature*, 332: 444–445.

deBlas, A.L., Vitorica, J. and Friedrich, P. (1988) Localization of the $GABA_A$ receptor in the rat brain with a monoclonal antibody to the 57,000 Mr peptide of the $GABA_A$ receptor/benzodiazepine receptor/Cl$^-$ channel complex. *J. Neurosci.*, 8: 602–614.

DeFelipe, J., Hendry, S.H.C., Jones, E.G. and Schmechel, D. (1985) Variability in the terminations of GABAergic chandelier cell axons on initial segments of pyramidal cell axons in the monkey sensory-motor cortex. *J. Comp. Neurol.*, 231: 364–384.

DeFelipe, J., Hendry, S.H.C. and Jones, E.G. (1986) A correlative electron microscopic study of basket cells and large GABAergic neurons in the monkey sensory-motor cortex. *Neuroscience*, 17: 991–1009.

DeFelipe, J., Hendry, S.H.C. and Jones, E.G. (1989) Visualization of chandelier cell axons by parvalbumin immunoreactivity in monkey cerebral cortex. *Proc. Natl. Acad. Sci. USA*, 86: 2093–2097.

DeFelipe, J., Hendry, S.H.C., Hashikawa, T., Molinari, M. and Jones, E.G. (1990) A microcolumnar structure of monkey cerebral cortex revealed by immunocytochemical studies of double bouquet cell axons. *Neuroscience*, 37: 655–673.

deLima, A.D. and Morrison, J.H. (1989) Ultrastructural analysis of somatostatin-immunoreactive neurons and synapses in the temporal and occipital cortex of the macaque monkey. *J. Comp. Neurol.*, 238: 212–227.

DeYoe, E.A., Hockfield, S., Garren, H. and Van Essen, D.C. (1990) Antibody labeling of functional subdivisions in visual cortex: Cat-301 immunoreactivity in striate and extrastriate cortex of the macaque monkey. *Vis. Neurosci.*, 5: 67–81.

Feldblum, S., Ackermann, R.F. and Tobin, A.J. (1990) Long-term increase of glutamate dcarboxylase mRNA in a rat model of temporal lobe epilepsy. *Neuron*, 5: 361–371.

Fitzpatrick, D., Itoh, K. and Diamond, I.T. (1983) The laminar organization of the lateral geniculate body and the striate cortex in the squirrel monkey, (Samiri sciureus). *J. Neurosci.*, 3: 673–702.

Fitzpatrick, D., Lund, J.S., Schmechel, D.E. and Towles, A.C. (1987) Distribution of GABAergic neurons and axon terminals in the Macaque striate cortex. *J. Comp. Neurol.*, 264: 73–91.

Frank, E., Gautvik, K. and Sommerschild, H. (1975) Cholinergic receptors at denervated mammalian motor end-plates. *Acta Physiol. Scand.*, 95: 66–76.

Freund, T.F., Martin, K.A.C., Smith, A.D. and Somogyi, P. (1983) Glutamate decarboxylase-immunoreactive terminals of golgi-impregnated axoaxonic cells and of presumed basket cells in synaptic contact with pyramidal neurons of the cat's visual cortex. *J. Comp. Neurol.*, 221: 263–278.

Graybiel, A.M. and Ragsdale, C.W., Jr. (1982) Pseudo-cholinesterase staining in the primary visual pathway of the macaque monkey. *Nature*, 299: 439–442.

Harweth, R.S., Smith, E.L. III, Duncan, G.C., Crawford, M.L.J. and von Noorden, G.K. (1986) Effects of enucleation of the fixating eye on strabismic amblyopia in monkeys. *Invest. Ophthalmol. Vis. Sci.*, 27: 245–254.

Hendrickson, A.E. (1982) The orthograde axoplasmic transport autoradiographic tracing technique and its implications for additional neuroanatomical analysis of the striate cortex. In: S. Palay and V. Chan-Palay, V. (Eds.), *Cytochemical Methods in Neuroanatomy*, New York: Alan Liss, pp. 1–16.

Hendrickson, A.E., Wilson, J.R. and Ogren, M.P. (1978) The neuroanatomical organization of pathways between the dorsal lateral geniculate nucleus and visual cortex in Old and New World monkeys. *J. Comp. Neurol.*, 182: 123–136.

Hendrickson, A.E., Hunt, S.P. and Wu, J.-Y. (1981) Immunocytochemical localization of glutamic acid decarboxylase in monkey striate cortex. *Nature*, 292: 605–607.

Hendry, S.H.C. (1991) Delayed reduction in GABA and GAD immunoreactivity of neurons in the adult monkey dorsal lateral geniculate nucleus following monocular deprivation or enucleation. *Exp. Brain Res.*, 86: 47–59.

Hendry, S.H.C. and Jones, E.G. (1986) Reduction in number of GABA immunostained neurons in deprived-eye dominance columns of monkey area 17. *Nature*, 320: 750–753.

Hendry, S.H.C. and Jones, E.G. (1988a) Activity-dependent regulation of GABA expression in the visual cortex of adult monkeys. *Neuron*, 1: 701–712.

Hendry, S.H.C. and Jones, E.G. (1988b) Synaptic organization of GABA and GABA/tachykinin immunoreactive neurons in layer IVCβ of monkey area 17. *Soc. Neurosci. Abstr.*, 14: 1123.

Hendry, S.H.C. and Kennedy, M.B. (1986) Immunoreactivity for a calmodulin-dependent protein kinase is selectively increased in macaque striate cortex afer monocular deprivation. *Proc. Natl. Acad. Sci. USA*, 83: 1536–1540.

Hendry, S.H.C., Houser, C.R., Jones, E.G. and Vaughn, J.E.

(1983) Synaptic organization of immunocytochemically identified GABA neurons in monkey sensory-motor cortex. *J. Neurocytol.*, 12: 639–660.

Hendry, S.H.C., Jones, E.G. and Emson, P.C. (1984a) Morphology, distribution, and synaptic relations of somatostatin- and neuropeptide Y-immunoreactive neurons in rat and monkey neocortex. *J. Neurosci.*, 4: 2497–2517.

Hendry, S.H.C., Jones, E.G., DeFelipe, J., Schmechel, D., Brandon, C. and Emson, P.C. (1984b) Neuropeptide-containing neurons of the cerebral cortex are also GABAergic. *Proc. Natl. Acad. Sci. USA*, 81: 6526–6530.

Hendry, S.H.C., Hockfield, S., Jones, E.G. and McKay, R.D.G. (1986) Monoclonal antibody that identifies subsets of neurons in the central visual system of monkey and cat. *Nature*, 307: 267–269.

Hendry, S.H.C., Schwark, H.D., Jones, E.G. and Yan, J. (1987) Numbers and proportions of GABA-immunoreactive neurons in different areas of monkey cerebral cortex. *J. Neurosci.*, 7: 1503–1519.

Hendry, S.H.C., Jones, E.G., Hockfield, S. and McKay, R.D.G. (1988a) Neuronal populations stained with the monoclonal antibody Cat-301 in the mammalian cerebral cortex and thalamus. *J. Neurosci.*, 8: 518–542.

Hendry, S.H.C., Jones, E.G. and Burstein, N. (1988b) Activity-dependent regulation of tachykinin-like immunoreactivity in neurons of monkey visual cortex. *J. Neurosci.*, 8: 1225–1238.

Hendry, S.H.C., Jones, E.G., Emson, P.C., Lawson, D.E.M., Heizmann, C.W. and Streit, P. (1989) Two classes of cortical GABA neurons defined by differential calcium binding protein immunoreactivities. *Exp. Brain Res.*, 76: 467–472.

Hendry, S.H.C., Fuchs, J., deBlas, A.L. and Jones, E.G. (1990) Distribution and plasticity of immunocytochemically localized GABA$_A$ receptors in adult monkey visual cortex. *J. Neurosci.*, 10: 2438–2450.

Hess, D.T. and Edwards, M.A. (1987) Anatomical demonstration of ocular segregation in the retinogeniculocortical pathway of the New World capuchin monkey (Cebus apella). *J. Comp. Neurol.*, 264: 409–420.

Horton, J.C. (1984) Cytochrome oxidase patches: a new cytoarchitectonic feature of primary visual cortex. *Phil. Trans. R. Soc. B (London)*, 304: 199–253.

Horton, J.C. and Hubel, D.H. (1981) Regular patchy distribution of cytochrome oxidase staining in primary visual cortex of macaque monkey. *Nature*, 292: 762–764.

Houser, C.R., Vaughn, J.E., Hendry, S.H.C., Jones, E.G. and Peters, A. (1984) GABA neurons in the cerebral cortex. In: E.G. Jones and A. Peters (Eds.), *Cerebral Cortex, Vol. 2*, New York: Plenum Press, pp. 63–89.

Hubel, D.H. and Wiesel, T.N. (1962) Receptive fields, binocular interaction and functional architecture in the cat's visual cortex. *J. Physiol. (London)*, 283: 101–120.

Hubel, D.H., Wiesel, T.N. and LeVay, S. (1977) Plasticity of ocular dominance columns in monkey striate cortex. *Phil. Trans. R. Soc. (London)*, 278: 131–163.

Humphrey, A.L. and Hendrickson, A.E. (1983) Background and stimulus-induced patterns of high metabolic activity in the visual cortex (area 17) of the squirrel and macaque monkey. *J. Neurosci.*, 3: 345–358.

Itaya, S.K., Itaya, P.W. and Van Hoesen, G.W. (1984) Intracortical termination of the retino-geniculo-striate pathway studied with transsynaptic tracer (wheat germ agglutinin-horseradish peroxidase) and cytochrome oxidase staining in the macaque monkey. *Brain Res.*, 304: 303–310.

Jones, E.G. (1975) Varieties and distributions of non-pyramidal cells in the somatic sensory cortex of the squirrel monkey. *J. Comp. Neurol.*, 160: 205–268.

Jones, E.G. and Hendry, S.H.C. (1984) Basket cells. In: A. Peters and E.G. Jones (Eds.), *Cerebral Cortex, Vol. 1*, New York: Plenum Press, pp. 309–366.

Jones, E.G. and Hendry, S.H.C. (1986) Co-localization of GABA and neuropeptides in neocortical neurons. *TINS*, 9: 71–76.

Jones, E.G., DeFelipe, J., Hendry, S.H.C. and Maggio, J.E. (1988) A study of tachykinin-immunoreactive neurons in monkey cerebral cortex. *J. Neurosci.*, 8: 1206–1224.

Jones, E.G., Benson, D.L., Hendry, S.H.C. and Isackson, P.J. (1991) Activity-dependent regulation of gene expression in adult monkey visual cortex. *Cold Sring Harbor Symp. Quant. Biol.*, in press.

Kaas, J.H., Merzenich, M.M. and Killackey, H.P. (1983) The reorganization of somatosensory cortex following peripheral nerve damage in adult and developing mammals. *Ann. Rev. Neurosci.*, 6: 325–356.

Katz, L.C., Gilbert, C.D. and Wiesel, T.N. (1989) Local circuits and ocular dominance columns in monkey striate cortex. *J. Neurosci.*, 9: 1389–1399.

Kisvarday, Z.F., Cowey, A. and Somogyi, P. (1986) Synaptic relationships of a type of GABA-immunoreactive neuron (clutch cell), spiny stellate cells and lateral geniculate nucleus afferents in layer IVC of the monkey striate cortex. *Neuroscience*, 19: 741–761.

Kosaka, T., Kosaka, K., Hama, K., Wu, J-Y and Nagatsu, I. (1987) Differential effect of functional olfactory deprivation on the GABAergic and catecholaminergic traits in the rat main olfactory bulb. *Brain Res.*, 413: 197–203.

Krnjević, K. (1984) Neurotransmitters in cerebral cortex. In: E.G. Jones and A. Peters (Eds.), *Cerebral Cortex, Vol. 2*, New York: Plenum Press, pp. 39–61.

Kuffler, S.W. (1943) Specific excitability of the endplate region in normal and denervated muscle. *J. Neurophysiol.*, 6: 99–110.

Kuljis, R.O. and Rakic, P. (1989) Neuropeptide Y-containing neurons are situated predominantly outside cytochrome oxidase puffs in macaque visual cortex. *Visual Neurosci.*, 2: 57–62.

LaGamma, E.F., White, J.D., Adler, J.E., Krause, J.E., McKelvy, J.F. and Black, I.B. (1985) Depolarization regulates adrenal preproenkephalin mRNA. *Proc. Natl. Acad. Sci. USA*, 82: 8252–8255.

LeVay, S., Wiesel, T.N. and Hubel, D.H. (1980) The development of ocular dominance columns in normal and visually deprived monkeys. *J. Comp. Neurol.*, 191: 1–51.

Lewis, D.A. and Lund, J.S. (1990) Heterogeneity of chandelier neurons in monkey neocortex: corticotropin-releas-ing-factor- and parvalbumin-immunoreactive populations. *J. Comp. Neurol.*, 293: 599–615.

Livingstone, M.S. and Hubel, D.H. (1984) Anatomy and physiology of a color system in the primate visual cortex. *J. Neurosci.*, 4: 309–356.

Lømo, T. and Rosenthal, J. (1972) Control of ACh sensitivity by muscle activity in the rat. *J. Physiol.*, 221: 493–513.

Lund, J.S. (1987) Local circuit neurons of macaque monkey striate cortex: I. Neurons of laminae 4C and 5A. *J. Comp. Neurol.*, 257: 60–92.

Lund, J.S., Hawken, M.J. and Parker, A.J. (1988) Local circuit neurons of macaque monkey striate cortex: II. Neurons of laminae 5B and 6. *J. Comp. Neurol.*, 276: 1–29.

Lynch, G., Matthews, D.A. and Mosko, S. (1972) Induced acetylcholinesterase-rich layer in rat dentate gyrus following entorhinal lesions. *Brain Res.*, 42: 311–338.

Marin-Padilla, M. (1969) Origin of the pericellular baskets of the pyramidal cells of the human motor cortex: A golgi study. *Brain Res.*, 14: 633–646.

Morris, B., Feasey, K.J., ten Bruggencate, G., Herz, A. and Höllt, V. (1988) Electrical stimulation in vivo increases the expression of proenkephalin mRNA and decreases the expression of prodynorphin mRNA in rat hippocampal granule cells. *Proc. Natl. Acad. Sci. USA*, 85: 3226–3230.

Mulligan, K.A., VanBrederode, J.F.M. and Hendrickson, A.E. (1989) The lectin Vicia villosa labels a distinct subset of GABAergic cells in macaque visual cortex. *Visual Neurosci.*, 2: 63–72.

Naegle, J.R. and Barnstable, C.J. (1989) Molecular determinants of GABAergic local-circuit neurons in the visual cortex. *TINS*, 12: 28–34.

Neve, R.L. and Bear, M.F. (1989) Visual experience regulates gene expression in the developing striate cortex. *Proc. Natl. Acad. Sci. USA*, 86: 4781–4784.

Olsen, R.W. and Tobin, A.J. (1990) Molecular biology of $GABA_A$ receptors. *FASEB J.*, 4: 1469–1480.

Omidi, K., Hendry, S.H.C., Jones, E.G. and Emson, P.C. (1988) Organization and plasticity of GABA neuronal sub-populations in monkey area 17, identified by coexistence of calcium binding proteins. *Soc. Neurosci. Abstr.*, 14: 188.

Peters, A., Proskauer, C.C. and Ribak, C.E. (1982) Chandelier cells in rat visual cortex. *J. Comp. Neurol.*, 206: 397–416.

Rakic, P., Goldman-Rakic, P.S. and Gallager, D. (1988) Quantitative autoradiography of major neurotransmitter receptors in the monkey striate and extrastriate cortex. *J. Neurosci.*, 8: 3670–3690.

Rockel, A.J., Hiorns, R.W. and Powell, T.P.S. (1980) The basic uniformity in structure of the neocortex. *Brain*, 103: 221–244.

Shatz, C.J., Lindström, S. and Wiesel, T.N. (1977) The distribution of afferents representing the right and left eyes in the cat's visual cortex. *Brain Res.*, 131: 103–116.

Shatz, C.J. and Stryker, M.P. (1978) Ocular dominance in layer IV of the cat's visual cortex and the effects of monocular deprivation. *J. Physiol. (London)*, 281: 267–283.

Shaw, C. and Cynader, M. (1986) Laminar distribution of receptors in monkey (Macaca fascicularis) geniculostriate system. *J. Comp. Neurol.*, 248: 301–312.

Shaw, C. and Cynader, M. (1988) Unilateral eyelid sutrue increases GABA$_A$ receptors in cat visual cortex. *Dev. Brain. Res.*, 40: 148–153.

Sillito, A.M. (1984) Functional considerations of the operation of GABAergic inhibitory processes in the visual cortex. In: E.G. Jones and A. Peters (Eds.), *Cerebral Cortex, Vol. 2*, New York: Plenum Press, pp. 91–117.

Somogyi, P. and Cowey, A. (1981) Combined golgi and electron microscopic study on the synapses formed by double bouquet cells in the visual cortex of the cat and monkey. *J. Comp. Neurol.*, 195: 547–566.

Somgyi, P. and Soltész, I. (1986) Immunogold demonstration of GABA in synaptic terminals of intracellularly recorded, horseradish peroxidase-filled basket cells and clutch cells in the cat's visual cortex. *Neuroscience*, 19: 1051–1065.

Somogyi, P., Cowey, A., Halász, N. and Freund, T.F. (1981) Vertical organization of neurones accumulating $^3$H-GABA in visual cortex of rhesus monkey. *Nature*, 294: 761–763.

Somogyi, P., Freund, T.F. and Cowey, A. (1982) The axo-axonic interneuron in the cerebral cortex of the rat, cat and monkey. *Neuroscience*, 7: 2577–2607.

Somogyi, P., Kisvárday, Z.F., Martin, K.A.C. and Whitteridge, D. (1983a) Synaptic connections of morphologically identified and physiologically characterized large basket cells in the striate cortex of cat. *Neuroscience*, 10: 261–294.

Somogyi, P., Cowey, A., Kisvárday, Z.F., Freund, T.F. and Szentágothai, J. (1983b) Retrograde transport of γ-amino[$^3$H]butyric acid reveals specific interlaminar connections in the striate cortex of monkey. *Proc. Natl. Acad. Sci. USA*, 80: 2385–2389.

Somogyi, P., Kisvárday, Z.F., Freund, T.F. and Cowey, A. (1984) Characterization by golgi impregnation of neurons that accumulate $^3$H-GABA in the visual cortex of monkey. *Exp. Brain Res.*, 53: 295–303.

Trusk, T.C., Kaboord, W.S. and Wong-Riley, M.T.T. (1990) Effects of monocular enucleation, tetrodotoxin, and lid suture on cytochrome-oxidase reactivity in supragranular puffs of adult macaque striate cortex. *Vis. Neurosci.*, 4: 185–204.

Wall, J.T., Kaas, J.H., Sur, M., Nelson, R.J., Felleman, D.J. and Merzenich, M.M. (1986) Functional reorganization in somatosensory cortical areas 3b and 1 of adult monkeys after median nerve repair: Possible relationships to sensory recovery in humans. *J. Neurosci.*, 6: 218–233.

Warren, R., Tremblay, N. and Dykes, R.W. (1989) Quantitative study of glutamic acid decarboxylase-immunoreactive neurons and cytochrome oxidase activity in normal and partially deafferented rat hindlimb somatosensory cortex. *J. Comp. Neurol.*, 288: 583–592.

Welker, E., Soriano, E., Dörfl, J. and Van der Loos, H. (1989) Plasticity in the barrel cortex of the adult mouse: transient increase of GAD-immunoreactivity following sensory stimulation. *Exp. Brain Res.*, 78: 659–664.

Werner, L., Winkelmann, E., Koglin, A., Neser, J. and Rodewohl, H. (1989) A golgi deimpregnation study of neurons in the rhesus monkey visual cortex (areas 17 and 18). *Anat. Embryol.*, 180: 583–597.

White, J.D., Gall, C.M. and McKelvy, J. (1987) Enkephalin biosynthesis and enkephalin gene expression are increased in hippocampal mossy fibers following a unilateral lesion of the hilus. *J. Neurosci.*, 7: 753–759.

Wong-Riley, M. and Carroll, E.W. (1984) The effect of impulse blockage on cytochrome oxidase activity in the monkey visual cortex. *Nature*, 307: 262–264.

R.R. Mize, R.E. Marc and A.M. Sillito (Eds.)
Progress in Brain Research, Vol. 90
© 1992 Elsevier Science Publishers B.V. All rights reserved

CHAPTER 23

# Molecular properties of GABAergic local-circuit neurons in the mammalian visual cortex

Colin J. Barnstable [1,2], Toshio Kosaka [3], Janice R. Naegele [1] and Yasuyoshi Arimatsu [4]

[1]Department of Ophthalmology and Visual Science and [2] Section of Neurobiology, Yale University School of Medicine, 333 Cedar Street, New Haven, CT 06510, USA, [3] Department of Anatomy, Faculty of Medicine, Kyushu University, Higashiku, Fukuoka 812 and [4] Laboratory of Neuromorphology, Mitsubishi Kasei Institute of Life Sciences, 11 Minamiooya, Machida-Shi, Tokyo, Japan

## Introduction

GABA is well established as the major inhibitory neurotransmitter in the mammalian CNS. In the visual and sensorimotor regions of the neocortex approximately 20% of neurons are thought to use GABA (Hendry and Jones, 1981; Gabbott and Somogyi, 1986). Almost all cortical GABAergic neurons studied so far form local inhibitory connections and thus are probably involved in modulatory actions that, for example, shape the receptive field properties of other cortical neurons. There is increasing evidence that distinct subpopulations of GABAergic neurons carry out separate functions, although the number of these and the ways in which their functional properties are related to other ways of classifying the cells is not yet clear.

It is likely that morphological and functional features unique to a particular subpopulation of GABAergic neurons are mediated by molecules unique to that subpopulation, and that identification of these molecules will ultimately provide a mechanistic basis for these features. In this chapter evidence is provided to justify this view. In addition to presenting the evidence, however, we would like to review briefly some of the other work on GABAergic neuron structure and function that provides a context in which to discuss our own work. Much of this material is covered in greater depth in other chapters.

## Morphological analysis of local circuit neurons

In many areas of cortex, including the visual cortex, neurons have been characterized extensively by the Golgi method. About seven distinct types of local circuit neuron have been classified on the basis of axonal arborizations and dendritic patterns (Jones, 1975; Lund et al., 1979; Peters and Regidor, 1981; Meyer and Ferres-Torres, 1984; Lund, 1987). Many of these types are now known to accumulate [$^3$H]GABA, or their terminals can be labelled immunocytochemically for GABA or the GABA synthesizing enzyme glutamic acid decarboxylase (GAD), indicating that they are GABAergic inhibitory neurons. The specific types are generally known by names given to reflect unique features of their axonal or dendritic branching patterns. For example, the large basket cells and small basket cells (also called "clutch" cells) are named for the pericellular endings they form on the cell bodies of pyramidal cells. Similarly, the chandelier cell type is named for the candelabra-like axonal endings formed on the initial axon segments of pyramidal cells. Other types include bipolar, double bouquet, horsetail and neurogliaform cells (also called "clewed" or

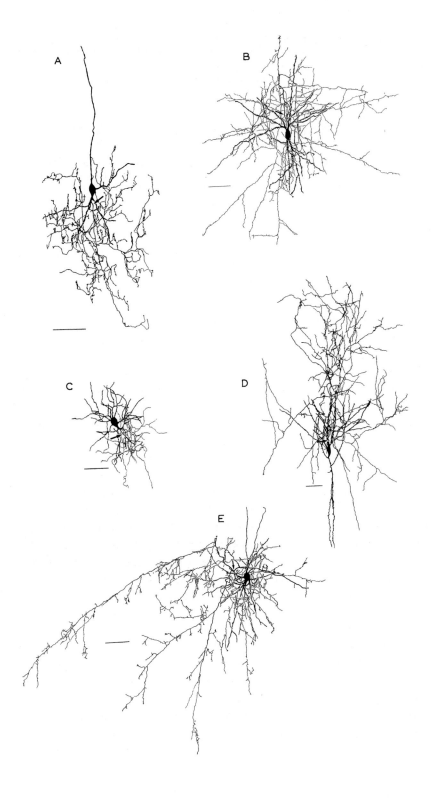

"spiderweb" cells). Neurogliaform cells have a distinctive local axon plexus which intertwines with short recurring dendrites, giving them the appearance of a loose ball of thread. While many of these names are now well accepted it is worth pointing out that many other names and classifications exist in the literature and that general agreement for all species does not yet exist (see discussion in chapters in Peters and Jones, 1984a).

Extensive Golgi studies have been carried out in the cat, monkey and rat (Peters and Jones, 1984b and references therein). In Fig. 1 are shown five types of local circuit neuron identified by Golgi staining of cat visual cortex (Meyer, 1983; Meyer and Ferres-Torres, 1984). The dendritic patterns of all the cell types are quite similar. The axonal arbors, however, show distinctive differences. Some cell types, for example the small basket cells, are often not completely stained in adult tissue because of myelination of their fine axons. This has resulted in very few of these cells being described in the literature. As well as the potential problem of incomplete staining of cells, the randomness of the Golgi method makes it difficult to obtain good quantitative estimates of cell numbers and distributions.

### Intracellular staining of GABAergic neurons

A number of GABAergic neurons have also been characterized by intracellular filling with horseradish peroxidase or the fluorescent dye Lucifer yellow. The difficulties of this approach are indicated by the report in Kisvarday et al. (1985), that three small basket, or "clutch", cells were filled during 4 years of work involving the filling of many hundreds of neurons. Thus, the numbers of cells from which conclusions can be drawn remains small, but they clearly include a number of physiological types. For example a neuron in layer 4c of cat cortex, with the characteristics of a GABAergic cell, was found to have a simple receptive field and to have an axonal arbor entirely confined to layer 4 (Gilbert and Wiesel, 1979). Two small basket cells were found in other experiments to have complex receptive fields and to have axonal arbors in layers 4a and 4b and to send axons into layers 5 and 6 (Kisvarday et al., 1985). Even from such limited data it can be concluded that GABAergic neurons have a range of physiological properties. More cells, however, are needed to be able to relate different physiological properties to different morphological subclasses.

### Synaptic interactions of GABAergic neurons

GABAergic neurons are found in all cortical layers and in the white matter. In visual cortex, a number of cells have been studied in great detail at the ultrastructural level. For example, serial section EM analysis of a layer 5/6 cell has provided evidence for intralaminar inhibitory circuits in cat area 17 (Kisvarday et al., 1987). Similarly, a recent study has documented the physiological and morphological characteristics of a layer 1 GABAergic neuron from kitten area 17 (Martin et al., 1989). For the purposes of this chapter, however, only a brief review of the features of layer 4 cells will be given.

---

Fig. 1. Some principal types of local-circuit neurons in layers II–III and IV of cat visual cortex, stained by Golgi impregnation. A. Neuron with chandelier-type axon forms very specfic synaptic contacts on the initial segments of nearby pyramidal cell axons. B. Multipolar neuron of layer IV with arcade axonal arbor. C. The neurogliaform cell type, also termed "clewed" or "spiderweb", is identified on the basis of both dendritic and axonal patterns. The short, recurving dentrites of this neurogliaform cell branch only near the soma and overlap closely with compact and highly branched axons. D. The bitufted dendrites of a neuron in layer IV with ascending axon plexus distinguish this type. E. Basket cells form semicircular axonal endings on somata of local and more distant pyradmidal and non-pyramidal cells. The nearly complete staining of this immature basket cell is a situation rarely observed in the mature cat, where most of the axon is myelinated and resists Golgi impregnation. Note that the right-hand portion of the axon has not been included (asterisk). Arrows indicate the initial axon segments. Scales are 100 $\mu$m. (Taken from Naegele and Barnstable, 1989.)

The inputs to the layer 4 GABAergic cells have been partially established but the data are far from complete. Studies of afferent input into layer 4 of area 17 from the LGN has established that most of the synaptic contacts are made with spiny stellate cells which are thought to be excitatory, but a significant proportion are made with the aspiny GABAergic cell types (Valverde, 1985). Separate sets of GABAergic neurons in layer 4 were shown to receive either X- or Y-type input from geniculocortical afferents. Those that received X-type were smaller (15 $\mu$m average diameter) than those that received Y-type inputs (24 $\mu$m average diameter) (Freund et al., 1985). It is likely that much geniculate input reaches the layer 4 GABAergic neurons through the intermediate step of the layer 4 spiny stellate cells.

Another source of input into layer 4 is from layer 6 pyramidal cells. Several studies have shown that most of the synapses made by the collaterals of layer 6 cells are onto dendritic shafts of layer 4 cells. The proportion of these that might be part of GABAergic cells is not clear. Using morphological criteria 36% of dendrites were identified as being from smooth stellate cells, which are generally assumed to be GABAergic (McGuire et al., 1984). By combining intracellular marking of a layer 6 cell with immunocytochemical labelling of sections with a GABA antiserum, it was estimated that only 14% of all postsynaptic targets were on dendritic shafts containing GABA, whereas 56% were on GABA negative dendritic shafts and 30% were on dendritic spines (Kisvardy et al., 1985). Assuming that the real number lies somewhere between 36 and 14%, or that the results represent some of the natural heterogeneity in layer 6 cells, it is clear that a major source of input to these cells comes from layer 6 pyramidal cells. Other important inputs to GABAergic neurons in area 17 are thought to come from other cortical and subcortical regions. For example, inputs from the prestriate cortex and pulvinar may regulate the activity of chandelier cells as part of a feedback regulatory loop (Ogren and Hendricksen, 1976; van Essen, 1984).

The synaptic contacts made by GABAergic neurons in visual cortex have been analysed in a few cases (Kisvarday et al., 1985, 1986). Serial section analysis of 321 synaptic boutons from two small basket cells in cat area 17 showed three types of synaptic target. 20–30% of boutons were on cell bodies, 35–50% on dendritic shafts and 30% were on dendritic spines. A random sample of 159 synapses made by three small basket cells whose cell bodies were in layer 4C$\alpha$ showed that they also contacted cell bodies (10–17%), dendritic shafts (43.8–58.5%) and spines (20.8–46.3%). In both sets of experiments postsynaptic cells were generally not GABAergic but included spiny stellate, star pyramid and pyramidal cells. This electron microscopic sampling was confirmed in a more complete light microscopic estimate of boutons and numbers of cells contacted. For one of the cells, 2733 boutons were counted in layer 4 and 143 in layers 5 and 6. Thus, 95% of the synaptic output of this cell was confined to layer 4. The two cells studied made contact with 454 and 345 neuronal cell bodies respectively, and over 90% of these contacts were in layer 4.

The synapses made by basket cells are found on different subcellular sites and probably carry out different functions. Those on spines probably modulate individual synaptic inputs, those on dendritic shafts can affect groups of inputs and those on cell bodies can affect the overall responsiveness of a cell. Thus, this cell type is likely to be part of several inhibitory circuits of different degrees of selectivity. A different type of function is thought to be carried out by the chandelier type of GABAergic neuron. Because these cells form synapses on the initial segment of pyramidal cell axons, they are probably responsible for regulating the output of particular cells. As mentioned above, substantial input to the chandelier cells is thought to come from regions that are targets of the pyramidal cells to which they are presynaptic. This sets up the possibility of feedback regulatory loops but such loops have yet to be demonstrated experimentally.

Studies of the type described above are arduous and have so far been able to provide few insights into the nature and function of GABAergic circuitry in visual cortex. Over the past few years we have begun an approach that we believe can add significantly to the methods already available so as to make it easier to identify cells of interest and ultimately to ask focussed and quantitative questions about the nature and function of particular types of circuits in visual cortex. This approach is based on the assumption that different functional subclasses of neurons in the visual cortex express unique molecules. With probes against these molecules it will be possible to define the distribution of cell types in a quantitative manner and also to combine labelling methods with other methods that allow estimates of the numbers of contacts between different types of cells to be made more rapidly than now possible.

## New molecular markers of GABAergic local circuit neurons

Production of monoclonal antibodies against cell types of one CNS region, the retina, has been an invaluable approach both for identifying new molecules in this tissue and for providing markers to study retinal development and function in culture (Barnstable, 1980, 1987, 1991; Akagawa and Barnstable, 1986; Sparrow et al., 1990). In particular, this work has shown that monoclonal antibodies can be generated against each of the major subclasses of neurons and glia present in the tissue. Some years ago we reasoned that a similar approach would also provide useful information in primary visual cortex.

Because we had no way of predicting whether detectable cell-type specific molecules would be cytoplasmic, or membrane associated, or both, we immunized mice with a homogenate of cat area 17. From the monoclonal antibodies prepared from these mice, two are of relevance for this chapter, VC1.1 and VC5.1 (Arimatsu et al., 1987). Both antibodies labelled subpopulations of neurons in area 17, with the labelled cells found

primarily in layer 4 with some in layers 5 and 6 (Fig. 2). While the labelled cells were clearly not pyramidal, little more could be discerned from this experiment because only the cell bodies and proximal dendrites were labelled. Double-labelling experiments revealed that within area 17, 83% of the cells that were labelled by VC5.1 were also labelled by VC1.1. All the VC1.1 positive cells were also VC5.1 positive leading to the conclusion that both antibodies were labelling essentially the same cell population.

Further double-labelling studies were performed with antibody VC1.1 and an antiserum recognizing GABA (Naegele et al., 1988). Because VC1.1 labelled membranes, and GABA is cytoplasmic, we were able to carry out enzyme-coupled immunocytochemistry using horseradish peroxidase and alkaline phosphatase, rather than the more usual two-color immunofluorescence.

The double-labelled neurons varied in both shape and size but they were generally medium to large, bipolar or multipolar cells. More than 98% of VC1.1 positive cells also contained GABA, indicating that essentially all the VC1.1 positive cells were GABAergic. In the sections studied, double-labelled cells represented approximately 35% of the total GABAergic population. Most of the GABA-IR neurons not labelled by VC1.1 were found in layer 1 and the upper half of layers 2 and 3, although some GABA + /VC1.1 − cells were found in layer 4 and layers 5 and 6. These results are presented diagrammatically in Fig. 3 which shows reconstructions of closely spaced sections in which all labelled cell bodies are marked. GABA-IR cell bodies were most numerous in superficial layers of area 17 and their numbers diminished in deeper layers (Fig. 3A). By contrast, VC1.1-immunoreactive, and double-labelled cells, were rare in layer 1 and and more frequent in middle and deeper layers (Fig. 3B). That all the cells labelled by VC1.1 were a distinct subset of GABAergic cells was also suggested by cell body size measurements. The diameters of GABA-IR cells cut in clear cross section ranged from 10 to 30 $\mu$m with a mean of 15.5

508

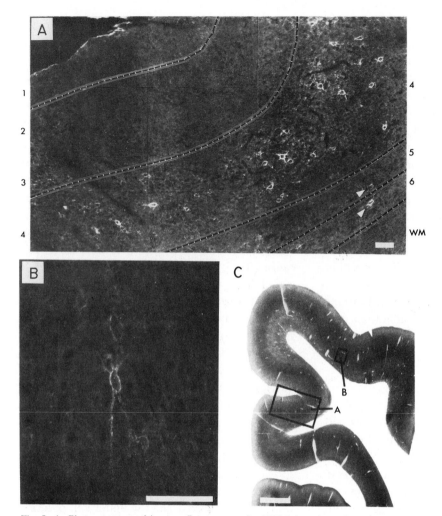

Fig. 2. A. Photomontage of immunofluorescence for VC5.1 in a frontal section of rostral area 17. Cortical layers (indicated by *numerals*) were determined by the staining pattern for cytochrome oxidase activity. B. Immunofluorescence photomicrograph for VC5.1 in area 18 in the same section as A. C. Cytochrome oxidase staining in a section adjacent to that shown in A and B. In area 17, layer 4 is distinctly identified by heavy staining for the enzyme. Areas corresponding to A and B are shown by rectangles. Scale: A and B, 100 $\mu$m; C, 1 mm. (Taken from Arimatsu et al., 1987.)

$\mu$m. The double labelled cells had diameters with a range from 12 to 26 $\mu$m with a mean of 18.0 $\mu$m.

Antibody VC5.1 appears to react only with cat tissue but VC1.1 reacts with many species. The pattern of reactivity in rat cortex is essentially the same as in cat. As shown in Fig. 4, most of the labelled cells are in layer 4, with a few in layers 2 and 3 and some in layers 5 and 6. The proportion of GABA-IR cells that were also VC1.1 immunoreactive differed somewhat between rat and cat. In rat occipital cortex only 13% of GABA-IR cells were labelled with VC1.1 and, as in cat, essentially all VC1.1 labelled cells were GABA-IR. The significance of these differences in the proportions of VC1.1 labelled GABA-IR cells is not clear because the areas used for cell counts was not identical and there are clear regional variations in the proportions of double labelled cells. For example, in rat the proportion varies from 13% in occipital cortex to 29% in parietal cortex.

Some of the patterns of immunocytochemical labelling given by VC1.1 described above, and some of the biochemical properties of the antigen recognized by VC1.1 (see below), were similar to reported patterns given by another antibody HNK-1 (Schwarting et al., 1987; Yamamoto et al., 1988). Antibody HNK-1 was originally generated against human natural killer cells (Abo and Balch, 1981). Subsequent studies have shown that it reacts with a carbohydrate epitope containing a sulphated glucuronic acid (Ariga et al., 1987). This carbohydrate moiety is expressed on a number of polypeptides that appear to have in common the property that they can be classified as cell adhesion molecules (reviewed in Naegele and Barnstable, 1991). Biochemical experiments have led to the estimate that 15–20% of the N-CAM polypeptides from mouse brain carry the HNK-1 epitope (Kruse et al., 1984).

The similarities between VC1.1 and HNK-1 prompted us to examine whether the two antibodies were recognizing the same cell groups in rat cortex (Kosaka et al., 1990; Naegele and Barnstable, 1991). Because both antibodies are mouse IgM, the usual methods of double-labelling could not be used. To overcome this problem, adjacent thick sections were taken and separately labelled with the two antibodies after which the paired surfaces were examined for cells cut in half by the sectioning. The result shown in Fig. 5 clearly shows identity of labelled cell bodies and even of larger dendrites cut in cross section (Kosaka et al., 1990).

### The biochemical basis of VC1.1 immunoreactivity

On immunoblots of cat cortex, antibody VC1.1 recognized a major band of 95–105 kDa and two other bands of approximately 145 kDa and 170 kDa (Arimatsu et al., 1987). (Other higher molecular weight molecules also reacted, some of which are discussed below, but these were not revealed by the gel system used in these early experiments.) On similar immunoblots of rat cortex only the 140 kDa and 170 kDa bands were strongly labelled. In both species a number of other, weakly labelled, bands were also detected.

Antibody VC5.1 labelled only immunoblots of cat tissue where two bands of 97 kDa and 150 kDa were detected. Subcellular fractionation studies showed other differences between the antigens recognized by VC1.1 and VC5.1. The VC1.1 antigens were integral membrane proteins whereas the VC5.1 antigens were soluble in aqueous buffers.

Another difference between the two sets of antigens was found following enzymatic digestion. Cat cortical membranes were digested with *N*-

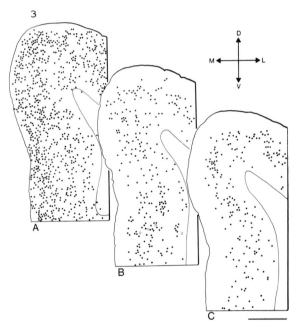

Fig. 3. Charts of computer-reconstructed sections showing positions of immunoreactive cell bodies in three different sections through the medial bank of cat area 17. Solid dots indicate the positions of all GABA-immunoreactive cells in a section stained with anti-GABA antiserum (A; n = 400). In B, stained with both VC1.1 and anti-GABA antiserum, all the double-labeled and GABA-/VC1.1+ cells are shown (GABA +/VC1.1+ cells, solid dots; n = 264; GABA-/VC1.1+ cells, open circles; n = 4). Quantitative comparison indicated that approximately 35% of GABAergic cells express the VC1.1 antigen. A control section stained only with VC1.1 is shown in C (n = 196). The 27% increase in the number of VC1.1-immunoreactive cells in B, as compared with C, may be a result of variability of immunoreactive staining from section to section. Scale: 1 mm. (Taken from Naegele et al., 1988.)

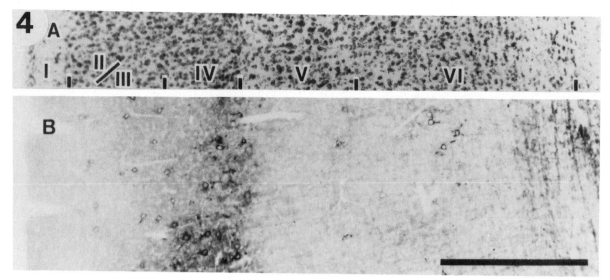

Fig. 4. A,B. Two adjacent sections of a part of rat cortex stained with cresyl-violet (A) and immunostained with monoclonal antibody VC1.1 (B), depicting the laminar distribution of VC1.1 positive cells. Scale: 500 μm. (Taken from Kosaka et al., 1989.)

glycosidase F which removes N-linked carbohydrate groups at their asparagine attachment site. Immunoblots of treated membranes showed that all VC1.1 immunoreactivity was removed but the

VC5.1 immunoreactivity was unaltered, indicating that VC1.1 antigens contain N-linked carbohydrate groups (Fig. 6).

The similarities between the immunocyto-

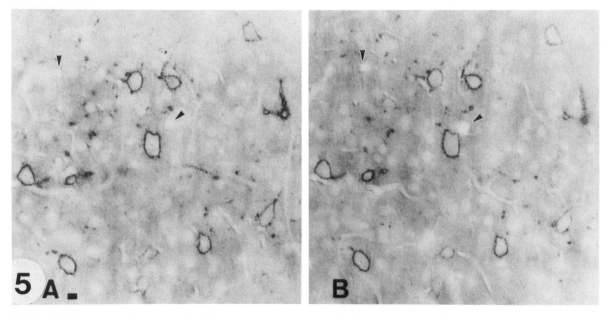

Fig. 5. A,B. Nomarski optics photomicrographs of paired surfaces of two 50 μm thick sections incubated with VC1.1 (A) and HNK-1 (B). Layer VI in the parietal cortex. There is no appreciable difference between VC1.1 and HNK-1 stainings. Arrowheads indicate profiles of blood vessels as landmarks. Scale: 10 μm. (Taken from Kosaka et al., 1990.)

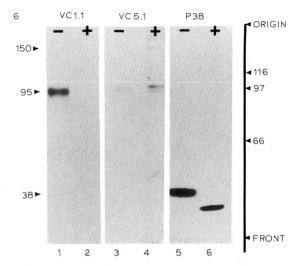

Fig. 6. Deglycosylation of cat cortical membranes results in a loss of VC1.1 immunoreactive bands on Western blots (lanes 1, 2). This effect was specific for N-linked carbohydrates since identical enzymatic treatment of cytosolic fractions (lanes 3, 4) or membrane fractions (lanes 5, 6) and subsequent staining with control antibodies, VC5.1 or anti-P38 (mAb 7.1b) against separate polypeptide determinants, did not alter the staining properties. (Taken from Naegele and Barnstable, 1991.)

chemical labelling given by antibodies VC1.1 and HNK-1 led us to examine whether the VC1.1 carbohydrate was expressed on molecules such as N-CAM. To detect N-CAM we used three monoclonal antibodies CB7.5, N-CAM-5D12 and N-CAM-0B11 (Neill and Barnstable, 1990; Naegele and Barnstable, 1991). Rat cortical membrane proteins were dissolved in detergent and antigens were precipitated with VC1.1 or an anti-N-CAM. When the precipitates were analysed on immunoblots, antigens precipitated by anti-N-CAM reacted with VC1.1 and vice versa (Fig. 7). Thus, the 140 kDa and 170 kDa bands recognized by VC1.1 are a subset of N-CAM molecules.

Comparison of the labelling patterns of VC1.1 and anti-N-CAM on sections of rat cortex and rat retina showed significant differences. Unlike the discrete labelling given by VC1.1 in cortex, anti-N-CAM gave a more general labelling of all layers and all regions. In retina VC1.1 labelled horizontal and amacrine cells in the inner nuclear layer and cells in the ganglion cell layer (Fig. 8A).

Anti-N-CAM, on the other hand-labelled all retinal layers including a uniform labelling of the inner plexiform layer (Fig. 8B). Combining the biochemical and immunocytochemical results suggests that whereas the N-CAM is expressed on most cells, the VC1.1 carbohydrate is attached to the N-CAM molecules of only a small subset of cells. The functional consequences of this are discussed later.

The heavy band at 95–105 kDa seen on immunoblots of cat tissue labelled with VC1.1 is probably due to expression of this carbohydrate on myelin associated glycoprotein (MAG), and the inclusion of white matter in the membranes used for the blots. Immunocytochemical labelling of cortical gray matter with an antibody against

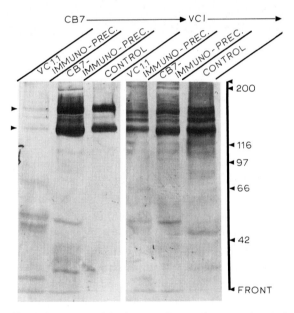

Fig. 7. Immunoprecipitation experiments demonstrating that VC1.1 precipitates N-CAM and anti-N-CAM precipitates VC1.1 reactive antigens. VC1.1 or anti-N-CAM (antibody CB7) were incubated with immunobeads (Biorad) and then with detergent solubilized membrane fractions from rat brain. Specifically bound material was analysed on SDS-polyacrylamide gels and transferred to nitrocellulose filters. Antigens precipitated by mAb VC1.1 reacted with both mAb CB7 (A) and VC1.1 (D). Similarly antigens precipitated by mAb CB7 reacted with both CB7 (B) and VC1.1 (E). Control lanes containing detergent solubilized membranes reacted with CB7 (C) and VC1.1 (F). Molecular weight standards are shown on the right. (Taken from Naegele and Barnstable, 1991.)

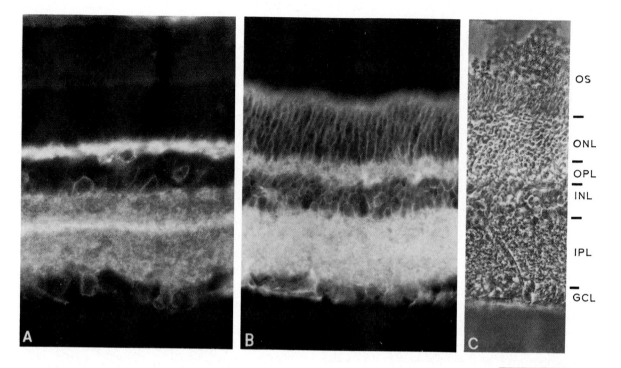

Fig. 8. In rat retina, the VC1.1 carbohydrate epitope is expressed on a subset of N-CAM molecules associated with horizontal and amacrine cells. A few ganglion cells are also immunoreactive (A). In contrast, most cell types and their processes exhibit N-CAM immunoreactivity (B). The VC1.1 epitope and N-CAM are also present in the fiber layers of the retina (OPL, IPL). A phase-contrast image of rat retina is shows in C. Scale: 50 μm. (Taken from Naegele and Barnstable, 1991.)

the polypeptide portion of L-MAG detected only small oligodendrocytes, not neurons (Naegele and Barnstable, 1991). Thus the VC1.1 labelling of GABAergic neurons is not due to its cross-reactivity with L-MAG.

Another well characterized monoclonal antibody, Cat-301, has been described as labelling GABAergic neurons in some cortical areas including visual cortex (Hendry et al., 1988). Cat-301 has been shown to react with a chondroitin sulphate proteoglycan, most probably with the polypeptide portion (Zaremba et al., 1989). The way in which Cat-301 outlined the cell bodies and proximal dendrites of neurons is very similar to the labelling pattern of VC1.1. Although the distributions of Cat-301 and VC1.1 immunoreactive neurons overlap in some areas, each antibody has a distinctive regional distribution of immunoreactivity (Zaremba et al., 1990). For example, in the

cat visual system, Cat-301 labels neuronal subsets in area 17 and the lateral geniculate nucleus (LGN) but not the retina. VC1.1, on the other hand, labels area 17 and the retina but not the LGN.

To test whether there might be any molecular relationship between the antigens recognized by the two antibodies, tissue was analysed on immunoblots using low percentage polyacrylamide gels and transfer conditions that permitted detection of large molecules (Zaremba et al., 1990). Cat-301 recognized high molecular weight material with the major band at approximately 680 kDa. VC1.1 recognized a band of 650–700 kDa as well as the lower molecular weight bands described earlier. The relationship between these high molecular weight bands was examined by exhaustive immunoprecipitation and immunoblotting. Cat-301 could remove part, but not all of the VC1.1 immunoreactivity from partially purified cortical proteoglycans. Similarly, VC1.1 could remove part, but not all, of the Cat-301 immunoreactivity. From these experiments it was concluded that some of the Cat-301 molecules also carried the VC1.1 carbohydrate epitope and that the VC1.1 carbohydrate was also expressed by other high molecular weight molecules. Although the range of these has yet to be defined, many of them appear to contain keratan sulphate moieties since material precipitated by VC1.1 could be stained with an anti-keratan sulphate antibody.

Because antibody Cat-301 does not react with rat cortex, all the above comparisons were done using cat tissue. The results are, however, likely to be true for rat as well because immunocyto-chemical labelling with monoclonal antibodies produced against chondroitinase ABC digested chondroitin sulphate proteoglycan gave a labelling pattern that was similar to that of VC1.1 (Kosaka et al., 1990). Direct comparison of sequential 0.5 $\mu$m sections showed a number of cells that were labelled with both VC1.1 and anti-chondroitin sulphate, but in addition a number of cells that were labelled with the anti-chondroitin sulphate only (see below). Thus, as in cat, VC1.1 is labelling a subset of the neurons that express chondroitin sulphate proteoglycans.

Subpopulations of GABAergic neurons have also been identified with the lectin VVA which recognizes $N$-acetyl-galactosamine (Nakagawa et

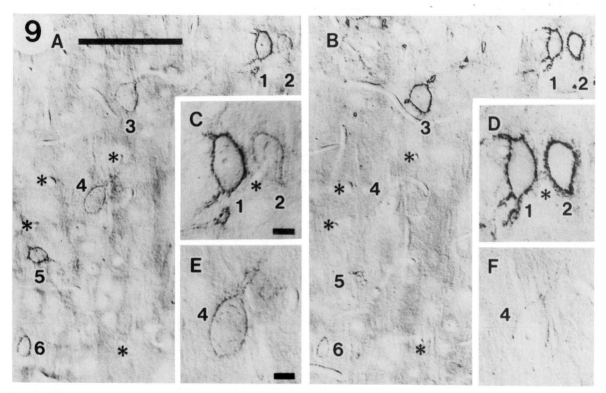

Fig. 9. A,B. Nomarski optics photomicrographs of paired surfaces of two 50 $\mu$m thick consecutive sections incubated with VVA (A) and VC1.1 (B). Layer IV of rat cortex. Various combinations of VVA and VC1.1 staining on the same cells. Cell 1 is intensely positive for both VVA and VC1.1 (A, B; C, D at higher magnification). Cells 2–6 are intermediately positive for VVA, but they are very different in the intensity of VC1.1 staining. Cells 2 (A,B; C,D at higher magnification) and 3 are intensely positive for VC1.1, cell 4 (A, B; E, F at higher magnification) only faintly positive for VC1.1 cell 5 negative for VC1.1 and cell 6 is intermediately positive for VC1.1. Asterisks indicate profiles of blood vessels as landmarks. Scale: A,B, 100 $\mu$m; C,E, 10 $\mu$m. (Taken from Kosaka et al., 1989.)

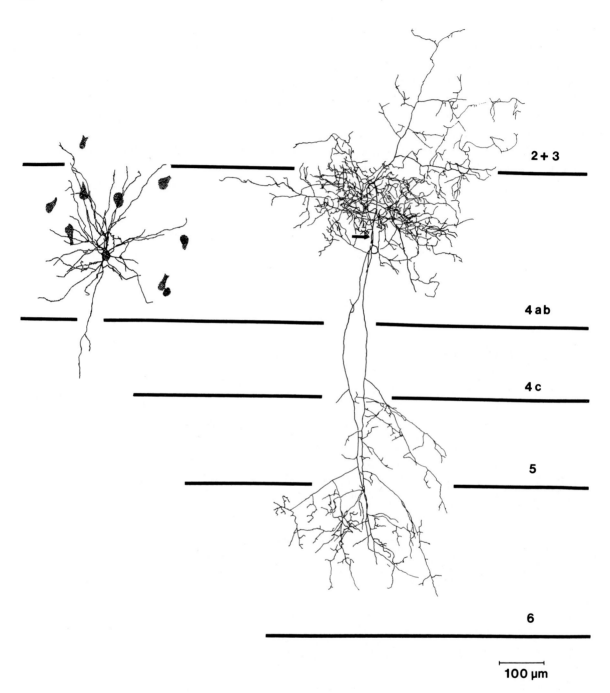

Fig. 10. VVA + basket-type local-circuit neuron intracellularly marked with Lucifer Yellow dye, in a living slice of cat area 17. VVA-Texas Red staining was subsequently performed on fixed, free-floating sections of the slice. The double-labelled neuron was identified by viewing the section with a combination FITC/texas Red filter cube. A. The cell body and dendrites of a VVA + basket cell are shown. Additional VVA + cell bodies in layer IVab (shown as meshwork pattern) received putative synaptic contacts from the basket cell axon. B. Serial reconstruction of the complete axonal arbor formed by the VVA + basket cell. The axon leaves the apical somatic pole (arrowhead) and issues a series of ascending and recurrent collaterals primarily in layer IVab. Sparser collateral branches extended into layer II + III and layers V and VI. Scale bar is 100 μm. (Taken from Naegele and Barnstable, 1989.)

al., 1986a,b; Kosaka and Heizmann, 1989; Naegele and Barnstable, 1989; Mulligan et al., 1989). The evidence so far available indicates that this sub-population is larger than that labelled by VC1.1. Double labelling studies in rat cortex using paired surfaces of adjacent sections (Fig. 9), showed a significant overlap in labelling (Kosaka et al., 1989). Most cells labelled with VC1.1 (256/281) were VVA positive. About 70% of VVA positive cells were also VC1.1 positive, although this percentage varies considerably with cortical area examined. This suggests that VVA lectin is recognizing more GABAergic cells than VC1.1. Similar results have also been obtained in cat area 17. In cat, preliminary biochemical studies have shown that VVA recognizes a number of bands on immunoblots. Two bands enriched in plasma membranes had apparent molecular weights of 72 kDa and 76 kDa (Naegele and Katz, 1990). It would therefore appear that VVA is recognizing a different set of cell surface molecules expressed on a distinct but overlapping subpopulation of cells as compared with VC1.1.

The type of GABAergic neurons labelled by VVA, or VC1.1, could not be identified from the labelling studies alone because only the cell body and part of the dendrites were labelled. To overcome this problem, single cells in layer 4 of coronal slices of cat area 17 were injected with Lucifer yellow (Naegele and Barnstable, 1989; Naegele and Katz, 1990). The slices were fixed, sectioned and labelled with fluorescent VVA. VVA positive cells in layer 4 that had been filled with Lucifer yellow were drawn with a camera lucida. An example of such a cell is shown in Fig. 10. Out of a total of 156 Lucifer yellow injected cells, 45 were non-pyramidal cells with smooth dendrites. Of these 19 were also labelled with VVA and were of two morphologies. The majority had axonal features characteristic of basket cells, and the remainder appeared to be neurogliaform cells. Twelve VVA positive basket cells shared a number of common features in their axonal arbors. All formed an arbor of 400–700 $\mu$m when viewed in the coronal plane. All had

most of their axonal processes in layer 4ab but they differed in the amount of arbor extending into layer 3. In addition, some of the neurons formed extensive projections in layers 5 and 6. These cells had axons that passed through layer 4c without branching or having any varicosities. All the cells had dendritic arbors in layer 4 with some extension up into more superficial layers.

The morphological features of the VVA positive layer 4 basket cells described above differed from the VVA negative basket cells that were filled with Lucifer yellow in these experiments. Most strikingly, the VVA negative basket cells had axonal arbors that included a dense plexus in layer 4c. In addition, few of these cells had descending processes that branched significantly in layers 5 and 6.

The other type of VVA positive neuron in layer 4 that was filled with Lucifer yellow was the neurogliaform cell. The dendrites and axon of these cells were extensively intertwined, as has been shown from Golgi studies of these cells. Most of their dendritic and axonal arbors were in layer 4 but also had descending axon collaterals in layers 5 and 6.

### The relationship between VVA, VC1.1 and parvalbumin

At the same time as we were characterizing some of the surface markers on cells in visual cortex, it was reported that many GABAergic neurons contained the calcium-binding protein parvalbumin (Celio, 1986; Demeulemeester et al., 1989; Kosaka and Heizmann, 1989). Since not all GABAergic neurons contained parvalbumin it was of interest to see how the subpopulation defined by this cytoplasmic marker was related to those we were defining by antibodies such as VC1.1 and the lectin VVA. Previous studies had shown an almost complete overlap between the subpopulations of GABAergic neurons labelled by parvalbumin and the lectin VVA. Since VC1.1 antibody labelled about 70% of VVA positive cells, it was not surprising that essentially all VC1.1 cells were

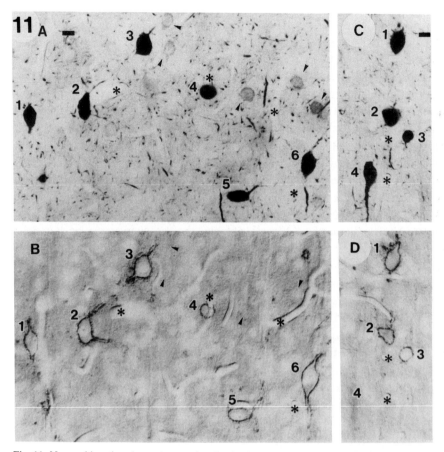

Fig. 11. Nomarski optics photomicrographs of paired surfaces of two 50 μm thick sections incubated with anti-PV serum (A) and VC1.1 (B). Parietal cortex. Asterisks indicate profiles of blood vessels as landmarks. Scale: 10 μm. *Left*. Layer IV. Cells 1–6 are positive for both PV and VC1.1 Some very faintly PV positive cells (arrowheads) are VC1.1 negative, although unstained profiles of these very faintly PV positive somata are barely discerned in B at this magnification. *Right*. Layer IV. Cells 1–3 are both PV and VC1.1 positive, whereas cell 4 is PV positive but VC1.1 negative. (Taken from Kosaka et al., 1989).

PV positive and that from 66 to 32%, depending on cortical region, of PV positive cells were positive for VC1.1 (Fig. 11).

In this work we also studied the overlap between VC1.1 labelling and the peptidergic subpopulations of GABAergic neurons. Since the PV positive subpopulation of GABAergic neurons had been shown not to contain peptides, it was also not surprising that the VC1.1 labelled cells were also generally not peptidergic (Kosaka et al., 1987). By analysing paired surfaces of adjacent sections, it was shown that only 2 out of 283 VC1.1 positive cells were positive for somato-

statin, 1 out of 254 for cholecystokinin and 0 out of 381 for VIP (Kosaka et al., 1989).

## Subpopulations of GABAergic cortical neurons

From all the results presented above we can begin to divide the GABAergic neurons of visual cortex into overlapping subpopulations. The markers used to delineate these populations are shown on five adjacent sections of rat cortex in Fig. 12. While this gives a good impression of the overall distributions of labelling, the reactivities of a single cell cannot be determined. To try and

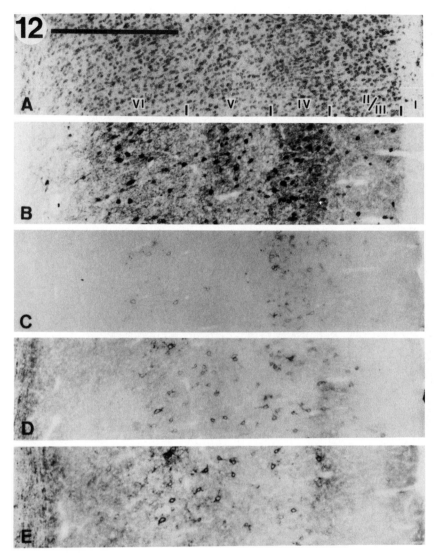

Fig. 12. A–E. Five adjacent sections of a part of the parietal cortex stainned with cresyl-violet (A), anti-PV (B), Mab HNK-1 (C), lectin VVA (D) and Mab 3B3 (E). Scale: 500 μm. (Taken from Kosaka et al., 1990.)

do this, we have carried out quadruple labelling. In Fig. 13 three consecutive 0.5 μm sections are shown labelled with anti-parvalbumin, HNK-1, VC1.1 and 3B3. Some cells are clearly positive for all four markers, others for only some of them.

A major subpopulation is defined by the cytoplasmic marker parvalbumin and cell surface labelling by the lectin VVA. The relationship between this subpopulation and the cells labelled by antibodies against chondroitin sulphate proteoglycans is less clear. Using antibody 3B3 in rat cortex revealed an over 90% overlap with the cells defined by VVA (Kosaka et al., 1990). In several species, and with several antibodies, it has been shown that while most of the cells expressing these chondroitin sulphate proteoglycans are GABAergic neurons, some are clearly pyramidal and thus presumably not GABAergic. The pro-

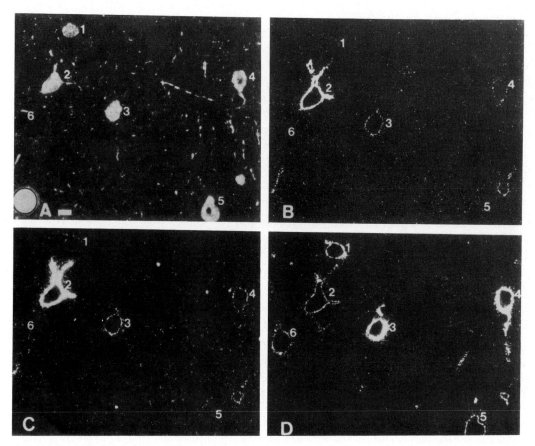

Fig. 13. Immunofluorescence labelling of 3 consecutive 0.5 μm thick sections of rat cortex; the first section has been double-labelled with anti-parvalbumin (A) and HNK-1 (B), the second with VC1.1 (C) and the third with 3B3 (D). Of 5 parvalbumin-positive cells, cell 2 is intensely HNK-1/VC1.1 positive but somewhat faintly 3B3 positive, whereas cells 3 and 4 are faintly HNK-1/VC1.1 positive but intensely 3B3 positive. Cells 1 and 5 are 3B3 positive but nearly negative for HNK-1/VC1.1. Cell 6 is 3B3 positive but parvalbumin negative. Scale: 10 μm. (Taken from Kosaka et al., 1990.)

portion of these cells varies with species, antibody used and cortical region examined, but is probably at least 10%.

A smaller subset of GABAergic neurons, included within the PV/VVA/chondroitin sulphate subset, is defined by expression of the VC1.1/HNK-1 carbohydrate epitope. An attempt to summarize these subpopulations is given in Fig. 14. The areas of overlap shown in the figure are determined from experimental data. There is substantial variation in the overlaps found in slightly different cortical regions, however, so that this diagram can only be taken as an approximation.

There are other groups of GABAergic neurons in visual and other cortical areas that do not overlap with the subsets defined above. As mentioned earlier the small subpopulation of GABAergic neurons that contain neuropeptides seems to be distinct from that defined by any of the above markers. Many of the GABAergic neurons that do not express parvalbumin contain another calcium-binding protein, calbindin (Demeulemeester et al., 1989; Hendry et al., 1989). Since most of the calbindin positive cells in visual cortex reside in layers 2 and 3, they probably also constitute a functionally different group. It would be predicted that this set of cells would also have

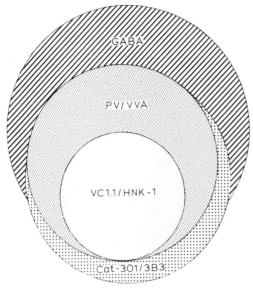

Fig. 14. A diagrammatic representation of the interrelationships of the subpopulations of neurons labelled with the markers described in this chapter. Although the relative areas of overlap are drawn to represent experimental findings, the differences found between different cortical areas make these relationships only approximate.

its unique array of cell surface molecules but these have yet to be identified. What is unclear at present is whether there are other molecules that cut across these definitions of subpopulations. For example, will we ever find a molecule expressed on 50% of the PV positive cells and 50% of the calbindin positive cells? Since the markers so far defined seem to fit well defined morphological and functional subclasses, this possibility seems unlikely.

**Conclusions**

In this chapter we have tried to show that reagents such as lectins and antibodies can be a valuable tool in the definition of GABAergic subpopulations of neurons in visual cortex. All the evidence so far available indicates that subpopulations defined previously by morphological or functional criteria can also be defined in molecular terms. This is not always in terms of a single molecule,

but often by the expression of a particular array of molecules. We have been able to achieve identification of cell types by single, double, and even quadruple labelling methods. Many of the markers we have defined are not expressed evenly over the cell surface, and none give good axonal labelling. Because definition of most GABAergic cell types is made on the basis of axonal morphology, we have had to combine intracellular dye injections with labelling methods to obtain unambiguous identification of cell types.

The VC1.1/HNK-1 carbohydrate epitope is expressed on cell adhesion molecules such as N-CAM. The restricted expression of this epitope suggests that its function may be to modify the function of N-CAM, and other adhesion molecules and there are several reports that support this idea. For example, HNK-1 antibodies have been reported to inhibit the migration of neural crest cells in developing chick (Bronner-Fraser, 1987). They have also been shown to inhibit neurite outgrowth. While antibody inhibition studies can be difficult to interpret, particularly when multivalent antibodies are used, the results do suggest a role in adhesive specificity for this epitope, though whether the effect is to enhance or reduce adhesion is not clear.

Earlier in this chapter some of the subcellular localization of synaptic inputs onto GABAergic neurons was described. It is not immediately obvious that the labelling patterns we have observed correlate with these synaptic patterns. Since the antigens seem to be expressed most strongly on cell bodies and proximal dendrites, perhaps they influence the formation or localization of presynaptic inputs. Since the formation of cortical laminae and synaptic circuitry can occur in organotypic cultures, this is now a testable hypothesis. One test of the validity of this hypothesis will be to determine the developmental patterns of expression of the epitopes discussed in this chapter. There is evidence that in the embryo an HNK-1 like epitope is found on a lipid as well as on polypeptides (Schwarting et al., 1987). The functional significance of this finding is not yet clear.

An extension of the hypothesis can be made from the finding of VC1.1 epitope on extracellular matrix molecules such as the Cat-301 chondroitin sulphate proteoglycan and on an as yet unidentified keratan sulphate proteoglycan. Since expression of the Cat-301 antigen occurs relatively late in development, and its expression can be modulated by neuronal activity, it has been suggested that its function is to stabilize synaptic interactions (Kalb and Hockfield, 1988). If so, then the localization in visual cortex would suggest that it is a specific set of synapses that is affected. Perhaps the VC1.1 epitope on N-CAM affects the specificity of synapse formation whereas the epitope on various extracellular matrix molecules modulates synaptic stabilization.

A carbohydrate epitope containing *N*-acetylgalactosamine and detected by VVA and other lectins has been found associated with certain forms of acetylcholinesterase and glycolipids at synaptic but not extra-synaptic regions of muscle fibers in many species (Scott et al., 1988). These authors suggested that the role of the carbohydrate might be to target molecules to the synapse by interactions with specific intracellular or extracellular binding proteins or lectins. It is not known whether such lectins for the HNK-1/VC1.1 carbohydrate epitope might also exist.

Since we have only been looking at a small subset of synapses on a small subset of cortical neurons, it will be of great interest to determine whether similar potential determinants of molecular specificity are to be found for other cell types and classes of synapses. If not then perhaps some of the molecules we have been examining will allow us to pick out those cells and synapses which undergo such modulations during development.

If, on the other hand, each cell type does have its characteristic array of molecules, it will have implications for studies trying to define cortical circuitry. Molecular markers for particular types of synaptic interaction would greatly simplify the quantitative analysis of these circuits. Such markers combined with appropriate cell markers or

even intracellular filling of cells would generate information much faster than currently possible. Although this is only hypothesis, at least it is a testable hypothesis. Also, as is often the case, the journey itself can be as interesting and rewarding as the arrival at the destination.

## Acknowledgements

Work described in this article has been supported by grants from the NIH and the Japanese Ministry of Education, Science and Culture, as well as by Research to Prevent Blindness, Inc. and the Darien Lions. CJB is a Jules and Doris Stein Research to Prevent Blindness, Inc. Professor and JRN is a Klingenstein Fellow in the Neurosciences.

## References

Abo, T. and Balch, C.M. (1981) A differentiation antigen of human NK and K cells identified by a monoclonal antibody (HNK-1). *J. Immunol.*, 127: 1024–1029.

Akagawa, K. and Barnstable, C.J. (1986) Identification and characterization of cell types in monolayer cultures of rat retina using monoclonal antibodies. *Brain Res.*, 383: 110–120.

Ariga, T., Kohriyama, T., Freddo, L., Latov, N., Saito, M., Kon, K., Ando, S., Suzuki, M., Hemling, M.E., Rinehart, Jr., K.L., Kusunoki, S. and Yu, R.K. (1987) Charactrization of sulfated glucuronic acid containing glycolipids reacting with IgM M-proteins in patients with neuropathy. *J. Biol. Chem.*, 262: 848–853.

Arimatsu, Y., Naegele, J.R. and Barnstable, C.J. (1987) Molecular markers of neuronal subpopulations in layers 4,5 and 6 of cat primary visual cortex. *J. Neurosci.*, 7: 1250–1263.

Barnstable, C.J. (1980) Monoclonal antibodies which recognise different cell types in the rat retina. *Nature*, 286: 231–235.

Barnstable, C.J. (1987) A molecular view of mammalian retinal development. *Mol. Neurobiol.*, 1: 9–46.

Barnstable, C.J. (1991) Molecular aspects of development of mammalian optic cup and formation of retinal cell types. *Prog. Retina Res.*, 10: 69–88.

Bronner-Fraser, M. (1987) Perturbation of cranial neural crest migration by the HNK-1 antibody. *Dev. Biol.*, 123: 321–331.

Celio, M.R. (1986) Parvalbumin in most γ-aminobutyric acid containing neurons of the rat cerebral cortex. *Science*, 231: 995–997.

Demeulemeester, H., Vandesande, F., Orban, G.A., Heizmann, C.W. and Pochet, R. (1989) Calbindin D-28K and parvalbumin immunoreactivity is confined to two separate neuronal subpopulations in the cat visual cortex, whereas partial coexistence is shown in the dorsal lateral geniculate nucleaus. *Neurosci. Lett.*, 99: 6–11.

Freund, T.F., Martin, K.A.C., Somogyi, P. and Whitteridge, D. (1985) Innervation of cat visual areas 17 and 18 by physiologically identified X- and Y-type thalamic afferents. II. Identification of postsynaptic targets by GABA immunocytochemistry and Golgi impregnantion. *J. Comp. Neurol.*, 242: 275–291.

Gabbott, P.L.A. and Somogyi, P. (1986) Quantitative distribution of GABA-immunoreactive neurons in the visual cortex (area 17) of the cat. *Exp. Brain Res.*, 61: 323–331.

Gilbert, C.D. and Wiesel, T.N. (1979) Morphology and intracortical projections of functionally characterised neurones in the cat visual cortex. *Nature*, 280: 120–125.

Hendry, S.H.C. and Jones, E.G. (1981) Sizes and distributions of intrinsic neurons incorporating tritiated GABA in monkey sensory-motor cortex. *J. Neurosci.*, 1: 390–408.

Hendry, S.H.C., Jones, E.G., Emson, P.C., Lawson, D.E.M., Heizmann, C.W. and Streit, P. (1989) Two classes of cortical GABA neurons defined by differential calcium binding protein immunoreactivities. *Exp. Brain Res.*, 76: 467–472.

Hendry, S.H.C., Jones, E.G., Hockfield, S. and McKay, R.D.G. (1988) Neuronal populations stained with the monoclonal antibody Cat-301 in the mammalian cerebral cortex thalamus. *J. Neurosci.*, 8: 518–542.

Jones, E.G. (1975) Varieties and distribution of non-pyramidal cells in the somatic sensory cortex of the squirrel monkey. *J. Comp. Neurol.*, 160: 205–268.

Kalb, R.G. and Hockfield, S. (1988) Molecular evidence for early activity-dependent development of hamster motor neurons. *J. Neurosci.*, 8: 2350–2360.

Kisvárday, Z.F., Cowey, A. and Somogyi, P. (1986) Synaptic relationships of a type of GABA-immunoreactive neuron (clutch cell), spiny stellate cells and lateral geniculate nucleus afferents in layer IVc of monkey striate cortex. *Neuroscience*, 19: 741–761.

Kisvárday, Z.F., Martin, K.A.C., Friedlander, M.J. and Somogyi, P. (1987) Evidence for intralaminar inhibitory circuits in the striate cortex of the cat. *J. Comp. Neurol.*, 260: 1–19.

Kisvárday, Z.F., Martin, K.A.C., Whitteridge, D. and Somogyi, P. (1985) Synaptic connections of intracellularly filled clutch cells: A type of small basket cell in the visual cortex of the cat. *J. Comp. Neurol.*, 241: 111–137.

Kosaka, T. and Heizmann, C.W. (1989) Selective staining of a population of parvalbumin-containing GABAergic neurons in the rat cerebral cortex by lectins with specific affinity for terminal *N*-acetylgalactosamine. *Brain Res.*, 483: 158–163.

Kosaka, T., Heizman, C.W. and Barnstable, C.J. (1989) Monoclonal antibody VC1.1 selectively stains a population GABAergic neurons containing a calcium binding protein parvalbumin in the rat cerebral cortex. *Exp. Brain Res.*, 78: 43–50.

Kosaka, T., Heizman, C.W., Tateishi, K., Hamaoka, Y. and Hama, K. (1987) An aspect of the γ-aminobutyric acidergic system in the cerebral cortex. *Brain Res.*, 409: 403–408.

Kosaka, T., Isogai, K., Barnstable, C.J. and Heizmann, C.W. (1990) Monoclonal antibody HNK-1 selectively stains a population of GABAergic neurons containing a calcium-binding protein parvalbumin in the rat cerebral cortex. *Exp. Brain Res.*, 82: 566–574.

Kruse, J., Keilhauer, G., Faissner, A., Sommer, I., Goridis, C. and Schachner, M. (1984) Neural cell adhesion molecules and myelin-associated glycoprotein share a common carbohydrate moiety recognized by monoclonal antibodies L2 and HNK-1. *Nature (London)*, 311: 153–155.

Lund, J.S. (1987) Local circuit neurons of macaque monkey striate cortex: I. Neurons of laminae 4C and 5A. *J. Comp. Neurol.*, 257: 60–92.

Lund, J.S., Henry, G.H., Macqueen, C.L. and Harvey, A.R. (1979) Anatomical organization of the primary visual cortex (area 17) of the cat. A comparison with area 17 of the Macaque monkey. *J. Comp. Neurol.*, 184: 599–618.

Martin, K.A.C., Friedlander, M.J. and Alones V. (1989) Physiological, morphological and cytochemical characteristics of a layer 1 neuron in cat striate cortex. *J. Comp. Neurol.*, 282: 404–414.

McGuire, B.A., Hornung, J.P., Gilbert, C.D. and Wiesel, T.N. (1984) Patterns of synaptic input to layer 4 of cat striate cortex. *J. Neurosci.*, 4: 3021–3033.

Meyer, G. (1983) Axonal patterns and topography of short-axon neurons in visual areas 17, 18 and 19 of the cat. *J. Comp. Neurol.*, 220: 405–438.

Meyer, G. and Ferres-Torres, (1984) Postnatal maturation of nonpyramidal neurons in the visual cortex of the cat. *J. Comp. Neurol.*, 228: 226–244.

Mulligan, K.A., van Brederode, J.F.M. and Hendrickson, A.E. (1989) The lectin Vicia villosa labels a distinct subset of GABAergic cells in macaque visual cortex. *Visual Neurosci.*, 2: 63–72.

Naegele, J.R. and Barnstable, C.J. (1989) Molecular determinants of GABAergic local circuit neurons in the cerebral cortex. *Trends Neurosci.*, 12: 28–34.

Naegele, J.R. and Barnstable, C.J. (1991) A carbohydrate epitope defined by monoclonal antibody VC1.1 is found on N-CAM and other cell adhesion molecules. *Brain Res.*, 559: 118–129.

Naegele, J.R. and Katz, L.C. (1990) Cell surface molecules containing *N*-acetylgalactosamine are associated with basket cells and neurogliaform cells in cat visual cortex. *J. Neurosci.*, 10: 540–557

Naegele, J.R., Arimatsu, Y., Schwartz, P. and Barnstable, C.J. (1988) Selective staining of a subset of GABAergic neurons in cat visual cortex by monoclonal antibody VC1.1. *J. Neurosci.*, 8: 79–89.

Nakagawa, F., Schulte, B.A. and Spicer, S.S., (1986a) Selective cytochemical demonstration of glycoconjugate-containing terminal *N*-acetylgalactosamine on some brain neurons. *J. Comp. Neurol.*, 243: 280–290.

Nakagawa, F., Schulte, B.A., Wu, J.Y. and Spicer, S.S., (1986b)

522

GABAergic neurons of rodent brain correspond partially with those staining for glycoconjugate with terminal *N*-acetylgalactosamine. *J. Neurocytol.*, 15: 389–396.

Neill, J.M. and Barnstable, C.J. (1990) Differentiation and dedifferentiation of rat retinal pigment epithelial cells. Expresion of RET-PE2, an RPE antigen and N-CAM during development and in tissue culture. *Exp. Eye Res.*, 51: 573–583.

Ogren, M.P. and Hendrickson, A.E. (1976) Pathways between striate cortex and subcortical regions in *Macaca mulatta* and *Saimiri sciureus*: evidence for a reciprocal pulvinar connection. *Exp. Neurol.*, 53: 780–800.

Peters, A. and Jones E.G. (1984a) *Cerebral Cortex, Vol. 1*, New York: Plenum Press, 565 pp.

Peters, A. and Jones, E.G. (1984b). Classification of cortical neurons. In A. Peters and E.G. Jones (Eds.), *Cerebral Cortex. Vol 1*, New York: Plenum Press, pp. 107–122.

Peters, A. and Regidor, J. (1981) A reassessment of the forms of nonpyramidal neurons in area 17 of cat visual cortex. *J. Comp. Neurol.*, 203: 685–716.

Schwarting, G.A., Jungalwala, F.B., Chou, K.H., Boyer, A.M. and Yamamoto, M. (1987) Sulfated glucuronic acid-containing glycoconjugates are temporally and spatially regulated antigens in the developing mammalian nervous system. *Dev. Biol.*, 120: 65–76.

Scott, L.J.C., Bacou, F. and Sanes, J.R. (1988) A synapse-specific carbohydrate at the neuromuscular junction: association with both acetylcholinesterase and a glycolipid. *J. Neurosci.*, 8: 932–944.

Sparrow, J.R., Hicks, D. and Barnstable, C.J. (1990) Cell commitment and differentiation in explants of embryonic rat retina. Comparison to the developmental potential of dissociated retina. *Dev. Brain Res.*, 51: 69–84.

Valverde, F. (1985) The organizing principles of the primary visual cortex in the monkey. In: A. Peters and E.G. Jones (Eds.), *Cerebral Cortex, Vol 3*, New York: Plenum Press, pp. 207–257.

Van Essen, D.C. (1985) Functional organization of primate visual cortex. In A. Peters and E.G. Jones (Eds.), *Cerebral Cortex, Vol 3*, New York: Plenum Press, pp. 259–329.

Yamamoto, M., Marshall, P., Hemmendinger, L.M., Boyer, A.B. and Caviness Jr., V.S. (1988) Distribution of glucuronic-acid and sulfate-containing glycoproteins in the central nervous system of the mouse. *J. Neurosci. Res.*, 5: 273–298.

Zaremba, S., Guimaraes, A., Kalb, R.G. and Hockfield, S. (1989) Characterization of an activity dependent neuronal surface proteoglycan identified with monoclonal antibody Cat-301. *Neuron*, 2: 1207–1219.

Zaremba, S., Naegele, J.R., Barnstable, C.J. and Hockfield, S. (1990) Multiple high molecular weight glycoconjugates in the cat CNS defined by monoclonal antibodies Cat-301 and VC1.1. *J. Neurosci.*, 10: 2985–2995.

R.R. Mize, R.E. Marc and A.M. Sillito (Eds.)
Progress in Brain Research, Vol. 90
© 1992 Elsevier Science Publishers B.V. All rights reserved

CHAPTER 24

# Development of GABA-containing neurons in the visual cortex

## John G. Parnavelas

*Department of Anatomy and Developmental Biology, University College London, England, UK*

### Introduction

Study of the development of GABA-containing neurons in the visual cortex is a study of the development of the cortical nonpyramidal neurons. The differentiation of the morphological and neurochemical features of these neurons have received considerable attention over the years and findings have been reviewed by a number of authors (Miller, 1988; Parnavelas et al., 1988). The aim of this chapter is to summarize the earlier findings and review more recent work published in this area. I shall concentrate on work in the visual cortex of the rat, which has been the focus of fairly extensive investigations, and only briefly mention observations in the visual cortex of other mammals.

### GABA-containing neurons in the adult visual cortex

In the mammalian cerebral cortex, GABA is almost entirely of intrinsic origin being localized in nonpyramidal neurons (Houser et al., 1984). These are the interneurons of the cortex distributed in all six layers (Parnavelas et al., 1977; Peters, 1985) (Fig. 1). The levels of GABA do not decline significantly after the cortex is undercut (Emson and Lindvall, 1979), although recent reports have documented the existence of GABA-ergic neurons in the posterior hypothalamus and

in the zona incerta that project to the cortex (Vincent et al., 1983; Köhler et al., 1985; Lin et al., 1990) as well as the presence of GABA in corticopetal cholinergic neurons in the basal forebrain (Fisher et al., 1988; Fisher and Levine, 1989). GABA-containing neurons in the visual and other areas of the cerebral cortex have been visualized by: (1) autoradiographic localization of [3H]GABA following its uptake (Chronwall and Wolff, 1978; Kisvárday et al., 1986); (2) immunocytochemical localization of glutamic acid decar-

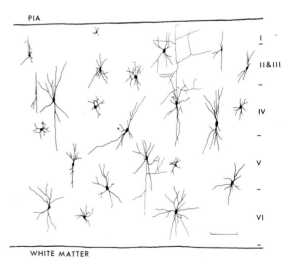

Fig. 1. Camera lucida drawings of nonpyramidal neurons in the different layers of the rat visual cortex. Their dendritic geometry is highly variable. Details of dendritic morphology (spines, varicosities) and the axonal trajectory of most cells are not included. Scale bar: 200 μm. (From Parnavelas et al., 1977, with permission.)

boxylase (GAD), the GABA-synthesizing enzyme, which is present in GABAergic neurons and their terminals in high concentrations (Ribak, 1978; Hendrickson et al., 1981; Bear et al., 1985; Lin et al., 1986); and (3) immunocytochemical localization of the transmitter itself (Ottersen and Storm-Mathisen 1984; Somogyi et al., 1984; Meinecke and Peters, 1987). Immunocytochemical methods are currently the most commonly used techniques for visualizing GABAergic elements in the cerebral cortex and elsewhere in the brain.

Ribak (1978) was the first to localize GAD in neurons and axon terminals in the visual cortex of the rat. He described labelled cells distributed throughout all cortical layers and numerous dark punctate structures both around cell bodies and in the intervening neuropil. The GAD-containing neurons were multipolar and bitufted in form with aspinous and sparsely spinous dendrites. As for the labelled punctate structures, electron microscopy showed that they were immunoreactive axon terminals forming Gray's type II or symmetrical (presumptive inhibitory) (Gray, 1969; Triller and Korn, 1982) synaptic contacts with somata and dendrites of pyramidal and nonpyramidal neurons, as well as with some axon initial segments.

In a more recent immunohistochemical analysis in the visual cortex of the rat, Lin et al. (1986) also reported GAD-positive cells throughout all cortical layers. However, these authors noted increased concentrations of both labelled somata and GAD-immunoreactive puncta in layer IV. In this study, GAD-stained cells formed approximately 15% of the neuronal population in the visual cortex and, in agreement with Ribak (1978), showed features typical of multipolar and bitufted nonpyramidal neurons. Our observations in the same cortical area of the rat are in fairly good agreement with the findings of Lin et al. (1986) (Figs. 2 and 3). Even more recently, an immunocytochemical study by Meinecke and Peters (1987), using an antibody against GABA, also revealed that approximately 15% of all neurons in the rat visual cortex are GABAergic. Further-

more, these authors were able to determine that, with the exception of a small proportion of the bipolar cell population, all cortical nonpyramidal neurons are indeed GABAergic. Comparable proportions of GABAergic neurons have been reported in the visual cortex of the cat (Gabbott and Somogyi, 1986) and primate (Fitzpatrick et al., 1987; Hendry et al., 1987).

It has been demonstrated that a substantial proportion of GABA-containing nonpyramidal neurons also contain one or more biologically active peptides (Jones and Hendry, 1986; Papadopoulos et al., 1987; Parnavelas et al., 1989). Peptides localized in cortical nonpyramidal neurons in the rat and other mammals include: somatostatin (somatotropin release inhibiting factor; SRIF), neuropeptide Y (NPY), vasoactive intestinal polypeptide (VIP), cholecystokinin (CCK) and corticotropin-releasing factor (CRF) (Parnavelas and McDonald, 1983; Peters, 1985; Jones and Hendry, 1986; Parnavelas et al., 1989). Substance P has also been localized in cortical interneurons in the monkey (Jones et al., 1988), but evidence for its presence in the rat neocortex is less compelling.

GABA-containing nonpyramidal neurons which are also immunoreactive for a neuropeptide may be divided into subpopulations on the basis of the coexisting peptide. This is supported by recent findings in the rat visual cortex which show that each subpopulation shows distinct cytological, synaptic and developmental features (Cavanagh and Parnavelas, 1988, 1989, 1990; Parnavelas et al., 1989). However, it must be emphasized that a fairly large proportion (up to 40%) of the GABAergic neurons in the rat cerebral cortex have not yet been demonstrated to contain a known neuropeptide.

### Genesis and migration

Earlier studies of histogenesis in the cerebral cortex have treated neurons as a single population (Angevine and Sidman, 1961; Berry and Rogers, 1965; Rakic, 1974). Some authors have

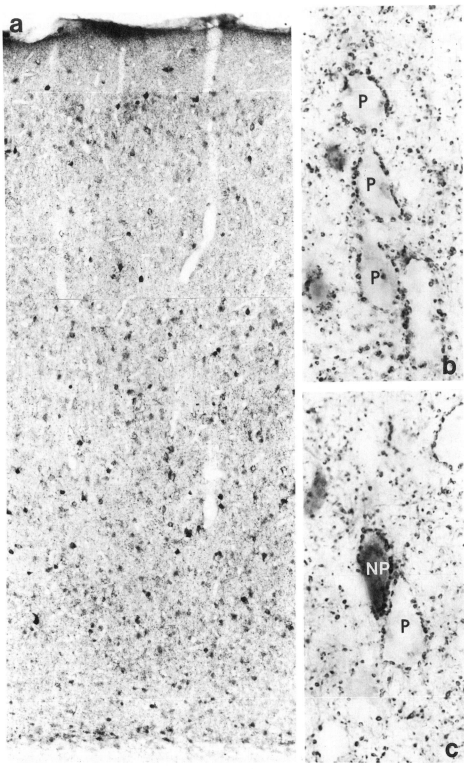

Fig. 2. a. Photomicrograph showing the distribution of GAD-labelled neurons and axon terminals in a 50 μm coronal section through the adult rat visual cortex. Pia is towards the top of the page ×160. b,c. GAD-positive axon terminals surrounding unstained pyramidal cell perikarya (P) (b) or an unstained pyramidal neuron (P) and a stained nonpyramidal neuron (NP) (c). ×1000. (From Parnavelas et al., 1989, with permission.)

attempted to distinguish between projection neurons and interneurons and have conveyed the notion that the production of the pyramidal cells precedes that of the nonpyramidal cells (see Jacobson, 1978). The issue remained unresolved

until investigators combined immunohistochemistry with [³H]thymidine autoradiography to specifically study the genesis of GABAergic neurons. In these studies, antisera to GAD were used in the rat visual cortex (Wolff et al., 1983)

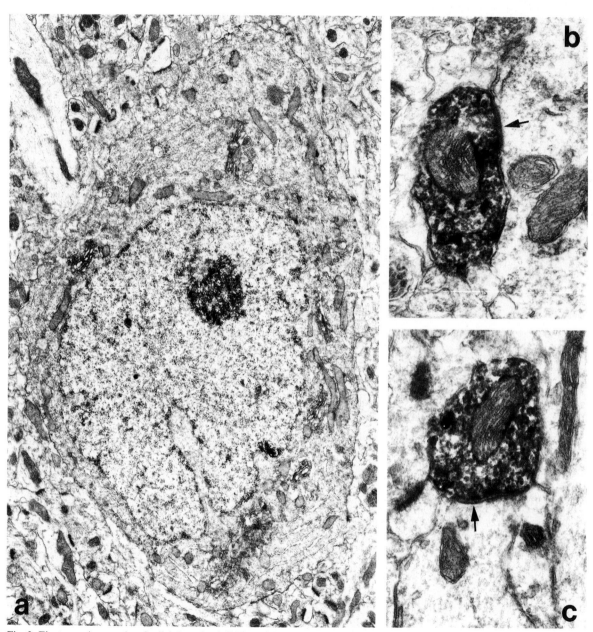

Fig. 3. Electron micrographs of a lightly stained GAD-positive nonpyramidal neuron in the rat visual cortex (a) and two intensely stained GAD-positive axon terminals forming type II axosomatic (b) and axodendritic (c) synapses (arrows). a, ×10000; b,c, ×41800. (From Parnavelas et al., 1989, with permission.)

and antisera to GABA itself were used in the visual cortex of the rat (Miller, 1985, 1988) and ferret (Peduzzi, 1988).

These combined studies have revealed that GABA-containing neurons in the rat visual cortex are born throughout the period of cortical neurogenesis, between embryonic day (E) 14 and E21, with peak production at E17 (Fig. 4). Their generation follows the same inside-out pattern as that of the projection neurons (Miller, 1986a). A similar pattern has been reported for the genesis of GABAergic neurons in the ferret visual cortex (Peduzzi, 1988) and in the somatosensory cortex of the mouse (Fairén et al., 1986). An earlier study in the rat visual cortex (Wolff et al., 1983) reported that the laminar position of GABAergic neurons was not related to their date of birth but these cells were diffusely distributed throughout

the cortex. The recent studies of Cavanagh and Parnavelas (1988, 1989, 1990), which examined the time of genesis of subpopulations of nonpyramidal neurons as defined by their neuropeptide content, have suggested that over the whole period of neurogenesis both layered and diffuse distributions take place. There appears to be an overall layered distribution but at E17, the peak production time, the distribution becomes diffuse.

Analysis in the rat visual cortex of the time of birth of nonpyramidal subpopulations, as defined by their neuropeptide content, has shown that these subpopulations are produced in succession during development (Cavanagh and Parnavelas, 1988, 1989, 1990). Thus, the peak of neurogenesis of SRIF neurons is at E15–E16, for NPY neurons at E17 and for VIP cells is at E19. These

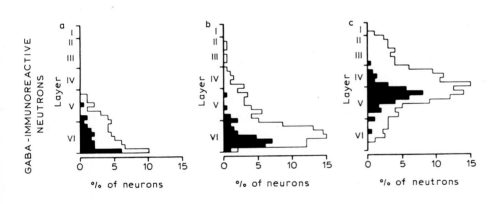

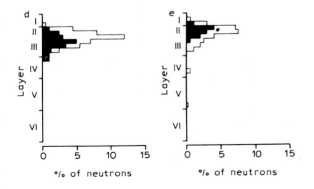

Fig. 4. Plots of the numbers of GABA-immunoreactive neurons double-labelled by injections of tritiated thymidine at E14 (a), E15 (b), E17 (c), E19 (d) and E20 (e). Double-labelled neurons with many silver grains over their nuclei (heavily-labelled neurons) and those with few silver grains over their nuclei (lightly-labelled neurons) are noted by solid bars and clear bars, respectively. Each graph is based on the mean data from two animals. From each animal, the distribution of double-labelled neurons in four 375 $\mu$m-wide vertical strips of cortex were compiled. (From Miller, 1985, with permission.)

findings suggest that either these subpopulations are all produced by a common precursor in the ventricular zone, where all cortical neurons are generated, or that there are multiple precursors which are activated at different times.

In addition to information about the genesis and neurochemical differentiation of small populations of cortical neurons, the combined immunohistochemical-autoradiographic studies have shown that, in common with other events in the developing brain, peptide-containing cells are initially overproduced and then decline in numbers to mature levels (Cavanagh and Parnavelas, 1988, 1989, 1990). Further evidence for this phenomenon is provided by the detailed studies of peptide-containing neurons in the developing visual cortex of the cat (Wahle and Meyer, 1987, 1989; Meyer and Wahle, 1988). Many of the cells which disappear are in inappropriate layers for their dates of birth. These cells are either eliminated because they are in the "wrong" layer or they serve some function during their ephemeral existence (Whale and Meyer, 1987). Evidence from experimental studies in the visual and somatosensory cortices of the rat suggests that SRIF cells, which would be eliminated in normal development, remain if sensory input is reduced or eliminated at birth (Jeffery and Parnavelas, 1987; Parnavelas et al., 1990). It is clear from these studies that sensory information is an important factor governing the density and distribution of at least one subpopulation of cortical nonpyramidal cells, the SRIF-containing neurons.

## Morphological differentiation

### Morphogenesis

The morphological maturation of nonpyramidal neurons in the rat visual cortex has been the subject of very detailed qualitative (Parnavelas et al., 1978; Hedlich and Winkelmann, 1982; Miller, 1986b, 1988) and quantitative (Parnavelas and Uylings, 1980; Miller, 1986b, 1988) investigations. The qualitative studies, which utilized Golgi-Cox and rapid Golgi methods, have shown that at birth very few immature nonpyramidal cells can be recognized, chiefly in the deeper part of the cortical plate. Over the next 8–10 days progressively more become recognizable, the most mature (excepting the Cajal-Retzius cells of layer I) occupying the infragranular layers. During this period, the number, size and extent of dendritic and axonal branching of these cells undergo considerable increases. Thereafter, differences in the state of maturation of nonpyramidal neurons at different cortical levels become less evident. So far as can be deduced from Golgi preparations, these cells acquire their mature perikaryal size, dendritic morphology and axonal ramification pattern more or less simultaneously in all layers at the end of the third postnatal week and at about the same time as pyramidal neurons acquire theirs. These conclusions are based on qualitative examinations, but quantitative analyses of Golgi-impregnated nonpyramidal neurons (Parnavelas and Uylings, 1980; Miller, 1986b, 1988) strongly support them (Figs. 5, 6). Although earlier studies did not distinguish between the different morphological types of nonpyramidal neurons, more recent investigations in the rat (Miller, 1986b) and cat visual cortex (Meyer and Ferres-Torres, 1984) have focussed on individual neuronal types as defined by their dendritic and axonal arborization patterns. These studies have shown that different nonpyramidal cell types undergo a differential sequence of maturation.

At the end of the third postnatal week, the number of spinous nonpyramidal neurons is greater and the spine density of some cells is higher than in the adult, falling to adult values during the fourth postnatal week (Parnavelas et al., 1978; Miller, 1986b). It would appear, therefore, that not only do most spinous nonpyramidal neurons become less spinous during the period 3–4 weeks postnatal, but that some neurons lose all or most of their spines to become spine-free nonpyramidal cells. These observations are in accordance with previous studies by LeVay (1973) who found the spine density of nonpyramidal

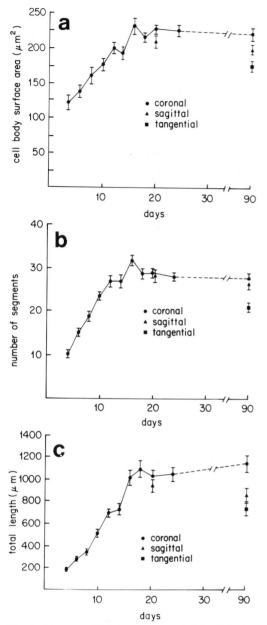

Fig. 5. Changes with increasing age of: (a) cell body surface area projected onto the plane of sectioning; (b) number of dendritic segments per neuron; (c) total dendritic length per neuron. All graphs show means ± S.E.M. per neuron. (From Parnavelas and Uylings, 1980, with permission.)

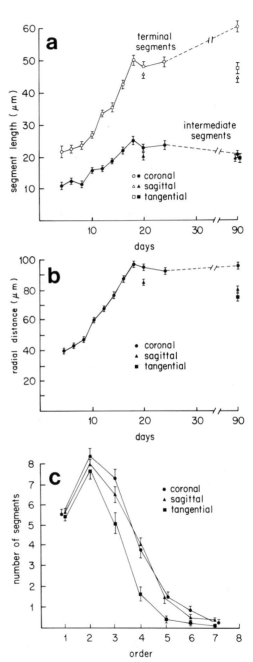

Fig. 6. a,b. Changes with increasing age of segment length (a) and radial distance of the terminal dendritic tips from the center of the cell body (b). Graphs show means ± S.E.M. per neuron. c. The number of dendritic segments of each order per neuron for nonpyramidal cells in coronal, sagittal and tangential sections at postnatal day 90. Shown are means ± S.E.M. (From Parnavelas and Uylings, 1980, with permission.)

neurons of the visual cortex to the higher in kitten than cat, and by Lund et al. (1977) who found that the maximal spine density of layer IV nonpyramidal cells in the monkey occurred at 8 weeks postnatal and was followed by a period of spine loss. This pattern of acquisition of dendritic spines by nonpyramidal neurons is different from that shown by pyramidal cells in the visual cortex (Parnavelas and Globus, 1976; Miller, 1988). The phenomenon of over-production with subsequent resorption of supernumerary spines, together with loss or redistribution of the synaptic contacts associated with them, is fairly common and probably of considerable significance in the development of the CNS (e.g., Cajal, 1960; Cragg, 1975; Lund et al., 1977; Ronnevi, 1977; Winfield, 1981; Meyer and Ferres-Torres, 1984).

The pattern of maturation seen in Golgi preparations is reflected in the ultrastructural appearance of the nonpyramidal neurons in the rat visual cortex (Parnavelas and Lieberman, 1979). An interesting feature to emerge from ultrastructural observations of the developing rat visual cortex is that, during the third and part of the fourth postnatal weeks, many of the nonpyramidal cells contain an extremely rich complement of cytoplasmic organelles. Not only do these cells appear to be more richly endowed with large orderly arrays of granular endoplasmic reticulum, ribosomes, Golgi apparatus and other cytoplasmic organelles than their counterparts at earlier developmental ages, but they also appear to be hypertrophic by comparison with nonpyramidal cells in mature animals. The presence in many of these cells of eccentric nuclei with prominent nucleoli and folded nuclear envelopes suggests that these cells are in a highly active state. It may be that this activity is directed towards the provision of materials to terminal regions of the cell processes in connection with the formation of large numbers of transient and/or permanent synaptic contacts. These observations, together with the finding in Golgi studies of transient dendritic spines during this period (shortly after eye opening), are entirely compatible with the suggestion that the early postnatal period is a period of great activity and plasticity in the nonpyramidal cell population (Jacobson, 1974, 1975).

## Synaptogenesis

The axons of nonpyramidal neurons form Gray's type II or symmetrical synapses within the cortical grey matter. These synapses are often associated with inhibition (Gray, 1969; Triller and Korn, 1982). Their formation during development of the visual cortex of the rat has been examined in considerable detail (Wolff, 1978; Blue and Parnavelas, 1983a,b; Miller, 1988).

Although synapses have been observed in the cerebral cortex of the rat during the last week of gestation (Wolff, 1978), their paucity in prenatal and newborn rats suggests that the process of synapse formation is essentially a postnatal event. During the first few days of postnatal life type II synapses are seen in the deeper part of the cortical plate, which is expected in view of the fact that nonpyramidal neurons are present predominantly in the deeper part of the visual cortex at these ages. They appear immature as judged by the irregular shape of the presynaptic and postsynaptic structures, the poorly defined membrane specializations and the presence of only a few synaptic vesicles. As the neuropil matures, type II synapses become distributed throughout the depth of the cortex, gradually show increased thickening of the presynaptic and postsynaptic specializations, and acquire more vesicles. However, it is not until the end of the fourth postnatal week that they appear qualitatively indistinguishable from type II synapses present in the adult material.

Quantitative analysis of synaptogenesis in the rat visual cortex (Blue and Parnavelas, 1983b) has shown that type II synapses increase in density slowly throughout most of the first postnatal week, dramatically in the second and third postnatal weeks, and then decline markedly between days 28 and 90 (Fig. 7). This pattern differs from that shown by the type I synapses which increase continuously during the first three weeks and achieve a density close to that of adult animals by day 20 (Fig. 7).

As illustrated in Fig. 7, the most marked increase in the density of the type II synapses in the visual cortex occurs between days 14 and 16, the time immediately after eye opening. This period of increased density of type II synapses coincides with the observed phase of hypertrophy of cortical nonpyramidal neurons. Furthermore, the number of synaptic vesicles contained in the axon terminals which form type II synapses are significantly higher during this period of hypertrophy (Fig. 8). These observations suggest that stimulation of the visual cortex following eye-opening may induce nonpyramidal neurons to form an excess number of type II synapses but only some, perhaps those positioned to be effective in the shaping of the receptive field propeties of cortical neurons, are maintained. This idea is similar to the concept of selective stabilization of developing synapses postulated by Changeux and Danchin (1976). According to these authors, a limited but significant redundancy in synaptic connectivity exists during development of the nervous system, and the specificity of the system is increased by reducing the redundancy of neuronal connections. The observed decrease in the density of type II synapses is a clear example of synapse elimination in the visual cortex. However, it is

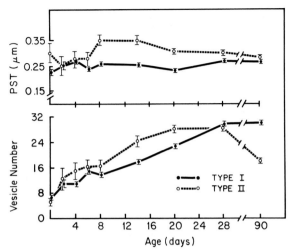

Fig. 8. Postsynaptic density lengths (PST) and the number of vesicles per terminal (vesicle number) for type I and type II axodendritic synapses at various ages between birth and 90 days. Mean ± S.E.M. values are shown. (From Blue and Parnavelas, 1983b, with permission.)

possible that the loss of these synaptic contacts reflects the probable elimination of significant proportions of peptide-containing subpopulations of nonpyramidal neurons (Parnavelas and Cavanagh, 1988).

### Neurochemical differentiation

Most GABA in the cerebral cortex is synthesized by the decarboxylation of glutamate, with GAD being the enzyme which catalyzes the reaction. Despite the relatively high level of GABA in neonatal cortex (about 50% of adult) and the presence of high-affinity GABA uptake system (about 30% of adult), GAD activity is low (about 5% of adult level) (Coyle and Enna, 1976; Coyle, 1982). Whereas the cortical content of GABA and the uptake of [$^3$H]GABA attain adult levels by the second postnatal week, GAD activity reaches adult levels one week later (Miller, 1988). However, low levels of GAD activity can lead to detectable concentrations of GABA, because the turnover of GABA is also low in prenatal and early postnatal ages due to low activity of GABA-transaminase, the enzyme which degrades

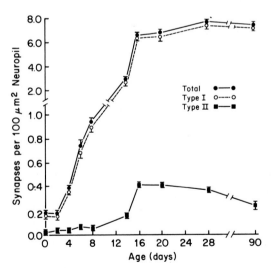

Fig. 7. Densities of axodendritic synapses for the total number (type I plus type II) and for each of the two synapse types in the visual cortex of rats at various postnatal ages. Mean ± S.E.M. values are shown. (From Blue and Parnavelas, 1983b, with permission.)

532

GABA (Coyle and Enna, 1976). For these reasons, it is thought that the GABAergic elements during early development can be best visualized with GABA immunohistochemistry.

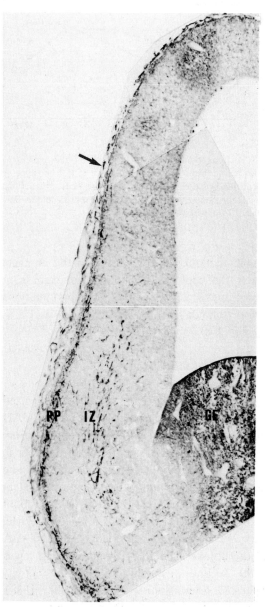

Fig. 9. Coronal section through the cortical anlage showing the distribution of GABA-immunoreactive elements in the primordial plexiform layer (PP) and in the intermediate zone (IZ) of a rat at E15. Arrow, dorsal extension of labelled neurons. GE, ganglionic eminence. ×100. (From Van Eden et al., 1989, with permission.)

[³H]GABA uptake (Chronwall and Wolff, 1980) and GAD immunohistochemistry (Wolff et al., 1984) demonstrated the first GABAergic cells in the neocortex of the rat at E15 and E16 respectively. These cells were initially located in the marginal zone and in the subplate zone, immediately below the cortical plate. However, immunohistochemical studies with antibodies directed against GABA (Van Eden et al., 1989; Cobas et al., 1991) have demonstrated a more widespread distribution of GABA-containing cells during early development. Furthermore, immunoreactive cells were detected earlier than with the previous methods. Specifically, these detailed studies of the prenatal development of GABAergic neurons in the neocortex of the rat first detected labelled cells in the primordial plexiform layer of the neocortical anlage at E14. At E15, the number of GABAergic cells is greatly increased appearing in the primordial plexiform layer as well as in the middle and lower portions of the intermediate zone (Fig. 9). Beginning at E16 and throughout the remaining period of gestation, GABA-containing neurons appear throughout all layers of the developing cortical anlage including the ventricular and subventricular zones (Fig. 10). After E19, while the number of GABAergic neurons in the cortical plate increases, those in the marginal zone and in the layers below the cortical plate diminish in number significantly. Thus, the early generated GABAergic neurons disappear by the time of birth. Both the study of Van Eden et al. (1989) and of Cobas et al. (1991) have suggested that the early GABAergic cells in the lower intermediate zone probably contribute to the population of interstitial cells of the adult white matter, many of which have been demonstrated to contain GABA. A very similar sequence of events have been described in a study of three embryonic stages of the developing visual cortex of the rhesus monkey (Huntley et al., 1988).

There is now a large body of evidence from a number of species which shows that many of the early born neurons in the developing neocortex

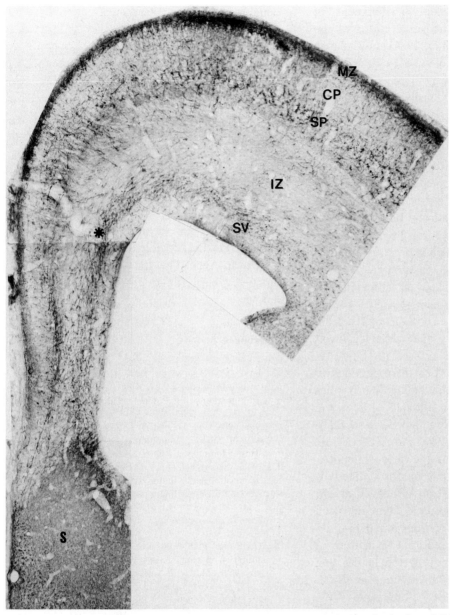

Fig. 10. Coronal section through the cortical anlage of a rat at E19 showing lamination of GABA-immunoreactive elements. Asterisk shows the population of labelled cells in the intermediate zone. MZ, marginal zone; CP, cortical plate; SP, subplate; IZ, intermediate zone; SV, subventricular zone; S, septal anlage. ×60. (From Van Eden et al., 1989, with permission.)

form a transient population which dies (Kostovic and Rakic, 1980; Luskin and Shatz, 1985; Chun et al., 1987; Valverde and Facal-Valverde, 1988; Al-Ghoul and Miller, 1989). A number of functions have been proposed for these neurons in the marginal zone (Edmunds and Parnavelas,

1982) and particularly in the subplate (Shatz and Luskin, 1986; Chun et al., 1987), but the most recent evidence (McConnell et al., 1989) suggests that the transient subplate neurons may form a scaffold essential for the establishment of permanent subcortical projections.

Studies of the postnatal development of GABAergic neurons in the visual cortex of the rat (Wolff et al., 1984; Miller, 1986a) have shown a progressive increase of GAD- or GABA-labelled neurons from layer VI to layer II over the first 2–3 weeks. The density of axonal label follows a similar pattern, and the adult distribution of GABAergic cell bodies and axons is attained by P30 (Miller, 1986a, 1988). Measurements of GAD activity in different layers of the visual cortex during development have shown that the enzyme activity is low during the first postnatal week, increases dramatically between days 8 and 18, and reaches adult levels by day 24 in all layers except layer IV which shows a continuous increase to adulthood (McDonald et al., 1987). A similar study which involved measurements of GAD activity in the cat visual cortex (Fosse et al., 1989) also showed a more or less steady rise from birth to 5–6 weeks when the adult level was reached.

The appearance of various neuropeptides in the GABA-containing nonpyramidal neurons has also been examined in considerable detail in the rat visual cortex (McDonald et al., 1982a–d; Shiosaka et al., 1982; Miller, 1988; Parnavelas et al., 1988). As mentioned earlier, the various subpopulations of nonpyramidal neurons as defined by their neuropeptide content are produced at different times during histogenesis. Thus, the peak of neurogenesis for SRIF neurons is at E15–E16, for NPY neurons at E17 and for VIP neurons at E19. These birthdates are reflected in the first detectable appearances of these neurons: SRIF cells appear in the cortex before birth, NPY neurons at about the time of birth and VIP cells towards the end of the first postnatal week. Finally, ultrastructural analyses in the visual cortex (Eadie et al., 1987, 1990) have shown that the time of genesis of the subpopulations is also reflected in the rate of acquisition of their nuclear, cytoplasmic and synaptic features.

## Conclusion

Cortical nonpyramidal neurons, nearly all of which contain GABA, comprise different neuronal subpopulations which are defined by morphological and/or neurochemical features. Recent studies have provided evidence which suggests that each subpopulation follows a unique pattern of development during life.

## Acknowledgements

The original work included in this review was supported by the Medical Research Council. I am grateful to Agnes Guy for typing the manuscript, and to Corbert Van Eden for providing Figs. 9 and 10.

## References

Al-Ghoul, W.M. and Miller, M.W. (1989) Transient expression of Alz-50 immunoreactivity in developing rat neocortex: a marker for naturally occurring neuronal death? *Brain Res.*, 481: 361–367.

Angevine, J.B. and Sidman, R.L. (1961) Autoradiographic study of cell migration during histogenesis of cerebral cortex in the mouse. *Nature*, 192: 766–768.

Bear, M.F., Schmechel, D.E. and Ebner, F.F. (1985) Glutamic acid decarboxylase in the striate cortex of normal and monocularly deprived kittens. *J. Neurosci.*, 5: 1262–1275.

Berry, M. and Rogers, A.W. (1965) The migration of neuroblasts in the developing cerebral cortex. *J. Anat.*, 99: 691–709.

Blue, M.E. and Parnavelas, J.G. (1983a) The formation and maturation of synapses in the visual cortex of the rat. I. Qualitative analysis. *J. Neurocytol.*, 12: 599–616.

Blue, M.E. and Parnavelas, J.G. (1983b) The formation and maturation of synapses in the visual cortex of the rat. II. Quantitative analysis. *J. Neurocytol.*, 12: 697–712.

Cavanagh, M.E. and Parnavelas, J.G. (1988) Development of somatostatin immunoreactive neurons in the rat occipital cortex: a combined immunocytochemical-autoradiographic study. *J. Comp. Neurol.*, 268: 1–12.

Cavanagh, M.E. and Parnavelas, J.G. (1989) Development of vasoactive-intestinal-polypeptide-immunoreactive neurons in the rat occipital cortex: a combined immunohistochemical-autoradiographic study. *J. Comp. Neurol.*, 284: 637–645.

Cavanagh, M.E. and Parnavelas, J.G. (1990) Development of neuropeptide Y (NPY) immunoreactive neurons in the rat occipital cortex: a combined immunohistochemical-autoradiographic study. *J. Comp. Neurol.*, 297: 553–563.

Changeux, J.-P. and Danchin, A. (1976) Selective stabilisation of developing synapses as a mechanism for the specification of neuronal networks. *Nature*, 264: 705–712.

Chronwall, B.M. and Wolff, J.R. (1978) Classification and location of neurons taking up [3]H-GABA in the visual cortex of rats. In: F. Fonnum (Ed.), *Amino Acids as Chemical Transmitters*, New York: Plenum Press, pp. 297–303.

Chronwall, B. and Wolff, J.R. (1980) Prenatal and postnatal development of GABA-accumulating cells in the occipital neocortex of rat. *J. Comp. Neurol.*, 190: 187–208.

Chun, J.J.M., Nakamura, M.J. and Shatz, C.J. (1987) Transient cells of the developing mammalian telencephalon are peptide-immunoreactive neurons. *Nature*, 325: 617–620.

Cobas, A., Fairén, A., Alvarez-Bolado, G. and Sánchez, M.P. (1991) Prenatal development of the intrinsic neurons of the rat neocortex: a comparative study of the distribution of GABA-immunoreactive cells and the GABA$_A$ receptor. *Neuroscience*, 40: 375–397.

Coyle, J.T. (1982) Development of neurotransmitters in the neocortex. *Neurosci. Res. Progr. Bull.*, 20: 479–507.

Coyle, J.T. and Enna, S.J. (1976) Neurochemical aspects of the ontogenesis of GABAergic neurons in the rat brain. *Brain Res.*, 111: 119–133.

Cragg, B.G. (1975) The development of synapses in the visual system of the cat. *J. Comp. Neurol.*, 160: 147–166.

Eadie, L.A., Parnavelas, J.G. and Franke, E. (1987) Development of the ultrastructural features of somatostatin-immunoreactive neurons in the rat visual cortex. *J. Neurocytol.*, 16: 445–459.

Eadie, L.A., Parnavelas, J.G. and Franke, E. (1990) Development of the ultrastructural features of neuropeptide Y-immunoreactive neurons in the rat visual cortex. *J. Neurocytol.*, 19: 455–465.

Edmunds, S.M. and Parnavelas, J.G. (1982) Retzius-Cajal cells: an ultrastructural study in the developing visual cortex of the rat. *J. Neurocytol.*, 11: 427–446.

Emson, P.C. and Lindvall, O. (1979) Distribution of putative neurotransmitters in the neocortex. *Neuroscience*, 4: 1–30.

Fairén, A., Cobas, A. and Fonseca, M. (1986) Times of generation of glutamic acid decarboxylase immunoreactive neurons in mouse somatosensory cortex. *J. Comp. Neurol.*, 251: 67–83.

Fisher, R.S. and Levine, M.S. (1989) Transmitter cosynthesis by corticopetal basal forebrain neurons. *Brain Res.*, 491: 163–168.

Fisher, R.S., Buchwald, N.A., Hull, C.D. and Levine, M.S. (1988) GABAergic basal forebrain neurons project to the neocortex: the localization of glutamic acid decarboxylase and choline acetyltransferase in feline corticopetal neurons. *J. Comp. Neurol.*, 272: 489–502.

Fitzpatrick, D., Lund, J.S., Schmechel, D.E. and Towles, A.C. (1987) Distribution of GABAergic neurons and axon terminals in the macaque striate cortex. *J. Comp. Neurol.*, 264: 73–91.

Fosse, V.M., Heggelund, P. and Fonnum, F. (1989) Postnatal development of glutamatergic, GABAergic, and cholinergic neurotransmitter phenotypes in the visual cortex, lateral geniculate nucleus, pulvinar, and superior colliculus in cats. *J. Neurosci.*, 9: 426–435.

Gabbott, P.L.A. and Somogyi, P. (1986) Quantitative distribution of GABA-immunoreactive neurons in the visual cortex (area 17) of the cat. *Exp. Brain Res.*, 61: 323–331.

Gray, E.G. (1969) Electron microscopy of excitatory and inhibitory synapses: a brief review. In: K. Akert and P.G. Waser (Eds.), *Mechanisms of Synaptic Transmission, Progress in Brain Research, Vol. 31*, Amsterdam: Elsevier, pp. 141–155.

Hedlich, A. and Winkelmann, E. (1982) Neuroentypen des visuellen Cortex der adulten und juvenilen Ratte. *J. Hirnforsch.*, 23: 353–373.

Hendrickson, A.E., Hunt, S.P. and Wu, J.-Y. (1981) Immunocytochemical localization of glutamic acid decarboxylase in monkey striate cortex. *Nature*, 292: 605–607.

Hendry, S.H.C., Schwark, H.D., Jones, E.G. and Yan, J. (1987) Numbers and proportions of GABA-immunoreactive neurons in different areas of monkey cerebral cortex. *J. Neurosci.*, 7: 1503–1519.

Houser, C.R., Vaughn, J.E., Hendry, S.H.C., Jones E.G. and Peters, A. (1984) GABA neurons in the cerebral cortex. In: E.G. Jones and A. Peters (Eds.), *Cerebral Cortex, Vol. 2, Functional Properties of Cortical Cells*, New York: Plenum Press, pp. 63–89.

Huntley, G.W., Hendry, S.H.C., Killackey, H.P., Chalupa, L.M. and Jones, E.G. (1988) Temporal sequence of neurotransmitter expression by developing neurons of fetal monkey visual cortex. *Dev. Brain Res.*, 43: 69–96.

Jacobson, M. (1974) A plentitude of neurons. In: G. Gottlieb (Ed.), *Studies on the Development of Behavior and the Nervous System, Vol. 2, Aspects of Neurogenesis*, New York: Academic Press, pp. 151–166.

Jacobson, M. (1975) Development and evolution of type II neurons: conjectures a century after Golgi. In: M. Santini (Ed.), *Golgi Centennial Symposium: Perspectives in Neurobiology*, New York, Raven Press, pp. 147–151.

Jacobson, M. (1978) *Developmental Neurobiology, 2nd Edn.*, New York, Plenum Press.

Jeffery, G. and Parnavelas, J.G. (1987) Early visual deafferentation of the cortex results in an asymmetry of somatostatin labelled cells. *Exp. Brain Res.*, 67: 651–655.

Jones, E.G. and Hendry, S.H.C. (1986) Co-localization of GABA and neuropeptides in neocortical neurons. *Trends Neurosci.*, 9: 71–76.

Jones, E.G., DeFelipe, J. and Hendry, S.H.C. (1988) A study of tachykinin-immunoreactive neurons in the monkey cerebral cortex. *J. Neurosci.*, 8: 1208–1224.

Kisvárday, Z.F., Cowey, A., Hodgson, A.J. and Somogyi, P. (1986) The relationship between GABA immunoreactivity and labelling by local uptake of [[3]H]GABA in the striate cortex of monkey. *Exp. Brain Res.*, 62: 89–98.

Köhler, C., Swanson, L.W., Haglund, L. and Wu, J.-Y. (1985) The cytoarchitecture, histochemistry and projections of the tuberomammillary nucleus in the rat. *Neuroscience*, 16: 85–110.

536

Kostovic, I. and Rakic, P. (1980) Cytology and time of origin of interstitial neurons in the white matter in infant and adult human and monkey telencephalon. *J. Neurocytol.*, 9: 219–242.

LeVay, S. (1973) Synaptic patterns in the visual cortex of the cat and monkey. Electron microscopy of Golgi preparations. *J. Comp. Neurol.*, 150: 53–86.

Lin, C.-S., Lu, S.M. and Schmechel, D.E. (1986) Glutamic acid decarboxylase and somatostatin immunoreactivities in rat visual cortex. *J. Comp. Neurol.*, 244: 369–383.

Lin, C.-S., Nicolelis, M.A.L., Schneider, J.S. and Chapin, J.K. (1990) A major direct GABAergic pathway from zona incerta to neorcortex. *Science*, 248: 1553–1556.

Lund, J.S., Boothe, R.G. and Lund, R.D. (1977) Development of neurons in the visual cortex (area 17) of the monkey (*Macaca nemestrina*): a Golgi study from fetal day 127 to postnatal maturity. *J. Comp. Neurol.*, 176: 149–188.

Luskin, M.B. and Shatz, C.A. (1985) Studies of the earliest generated cells of the cat's visual cortex: cogeneration of subplate and marginal zones. *J. Neurosci.*, 5: 1062–1075.

McConnell, S.K., Ghosh, A. and Shatz, C.J. (1989) Subplate neurons pioneer the first axon pathway from the cerebral cortex. *Science*, 245: 978–982.

McDonald, J.K., Speciale, S.G. and Parnavelas, J.G. (1983) The laminar distribution of glutamate decarboxylase and choline acetyltransferase in the adult and developing visual cortex of the rat. *Neuroscience*, 21: 825–832.

McDonald, J.K., Parnavelas, J.G., Karamanlidis, A.N., Brecha, N. and Koenig, J.I. (1982a) The morphology and distribution of peptide-containing neurons in the adult and developing visual cortex of the rat. I. Somatostatin. *J. Neurocytol.*, 11: 809–824.

McDonald, J.K., Parnavelas, J.G., Karamanlidis, A.N. and Brecha, N. (1982b) The morphology and distribution of peptide-containing neurons in the adult and developing visual cortex of the rat. II. Vasoactive intestinal polypeptide. *J. Neurocytol.*, 11: 825–837.

McDonald, J.K., Parnavelas, J.G., Karamanlidis, A.N., Rosenquist, G. and Brecha, N. (1982c) The morphology and distribution of peptide-containing neurons in the adult and developing visual cortex of the rat. III. Cholecystokinin. *J. Neurocytol.*, 11: 881–895.

McDonald, J.K., Parnavelas, J.G., Karamanlidis, A.N. and Brecha, N. (1982d) The morphology and distribution of peptide-containing neurons in the adult and developing visual cortex of the rat. IV. Avian pancreatic polypeptide. *J. Neurocytol.*, 11: 985–995.

Meinecke, D.L. and Peters, A. (1987) GABA immunoreactive neurons in rat visual cortex. *J. Comp. Neurol.*, 261: 388–404.

Meyer, G. and Ferres-Torres, M. (1984) Postnatal maturation of nonpyramidal neurons in the visual cortex of the cat. *J. Comp. Neurol.*, 228: 226–244.

Meyer, G. and Wahle, P. (1988) Early postnatal development of cholecystokinin-immunoreactive structures in the visual cortex of the cat. *J. Comp. Neurol.*, 276: 360–386.

Miller, M.W. (1985) Cogeneration of retrogradely labeled corticocotical projection and GABA-immunoreactive local circuit neurons in cerebral cortex. *Dev. Brain Res.*, 23: 187–192.

Miller, M.W. (1986a) The migration and neurochemical differentiation of γ-aminobutyric acid (GABA)-immunoreactive neurons in rat visual cortex as demonstrated by a combined immunocytochemical-autoradiographic technique. *Dev. Brain Res.*, 28: 41–46.

Miller, M.W. (1986b) Maturation of rat visual cortex. III. Postnatal morphogenesis and synaptogenesis of local circuit neurons. *Dev. Brain Res.*, 25: 271–285.

Miller, M.W. (1988) Development of projection and local circuit neurons in neocortex. In: A. Peters and E.G. Jones (Eds.), *Cerebral Cortex, Vol. 7, Development and Maturation of Cerebral Cortex*, New York, Plenum Press, pp. 133–175.

Ottersen, O.P. and Storm-Mathisen, J. (1984) Neurons containing or accumulating transmitter amino acids. In: A. Björklund, T. Hökfelt and M.J. Kuhar (Eds.), *Handbook of Chemical Neuroanatomy, Vol. 3, Chemical Transmitters and Transmitter Receptors in the CNS, Part II*, Amsterdam: Elsevier, pp. 141–246.

Papadopoulos, G.C., Parnavelas, J.G. and Cavanagh, M.E. (1987) Extensive coexistence of neuropeptides in the rat visual cortex. *Brain Res.*, 420: 95–99.

Parnavelas, J.G. and Globus, A. (1976) The effect of continuous illumination on the development of cortical neurons in the rat: a Golgi study. *Exp. Neurol.*, 51: 637–647.

Parnavelas, J.G. and Lieberman, A.R. (1979) An ultrastructural study of the maturation of neuronal somata in the visual cortex of the rat. *Anat. Embryol.*, 157: 311–328.

Parnavelas, J.G. and Uylings, H.B.M. (1980) The growth of non-pyramidal neurons in the visual cortex of the rat: a morphometric study. *Brain Res.*, 193: 373–382.

Parnavelas, J.G. and McDonald, J.K. (1983) The cerebral cortex. In: P.C. Emson (Ed.), *Chemical Neuroanatomy*, New York: Raven Press, pp. 505–549.

Parnavelas, J.G. and Cavanagh, M.E. (1988) Transient expression of neurotransmitters in the developing neocortex. *Trends Neurosci.*, 11: 92–93.

Parnavelas, J.G., Lieberman, A.R. and Webster, K.E. (1977) Organization of neurons in the visual cortex, area 17, of the rat. *J. Anat.*, 124: 305–322.

Parnavelas, J.G., Bradford, R., Mounty, E.J. and Lieberman, A.R. (1978) The development of non-pyramidal neurons in the visual cortex of the rat. *Anat. Embryol.*, 155: 1–14.

Parnavelas, J.G., Papadopoulos, G.C. and Cavanagh, M.E. (1988) Changes in neurotransmitters during development. In: A. Peters and E.G. Jones (Eds.), *Cerebral Cortex, Vol. 7, Development and Maturation of Cerebral Cortex*, New York: Plenum Press, pp. 177–209.

Parnavelas, J.G., Dinopoulos, A. and Davies, S.W. (1989) Central visual pathways. In A. Björklund, T. Hökfelt and L.W. Swanson (Eds.), *Handbook of Chemical Neuroanatomy, Vol. 7, Integrated Systems of the CNS, Part II*, Amsterdam: Elsevier, pp. 1–164.

Parnavelas, J.G., Jeffery, G., Cope, J. and Davies, S.W. (1990)

Early lesion of mystacial vibrissae in rats results in an increase of somatostatin-labelled cells in the somatosensory cortex. *Exp. Brain Res.,* 82: 658–662.

Peduzzi, J.D. (1988) Genesis of GABA-immunoreactive neurons in the ferret visual cortex. *J. Neurosci.,* 8: 920–931.

Peters, A. (1985) The visual cortex of the rat. In: A. Peters and E.G. Jones (Eds.), *Cerebral Cortex, Vol. 3, Visual Cortex,* New York: Plenum Press, pp. 19–80.

Rakic, P. (1974) Neurons in rhesus monkey visual cortex: systematic relation between time of origin and eventual disposition. *Science,* 183: 425–427.

Ramón y Cajal, S. (1960) *Studies on Vetebrate Neurogenesis* (translated by L. Guth), Springfield, Illinois: Charles C. Thomas, pp. 325–335.

Ribak, C.E. (1978) Aspinous and sparsely-spinous stellate neurons in the visual cortex of rats contain glutamic acid decarboxylase. *J. Neurocytol.,* 7: 461–478.

Ronnevi, L.-O. (1977) Spontaneous phagocytosis of boutons on spinal motoneurons during early postnatal development. An electron microscopical study in the cat. *J. Neurocytol.,* 6: 487–504.

Shatz, C.J. and Luskin, M.B. (1986) The relationship between the geniculocortical afferents and their cortical target cells during development of the cat's primary visual cortex. *J. Neurosci.,* 6: 3655–3668.

Shiosaka, S., Takatsuki, K., Sakanaka, M., Inagaki, S., Takagi, H., Senba, E., Kawai, Y., Iida, H., Minagawa, H., Hara, Y., Matsuzaki, T. and Tohyama, M. (1982) Ontogeny of somatostatin-containing neuron system of the rat: immunohistochemical analysis. II. Forebrain and diencephalon. *J. Comp. Neurol.,* 204: 211–224.

Somogyi, P., Hodgson, A.J., Smith, A.D., Nunzi, M.G., Gorio, A. and Wu, J.-Y. (1984) Different populations of GABAergic neurons in the visual cortex and hippocampus of cat contain somatostatin- or cholecystokinin-immunoreactive material. *J. Neurosci.,* 4: 2590–2603.

Triller, A. and Korn, H. (1982) Transmission at a central inhibitory synapse. III. Ultrastructure of physiologically identified and stained terminals. *J. Neurophysiol.,* 48: 708–736.

Valverde, F. and Facal-Valverde, M.V. (1988) Postnatal development of interstitial (subplate) cells in the white matter of the temporal cortex of kittens: a correlated Golgi and electron microscopic study. *J. Comp. Neurol.,* 269: 168–192.

Van Eden, C.G., Mrzljak, L., Voorn, P. and Uylings, H.B.M. (1989) Prenatal development of GABA-ergic neurons in the neocortex of the rat. *J. Comp. Neurol.,* 283: 213–227.

Vincent, S.R., Hökfelt, T., Skirboll, L.R. and Wu, J-Y. (1983) Hypothalamic γ-aminobutyric acid neurons project to the neocortex. *Science,* 220: 1309–1311.

Wahle, P. and Meyer, G. (1987) Morphology and quantitative changes of transient NPY-ir neuronal populations during early postnatal development of the cat visual cortex. *J. Comp. Neurol.,* 261: 165–192.

Wahle, P. and Meyer, G. (1989) Early postnatal development of vasoactive intestinal polypeptide- and peptide histidine isoleucine-immunoreactive structures in the cat visual cortex. *J. Comp. Neurol.,* 282: 215–248.

Winfield, D.A. (1981) The postnatal development of synapses in the visual cortex of the cat and the effects of eyelid closure. *Brain Res.,* 206: 166–171.

Wolff, J.R. (1978) Ontogenetic aspects of cortical architecture: lamination. In: M.A.B. Brazier and H. Petsche (Eds.), *Architectonics of the Cerebral Cortex,* New York: Raven Press, pp. 159–173.

Wolff, J.R., Chronwall, B.M. and Rickmann, M. (1983) "Diffuse disposition mode" provides rat visual cortex with nonpyramidal and GABA-ergic neurons. *4th Intern. Congr. Intern. Soc. Dev. Neurosci.* Abstr. p. 54.

Wolff, J.R., Böttcher, H., Zetzsche, T., Oertel, W.H. and Chronwall, B.M. (1984) Development of GABAergic neurons in rat visual cortex as identified by glutamate decarboxylase-like immunoreactivity. *Neurosci. Lett.,* 47: 207–212.

# Subject Index